NEUROBEHAVIORAL TERATOLOGY

Joseph Yanai (EDITOR)

Department of Anatomy and Embryology, Hadassah Medical School, The Hebrew University, Jerusalem, Israel

ELSEVIER 1984

Amsterdam · Oxford · New York

ISBN 0-444-80516-8

Published by:
Elsevier Science Publishers BV, PO Box 211,
1000 AE Amsterdam, The Netherlands

Sole distributors for the USA and Canada:
Elsevier Science Publishing Company, Inc.,
52 Vanderbilt Avenue, New York, NY 10017,
USA

Library of Congress Cataloging in Publication Data
Main entry under title:

Neurobehavioral teratology.

    Includes bibliographies and index.
    1. Fetus--Effect of drugs on. 2. Central nervous
system--Effect of Drugs on. 3. Psychotropic drugs--
Toxicology. 4. Abnormalities, Human--Etiology.
5. Developmental psychobiology. I. Yanai, Joseph.
[DNLM: 1. Abnormalities, Drug-induced. 2. Behavior--
Drug effects. 3. Nervous system diseases--Etiology.
4. Teratogens. QS 679 N494]
RG627.6.D79N48 1984   616.8'0443   83-25492
ISBN 0-444-80516-8

Cover drawing: J. Dyer
Printed in the Netherlands

Preface

TERATOLOGY, the study of abnormalities arising during prenatal development, is not usually associated with minor abnormalities of the central nervous system (CNS) and resulting behavior, although teratological studies of gross CNS malformations have been published. While sporadic studies have been conducted on the behavioral and CNS effects of prenatal exposure to various insults, only since the sixties have increasing interest and research been devoted to the issue. The new field was then defined by *Werboff* and *Gottlieb* (1963), who coined the term 'behavioral teratology'. Behavioral teratology studies have increased rapidly in the last decade. Several theoretical publications defined the field and put forth the rationale for its dependent existence (*Barlow* and *Sullivan*, 1975; *Coyle* et al., 1976; *Hutching*, 1978). Among the unique characteristics proposed in the definition of behavioral teratology, differentiating it from its mother field teratology, was the appearance of behavioral alterations in the absence of gross structural deformity. (However, this concept should now be revised, since with finer and quantitative scrutiny, not only behavioral but also the underlying neuromorphological and neurochemical changes can often be demonstrated.) In addition, congenital behavioral alterations occur after insults below teratogenic levels and the critical periods in behavioral teratology extend to late pregnancy, commonly considered not susceptible to congenital malformation. Behavioral teratology also possesses several unique methodological prob-

v

lems, among them the need to study adult offspring rather than fetuses, and the need to analyse behavioral deviation quantitatively, since often teratogenicity is expressed not by behavioral abnormality but by a quantitative reduction in performance within a range still considered normal. It is for all these reasons that behavioral teratology rapidly developed as an independent field and has become well established. Section or satellite meetings on behavioral teratology have been part of Teratology Society meetings since 1977, and the Behavioral Teratology Society was founded in 1979. The independence of the field was recognized by scientific journals that devoted a section to behavioral teratology *(Teratology)* or became largely devoted to the field *(Neurobehavioral Toxicology and Teratology)*. The title of this volume does not imply that we intend to add yet another field to the study of development, a science already overburdened with numerous subfields. Rather, *Neurobehavioral Teratology*, while providing an update on behavioral teratology, points to the direction that contemporary research into behavioral teratology should take, that is, the study of the mechanisms underlying the effects on behavior of early insults. Most early studies of behavioral teratology were descriptive only, fulfilling the necessary first requirement in a new field. The obvious next step is to ascertain the pathways from the early input to the behavioral alterations which will, hopefully, facilitate future studies on the prevention or reversal of the effect of early exposure to the substance, especially in those cases when exposure is deemed necessary or unavoidable. Indeed, many of the studies presented in this volume investigate or discuss biochemical and/or neuromorphological changes which could mediate the behavioral alterations. In most chapters, the neural changes are presented concomitantly with behavioral alteration, but this does not necessarily imply causality. Perhaps this is indicative of the current state of the field of behavioral teratology. It appears that in the normal progression of fields of behavioral study, where description of behavioral events is followed by association between behavioral and neural events and finally establishment of causal (lineal) relationships, behavioral teratology finds itself in the second of these phases, about to move to the third. It is difficult to establish causal relationships because prenatal insults generally affect numerous processes in the brain, resulting in multiple behavioral alterations. A partial solution may be found in using input known to have a specific effect, such as neuroleptics, which block dopamine receptors (see *Spear*'s Chapter 14), but even neuroleptics probably produce several other non-specific changes. On the behavioral end, it may be advantageous to study changes specific to a particular process, such as changes in behavioral responses to dopamine agonist after prenatal exposure to dopamine blocker (*Spear*'s Chapter 14), or changes in brain response to barbiturate after prenatal exposure to barbiturate (*Yanai*'s Chapter 5). Another approach is to use as the dependent variable behavior most specific to a certain area of the brain (e.g. hippocampal behaviors in *Yanai*'s Chapter 5), although it is clear that region-specific behavior is only a relative term, since other regions in the brain often contribute to the behavior in question. It can be seen that even with all partial solutions available, the problem of specificity of the effect cannot be resolved completely.

Another methodological consideration in behavioral teratology research is the possible indirect effect of the administered substance. For example, hypnotics in large doses may induce undernutrition since sedated pregnant females may not be able to consume normal amounts of food. Pair-fed controls provide only a partial solution, since many administered substances may affect absorption of nutrients.

Neonatal exposure to neuroteratogen in certain small rodents is often thought equivalent to late pregnancy in humans. If administered to the nursing dam, the substance may affect milk production or maternal behavior. Direct administration to neonates offers a possible solution, but the affected pups may not be able to suckle enough milk or properly display the cues necessary to elicit maternal care. There are also factors that fall between direct and indirect effects; for example, various drugs affect uteral contraction, body temperature, nutrient metabolism, oxygen intake, etc. With the development of new techniques, some of these indirect effects may be controlled. Rat pups can be raised without their mothers (*Diaz* et al., 1977), and embryos may develop in vitro (*Ornoy* and *Zusman*'s Chapter 4). The latter technique cannot, obviously, be applied to studies on adult behavior, but it can provide control for neural changes during embryonic development.

In certain cases, the results of early administration serve as evidence against indirect effects when results are contrary to known consequences of the indirect effect, or when the results are specific to the substance applied (both situations are discussed in *Yanai*'s Chapter 5). Yet it appears that the issue of indirect effect will remain a problem complicating neurobehavioral teratology research for some time to come.

The issue, too, of comparable dose between animal model and human is ever a subject of heated controversy. It is claimed by laymen and even by peers that the doses in most studies are too high to pertain to human situations. On the other hand, the findings on the teratogenic properties of thalidomide in rats were ignored since the dosage used in the studies was considered high in human terms (*Cohen*, 1966). Although in certain neuroteratogens the effective doses are comparable in humans and laboratory animals, for most other substances dose-for-dose comparison is not applicable, since small rodents possess a higher metabolic or excretion rate for many substances than humans, resulting in lower blood-substance concentrations. Equalizing animals' blood levels with those of humans does not offer a satisfactory comparison since animal sensitivity to various substances may differ from the human. It appears that the most appropriate method of standardisation is to administer to experimental pregnant animals doses that produce physiological effects similar to those in humans, even if this implies administration of higher doses, that is, not comparable doses, but comparably effective doses.

This book is divided into six sections. The first section gives an overview of the field and presents some of its major methodological issues. In the first chapter *Brown* and *Fishman* present an overview of neurobehavioral teratology as it relates to many of the major substances that pregnant women are exposed to. These include mainly drugs of use and abuse, psychoactive as well as others, but also various neuroteratogens such

VIII

as stress and hypoxia. Some of these factors are the subjects of individual chapters in this volume. However, a major aim of the overview is to discuss substances which are not covered in specific chapters, whether because research into their neurobehavioral teratogenicity is sparse or for any other reason. Examples of substances discussed there are nicotine, caffeine and aspirin. *Swaab* and *Mirmiran* (Chapter 2) further survey the field and discuss the neurobehavioral teratogenicity of various psychoactive drugs, hormones and peptides.

While animal studies can be well controlled, studies of human neurobehavioral teratology clearly can derive their data only from existing incidence in the population. Because of this limitation the role of epidemiological studies is central in human neurobehavioral teratology. In Chapter 3, *Klingberg* et al. discuss the epidemiological approach to human congenital CNS and behavioral defects.

The possible indirect effect of neuroteratogens has necessitated the development of control methods enabling demonstration of direct effects of substances on the developing CNS. Accordingly, *Ornoy* and *Zusman* (Chapter 4) discuss the potential effectiveness of in vitro embryo cultures as a control in neuroteratological research.

Other methodological issues are dealt with in several of the chapters in other sections. Thus, after early exposure to various neuroteratogens, the expression of certain resulting neural and behavioral deficits is dependent on the developmental stage of the CNS. This phenomenon is discussed by *Spear* in Chapter 14. In human neurobehavioral teratology studies, the apparent randomised control may actually be biased by self-selection and other factors. Ethical considerations also make the necessary control difficult to achieve. These issues are discussed by *Cuckle* in Chapter 17.

The use and abuse of drugs during pregnancy is extremely common, especially if ethanol is included in this classification. Thus, drug use and abuse is a major contributor to neurobehavioral birth defects. Barbiturate and other anticonvulsants are among the drugs whose use during pregnancy or early childhood cannot always be avoided since the substitutes may also be teratogenic. In the first section, devoted to drugs of use and abuse (Section II), *Yanai* (Chapter 5) discusses the animal work on the effect on CNS of early exposure to barbiturate, and *Wallace* (Chapter 6) discusses the human studies on both phenobarbital and other anticonvulsants. Benzodiazepines, especially diazepam (valium), are also commonly used. The neurobehavioral consequences of their consumption during pregnancy in both humans and animals are presented by *Grimm* (Chapter 7).

Fetal alcohol syndrome is the most common and most extensively studied outcome of early substance exposure. Although the syndrome is of major significance, it has already been described thoroughly (e.g. *Abel*, 1981), and therefore will not receive further attention here. Rather, preference is given to presenting a less conventional approach to fetal alcohol syndrome, that is, the ascertainment of fine neuromorphological deficits, as described by *Volk* (Chapter 8).

Opioid abuse is an increasing problem aggravated by the fact that methadone, its less harmful, recommended alternative, may also be a neuroteratogen. It has been estimated that one out of every 1000 babies is born in the United States to an opioid-consuming mother (*Zagon* and *McLaughlin*, Chapter 9). Appropriately, therefore, most of the second section on drugs of use and abuse is devoted to opioids (Section III). An overview of opioid neurobehavioral teratology in humans and animals is provided by *Zagon* and *McLaughlin* (Chapter 9). *Kirby* (Chapter 10) discusses the specific alterations in animal responsiveness to opioids after prenatal morphine administration. The recognition of the growing problem of opioid addiction led to the establishment of large research projects into the issue by several groups. The results are discussed comprehensively in Chapter 11 by *Hans* et al. Marihuana consumption has become popular and, significantly, mostly during child-bearing age. Neural and behavioral sequelae of prenatal marihuana exposure both in the animal model and human situations is discussed by *Fried* in Chapter 12.

Recent evidence points to the fact that substances known as neurotransmitters also play a role in neural development (Section IV). As described by *Lauder* and *Krebs* (Chapter 13), abating neurotransmitter substances by neurotoxins, and possibly by drugs, perturbs specific neural development processes. In the same section *Spear* (Chapter 14) describes effects of early treatments, specifically neurotoxin (6-OHDA) and receptor blocker, that alter the sensitivity of dopamine receptors on behaviors related to the dopaminergic system. This approach appears promising, since both the early input and the postnatal output (behavior) are specific. Thus, the inherent methodological problems in neurobehavioral teratology of the generality of both input and output may largely be avoided.

There is a growing awareness that hormonal levels can affect neural and behavioral development. Section V considers this matter in detail. Such effects may have far-reaching ramifications, since the maternal emotional state during pregnancy affects, for example, glucocorticoid levels, and as shown by *Bohn* (Chapter 16), glucocorticoid levels determine the development of the CNS. The chapter presents primarily animal studies, but the situation in humans is also discussed. The effect of hypo- and hyperthyroidism on the CNS, mainly in animals but also in humans, is discussed by *Legrand* (Chapter 15). Section V also presents the role of vitamin deficiency in the induction of neural tube defects in humans (*Cuckle*, Chapter 17). It seems pertinent to mention in this context the neuropeptides which have received increasing attention in recent years. Their possible neurobehavioral teratogenicity is described in part of *Swaab's* chapter (Chapter 2) in Section I.

Heavy metals fall under a different classification to the other substances described here. Essentially they are environmental pollutants spread by humans, but may also derive from natural sources. The last section (Section VI) is devoted to neural and behavioral sequelae of early exposure to heavy metals. *Chang* and *Annau* (Chapter 18) describe the effect of methylmercury, while *Silbergeld* (Chapter 19) describes the effect of lead. Each chapter deals with both animal models and human studies.

Joseph Yanai

x

References

Abel, E.L. (ed.) (1981) Fetal Alcohol Syndrome: Vol. I, An Annotated and Comprehensive Bibliography. CRC Press, Boca Raton.

Barlow, S.M. and Sullivan, F.M. (1975) Behavioral teratology. In: Teratology: Trends and applications (Berry, C.L. and Poswillo, D.E., eds.) Springer-Verlag, New York, pp. 103–120.

Cohen, R.L. (1966) Experimental and clinical chemateratogenesis, Adv. Pharmacol. 4, 263–349.

Coyle, I., Wayner, M.J. and Singer, G. (1976) Behavioral teratogenesis: A critical evaluation, Pharmacol. Biochem. Behav. 4, 191–200.

Diaz, J., Schain, R.J. and Baily, B.G., (1977) Phenobarbital-induced brain growth retardation in artificially reared rat pups. Biol. Neonate 32, 77–82.

Hutchings, D.E. (1978) Behavioral teratology: Embryopathic and behavioral effects of drugs during pregnancy. In: Studies on the Development of Behavior and the Nervous System. Vol. 4, Early Influences (Gottlieb, G., ed.) Academic Press, New York, pp. 7–34.

Werboff, J. and Gottlieb, J.S. (1963) Drugs in pregnancy: behavioral teratology. Obstet. Gynecol. Surv. 18, 420–423.

Dedication

To Shanie

Contents

2   POSSIBLE MECHANISMS UNDERLYING THE TERATOGENIC EFFECTS OF MEDICINES ON THE DEVELOPING BRAIN

3   THE ETIOLOGY OF CENTRAL NERVOUS SYSTEM DEFECTS

4   IN VITRO EMBRYO CULTURES AS A METHOD FOR THE STUDY OF CENTRAL NERVOUS SYSTEM MALFORMATIONS

SECTION II DRUGS OF USE AND ABUSE.
A. BARBITURATES AND OTHER ANTICONVULSANTS, BENZODIAZEPINES AND ALCOHOL

7   A REVIEW OF DIAZEPAM AND OTHER BENZODIAZEPINES IN PREGNANCY

8   NEUROHISTOLOGICAL AND NEUROBIOLOGICAL ASPECTS OF FETAL ALCOHOL
     SYNDROME IN THE RAT

SECTION III DRUGS OF USE AND ABUSE.

B. OPIOIDS AND MARIHUANA

SECTION **IV** SUBSTANCES ACTING ON
NEUROTRANSMITTERS AND THEIR RECEPTORS

13 NEUROTRANSMITTERS IN DEVELOPMENT AS POSSIBLE SUBSTRATES FOR DRUGS OF
    USE AND ABUSE

14 AGE AT THE TIME OF TESTING RECONSIDERED IN NEUROBEHAVIORAL
    TERATOLOGICAL RESEARCH

SECTION **V** HORMONES AND VITAMINS

15 EFFECTS OF THYROID HORMONES ON CENTRAL NERVOUS SYSTEM DEVELOPMENT

SECTION VI HEAVY METALS

18 DEVELOPMENTAL NEUROPATHOLOGY AND BEHAVIORAL TERATOLOGY OF METHYLMERCURY

19 BEHAVIORAL TERATOLOGY OF LEAD

Contributors

THE numbers in this alphabetical list indicate the chapter to which the author contributed. Full postal addresses are to be found on the opening page of each chapter.

Section I
OVERVIEW AND METHODOLOGY

F OR further discussion on methodological issues see the Preface by Yanai, Chapter 14 in Section IV by Spear and Chapter 17 in Section V by Cuckle.

Neurobehavioral Teratology
edited by Joseph Yanai
© Elsevier Science Publishers BV 1984

1

AN OVERVIEW AND SUMMARY OF THE BEHAVIORAL AND NEURAL CONSEQUENCES OF PERINATAL EXPOSURE TO PSYCHOTROPIC DRUGS

Roger M. Brown[1] and Rachelle H.B. Fishman[2]

[1] National Institute on Drug Abuse, Rockville, MD 20857, USA and [2] Hadassah Medical School of the Hebrew University of Jerusalem, Jerusalem 91010, Israel

DRUGS used by pregnant women may be prescribed by a physician, self-prescribed, or taken to support a drug habit. Psychotropic drug use among women of child-bearing age, which is greater than among men of comparable age (Finnegan, 1979), is important because the effect of the use of many drugs by the mother on fetal development is generally unknown. There is a striking lack of information on subtle drug-induced changes in the functional capacity of the central nervous system.

This chapter is concerned with preclinical studies of the behavioral consequences of perinatal psychotropic drug exposure as well as possible centrally mediated mechanisms underlying drug-induced behavioral alterations. Sufficient data exist in some areas of study to warrant the preparation of a summary table of major findings. These are presented at the end of each section. In the tables the gestational age in days (GD) of maternal drug treatment is provided, as well as the postanal age in days (P) of the offspring when the testing was conducted.

Opiates (Table 1.1)

A 1977 survey of young adults 18 to 25 years of age indicated that among the various

Table 1.1. Opiates

Treatment	Symptoms in offspring

I. FUNCTIONAL ALTERATIONS

1. *Developmental milestone and reflex ontogeny*

| *Methadone*, 5 mg/kg, ip, to rats prior to and throughout pregnancy and nursing | Crossfostering studies indicated a *delay* in:
a) reflex ontogeny (tailhanging, startle, and visual orientation)
b) eye opening, incisor eruption, ear opening
c) locomotion
(Zagon and McLaughlin, 1978) |

2. *Activity, acquisition, performance*

Heroin, 5 mg/kg, ip, to female rats prior to and throughout pregnancy and nursing	*Increased activity* at P21 in: a) activity cage b) activity wheel c) step-down latency (Lasky et al., 1977)
Morphine, increasing doses reaching 45 mg/kg, sc, to pregnant rats from GD 5 to 18	*Increased activity* in open field P30 and P70 and activity cage (P70) (Davis and Lin, 1972)
Morphine, increasing doses reaching 40 mg/kg, sc, to pregnant rats from GD 7 to 21	Fostering to surrogate mothers indicated drug related: *Hyperactivity* from P10 to P30 (Sobrian, 1977)
Methadone, 5 mg/kg, ip, to rats prior to and throughout pregnancy and nursing	Crossfostering studies indicated that animals were: a) *Hyperactive* at P45 and 60 (lactation-exposed animals) (Zagon and McLaughlin, 1979) b) *Impaired* in the acquisition of *active avoidance* and *discrimination learning* at P120 (Zagon et al., 1979)
Methadone, 5 then 10 mg/kg, po, to pregnant rats from GD 8 to delivery	*High response rate* on VI 40 (males not females) at P60 *Positive behavioral contrast* on learning S + S − discrimination (females, not males) (Hutchings et al., 1979)
Met-enkephalin, 80 μg/kg, sc, to rat pups from P1 to P7	*Facilitated maze learning* at P90 (Kastin et al., 1980)

3. *Drug tolerance/sensitivity*

Morphine, up to 10 mg/kg, sc, to pregnant rats from GD 5 to 12	Crossfostering studies indicated: *Tolerance to morphine analgesia* using hot plate test (up to 11 weeks) (O'Callaghan and Holtzman, 1976)
Morphine, up to 8 mg/kg, sc, to rat pups from P1 to 21	*Tolerance to morphine analgesia* at P80 using hot plate test (Zimmerman et al., 1974; see also Sonderegger and Zimmerman, 1978)
Beta-endorphin, 50 μg, sc, to rat pups from P2 to 7	*Elevated threshold for tail flick test* at P90 (Sandman et al., 1979) Treatment correlated with *reduced beta-endorphin-like immunoreactivity* in several brain regions (Moldow et al., 1981)

II. NEUROBIOLOGICAL FINDINGS

Methadone, 5 mg/kg, ip, to pregnant rats prior to and throughout pregnancy and nursing	Crossfostering studies indicated: *reduced size of brain and cerebellum* at P21 (Zagon and McLaughlin, 1977a, 1977b) At 60 days of age: *reduced total DNA content* ('cell number') *reduced DNA concentration* ('cell packing density') *increased protein/DNA* ('cell size') (Zagon and McLaughlin, 1977c, 1978)
Methadone, 1 to 5 mg/kg, sc, to pregnant from GD 13 to delivery	Crossfostering studies indicated abnormal *cerebral cortex:* a) reduced thickness with 'catch-up' by 3rd week b) reduced cell count *hippocampus:* increased cell population in Cajal fields (decreased neuropil) (Ford and Rhines, 1979) Compared to *pair-fed* controls: reduced forebrain NE and DA levels until P40. reduced in vitro NE uptake (V_{max}) (McGinty and Ford, 1980)
Methadone, up to 5 mg/kg, sc, to pregnant rats from GD 10 through nursing	Crossfostering studies indicated a *reduction in:* a) *Tyrosine hydroxylase activity* from P2-17 (Lau et al., 1977) b) *Synaptosomal uptake of* NE, DA, 5-HT c) *Vesicular NE uptake* (Slotkin et al., 1979) d) *Maturational pattern of ornithine decarboxylase* (Slotkin et al., 1976) (see also Butler and Schanberg, 1975)

drugs asked about, experience with opiates placed second only to the use of marijuana (Richards, 1981). In New York City, approximately 25% of the persons enrolled in methadone clinics during the 1970s were women of child-bearing age (Newman, 1974); approximately 80% of pregnant drug-dependent women in New York City, as well as Philadelphia, were reported to be taking methadone alone or in combination with other narcotics (Finnegan, 1979). Well over 50% of the infants born to mothers who continue narcotic abuse during pregnancy show symptoms of the *neonatal narcotic abstinence syndrome*. In addition to the abstinence syndrome, the symptoms of which may last for weeks following birth (Zelson, 1973), later behavioral disturbances also often develop, including hyperactivity and brief attention span (Ramer and Lodge, 1975; Strauss et al. 1976; Wilson et al. 1973).

Animal studies further emphasize the long-term consequences of pre/postnatal narcotic exposure: relatively permanent behavioral deficits and neurobiological complications often accompany early narcotic exposure. Zagon and McLaughlin (1978a) reported a 1–3 day delay in the appearance of certain developmental landmarks (eye opening, incisor eruption and ear opening) in the pups of pregnant rats exposed to methadone throughout pregnancy. In addition, these pups, and those exposed during the nursing period, exhibited markedly retarded development of certain reflex behaviors (including tail hanging reflex, startle response and the visual orientation reflex) as well as walking, which was seen in only 31–35 % of the animals by day 13, compared to 100 % of the controls.

Animal experiments have also shown excessive enhanced activity in offspring of mothers treated with heroin (Laskey et al., 1977), morphine (Davis and Lin, 1972; Sobrian, 1977) or methadone (Zagon and McLaughlin, 1979) during pregnancy.

The offspring of opiate-treated pregnant rats have been reported to differ from controls in the learning of an active avoidance or discrimination task (Zagon et al. 1979; Hutchings, et al. 1979). Zagon et al. (1979) found that rats exposed to methadone during the gestation period were severely inhibited in learning both active avoidance and appetitive discrimination behaviors, while animals exposed to drug during the nursing period showed only impairment of the acquisition of the discrimination. Interestingly, animals exposed during both the gestational and the nursing periods were less behaviorally disrupted than might be expected on the basis of duration of drug exposure alone. These animals showed an impaired active avoidance behavior only. Several studies by Zagon and coworkers have found a relative protection induced by drug exposure during gestation plus nursing periods when compared to either period alone (Zagon and McLaughlin, 1978; Zagon et al. 1979; Zagon and McLaughlin, 1978a, b.). Thus, continuous exposure to methadone might confer some degree of tolerance on neural tissue, thereby allowing developmental processes to proceed undisturbed (Zagon and McLaughlin, 1977, 1978a, b).

Hutchings et al. (1979) observed a sex difference in rats in the response of methadone offspring to a VI 40 schedule of water reinforcement. Treated male offspring responded at a higher rate than did control males or treated females. In contrast, with the introduction of S + S − components, the treated females, but not the males, showed a positive behavioral contrast phenomenon. That is, the females increased responding during the S + component as they learned that responding during the S − phase was not reinforced. Unlike males, the treated female offspring also showed a greater response suppression in the VI component upon introduction of noncontingent shock. The general increase in overall rate of responding by the methadone offspring did not impair the acquisition of performance of these tasks; however, preliminary data suggested that acquisition of a task contingent upon a low rate of responding was impaired.

Not only can opiates influence behavioral development, but when the endogenously occurring opioid compound, met-enkephalin, is administered to neonates, there is a facilitation of the acquisition of maze performance in adulthood. Opioids may thus activate maze learning behavior as well as influence brain organization during neonatal development (Kastin et al. 1980).

Early drug exposure also affects the later action of opiate/opioid compounds. O'Callaghan and Holtzman (1976) found no group differences in morphine concentration in brain or plasma at the time when rat offspring, perinatally exposed to morphine, were clearly tolerant to the analgesic actions of morphine. This long-term tolerance to morphine must occur at the neural level, since differences in drug metabolism were not apparent. Nor can behavioral (i.e. learned) tolerance explain these data, since the morphine-treated offspring showed tolerance during the first test session.

Males and females develop perinatally induced tolerance differentially, implying an endocrine involvement in the physiological response to morphine. O'Callaghan and Holtzman (1976) found a cross tolerance to levorphanol in rat offspring with perinatally induced morphine tolerance; but, the analgesic effect of levorphanol was greater in both the nontolerant as well as tolerant male offspring when compared to the females, regardless of the maternal drug treatment. The mediating endocrines may not be sexual per se. Zimmerman et al. (1974) observed that female rats exposed prenatally to morphine showed increased plasma corticosterone levels in response to naloxone for as long as 180 days of life. In spite of this adrenal steroid – stress – response, there was no sign of precipitated abstinence as a result of the naloxone treatment. Neither control nor treated males showed this hormonal response, even when the dose of naloxone was doubled.

Prepubertal administration of beta-endorphin to rats increased their analgesic capacity. Adults responded at elevated threshold to thermal stimuli, as measured by the tail flick test. Naloxone failed to reverse the analgesia, suggesting to Sandman et al. (1979) a relatively permanent alteration in opioid receptor development. Upon examination a reduced beta-endorphin-like immunoreactivity in several brain structures, including limbic regions, areas of neocortex, hypothalamus and striatum, was found (Moldow et al. 1981). The reduced levels might result from increased peptide degradation, reduced synthesis, or possibly interaction with the neurotransmitter dopamine, which is particularly rich in these brain regions.

Structural and biochemical alterations of the brain have also been seen as a consequence of early opiate exposure. Whole brain and cerebellar size and weight were reduced in methadone exposed rat offspring at P21; the severity was related to duration of the maternal treatment (Zagon and McLaughlin, 1977a, 1977b; McGinty and Ford, 1980). Whole brain and cerebellar DNA and protein content were reduced. If DNA content is taken to reflect cell number, protein per unit DNA to reflect cell size, and DNA concentration to estimate cell packing density (Zagon and McLaughlin, 1977c, 1978; see also Fish and Winick, 1969) then reduction in brain size is due to a real loss of neurons. Offspring of methadone-treated dams had reduced cortical thickness and cell count. In the Cajal fields of the hippocampus there was an apparent increase in the number of cells, presumably due to a reduced neuropil with a corresponding increase in neuron density (Ford and Rhines, 1979).

A reduction in norepinephrine (NE) and dopamine (DA) neurotransmitter levels was reported in the forebrain of methadone-exposed offspring. This reduction in catecholamines was observed early in postnatal life; recovery occurred by about 40 days of age. Such a delay in maturation of neurotransmitter levels in vivo was paralleled by reduced high affinity NE uptake in vitro (McGinty and Ford, 1980). McGinty and

Ford (1980) proposed that since forebrain structures were altered more than hindbrain regions, the rate at which neuronal processes in the hindbrain reach their cellular targets in the forebrain may be inhibited by drug exposure resulting in a deficit in the number of forebrain terminals or a depressed functional capacity of the catecholamine neurons reaching the forebrain during the early postnatal period. Slotkin and coworkers (1979; 1980) found similar effects. They showed less noradrenergic synaptogenesis as reflected by a reduction in synaptosomal NE uptake (a measure of the number of synaptic terminals), reduced tyrosine hydroxylase activity (a measure of biosynthetic capacity) (Lau et al. 1977), and reduced vesicular uptake and dopamine-beta-hydroxylase activity (measures of transmitter storage capability). The delayed rate of synaptogenesis was also seen for DA and 5-hydroxytryptamine (5-HT) neurons. Slotkin (1979) suggested that the effects of methadone were not on a specific neuronal element, but on a general developmental process. To test this hypothesis, the influence of methadone on brain ornithine decarboxylase (ODC) activity was examined. ODC catalyzes the rate limiting step in the synthesis of polyamines, which are found at maximal levels during periods of rapid cellular growth and differentiation (see Slotkin, 1979). Both morphine (Butler and Schanberg, 1975) and methadone (Slotkin et al. 1976) administration during pregnancy produced a delay in the maturational profile of ODC activity in the brains of the offspring, which in general, preceded or coincided with a deficit in development of catecholamine biosynthetic capacity.

It remains to be determined whether opiates act directly through ODC to alter protein synthesis or whether the change in ODC activity is a reflection of an even broader modification of protein synthesis. Nevertheless, it is of interest that the delay in maturation of synaptogenesis and neurotransmitter development closely parallels the delay in behavioral ontogeny noted by Zagon and McLaughlin (1978a, b).

Lysergic acid

Although early reports suggested physical anomalies in children as a consequence of maternal lysergic acid (LSD) use (Hecht et al. 1968; Carakushansky et al., 1969), parental drug consumption in these reports was not confined to LSD, so the causal factor in presumed LSD-induced teratogenicity is still unknown. A review of the early human and animal literature indicates very weak evidence for either chromosomal damage or teratogenesis as a result of LSD use (see Long, 1972).

Only a few studies have examined the perinatal effects of LSD on brain growth and functional development. Treating pregnant rats with 100 μg/kg on GD 18–21 was reported to result in hyperactive offspring whose brains contained low serotonin content with elevated concentrations of 5-hydroxyindolacetic acid (5-HIAA). This biochemical finding suggests that prenatal exposure to LSD increases serotonin turnover at least over the first 80 days of life (Nair, 1974). Another study in mice showed that postnatal (PI) exposure to 50 micrograms per kg LSD resulted in reduced brain weight in male mice at 8 weeks of age (Goodrich et al., 1974); no deficits of exploratory behavior were found in these animals (Goodrich et al., 1974). Mice injected on P7, but not on P1, were found to have elevated serotonin concentrations in the mesencephalon/diencephalon at 8 weeks of age (Baker and Hoff, 1975). Thus, perinatal LSD exposure appears to produce long lasting changes in brain biochemistry although their functional correlates have not yet been established.

On a phenomenological basis, hallucinogenic agents might be expected to exert an effect on the visual system. One experimental approach has utilized the finding that in kittens, but not adult cats, depriving one eye of vision for a short period of time reduces the number of cells in the visual cortex that can be activated by both eyes, i.e. monocular deprivation reduces the number of binocularly driven cells (Hubel and Wiesel, 1970; Hubel, 1979). Because LSD exerts an effect on monoamines, which play an important role in modulating this cortical plasticity (Kasamatsu and Pettigrew, 1976), LSD was tested for its effect on monocular deprivation. Adult cats were given intraventricular LSD over a week period simultaneously with monocular deprivation. This treatment was found to increase the number of monocularly driven cells in the striate cortex, suggesting a drug-induced reinstatement of the cortical plasticity which is normally observed only in younger animals (McCall et al., 1979). No reports have examined the perinatal effect of hallucinogens on later visual cortical information processing; however, the above preliminary findings suggest that such an investigation would be productive.

Cannabinoids: marihuana and tetrahydrocannabinol (Table 1.2)

Developmental consequences of marihuana use are of major interest because of the prevalence of its use, particularly by young adults (Richards, 1981; Miller and Cisin, 1980). Although marihuana has been cited as a potential teratogen in humans (Carakushansky et al., 1969; Hecht et al., 1968), in all cases LSD and other drugs had also been used. In a recent prospective study of 291 pregnant women, 20% of whom reported marihuana use before or during pregnancy, no birth deformities were noted. Babies born to these mothers were examined 60 to 80 hours postpartum and while medical indices (weight, head circumference, crown–head length, Apgar status) did not differ between the offspring of non-users, behavioral differences were found. Babies born to heavy marihuana smokers (more than 5 joints per week) showed alterations in visual responding and habituation to a light stimulus. In addition, they had an increased incidence of tremors and startles, and the shrill, high-pitched cry, 'cri de chat', which has been reported among neonates born to opiate- or barbiturate-dependent mothers, and which is generally considered to be a symptom of drug withdrawal (Zelson et al., 1973; Finnegan, 1979). Similarly, Golub et al. (1981) reported a visual response abnormality in the offspring of monkeys chronically exposed to delta-9-tetrahydrocannabinol (THC) during gestation and throughout lactation. At 1 and 2 years

Table 1.2. Marihuana

Treatment	Symptoms in offspring

I. FUNCTIONAL ALTERATIONS

1. *Developmental milestones and reflex ontogeny*

Treatment	Symptoms in offspring
Pregnant rats exposed to *cannabis smoke* from GD 1 to 19	Crossfostering indicated: drug-induced *delay in incisor eruption and eye opening* (Fried, 1976)
THC, 10 mg/kg, sc, given to pregnant rats on GD 10, 11, 12	Crossfostering studies indicated: *delay in tooth eruption* *retarded development of cliff avoidance and visual placing* (Borgen et al., 1973)

2. *Activity, acquisition, performance*

Treatment	Symptoms in offspring
Neonates of mothers who were heavy users of *marihuana*	Symptoms among the infants at 60–80 h postpartum: a) *Visual attention deficits* b) *Trimors and startles* c) *Cri-de-chat* (Fried, 1980)
THC, 2.4 mg/kg, po, to pregnant rhesus monkeys throughout pregnancy and lactation	*Attention deficit disorder* at 1–2 years of age. More time directed toward attending to novel stimuli (Golub et al., 1981)
Cannabis extract, 250 mg/kg, sc, given to pregnant rats from GD 8 to 11	*Impaired maze learning* at P65 (Gianutsos and Abbatiello, 1972)
Cannabis extract, 150 mg/kg, po, given to pregnant rats from GD 2 to 21	A design utilizing pair-fed controls indicated: *Impairment of rotorod performance* at P75 (Abel, 1979)
THC given to postnatal mice in a dose of 10 mg/kg, ip, from P20 to P60	*Conditioned avoidance testing* beginning at P60: a) *Enhanced acquisition* b) *Impaired retention* c) *Reduction in performance over time* (Radouco-Thomas et al., 1976)
THC, 2 mg/kg, po, given to pregnant rats from GD 3 to delivery	*Impaired passive avoidance acquisition* at P21 *Enhanced dominance* in push-tube competition at P90 (No passive avoidance deficit observed). (Vardaris et al., 1976)

3. *Drug tolerance/sensitivity*

Treatment	Symptoms in offspring
Pregnant rats exposed to *cannabis* smoke from GD 1 to 19	Crossfostering studies indicated: *Prenatal exposure: enhanced THC sensitivity* at P90 *Postnatal exposure: enhanced THC tolerance* at P90 (Fried, 1976; Barnes and Fried, 1974)

4. *Sexual behavior*

Treatment	Symptoms in offspring
THC or *Cannabinol* (CNB) 50 mg/kg, po, to pregnant mice on GD 20 and for 6 days following delivery	Adults: Both THC and CNB reduced male sexual behavior THC treatment: elevated plasma LH concentration CNB treatment: reduced plasma FSH concentration (Dalterio and Bartke, 1979) (See also: Fried and Charlebois, 1979)
Pregnant rats exposed to *marihuana* smoke for 9 min/day	Crossfostering studied indicated: *Reduced reproductive organ weight* in both males and females at P180 (Fried and Charlebois, 1979)

of age, the human infants in the above studies were found to direct significantly more attention toward novel objects than familiar stimuli, unlike the unexposed controls.

Preclinical studies have been hampered by difficulties with drug administration and experimental design (viz. the review by Abel, 1980). Cannabinoids have extremely low water solubility, thus the vehicle itself as well as route of administration are critically important factors in outcome and must be controlled for.

THC or marihuana extract administered orally has not been found to be teratogenic in several species (Wright et al., 1976; Fleischman et al., 1975). High doses of cannabinoids reduce food intake (Manning et al., 1971; Abel, 1980; Abel et al., 1980), so an experimental design including cross fostering and pair feeding must be used to distinguish between drug effects and malnutrition or poor maternal care. As a case in point, Abel et al., (1979) cross fostered unexposed pups at birth to dams which had received marihuana extract while pregnant. The offspring, themselves never directly exposed to the drug, showed a maternal dose-related decrease in postnatal growth and a reduction in rearing behavior in an open field.

In one study, a delay in incisor eruption and eye opening, i.e. developmental landmarks, was noted in rat offspring whose mothers had been exposed to marihuana smoke for 9 minutes per day throughout most of the gestational period; however, there were no group differences in the development of reflex behavior, such as the righting reflex, free-fall righting, cliff avoidance, and visual placing (Fried, 1976). In another study, the offspring of pregnant rats receiving higher doses of THC on GD 10–12 also showed a delay in incisor eruption but not in eye opening. These animals showed some retardation in the ontogeny of cliff avoidance and visual placing, while no delay in other reflexes (righting, free-fall righting, negative geotaxis) was observed (Borgen et al., 1973).

An early study suggested that high doses of marihuana could lead to learning disabilities. Pregnant rats were given cannabis resin early in gestation. At P65 the offspring were impaired in maze learning: they made more errors and spent less time in the maze (Gianutsos and Abbatiello, 1972). On the other hand, a study utilizing pair-fed controls (Abel, 1979) failed to distinguish the effect of in utero drug exposure from malnutrition on a variety of procedures including open field behavior, spontaneous alternation, learning and retention of a brightness discrimination, and shock avoidance. Impaired rotorod performance may (Abel, 1979) or may not (Abel et al., 1981) be drug related.

Mice were treated neonatally from P20 to P60 with THC and then trained to avoid shock in a shuttle box at 2–3 days after termination of treatment and again at 100 and 200 days later (Radouco-Thomas et al., 1976). Treatment enhanced acquisition of the response in two strains (C57BL6 and DBA/2J) and impaired acquisition in another (A/J strain). When the C57BL6 strain was given 5 daily sessions at P80, and again at P180, the treated animals showed large decrements in performance between the fifth session at P80 and the first session at P180, presumably due to a retention deficit. All treatment groups showed a deterioration of shock avoidance performance over time, which may be related to the 'amotivational syndrome' (Kolansky and Moore, 1972), to a drug-induced facilitation of the aging process (since other signs of aging appeared earlier in the treated animals (Radouco-Thomas et al., 1976)), or to changes in neural processing of pain (shock) and motor (avoidance) behavior because the amotivation is not seen in agonistic situations.

Vardaris et al. (1976) used a push tube to test the offspring of THC-treated female rats. A treated pup and a control were released simultaneously into opposite ends of a tube. The test was completed when one of the pair was forced out of the tube, the 'loser'. By P90, the prenatally treated offspring were winners 94% of the time. However, the treated offspring at P21 were slower to aquire a 1-trial passive avoidance response, while at P90 no passive avoidance deficit was observed. A difference in procedure between these two age groups, however, could have compromised the comparison.

The use of cross-fostering methods allowed Fried (1976) to note a difference in functional outcome with respect to multiple exposures to THC during different periods of development. Animals exposed in utero demonstrated enhanced sensitivity to the later administration of THC. On the other hand, animals exposed to the cannabinoids during lactation developed tolerance to THC more rapidly than controls (Fried, 1976; Barns and Fried 1974).

Since high doses of marihuana affect reproduction capability in adult male rodents (Dalterio et al., 1977; Fried and Charlebois, 1979) and in some human studies (Hembree et al., 1979), the effects of cannabinoids upon male sexual differentiation in the fetus were studied. Pregnant mice were given either THC or the non-psychoactive marihuana component cannabinol (CBN) on GD 20 and for 6 days following delivery. The exposed offspring showed reduced male sexual behavior, but probably via different central mechanisms. THC exposure was associated with an elevated plasma LH level, while CBN treatment was related to a reduced plasma FSH value (Dalterio and Bartke, 1979). Prenatally THC-exposed adult male mice also had smaller vas deferens and were peripherally less sensitive to norepinephrine and enkephalins (Dalterio et al., 1980). Similar results were obtained by Fried and Charlebois (1980) who exposed pregnant rats to marihuana smoke for 9 minutes per day throughout gestation. At P180, male and female offspring were less fertile as reflected by reduced gonad weights. Those females which did conceive showed more resorptions than controls, but no gross malformations or stunting in the live offspring.

In summary, perinatal marihuana/THC exposure has been shown to result in behavioral disturbances in experimental animals and at high doses with regular use in humans. Attention disturbances seem to be the major developmental finding in human infants. In experimental animal work, many studies in the past have been hampered by difficulties associated with drug solubility and vehicle toxicity. Nevertheless, it appears that at high enough doses marihuana/THC can postpone developmental milestones and behavioral ontogeny. Particular attention should be addressed to lasting disturbances in learning, retention and reproductive behavior, controlling for nutrition, multiple drug exposure and socioeconomic class. The mechanisms underlying the behavioral findings are generally unknown, although the neuroendocrine system appears to be a likely candidate in deleterious marihuana/THC action.

Barbiturates (Table 1.3)

Research investigating the possible behavioral consequences of pre- or postnatal barbiturate exposure is important because of the large number of women taking barbiturates during pregnancy as sedatives, hypnotics, anticonvulsants and even antianxiety agents (Hill, 1973). In addition to the licit use, the nonprescription use of the barbiturates is likewise considerable (Cooper, 1978). Data obtained from the Collaborative Perinatal Project (Heinonen et al., 1977) indicate that, of the pregnant women interviewed in the survey, 25% took barbiturates at some time during their pregnancy. Another study (Cooper, 1978) reported the existence of a high rate of barbiturate consumption among 22–25 year old young adults. The reports and descriptions of the signs and symptoms of barbiturate withdrawal are by no means minor (Bleyer and Marshall, 1972; Desmond et al., 1972; Finnegan, 1979), and there are mixed reports in the clinical literature suggesting behavioral disturbances following pre- and postnatal barbiturate exposure (viz. the review of Fishman and Yanai, 1983).

Preclinical studies strongly implicate neuropathological consequences in the offspring following barbiturate exposure of the mother. There is strong evidence for neurobiological complications, some with behavioral correlates.

The offspring of phenobarbital treated mice generally show no physical abnormalities; however, development of certain reflexes over the first 20 days of life (hindlimb placing, accelerated righting, straight line walking, bar holding, and crossed extensor) but not others (righting reflex, forelimb grasping, or vibrissae placing) has been shown to be retarded (Zemp and Middaugh, 1975). Hyperactivity in an open field procedure (i.e. increased square crossing) at P75 is one long-lasting effect. At P90, the treated mice did not differ from controls in the acquisition of a passive avoidance response; however, they showed poorer retention of the response 24 hours later. In a final series of behavioral tests, the animals were trained in an operant task consisting of a series of progressive fixed ratio schedules from FR 1 through FR 40. There were no group differences in either acquisition or response rate until FR 20 when the phenobarbital-exposed offspring responded less rapidly than control. This response decrement became even more pronounced under the FR 40 schedule (Middaugh et al., 1975; Zemp and Middaugh, 1975). The authors ascribed the results of the passive avoidance test to a reduction in fear and the impaired fixed ratio performance to an attentional deficit. Both of these results, however, could also equally as well result from increased activity as observed in the open-field situation.

That early barbiturate exposure produces long-lasting changes in brain sensitivity is illustrated by the finding that prenatal phenobarbital exposure results in a tolerance

14

Table 1.3. Barbiturates

Treatment	Symptoms in offspring
I. FUNCTIONAL ALTERATIONS	
1. *Developmental milestones and reflex ontogeny*	
Phenobarbital, 40 mg/kg, sc, to pregnant mice from GD 13 to delivery	*Retarded reflex development* (hindlimb placing, accelerated righting, straight line, walking, bar holding, crossed extensor) (Zemp and Middaugh, 1975)
2. *Activity, acquisition, performance*	
Phenobarbital, 40 mg/kg, sc, to pregnant mice from GD 15 to 21	at P75: *Increased locomotion* *Impaired passive avoidance acquisition* *Reduced FR 40 response rate* (Middaugh, 1975)
3. *Drug tolerance/sensitivity*	
Phenobarbital, 3 g/kg food given to pregnant mice from GD 9 to 18	*Enhanced tolerance to:* a) *Barbiturates* (Yanai and Tabakoff, 1979) b) *Ethanol* (Yanai and Tabakoff, 1980)
4. *Sexual behavior*	
Pentobarbital, 50 or 100 μg given to hamster pups on P2 to 4	Masculinization of males blocked during a critical period (Clemens et al., 1979)
Phenobarbital, 40 mg/kg, sc, given to pregnant rats from: GD 12–19	*Female* sexual behavior and cyclicity impaired at P60 (Gupta et al., 1980)
GD 17–20	*Male* sexual behavior impaired at P60 (Gupta et al., 1982)
II. NEUROBIOLOGICAL FINDINGS	
1. *Biochemistry*	
Phenobarbital, 80 mg/kg, sc, given to pregnant mice from GD 13 to delivery	Whole brain determinations: *DNA:* Reduced (P5–14) followed by increased (P21, P28) levels *RNA:* Reduced concentration (P5–P28) *Protein:* Reduced concentration (P5–P28) (Zemp and Middaugh, 1975)
Phenobarbital, 60 mg/kg, sc, to rat pups from P3 to P21	Whole brain determinations at P21: *Reduced RNA, DNA, protein and cholesterol* (Schain and Watanabe, 1975) (See also: Diaz et al., 1977)
Phenobarbital, 40 mg/kg, sc, given to pregnant rats from GD 12 to 19:	*Females: Increased* plasma estrogen and progestone and *Reduced LH* (Gupta et al., 1980)
GD 17 to 20:	*Males: Reduced* brain and plasma testosterone (Gupta et al., 1982)
Phenobarbital, 50 mg/kg, sc, P2 to P21	*Eliminated* peak thyroxine levels in mice (Fishman et al., 1982)

2. *Neuroanatomy*

Phenobarbital, 50 ,g/kg, sc, to rat pups from P2 to P21	*Brain weight at P50:* Reduced 8% *Cerebellum:* Both *Purkinje* and *granule cells* reduced 33% *Hippocampus:* 33% fewer *pyramidal* cells and 25% fewer *granule* cells *Cortex:* Reduced area (Bergman and Yanai, 1981; Yanai et al., 1981) *Cerebellum:* Significant ultrastructural deficits thruout cortex (Fishman et al., 1983)
Phenobarbital, 3 gm/kg food to pregnant rats from GD 9 to 18	*Brain weight* at P50: Reduced 8% *Cerebellum: Purkinje cells* reduced 30%, no change in granule cells *Hippocampus:* 15% fewer *pyramidal cells*, no change in granule cells *Cortex:* No change (Yanai et al., 1979)

to the hypothermic and hypnotic action of pentobarbital or ethanol at P50 (Yanai and Tabakoff, 1979, 1980). The tolerance induced by barbiturate exposure resides in the brain tissue; the duration of sleeping time induced by either pentobarbital or alcohol was reduced in spite of higher than control brain levels of these drugs upon awakening. The authors suggest that the mechanisms underlying brain changes induced by drug exposure are different in the developing organism because the changes induced by prenatal exposure last into adulthood while the effects due to chronic drug exposure in the adult rapidly diminish (Yanai and Tabakoff, 1980).

Perinatal barbiturate exposure has also been reported to disrupt adult sexual behavior. Male hamsters given 50 or 100 μg of pentobarbital on P2 to P4 showed reduced sexual performance at 60 days of age. These defects were probably not due to low circulating androgen because there was no reversal of the behavior following administration of testosterone propionate. Further, since pentobarbital blocked masculinization of androgen-treated females, the effect of the barbiturate was considered to interfere with normal masculinization of the brain during a critical period (Clemens et al., 1979). This investigator found pentobarbital to have no effect on normal female sexual behavior. However, in another species, female rats exposed in utero to phenobarbital were reported to have severe deficits in reproductive function, including a delay in the onset of puberty, disorders of the estrous cycle (persistent and/or constant estrous), and infertility. These physiological alterations were associated with a subnormal plasma LH concentration, a lack that suggests a possible defect in hypothalamic-hypophyseal regulation of trophic hormone secretion. Although in normal adults this type of effect is reversible once the drug clears the system, hormonal changes due to early (prenatal) phenobarbital exposure still are apparent in the offspring three to four months later (Gupta et al., 1980). Males were also affected by in utero phenobarbital exposure. In offspring of phenobarbital-treated mothers, reduced testosterone titer was found in plasma as well as brain as late as 120 days of age (Gupta et al., 1982).

Barbiturates may affect other hormonal systems. Fishman et al. (1982) showed a significant phenobarbital-related decline in serum thyroxine which occurs at the time of the brain growth spurt and may be related to neuronal damage.

Biochemical measures following early barbiturate exposure have focused largely on whole brain nucleic acid and protein content. Most studies have found a reduction in the concentration of DNA, RNA and protein following early phenobarbital treatment. Zemp and Middaugh (1975) reported a reduced DNA content from P1 through P14 followed by an increased concentration from P21 through P28. A continual reduction in RNA and protein was observed throughout these same time periods. The data were interpreted as a drug-induced reduction in brain cell size accompanied by either an increase in gliosis or in neuronal number. Similar findings have been reported by Schain and Watanabe (1975). Since postnatal barbiturate administration may produce sedation which could impair feeding, Diaz et al. (1977) utilized a chronic intragastric feeding cannula to prevent drug-induced undernutrition. Their results were similar to the results of prenatal exposure, i.e. brain growth was retarded not only in weight but also in levels of RNA, DNA, protein and cholesterol. Yanai et al. (1982) showed that early phenobarbital interferes with dopamine-mediated behavior, implying a long-lasting defect in this neurotransmitter system.

Morphological studies have confirmed the biochemical suggestion of drug-induced cell loss. When phenobarbital was given to pregnant mice in the diet, the offspring, at P50, had a reduction of 30 and 15 % in the prenatally forming cerebellar Purkinje cells and hippocampal pyramidal cells, respectively. Neonatal treatment, on the other hand, produced the expected loss in the postnatally forming cerebellar and hippocampal granule cells, but in addition 30 % of the cerebellar Purkinje cells and the hippocampal pyramidal cells were also destroyed (Bergman and Yanai, 1981). Since these latter cells are formed well before the drug exposure (see Rodier, 1977), and therefore would be expected to be less vulnerable to the drug, the data indicate that phenobarbital may not only destroy proliferating neurons but also cause considerable damage to neurons which are relatively advanced in their stage of development (Bergman and Yanai, 1981; Bergman et al., 1980). Further studies will be required to determine the extent of the period of neuronal susceptbility to phenobarbital as well as the nature of the underlying mechanism. The neuronal degenerative effects of the early phenobarbital exposure are still seen in adult mice. Electron microscopic studies showed evidence of defects which implied that degenerative processes were continuing even though drug exposure was long past (Fishman et al., 1982b). Yanai et al. (1981) showed that the neuronal deficits produced by early drug exposure correlated with audiogenic seizure susceptibility. Future investigations will surely continue to relate more specific anatomical findings to behavioral events.

Alcohol (Table 1.4)

The cluster of symptoms comprising the fetal alcohol syndrome (FAS) is estimated to be associated with one out of 750 births (see Streissguth et al., 1980). Central nervous system involvement includes retarded or delayed motor development, hypotonia, mild to moderate mental retardation, irritability in infancy (including heightened sensitivity to sound), reduced habituation to repetitive stimuli, and hyperactivity in childhood. Growth deficiency, small brain size at autopsy, and particular facial characteristics are the primary diagnostic criteria in newborn (Hanson et al., 1976; Jones et al., 1973; Clarren and Smith, 1978; Streissguth et al., 1980). FAS symptomatology has been found to be directly related to the amount of maternal alcohol intake (Quellette et al., 1977).

In general, animal models of FAS have replicated many of the clinical findings including growth deficits, hyperactivity, and learning disabilities. When alcohol was administered to rat pups through an intragastric cannula to meet all daily nutritional requirements independent of the alcohol regimen, brain growth, particularly that of the cerebellum, was reduced in spite of a normal body growth (Diaz and Sampson, 1980). This confirmed nutrition as an important variable in the reduction of somatic growth of offspring born to alcohol consuming mothers. In line with disturbed brain development was altered reflex ontogeny. Ten days following termination of postnatal alcohol treatment the negative geotaxis and free-fall righting reflexes were impaired, as was general motor coordination (Diaz and Sampson, 1980). Alcohol exposure throughout gestation has been reported by some investigators (Martin et al., 1978) to delay developmental milestones in rats (such as the age of ear flap uncurling and eye opening) but not others (Da Silva et al., 1980), who did, however find impaired maternal behavior (such as pup retrieval and nest rebuilding). This highlights the difficulty of separating alcohol-induced brain damage from maternal neglect (see Abel, 1980).

Increased locomotor activity is one long-lasting outcome of prenatal alcohol treatment (Bond and DiGiusto, 1976; Krsiak et al., 1977; Martin et al., 1978). Martin et al. (1978) showed by cross-fostering that maternal factors were not responsible for enhanced wheel-running in the offspring at P60. Similarly, Bond and DiGusto (1976) found treated rat pups more active in an open field at P45–50; nutritional differences were an unlikely explanation for the results since experimental and control groups did not differ in weight. Species or strain susceptibility does exert an influence on the locomotor effect of prenatal alcohol exposure, since in C57 mice, treated offspring had decreased open field activity while treated DBA offspring were not affected on this variable (Yanai and Ginsburg, 1979).

Clinical findings have suggested a relationship between alcoholism in parents and hyperactivity in their children, and further that hyperactivity in childhood may be predisposing to adult alcoholism (Goodwin et al., 1975). In support of this, Bond and DiGuisto (1976) found that the rat offspring of alcohol-treated mothers were both

18

hyperactive and they showed a preference for low concentration alcohol solutions when given a choice between alcohol and water. Riley et al. (1979a), who found that rat offspring of alcohol-treated mothers consumed more of an aversive lithium chloride solution than controls, suggested that the treated animals might have a deficit in response inhibition. Consistent with this hypothesis is the co-existing deficit in passive avoidance learning, i.e. inability to withhold a response (Riley et al., 1979a) and a tendency to persevere when alternation is the correct response (Riley et al., 1979b).

Table 1.4. Alcohol

Treatment	Symptoms in offspring
I. FUNCTIONAL ALTERATIONS	
1. *Developmental milestones and reflex ontogeny*	
Rat pups given intragastric infusion of approximately 5% ETOH from P4 to 8	At P18 there was: 1) *Reduced brain growth* (Body weight was not affected) 2) *Impaired reflex development* i) Negative geotaxis ii) Free-fall righting 3) *Motor incoordination* (Diaz and Samson, 1980)
Pregnant rats given 8.5 g/kg of 20% ETOH, po, from GD 1 throughout pregnancy and nursing	Crossfostering studies indicated at P1–14: *Delay* in *ear flap uncurling* and *eye opening* (incisor eruption and righting reflex developed normally) (Martin et al., 1978)
Pregnants rats were given 10% or 20% ETOH, po, from GD 1 throughout nursing	Crossfostering studies indicated at P1–14: There was normal reflex ontogeny but poor maternal behavior (Da Silva et al., 1980)
2. *Activity, acquisition, performance*	
Pregnant rats given 8.5 mg/kg 20% ETOH, po, from GD 1 through nursing	Crossfostering studies indicated hyperactivity at P60 (Martin et al., 1978)
Pregnant rats given 6.5% ETOH (14 g/kg) in diet from GD 1 to delivery	*Hyperactivity* at P45–50 (females) in an open field *Alcohol preference* was observed at P65–70 (Bond and DiGiusto, 1976)
Pregnant rats given a diet of 35% ETOH-derived calories from GD 5 to 20	*Enhanced consumption of lithium chloride solution* at P4–10. Also, *Impaired:* a) *Passive avoidance acquisition* (P18, P41–53) (Riley et al., 1979a) b) *Alternation in a T-maze* (P20) c) *Reversal learning* (P20–21) (Riley et al., 1976b)
3. *Drug tolerance/sensitivity*	
Pregnant rats given 3 g/kg 8% ETOH daily from GD 1 to delivery	Fostering studies demonstrated: *Tolerance to ETOH, pentobarbital, diazepam* but not to morphine, chlorpromazine, amphetamine (female offspring) (Abel et al., 1981)

4. *Social behavior*

Pregnant mice given 20% ETOH, po, from GD 1 to delivery	At 11 weeks of age, in isolated mice: 1) more aggression 2) more activity 3) reduced whole brain serotonin (Krsiak et al., 1977)
Pregnant mice given 5% ETOH, po, throughout gestation and lactation. At P21–30, pups given ETOH (5%) in drinking water	At 3–4 weeks of age: *reduced social investigation* As adults: *increased 'flight' behavior* (Ewart and Cutler, 1979)

II. NEUROBIOLOGICAL FINDINGS

1. *Biochemistry*

Pregnant rats were given 6% ETOH in their diet from GD 1 to delivery, or to mothers during the nursing period (P1 to 10)	*Increased histamine* in fetal (GD 18) and neonatal (P10) brain (Rawat, 1980) At P10, there was: 1) *Decreased ACh* levels 2) *Increased GABA* and *glutamate* concentration 3) *Decreased GAD* and *GAT* activities (Rawat, 1977)
Pregnant rats given 5% ETOH in diet from GD 10 through delivery	*Increased caudate tyrosine hydroxylase activity* (P8 through 22) (Branchey and Friedhoff, 1973)
Pregnant rats given 6.8% ETOH in diet from GD 13 through delivery (about 11 g/kg/day)	Postnatally (P1–15): a) *Reduced synaptosomal 5-HT uptake* (Slotkin et al., 1980) b) *Increased synaptosomal tyramine uptake* (Thadani et al., 1977a) c) *Perturbed ornithine decarboxylase activity,* especially in the cerebellum (Thadani et al., 1977b)

2. *Neuroanatomy*

Pregnant rats consumed approximately 12 g/kg per day ETOH from GD 1 to 21	*Aberrant hippocampal mossy fiber topography* (found in 60 day old offspring) (West et al., 1981)

Social interaction can also be influenced by maternal alcohol intake. Prenatally treated mice show reduced duration and frequency of social investigation (sniff, explore) at the juvenile stage of development; adult males show increased incidence of 'flight' behavior (Ewart and Cutler, 1979). Prenatal alcohol potentiated the aggression induced by a period of isolation. This was accompanied by a reduction in whole brain serotonin levels with no change in whole brain norepinephrine or dopamine (Krsiak et al., 1977).

In utero exposure to alcohol also influences central mechanisms underlying drug tolerance. Female, but not male rats which had received in utero alcohol throughout gestation were tolerant, as adults, to the hypothermic effect of alcohol and cross-tolerant to pentobarbital, and diazepam, but not to morphine, chlorpromazine, or amphetamine (Abel et al., 1981).

Perinatal alcohol exposure has been correlated with reduced whole brain acetylcholine levels, as well as increased GABA and glutamate concentrations accompanied by reduced glutamate decarboxylase and GABA-aminotransferase activities (Rawat, 1977). Whole brain histamine was found elevated in fetal and neonatal rat but only during alcohol exposure and not associated with an increase in histidine decarboxylase activity; hence, it was speculated that alcohol had an effect on histamine release rather than synthesis (Rawat, 1980).

Alcohol-induced disturbance in monoaminergic function has been reported by several workers. Rat offspring of mothers who were consuming 5% alcohol had increased tyrosine hydroxylase activity in caudate nucleus when tested at P8, P15 and P22. This may be a unique response to prenatal treatment since caudate tyrosine hydroxylase activity was not altered in adult animals following 15 days of ethanol administration, and actually a decrease in enzyme activity was noted following more prolonged alcohol exposure (Branchey and Friedhoff, 1973). Other studies reported no treatment differences in whole brain tyrosine hydroxylase activity, rather that alcohol treatment increased tyramine uptake into synaptosomes (Thadani et al., 1977). Using tyramine uptake as an indicator of synaptogenesis, the alcohol-induced increase in uptake was interpreted to indicate that ethanol shifts the time course of development of noradrenergic neurons to earlier periods. In contrast, whole brain serotonin levels are reduced by prenatal alcohol exposure (Krsiak et al., 1977), consistent with the finding of a deficit in serotonin synaptosomal uptake (Slotkin et al., 1980). Ornithine decarboxylase activity was found to differ markedly in brains of neonates prenatally exposed to alcohol. The cerebellum was most affected with the pattern of change depending on the duration of exposure and the age at the start of treatment (Thadani et al., 1977).

Prenatal alcohol exposure has been shown to alter the cytoarchitecture of hippocampal neurons. The larger pyramidal cells (targets for granule cell mossy fiber axons) are formed during the prenatal period, before the smaller granule cells differentiate, postnatally. There was a change in mossy fiber topography which consisted of aberrant fibers entering the pyramidal region in subfield CA3a. The functional implications of the hypertrophied mossy fiber distribution remains to be elucidated. The subtle change in neuroanatomical connections may be secondary to some other, possibly hormonal, action since similar hippocampal malformations have been reported following prenatal thyroxine exposure (Lauder and Mugnaini, 1977).

Amphetamine (Table 1.5)

According to a 1979 survey, 18% of American young adults interviewed (Fishburne and Cisin, 1979) have experimented with amphetamine. A report from Scandanavia indicated that complications due to amphetamine use during pregnancy are few, although six out of 17 infants were preterm and three were small for their gestational age (Ericksson et al., 1978). A single-case report describes a pregnant woman who took an average daily divided dose of 140 mg amphetamine for narcolepsy, yet gave birth to a normal girl. Follow up studies of the child over 18 months revealed no complications and normal growth and development (Briggs et al., 1975).

Amphetamine is often used in the treatment of childhood hyperactivity, now termed attentional deficit disorder with hyperactivity (American Psychiatric Association, 1980). Data indicate that chronic amphetamine treatment (more so than methylphenidate) retards growth in terms of weight but not height, although any slowing of growth at the beginning of treatment is compensated for later (Safer et al., 1972; Gross, 1976; McNull et al., 1977; Roche et al., 1979). The developmental effects of the amphetamines are of interest because of the prevalence of amphetamine consumption in women of childbearing age and because of its use in the treatment of childhood disorders.

In general, perinatal amphetamine treatment has resulted in hyperactivity and growth retardation (Zemp and Middaugh, 1975; Martin et al., 1976; Hitzeman et al.,

Table 1.5. Amphetamine

Treatment	Symptoms in offspring
Pregnant rats given 1–5 mg/kg *methamphetamine*, sc, from GD 1 to 21	Dose-related *delay in eye opening* (on day 14) (Martin, 1975)
Pregnant mice given d-*amphetamine*, 5 mg/kg, ip, from GD 13 to delivery	*Increased activity* in open field (P75) *Higher whole brain NE and DA levels* (P30) (Zemp and Middaugh, 1975)
Pregnant rats received 5 mg/kg *methamphetamine*, sc, 2 × daily from GD 1 through weaning	*Increased activity* in activity wheel at (P90) (Martin et al., 1970) *Hyperactivity persisted throughout lifetime* (Martin and Martin, 1981) *Growth retardation* throughout lifetime (Martin et al., 1979)
Pregnant rats given 3 mg/kg d-*amphetamine*, sc, 2 × daily from GD 5 through delivery	*Reduced habituation* to activity cage produced *hyperactivity* *Reduced NE* in diencephalon and brainstem (Hitzemann et al., 1976)
Pregnant rats given 0.5 mg/kg d,l-*amphetamine*, sc, 2 × daily from GD 5 through delivery	*Enhanced CAR acquisition and retention* at 90 days of age (Nasello et al., 1974) *Increased conversion of tyrosine to NE and DA* *Increased tyrosine hydroxylase activity* (Nasello and Ramirez, 1978)
Pregnant rats received *methamphetamine* in in drinking water (80 mg/l) throughout gestation and nursing	9 months after weaning: *NE levels: increased* in hippocampus; *decreased* in thalamus *Normetanephrine levels increased* in cortex, hippocampus; *decreased* in brainstem (Tonge, 1973a) 5-*HT levels increased* in cortex, hippocampus, and *decreased* in hypothalmus, brainstem 5-*HIAA levels increased* in cortex, hippocampus (Tonge, 1973b)

1976; Martin et al., 1979; Martin and Martin, 1981), with dose-related delays in developmental landmarks, such as eye opening in rat offspring (Martin, 1975). Zemp and Middaugh (1975) reported hyperactivity at P75 when total activity, including locomotion, rearing and grooming, was measured in open field. The treated mice had higher whole brain concentrations of norepinephrine and dopamine (Zemp and Middaugh, 1975). Prenatal methamphetamine treatment produced hyperactivity in offspring which persisted for at least 1 year (Martin et al., 1976), and even throughout most of the lifespan of the rats (Martin and Martin, 1981).

Hitzeman et al. (1976) found that the d-amphetamine-induced hyperactivity was related to an inability to acclimatize to new surroundings. Treated offspring were more active than controls only during the early segments of the session and only if activity was measured immediately after placing the animals into a new cage. In these animals, norepinephrine content was reduced in the diencephalon and brainstem, but only minimal alterations in dopamine or serotonin were found (Hitzeman et al., 1976).

Of functional interest, P45 and P90 offspring of mothers receiving d,l-amphetamine during gestation performed better than controls in a shuttle box on both acquisition and retention measurements (Nasello et al., 1974). Neurochemically, at P90–120, the treated animals showed no apparent differences in whole brain concentrations of norepinephrine or dopamine, but did show increased brain tyrosine hydroxylase activity and a higher rate of conversion of tyrosine to dopamine and norepinephrine (Nasello and Ramirez, 1978).

The neurochemical changes resulting from prenatal exposure of rats to methamphetamine are still seen 9 months after termination of treatment. Dopamine level was increased in cortex while norepinephrine concentration was increased in hippocampus and hypothalamus, and decreased in thalamus. Since normetanephrine concentrations were also altered, i.e. increased in cortex and hippocampus and reduced in brainstem, the metabolism of norepinephrine in general might be disturbed (Tonge, 1973a), consistent with the biochemical findings of Nasello and Ramirez (1978) and indicating more rapid norepinephrine turnover as a result of perinatal amphetamine treatment. Indoleamine metabolism was also measured: serotonin levels were higher in cortex and hippocampus and reduced in hypothalamus and brainstem. These changes roughly parallel increases in cortical and hippocampal 5-HIAA levels, suggesting enhanced serotonin turnover (Tonge, 1973b).

Thus, the data available indicate that perinatal amphetamines influence the developing fetus to alter behavioral and developmental processes, particularly hyperactivity and growth retardation. Considering the known devastating effects of amphetamine on the integrity of monoamine systems in adult animals (Ellison et al., 1978; Trulson and Jacobs, 1979; Wagner et al., 1980), it is surprising that the magnitude of changes in neurotransmitter systems following early exposure seems much less pronounced. The dynamics of these neurochemical alterations and their relation to functional development requires further study. Potential influence of the drug's action on central structural organization of the developing brain deserves attention.

Methylxanthines

The potential teratogenic effect of the methylxanthines (caffeine, theophylline and theobromine) is of concern first because of the widespread consumption of these compounds (e.g. in coffee, tea, cocoa) by society in general and second because caffeine is a demonstrated mutagen in lower species (Goldstein et al., 1974). Furthermore, doses of methylxanthines have been used to induce respiration in premature newborns (Armanda et al., 1977), and this procedure could possibly result in an alteration in postnatal brain development.

Different subjective and objective effects between boys and men have been found following caffeine administration, indicating an age-dependent site of action for this stimulant (Rapoport et al., 1981). There exist few if any studies that are concerned with the behavioral consequence of perinatal methylxanthine exposure. One study showed that daily 50–75 mg/kg caffeine per os, GD 3–19, resulted in offspring at 9 weeks whose body and gonad weight was decreased and active avoidance impaired. At lower doses, results were similar but inconsistent (West et al., 1982). Experimental toxicology studies in rats indicate that fresh coffee in neither fetal toxic nor teratogenic, with the possible exception of a delay in ossification of the rib cage (Nolen, 1981). In another study, caffeine itself was minimally embryotoxic even at high doses, but it markedly potentiated the teratogenic effect of cytotoxic agents such as nucleic-acid-synthesis inhibitors (Ritter et al., 1982). Thus an investigation into the interaction of caffeine with other potential behavioral/neurological teratogens might be beneficial. Developmentally, high-dose caffeine has been found to delay or interfere with postnatal myelination of brain tissue (Fuller and Wiggins, 1981). The need for an evaluation of correlative methylxanthine-induced behavioral teratology is obvious, and such studies should be strongly encouraged. High-dose caffeine has been found to delay or interfere with postnatal myelination of brain tissue (Fuller and Wiggins, 1981). The need for an evaluation of correlative methylxanthine-induced behavioral teratology is obvious, and such studies should be strongly encouraged.

Nicotine

It is generally believed that tobacco smoking during pregnancy leads to intrauterine growth retardation and smaller infants than those from non-smoking mothers (Ericksson et al., 1979; Meyer et al., 1974; Butler and Goldstein, 1973; Naeye, 1978). In humans, nicotine or some combustion product(s) may affect the fetus indirectly as a result of chronic hypoxia (Dow et al., 1975; Cole et al., 1972) or directly by stimulating the autonomic nervous system (Manning et al., 1975; Quigley et al., 1979), an effect dependent upon the degree of receptor maturation. Hyperactivity has also been observed in the infants of smoking mothers (see Longo, 1977). Follow-up studies of the offspring of smoking mothers show that, at 11 years of age, their children were not up to normal standards in reading or mathematical ability, even when factors such as social class or family size were taken into account (Ericksson et al., 1979; Butler and Goldstein, 1973; Longo, 1977).

Studies with animals have provided evidence to support the clinical suggestions of potential nicotine behavioral teratology. Sonawane (1982) reported significant weight reduction at birth and later abnormalities in both male and female reproductive anatomy and functions. Pregnant rats given 3 mg/kg nicotine, s.c., twice daily from GD 1 through weaning gave birth to pups which were hyperactive on an activity wheel at P 52–57. Offspring of pregnant mothers exposed to hypoxia showed similar behaviors (Martin and Becker, 1970), suggesting that hypoxia induced by nicotine may be an important factor in the etiology of the behavioral deficits.

Animals exposed pre- and postnatally to nicotine were less able than saline controls to learn a spatial alternation problem at P80 as a result of increased perserveration errors. The same animals were also less able to learn a discrimination reversal (Martin and Becker, 1971). It is yet to be determined if the behavioral symptoms in the nicotine-exposed offspring are due to hypoxia, or to some other indirect mechanism, or to direct stimulation of nicotinic receptors.

Nicotine had direct influence on developing neurons. One study found that the postnatal injection of 3 to 4 mg/kg of nicotine, s.c., on P1 and P2 facilitated the development of [^{3}H]NE uptake mechanisms, suggesting a growth-enhancing effect of nicotine on central noradrenergic nerve terminals (Jonsson and Hallman, 1980). On the other hand, prenatal nicotine exposure increased neuronal death in brain stem (Kraus et al., 1981). Postnatal nicotine has also been shown to antagonize the monoamine-depleting action of 6-hydroxydopamine (Jonsson and Hallman, 1980), possibly the result of a growth-promoting effect of nicotine-induced neuronal activation (Jonsson and Hallman, 1980; 1982).

Tricyclic antidepressants (Table 1.6)

Experimental studies have produced evidence for developmental and behavioral disturbances in rat offspring following maternal imipramine administration. Reports include drug-induced delays in eye opening (Broitman and Donoso, 1978), incisor eruption, and negative geotaxis, as well as cliff-avoidance reflexes (Coyle, 1975). Adults were more emotional after perinatal drug exposure (Broitman and Donoso, 1978; Mirmiran et al. 1981). Chlorimipramine given to neonates suppressed active (REM) sleep in infants but increased its duration and intensity in adults. Perinatal imipramine treatment suppressed adult exploratory activity and reduced male sexual behavior (Mirmiran et al., 1981). One possibility is that these drugs might increase synaptic serotonin concentration via uptake blockade which would be compensated for by either decreased receptor sensitivity or reduced serotonin availability.

The importance of environmental factors in revealing perinatal drug influences has

Table 1.6. Tricyclic antideprissants

Treatment	Symptoms in offspring
On the day of delivery, the lactating rats were given *imipramine* in the drinking water (180 mg/l or about 10 mg/kg). Treatment continued through weaning	*Delayed eye opening* (Maternal food and water intake was reduced. Reduction of milk intake by pups) (Broitman and Donoso, 1978)
Pups given 15 mg/kg *chlorimipramine*, ip, 2 × daily from P2 to 8	*Active (REM) sleep depressed in infants and enhanced in adults* *Reduced exploratory activity* *Reduced sexual behavior* (Mirmiran et al., 1981)
Pregnant rats given 5 mg/kg *imipramine*, po, prior to and through gestation	Cross fostering studies indicated *defects in reflex ontogeny and developmental milestones* (P9–21): a) *Delay in incisor eruption* b) *Retarded development of cliff avoidance and negative geotaxis* (Coyle, 1975) Pups reared in *impoverished environment:* Controls and experimentals were equally *poor in maze solving* Pups reared in *enriched environment:* Imipramine offspring *inferior* to controls in maze solving (Coyle and Singer, 1975a) Imipramine-treated pups did not respond to the enriched environment with increased cortical thickness (Coyle and Singer, 1975b)

been demonstrated by Coyle and Singer (1975a; 1975b). The offspring of imipramine-treated rat mothers were fostered at birth to non-treated females. At weaning, the pups were assigned to a deprived or enriched environmental condition. Increased learning ability with correlated changes in brain morphology and biochemistry has been found following rearing in an 'enriched environment' (see Rosenzweig et al., 1972). Imipramine-treated offspring and controls raised in an impoverished environment were equally poor in performing a maze problem; however, among the groups raised in the enriched environment, the imipramine group did much worse than the controls (Coyle and Singer, 1975a). Histologically, the placebo group, but not the imipramine group, showed a greater cortical thickness in response to the enriched enviromental rearing conditions. Thus some of the negative effects of prenatal drug exposure may not become fully apparent until the influences of environmental interactions are taken into account.

Neuroleptics (Table 1.7)

The study of neuroleptics on central nervous system development is of interest because

(1) most of these studies have utilized a procedure in which the nursing offspring receives the drug through the mother's milk (see Beeley, 1981) and (2) the neuropharmacological actions of these drugs on the nature of dopaminergic receptor systems have been well characterized (see Snyder et al., 1974; Carlsson, 1978). In an early study, haloperidol was given to nursing rabbit mothers for 7 days following delivery.

Table 1.7. Neuroleptics

Treatment	Symptoms in offspring
Lactating rabbits given 1 mg/kg *haloperidol* in drinking water from day 1 to 7 after delivery	At 8 days: the experimentals were *unable to elevate themselves* and showed *uncoordinated movements* At 4 weeks: *Muscular dysfunction in hind limbs* (Lundborg, 1972)
Lactating rats given 1 mg/kg *penfluridol*, po, on days, 1, 3, and 5 after delivery	At 4 weeks: *Impaired acquisition of a conditioned avoidance response* (Ahlenius et al., 1973) Other behavioral tests indicated: a) Normal reflex development b) *hyperactivity* at 4 weeks; *hypoactivity* at 8 and 12 weeks c) *reduced habituation* (8 and 12 weeks) d) *increased defecation* (Ahlenius et al., 1977) Monoamine synthesis: *Decreased dopa accumulation in limbic forebrain* and hemispheres. (striatum normal). Decreased 5-HTP accumulation in limbic forebrain and brainstem (Engel and Lundborg, 1974) Following synthesis inhibition with *AMpT*: *Reduced dopamine fall-off in limbic forebrain* (not in striatum) (Engel and Lundborg, 1976) *Increased [^3H]spiroperidol binding in limbic forebrain*, but not in striatum (Engel and Lundborg, 1979)
Lactating rats given 0.5 mg/kg *pimozide*, ip, on days 1–7 after delivery	At 4 weeks, *amphetamine pretreatment* improved the acquisition of: a) *Conditioned avoidance response* b) *Discriminated avoidance* (Ahlenius et al., 1975)
Pregnant rats given 0.25 mg/kg *haloperidol*, sc, twice daily, from GD 1 through weaning	*High* vs. *low dose of apormorphine:* a) *Reduced sensitivity to low dose* b) *Both groups equally affected by high doses* (Shalaby and Spear, 1980)
Haloperidol (pre- vs. Postnatal): *Prenatal treatment:* Pregnant rats given 2.5 mg/kg, ip, from GD 5 to 21 *Postnatal treatment:* Lactating females given 2.5 mg/kg, ip, from P1 to weaning	At 35 days of age: *Reduced [^3H]spiroperidol binding* (reduced number of receptors) *Reduced sensitivity to apomorphine (stereotypy)* *Increased [^3H]spiroperidol binding* *Increased sensitivity to apomorphine (stereotypy)* (Rosengarten and Friedhoff, 1979; see also Spear et al., 1980)

At 4 weeks of age, the treated offspring were unable to elevate themselves above the floor surface and attempts to raise their heads resulted in head tremors. Further, they could only move by crawling or with uncoordinated steps. By 8 weeks of age, their condition improved but the muscular dysfunction in the hind limbs was still observable (Lundborg, 1972). Increased homovanillic acid, a dopamine metabolic product, in the brains of the nursing offspring indicated that a sufficient amount of the drug had passed from the mother's milk to the infant to exert a pharmacological effect on the developing brain (Lundborg and Roos, 1974).

When penfluridol was given to lactating rat mothers during the early nursing period, the offspring were impaired in the acquisition of a conditioned avoidance response (CAR) at 4 weeks of age, the earliest age at which rats normally learn shuttle box performance (Ahlenius et al., 1973). Later studies showed that the treatment effect was not on gross motor or reflex development (Ahlenius et al., 1977), although the animals were hyperactive in an open field at 4 weeks of age, and hypoactive at 8 and 12 weeks; they were also unable to habituate to a novel environment.

Catecholamine dynamics were examined in these animals because an intact dopamine system is required to maintain conditioned avoidance behavior in the shuttle box (see Seiden and Dykstra, 1977). Brain catecholamine and indoleamine synthesis was estimated by measuring the accumulation of DOPA and 5-HTP, respectively, following inhibition of aromatic amino acid decarboxylase activity with NSD 1015. A significant decrease in DOPA accumulation was found in the dopamine-dominant limbic forebrain and in the hemispheres but no difference was found in striatum or other regions examined. Serotonin synthesis was reduced in limbic forebrain as well as brainstem (Engel and Lundborg, 1974). The limbic forebrain was further implicated as a target for neonatal penfluridol administration: a decreased impulse flow, as measured by a fall-off of dopamine following synthesis inhibition with alpha-methyl-p-tyrosine, was observed in limbic forebrain, but not striatum (Engel and Lundborg, 1976) as was a selective increase in [³H]spiroperidol binding (Engel and Lundborg, 1979). The authors hypothesized that disturbed dopaminergic limbic neurons with intact striatal dopamine system might be the result of an earlier maturation of the limbic forebrain structures making them vulnerable at the time of the neuroleptic treatment (Engel and Lundborg, 1974; 1976). The disturbed dopamine biodynamics might be due to altered feedback mechanisms (Engel and Lundborg, 1976).

If the behavioral deficits resulting from neonatal neuroleptic treatment are due to central catecholamine neuron dysfunction, then drugs which enhance catecholaminergic activity should counteract on the behavioral defect. This was shown to be the case. Offspring of rat mothers treated with pimozide were normally inferior in learning the CAR). However, if pretreated with amphetamine, prior to testing, the 'pimozide' animals did not differ from controls (Ahlenius et al., 1975). Amphetamine also facilitated the acquisition of a discriminated avoidance paradigm indicating that the improved CAR performance was not entirely due to stimulant-facilitated increase in locomotor activity (Ahlenius et al., 1975).

Spear et al. (1980) gave pregnant rats haloperidol throughout gestation and weaning and found the offspring to be hyporesponsive to the locomotor-stimulating effect of amphetamine, suggesting a functional decrease in the sensitivity of the dopamine receptors to stimulation. In another experiment, offspring of haloperidol-treated mothers were assessed for their response to low versus high doses of apomorphine (Shalaby and Spear, 1980), since low doses stimulate dopaminergic autoreceptors (depressing activity) while high doses stimulate dopaminergic postsynaptic receptor responses (enhancing activity) (see Ernst, 1977; Strombom, 1975). Only the control animals showed reduced matrix crossing and rearing behavior in an open field in response to low doses of apomorphine. However, both treated and control animals were equally affected by high apomorphine doses. It would appear that dopaminergic presynaptic (autoreceptor) sensitivity is reduced by the neuroleptic treatment while dopaminergic postsynaptic mechanisms remain intact (Shalaby and Spear, 1980). In addition, the cholinergic system also appears to be involved as the treated animals were hypersensitive to arecoline-induced catalepsy (Shalaby and Spear, 1980).

These results are directly opposite to those of chronic neuroleptic treatment of adult animals in which supersensitivity to the locomotor-stimulating actions of dopaminergic agonists develops (see Spear et al., 1980). Rosengarten and Friedhoff (1979) also found that haloperidol administered prenatally resulted in offspring that were less sensitive to apomorphine-induced stereotypy and whose striatal membranes bound less spiroperidol, while haloperidol administered postnatally increased both spiroperidol binding and the behavioral response to apomorphine.

In summary, offspring exposed to chronic neuroleptic treatment during the perinatal period show: (a) impaired acquisition of the conditioned avoidance response, (b) reduced dopamine synthesis and utilization in limbic forebrain structures, and (c) reduced dopaminergic sensitivity. A striking feature of chronic neuroleptic treatment in the perinatal period is the production of behavioral and neurochemical consequences opposite to that seen following chronic treatment in the adult.

Diphenylhydantoin

The fetal hydantoin syndrome in its full expression includes congenital heart disease, cleft lip and/or palate, trigonocephaly or microcephaly and various minor signs such as low-set abnormal ears, low posterior hair line, and unusual facies. A reduction in intellectual ability is a common finding in the affected children (Speidel and Meadow, 1972; Annegers et al., 1974; Hanson et al., 1976). Thus, epileptic women receiving hydantoin therapy are at risk for producing abnormal children should they become pregnant.

It is fairly well established that the fetal hydantoin syndrome is due to drug therapy itself and not to the convulsions or epilepsy per se since the incidence of anomalies for epileptic patients not on drug therapy is no different than for nonepileptic indivuduals

(Hill and Stern, 1979; Monson et al., 1973; Annegers et al., 1974). This circumstance has been validated in animal studies by taking advantage of an inbred strain of mice which has an autosomal recessive gene which confers a seizure disorder. The incidence of animals born with malformations was found to increase with the maternal drug dosage, and the pregnant mice whose seizure disorder was not drug-treated produced normal offspring in spite of daily seizure episodes (Finnell, 1981).

Experimentally, diphenylhydantoin given to pregnant rats through most of the gestational period has been found to result in offspring whose physical development is minimally affected but whose behavioral development is retarded or subnormal (Elmazar and Sullivan, 1981). No differences were noted between diphenylhydantoin-treated offspring and cross-fostered controls with respect to timing of ear opening, tooth eruption or eye opening, but the treated animals were delayed in ossification of forepaws. Although the prenatal drug exposure had no effect on the development of crawling, walking, or exploratory behavior/habituation, the treated animals were delayed by 6 to 15 days in the development of the mid-air-righting reflex and were significantly worse than controls on rotorod performance and on walking elevated-parallel rods (Elmazar and Sullivan, 1981). Elmazar and Sullivan (1981) suggested that possibly a delayed cerebellar maturation might be responsible for the lack of motor coordination in the behavioral studies, but no gross structural brain changes were observed in treated offspring at P90 other than reduced brain and cerebellar weight.

In support of the hypothesis for cerebellar damage, Origuchi et al. (1975) observed no evidence at the light microscopic level for diphenylhydantoin induced cerebellar damage, but closer examination using the electron microscope revealed dose-related cytological alterations in cerebellar Purkinje cells including increased lipofuscin granules and irregularities in the shape and distribution of mitochondria. At higher drug doses, the ultrastructural damage was more severe and included morphological alterations in the granule cell layer.

The process underlying the hydantoin-induced behavioral/neurological damage is believed to involve some type of folic acid antagonism since the drug reduces plasma folate levels (Speidel and Meadow, 1972; Netzloff et al., 1979). It is possible that important biochemical processes, such as one carbon transfer, are negatively influenced by diphenylhydantoin. The mechanism is complicated however; the success of reversing diphenylhydantoin-induced anomalies with folic acid supplements has produced variable success rates (Kernis et al., 1973; Marsch and Fraser, 1973; Sullivan and McElhatton, 1975).

Antagonists of folic acid are known to reduce cellular respiration (Netzloff et al., 1977). Hyperoxia has been reported to reduce the incidence of hydantoin-induced cleft lip and palate in mice (Millicovsky and Johnston, 1981) so (like with early nicotine exposure) drug-induced hypoxia may be a considerable factor in diphenylhydantoin teratogenesis.

Aspirin

In a study of over 14 000 exposures to aspirin taken by pregnant women no evidence was found that the aspirin (salicylate) was responsible for any physical malformations (Heinonen et al., 1977). In experimental studies, however, doses of aspirin that were insufficient to produce gross brain malformations produced behavioral impairments (Butcher et al., 1972). Aspirin given to pregnant rats on GD 8, 9, and 10 was found to impair the ability of the offspring to escape from a water maze at 53 days of age. No gross abnormalities were found and the offspring were not impaired in their ability to learn to swim (Butcher et al., 1972).

Studies have suggested that it is the chelating property of aspirin which may be responsible for its teratogenic effects (Koshakji and Schulert, 1973). Aspirin can form a complex with metals which are critical for certain enzyme reactions. However, pre-

Table 1.8. Environmental influences on CNS development

	Treatment	Symptoms in offspring
I.	*Stress*	
	Pregnant rats given shock-escape training from GD 7 to 13 or GD 14 to 20	*Reduced emotionally* in openfield (Hutchings and Gibbon, 1970)
	Pregnant rats were restrained for 9 h from GD 18 to 20:	*Delayed ear opening*, also *auditory startle* and *cliff avoidance* (Barlow et al., 1978)
	from GD 12 to 14:	*Delayed ear opening*, and *righting* and *free-fall righting reflexes* Inability to reverse a learned response *(symptoms prevented by maternal diazepam treatment)* (Barlow et al., 1979)
	On P1, rat pups placed on ice for 15 min, then under heat lamp for 15 min	At P240: *reduced emotionally* *increased activity* *elevation of whole brain 5-HT* (Giulian et al., 1974)
	Rat pups separated from mother on P10	*Reduced brain ornithine decarboxylase activity* (Butler and Schanberg, 1977)
II.	*Hypoxia*	
	Rat pups exposed to 4.5 h of 6% oxygen on P1	At 4 weeks: *Impaired CAR acquisition* *Reduced monoamine synthesis* (DOPA/5-HTP accumulation) (Hedner et al., 1979)
	Pregnant rats exposed to 13% oxygen for 2 h from GD 6 to 20	*Impaired maze performance* (McCullough and Blackman, 1976)
	Pregnant rats exposed to 4% oxygen for 5 min (brought to ground level over a 40 min period) from GD 1 to delivery	*Hyperactivity* (Martin and Becker, 1970) *Non-contingent responding* *Poor discrimination reversal* (Martin and Becker, 1971)

III. *Nutrition*

A. *Behavior*

Mice reared in groups of 20/litter	*Impaired acquisition of CAR* at 2 months (Leathwood et al., 1974)
Pregnant rats were underfed during the gestation period. Pups cross-fostered at birth	*Increased social behavior* (Whatson and Smart, 1978)
Pregnant rats were food deprived from GD through lactation. Pups cross-fostered at birth	*More efficient in maze solving* *Poor motor coordination* *Reduced forebrain and cerebellar weight* (Smart et al., 1973)
Pregnant rats maintained on low protein	*Attenuated apomorphine-induced stereotypy* (Leahy et al., 1978)

B. *Neurochemistry*

Pregnants rats were fed low protein (12 %) diet throughout gestation and lactation	At weaning (P21): *Reduction in body weight greater than brain weight* *Less amino acid incorporation into protein in muscle than brain* *Less amino acid transport in muscle than brain* (Freedman et al., 1980)
Pregnant rats fed low protein (8 %) diet from GD 14 through lactation. Pups crossfostered at birth	At 24 days of age: *Reduced NE and DA levels* in whole brain *Higher tyrosine hydroxylase activity* *NE uptake not affected* (Shoemaker and Wurtman, 1971) No change in brain tyrosine content *Slowed NE turnover* (fall-off of [^{3}H]NE) (Shoemaker and Wurtman, 1973)
Pregnant rats fed reduced protein (8 %) diet from GD 14 through lactation. At birth pups were cross-fostered. Pups fed reduced protein diet for 50 days following weaning	At 140 days of age: *Increased conversion of tyrosine to NE* *Increased tyrosine hydroxylase activity* (Marichich et al., 1979) *Reduced number of alpha and beta noradrenergic receptors* (Keller et al., 1981)
At birth, rat pups placed in crowded (18 pups) litter	*DNA* used to estimate *cell number* and *protein/DNA* used to estimate *cell size* (from P6 to 21): Cerebelum: *Reduced DNA* after P6 Hippocampus: *Reduced DNA* after P14 Brainstem: *DNA not altered, protein/DNA reduced after P10* (Fish and Winick, 1969)

C. *Neuroanatomy*

Pregnant rats maintained on 50 % of normal diet during gestation and lactation	At 30–90 days: a) *Reduced brain and cerebellar weight* b) *Reduced cerebellar molecular cell layer and Purkinje cell number* (Barnes and Altman, 1973) At P20: *impaired synapse formation* (Jones and Dyson, 1976)
Pregnant rats fed 57 % of normal diet from GD 9 through delivery and lactation At birth, rat pups placed in crowded (18/pups litter) nursing groups	At 30 weeks of age: *Cerebellum:* areal deficit in molecular and granular layers (and in granule cell and Purkinje cell numbers) *Cortex:* Loss of glial cells (Dobbing et al., 1971)

treatment with ferrous sulfate, which might be expected to antidote the chelating effect of aspirin, was actually found instead to potentiate the behavioral teratological action (Kimmel et al., 1974). Thus, another or additional mechanisms must be sought. One possibility is the strong inhibition of prostaglandin synthesis by aspirin (Ferreira, 1979).

Environmental influences on brain development (Table 1.8)

The degree to which the fetus and neonate are affected by environmental manipulations is important for both clinical and theoretical reasons in understanding how the brain develops and uses environmental information for formation of neuronal circuitry, for pharmaco-physiological settings, and information/behavior processing (viz. e.g. Rosenzweig et al., 1972; Coyle and Singer, 1975a, 1975b). If left uncontrolled in an experimental design, environmental influences might confuse data interpretation. A case in point is the finding by Hutchings et al. (1979) that the stress of an intubation procedure itself can produce developmental consequences. The importance of adequate design in developmental psychopharmacology has been discussed by several investigators (Kornetsky, 1970; Spyker, 1975; Coyle et al., 1976; Abel, 1980a, 1980b). Environmental variables which might affect development include the following.

Stress
Hutchings and Gibbon (1970) showed that offspring of rats who had undergone shock-escape training were considerably less emotional than non-handled controls at P28. When pregnant mice were immobilized by restraint, offspring were retarded in the development of certain milestones, such as ear opening, and delayed in the onset of startle and cliff avoidance reflexes (Barlow et al., 1978). Since diazepam is generally used in humans to reduce stress and 'anxiety', it was administered during immobilization. Diazepam did not prevent the stress-induced rise in maternal plasma corticosterone levels, but it did counteract most of the developmental behavioral consequences otherwise seen in their offspring (Barlow et al., 1979). In this case, the diazepam could have been acting directly on the fetuses (viz. Chapter 7) to counteract the maternal stress.

A single 15-minute cold exposure on the first day of life was sufficient to reduce emotionality and increase open field activity in rats at P240. This stress during the period from P1 to P6 resulted in increased whole brain serotonin, which was not mediated by the adrenal response since increased brain serotonin content was also found in adrenalectomized animals (Giulian et al., 1974). A 'stress' of separation from the mother for a period as brief as 1 hour was sufficient to disrupt ornithine decarboxylase activity in the brain of the P10 rat pup in comparison to handled littermates, controlling for nutrition and temperature change. Return to the mother reversed the decline in enzyme activity via a short-lived overshoot followed by normalization within a few hours (Butler and Schanberg, 1977). Thus, maternal deprivation might be an important factor in the speculated role of polyamine biosynthesis in brain synaptogenesis (see Slotkin and Thadani, 1980).

Hypoxia

Brain tissue is extremely oxygen sensitive, so any drug or procedure (e.g. as indicated above) which reduces the oxygen supply could lead to neurological and/or behavioral impairments. Rat pups exposed once on the first day of life to 6% oxygen for 4.5 hours were inferior in the acquisition of a conditioned avoidance response at P28. The behavioral impairment was accompanied by a reduction in monoamine biosynthesis (Hedner et al., 1979). Intact dopamine neurotransmission has been shown to be necessary for maintenance of conditioned avoidance responses (Seiden and Dykstra, 1977); but, it is unclear if the behavioral disturbance causes or affects the biochemical changes.

Two-hour daily exposures of pregnant rats to 13% oxygen during the last 14 days of pregnancy led to offspring that made more errors on a maze problem at P8 than controls (McCollough and Blackman, 1976). Gradually equilibrating pregnant rats to a 5-minute exposure to 4% oxygen resulted in offspring that were hyperactive when tested at P50 (Martin and Becker, 1970). The same offspring also made more responses on a non-contingent lever during a fixed ratio paradigm, used less collateral behavior to mediate responding on a discrimination reversal learning schedule, and were more stimulus bound which impeded the solution of a discrimination reversal problem (Martin and Becker, 1979).

Malnutrition

Rearing mice in large litters was sufficient to result in impaired acquisition of a conditioned avoidance response when tested at 2 months of age; no improvement was noted in learning ability following 2 to 6 months of nutritional rehabilitation (Leathwood, et al., 1974). Nursing by malnourished rat mothers had more severe effects on behavioral development than did exposure to malnutrition in utero. On the other hand, offspring nursed by malnourished dams solved a maze problem for food more efficiently and responded more rapidly on a VI schedule than did non-deprived controls. The data were interpreted as indicating greater food motivation (Smart et al., 1973). These conditions also produced a higher frequency of social interaction than among control animals (Whatson and Smart, 1978). The lactation-deprived group had lower forebrain and cerebellar weights than gestation-deprived or control groups, although the DNA content of the forebrain was lower in the gestation-malnourished animals (Smart et al., 1973). It is generally accepted that the effects of malnutrition are greater during the early postnatal period than the gestational period because the brain undergoes a rapid growth spurt which makes the differentiating brain structures more vulnerable to environmental insult (Dobbing and Sands, 1971; see also Fish and Winick, 1969; Rodier, 1977).

Hyperactivity has been associated with postnatal malnutrition primarily in male mice, including less responsiveness to amphetamine (Loch et al., 1978). Altered catecholamine metabolism was suggested by the behavioral data (Leahy et al., 1978), but no malnutrition-induced changes were found in norepinephrine-mediated behaviors; on the other hand, malnourished animals were less sensitive to apomorphine challenge (as shown by a significant reduction in the degree of stereotypy) which suggests (with the reduced response to amphetamine) that dopamine receptors might have been made hyposensitive as a result of early malnutrition.

'Brain sparing' is a concept that was derived from the observation that body growth is more affected by early malnutrition than brain growth. For example, Freedman et al. (1980) found that malnutrition during the preweaning period resulted in a 50% deficit in body weight but only a 12% reduction in brain weight. Further, amino acid incorporation into muscle protein was severely reduced while synthesis of brain protein was hardly influenced. The less reduced protein synthesis may likely be due to compensatory alterations in amino acid transport (Freedman et al., 1980). At P24, the brains of malnourished offspring concentrate tyrosine at the expense of the body (Shoemaker and Wurtman, 1973); nevertheless, whole brain levels of norepinephrine and dopamine were significantly reduced following severe lactation-induced deprivation (Shoemaker and Wurtman, 1971). The uptake of intracisternally administered tritiated norepinephrine was not less than controls implying that the number of noradrenergic neurons was not decreased by malnutrition (Shoemaker and Wurtman, 1971; 1973). Yet the activity of tyrosine hydroxylase was increased and norepinephrine turnover rate reduced. So, it may be that during development brain catecholamines are conserved when the nutritional supply limits their biosynthesis (Shoemaker and Wurtman, 1973).

Following 90 days of nutritional recovery from neonatal malnourishment, whole brain tyrosine hydroxylase activity was still increased, as was the conversion of tyrosine to norepinephrine and dopamine. Thus, even following a period of recovery, early undernutrition leads to activation of catecholaminergic systems in adulthood (Marichich et al., 1979). Consistent with this interpretation is the finding of a starvation-induced reduction in the number of brain noradrenergic alpha and beta binding sites (Keller et al., 1982). A permanent activation of noredrenergic neurons as observed in the recovered adults would be expected to lead to receptor subsensitivity as a result of a homeostatic mechanism to counterbalance a greater neurotransmitter release.

Fish and Winnick (1969) used protein and nucleic acid determination to indicate regional brain growth and the influence of malnutrition. DNA content was taken as an estimate of cell number and the protein/DNA ratio as an indicator of cell size. The rate and duration of cell division varies within different brain structures. The development of the cerebellum, which grows rapidly by cell division postnatally, was stunted by malnutrition at an early age (P6). Cell division in the cerebrum was slower and was not influenced by malnutrition until P14. In the brainstem, there was little postnatal cell division and DNA content was not altered by malnutrition. The protein/DNA ratio, however, was affected since the nutritional deficit prevented the normal cell hyperplasia which occurs in this structure. Thus, the effects of malnutrition depend on the state of growth of a particular brain region when the nutritional deficit is imposed.

Anatomically, the cerebellum has been studied because of its postnatal period of vulnerability and its well-defined developmental profile. Malnutrition reduced cerebellar weight, area measurement of the molecular layer, and the number of Purkinje cells (Barnes and Altman, 1973; Dobbing et al., 1971). Synaptogenesis is also influenced by undernutrition. The thickness of presynaptic neuron terminal densities was reduced in the occipital cortex (Jones and Dyson, 1976) and fewer synaptic terminals were found in a visual cortical region (Cragg, 1972).

In summary, environmental factors such a stress, hypoxia and undernutrition lead to behavioral alterations including delays in developmental landmarks and reflex ontogeny as well as impaired learning and performance. These environmental influences also lead to perturbations in monoamine, polyamine, nucleic acid, and protein metabolism. Subtle changes in neuronal structure have also been reported following malnutrition. Nutritional studies emphasize the vulnerability of brain structures during the brain growth spurt and brain sparing with respect to somatic damage.

Animal models for 'attention deficit disorder' with hyperactivity (Table 1.9)

The American Psychiatric Association (1980) has recently classified as 'attention deficit disorder' (ADD) the syndrome previously known as minimal brain dysfunction, hyperactive child syndrome, hyperkinetic syndrome, etc. ADD is the new preferred nomenclature since attention deficits are prominent and persist even though excessive motor activity frequently diminishes in adolescence. ADD onset usually occurs by three years of age, but may not come to professional attention until the child enters school. The disorder is more common in males than females, and, the condition is treated, paradoxically, with psychostimulants such as amphetamine.

An animal model of ADD should satisfy three criteria: it should (1) replicate the cardinal feature of the syndrome (i.e., attentional difficulties, learning problems, impulsivity, hyperactivity); (2) bear some temporal relationship, in terms of onset and duration, to the pathogenesis in humans; and (3) respond consistently to psychostimulant medication or other therapeutic intervention.

Neurotoxins (6-hydroxydopamine)
In normal rat pups little locomotor activity is observed during the first week of life. From about P12 to P22 days, activity increases, peaking at 2 to 3 times the level observed during the first week of life. Activity then declines to approach the usually low adult levels by P25–27 (Bolles and Woods; 1964; Campbell et al., 1969; Altman and Sudarshan, 1975).

A model of ADD was developed by Shaywitz and coworkers. First, treatment of 5 day old rat pups with 6-hydroxydopamine (6-OHDA) resulted in hyperactivity, reflected by gross increases of behavior such as walking, sleeping, rearing and climbing. Second, treated pups developed locomotor activity earlier than controls and of a greater intensity, but by P26, activity was comparable to the low level of control animals (Shaywitz et al., 1976a). Third, in contrast to controls, administration of amphetamine led to a reduction in total activity in the 6-OHDA lesioned animals (Shaywitz et al., 1979b). Finally, even after activity had normalized, the inability to learn a conditioned avoidance response persisted into adulthood (Shaywitz et al., 1976a).

Lesions induced by 6-OHDA also produced an inability to habituate to unfamiliar stimuli (Shaywitz and Pearson, 1978; Stoff et al., 1978; Thieme et al., 1980) which,

Table 1.9. Potential animal models for 'attention deficit disorder with hyperactivity'

Cardinal feature of syndrome	Temporal relationship to human pathogenesis	Response to therapy	Reference
1. *Neurotoxins (6-OHDA)*			
Hyperactivity in rats	Hyperactive at 2–3 weeks of age, not at 4 weeks		Shaywits et al., 1976a
Impaired habituation in rats		Amphetamine reversal (Supersensitivity to apomorphine, no amphetamine reversal)	Shaywitz et al., 1976b Thieme et al., 1980
Impaired habituation with hyperactivity in rats	Hyperactive at P15–22		Stoof et al., 1978
Hyperactivity in rats	Duration or magnitude of hyperactivity related to: a) dose of 6-OHDA b) degree of DA depletion c) age when damage occurred		Miller et al., 1981 Erinoff et al., 1979
Hyperactivity in rats	Age and sex related		Concannon and Schechter, 1981
Hyperactivity and impaired passive avoidance (Lesion of ventral mesencephalic tegmentum; A10 dopaminergic cell group)		Amphetamine reversal	LeMoal et al., 1977
2. *Neuroleptics*			
Hyperactivity in rats		(No amphetamine reversal)	Schechter and Concannon, 1982
Impaired learning of conditioned avoidance response in rats		Improvement with amphetamine pretreatment	Ahlenius et al., 1975

3. *Undernutrition*
   Hyperactivity due to reduced habituation in activity cage in male, but not female, mice — Attenuated locomotor response to amphetamine — Loch et al., 1978

4. *Lead*
   Hyperactivity in mice — Improvement with amphetamine treatment — Silbergeld and Goldberg, 1974; 1975

5. *Other possible causitive drugs*
   A. *Opiates*
      Hyperactivity of rat offspring exposed to *heroin*. — Lasky et al., 1977
      Hyperactivity in rat offspring exposed to *morphine* — Exaggerated ontogeny of locomotion. At control level by 5th week. — Sobrian, 1977
      Hyperactivity in rat offspring exposed to *methadone* — Zagon and McLaughlin, 1979
   B. *Barbiturates*
      Hyperactivity in response to phenobarbital — Zemp and Middaugh, 1975
   C. *Marihuana/THC*
      Prolonged attention to novel stimuli in rhesus monkey offspring — Golub et al., 1981
      Human neonates either failed to habituate or failed to react to a visual stimulus — Fried, 1980
      Hyperactivity in rats — From P9 to P13, not at P21 — Borgen et al., 1973
   D. *Alcohol*
      Hyperactivity in rats — Martin et al., 1978; Bond and DiGiusto, 1976
      Hyperactivity in mice — Krsiak et al., 1977
   F. *Amphetamine*
      Impaired ability to habituate in rats — Hitzemann et al., 1976
      Hyperactivity in rats — Zemp and Middaugh, 1975; Martin and Martin, 1981
   F. *Hypoxia*
      Hyperactivity in rats — Martin and Becker, 1970

relative to controls, resulted in increased locomotor activity in a novel environment. However, Thieme et al., (1980) were unable to detect a paradoxical response to amphetamine following dopamine lesions although they noted apomorphine super-sensitivity.

Erinoff et al. (1979) found that the age at which damage is produced is critical for an effect of 6-OHDA on locomotor activity. Lesions at P3 to P6 or P11 to P14 resulted in hyperactivity while lesions at P46 to P48 did not. It was suggested that the key element in induction of hyperactivity is the destruction of dopamine fibers prior to the normal age of locomotor decrement. Although Erinoff et al. (1979) found that 6-OHDA-induced hyperactivity could persist into adulthood, Shaywitz et al. (1976) reported that the hyperactivity abated with maturation. Miller et al. (1981) provided further dose-response information with the report that the extent and duration of neo-natal hyperactivity is correlated with the dose of neurotoxin which itself is directly related to the degree of dopamine depletion. Concannon and Schechter (1981) found that the ontogeny of the locomotor response as well as the effect of 6-OHDA was gender related, implying mediation via hormonal intervention, and consistent with human findings.

Although most studies have used procedures which depleted whole brain dopa-mine, at least one study used more discrete electrolytic and neurotoxin-induced lesions of the ventral mesencephalic tegmentum involving the A10 dopaminergic cell group. This produced a syndrome which included locomotor hyperactivity and hyperreacti-vity, inability to suppress a previously learned response, loss of alternation behavior in a T-maze, and reduced hyperactivity upon treatment with amphetamine or apo-morphine (LeMoal et al., 1977).

Since catecholamine containing neurons are destroyed following treatment with 6-OHDA, the above studies strongly imply a dopaminergic component in the hyperac-tivity and learning deficits induced by the neurotoxin. The mechanism underlying the paradoxical response to amphetamine is generally thought to involve the release of dopamine onto supersensitive receptors (see discussions by Shaywitz et al., 1976a; Concannon and Schechter, 1981).

Neuroleptics

The tardive dyskinesia-like syndrome resulting from chronic administration of halo-peridol is similar to the hyperactivity associated with ADD (Schechter and Concan-non, 1982); but, although hyperactivity is produced, neither amphetamine nor methylphenidate reverse it. Thus it was concluded that neuroleptic treatment does not constitute an appropriate model for the human syndrome. However, Ahlenius et al. (1975) found that the impaired acquisition of a conditioned avoidance response result-ing from neonatal neuroleptic treatment, was reversed by pretreating the offspring with amphetamine. Further, the improvement was not simply due to amphetamine-induced facilitation of locomotor activity because improvement was noted for a discrim-ination problem as well. Clinically, in children, low doses of stimulants produce not only a paradoxical calming of hyperactivity, but also improve attention span, learning, and retention.

Undernutrition

Another possible model for childhood ADD is undernutrition. Mice reared in large litters were hyperactive at P35–37. The increased activity in male mice was primarily a result of reduced habituation. Those offspring showing growth retardation also showed amphetamine-induced activity decrements, sometimes below the normal baseline level (Loch et al., 1978).

Lead

Young animals exposed to lead, by addition of lead acetate to their drinking water, demonstrate hyperactivity (Silbergeld and Goldberg, 1974). Amphetamine and methylphenidate both decrease, while phenobarbital increases, the lead-induced hyperactivity. In fact, lead produced an altered response to a variety of pharmacological agents (Silbergeld and Goldberg, 1975).

Consistent with a proposed involvement of brain catecholamines in hyperactivity, lead treatment was found to alter dopamine turnover, as indicated by measuring a dopamine metabolite, and dopaminergic activity was reduced in the neostriatum and enhanced in the nucleus accumbens (Lucchi et al., 1981). Golter and Michaelson (1975) found no effect of lead on dopamine levels, but did observe an increase in brain norepinephrine concentration. Measures of catecholaminergic dynamics have yet to be made, however.

Other possible causative agents

Behavioral data discussed in this overview have indicated that perinatal exposure to certain drugs frequently results in hyperactivity in the offspring. Whether this symptom is related to ADD remains to be determined. This possibility should be kept in mind, however, for future investigations. Drugs of potential importance in this regard include:

(a) *Opiates.* Hyperactivity has been reported in offspring of mothers exposed to heroin (Laskey et al., 1977), morphine (Sobrian, 1977), and methadone (Zagon and McLaughlin, 1979). Of particular interest is the report of Sobrian (1977) who demonstrated an age related exaggeration of the ontogeny of locomotor responses following morphine exposure.

(b) *Barbiturates.* Increased locomotor activity was observed following prenatal phenobarbital exposure by Zemp and Middaugh (1975).

(c) *Marihuana/THC.* Increased locomotor activity has been reported following prenatal THC exposure (Borgen et al., 1973), changes in attention have been noted in rhesus monkey offspring (Golub et al., 1981) as well as human infants (Fried, 1980).

(d) *Alcohol.* The relationship of childhood hyperactivity and alcoholism in the par-

40

ents has been previously mentioned. Few studies have yet utilized an animal model for attention deficit disorder with alcohol as the causative agent although hyperactivity is reported following perinatal alcohol administration (Bond and DiGuisto, 1976; Krsiak et al., 1977; Martin et al., 1978). Streissguth et al. (1980) pointed out the prevalence of the fetal alcohol syndrome in families of lower socioeconomic status. Thus, there might be a relationship between malnutrition, alcoholism and childhood hyperactivity (see Loch et al., 1978); Streissguth et al., 1980).

(e) *Amphetamine.* Increased locomotor activity results from early amphetamine exposure (Zemp and Middaugh, 1975; Martin and Martin, 1981) as does an impaired ability to habituate to a novel environment (Hitzeman et al., 1976). In light of the ability of amphetamine to damage dopaminergic neurons (Ellison et al., 1978; Wagner et al., 1981) and the involvement of abnormal dopamine systems in hyperactivity (above discussion), a role for an involvement of perinatal amphetamine exposure in the etiology of attention-deficits and hyperactivity might be profitably examined.

(f) *Hypoxia.* Perinatal hypoxia exposure results in offspring which are not only hyperactive (Martin and Becker, 1970) but also emit more non-contingent responses ('impulsivity'?) on a fixed ratio paradigm (Martin and Becker, 1971). Hypoxia might be of interest in relation to the development of ADD, particularly in view of its ability to impair dopamine metabolism (see Hedner et al., 1979).

Summary/Conclusions

Deleterious effects on the behavior of adult animals have been described as a consequence of pre- and/or postnatal drug exposure. In many cases, these have been correlated with deviations in neurobiological processes.

(1) Opiates have been found to delay the time of appearance of developmental milestones including behavioral maturation. Offspring are frequently hyperactive and impaired in the acquisition of avoidance and discrimination tasks. Brain growth rate is reduced and the appearance of biochemical markers of synaptogenesis is delayed.

(2) LSD has been considered to be teratogenic in humans, but studies are confounded by multiple drug use. Following perinatal exposure in rats, offspring are hyperactive, have reduced brain weight, and increased serotonin turnover, LSD also has been shown to affect neuronal plasticity.

(3) Marihuanal/THC at high doses has been found to retard the occurrence of developmental milestones and behavioral ontogeny. Learning impairments have also been reported, perhaps related to attention deficits that have been found in both humans and in non-human primates following high chronic exposure during pregnancy. The mechanisms underlying the developmental effects of marihuana have been confounded

Table 1.10. Not all perinatal drug effects are negative

1. Mice given a cytotoxic agent (5-azacytidine) on E14 learned an active (dark to light side) faster than controls	(Rodier et al., 1979)
2. Perinatal drug exposure may induce drug tolerance in the adult:	
a) Prenatal exposure of mice to phenobarbital induced tolerance to pentobarbital and alcohol	(Yanai and Tabakoff, 1979; 1980)
b) THC given postnatally to rat pups facilitated the development of THC tolerance in adults	(Fried, 1976; Barnes and Fried, 1974)
c) Prenatal alcohol leads to adult rats showing tolerance to alcohol, pentobarbital, and diazepam	(Abel, 1981)
3. Rat offspring of mothers given THC were more dominant in push-tube competition	(Vardaris et al., 1976)
4. Neonatal THC enhanced the acquisition of a conditioned avoidance response in mice	(Radouco-Thomas et al., 1976)
5. Neonatal administration of Met-enkephalin facilitated problem solving in a maze	(Kastin et al., 1980)
6. Prenatal amphetamine exposure in rats resulted in:	
1) facilitated acquisition of a conditioned avoidance response	(Nasello et al., 1974;
2) increased catecholamine turnover	Nasello and Ramirex, 1978; see also Martin, 1975)
7. Neonatal malnutrition in rats leads to increased social interaction	(Whatson and Smart, 1978)
as well as facilitated maze solving behavior for food	(Smart et al., 1973)

by methodological considerations. Neuroendocrine alterations have been reported which may last into adulthood.

(4) Barbiturates have been shown to retard behavioral ontogeny in animals, produce hyperactivity in young children, and to impair acquisition of learning tasks. In addition, early exposure leads to both barbiturate and alcohol tolerance, as well as disruption of sexual behavior of both male and female offspring at adulthood. Brain weight reduction is found following prenatal or postnatal drug exposure, with reduction in neuronal populations. The type of cerebellar or hippocampal cells affected depends on the time of drug exposure with respect to neuronal differentiation.

(5) Alcohol treatment in animals has been found to replicate many of the clinical features of the fetal alcohol syndrome. Maternal alcohol consumption during pregnancy results in offspring with delayed synaptogenesis, reduced brain growth rate and size, slowed reflex development, motor incoordination, and long-lasting hyperactivity. Neurobiological consequences include altered neurotransmitter dynamics, and changes in development of tolerance in adults following exposure to pentobarbital and diazepam as well as alcohol. Amphetamine exposure has been shown to result in growth retardation, and behavioral impairment. Offspring are hyperactive and less able than controls to habituate to novel stimuli. Neurochemical data suggest brain site-specific changes in monoamine dynamics in adult offspring exposed prenatally.

(7) Methylxanthines (caffeine, theophylline and theobromine) have been found to

Table 1.11. Drug effects are age dependent

1. In rats prenatally exposed to haloperidol, at 35 days of age there is: *decreased* [³H]spiroperidol binding and *decreased* sensitivity to apomorphine Following neonatal exposure, at 35 days of age there is: *increased* [³H]spiroperidol binding and *increased* sensitivity to apomorphine	(Rosengarten and Friedhoff, 1979; see also Spear et al., 1980)
2. Binding of [³H]diazepam to cortex is *decreased* in rats exposed in utero to diphenylhydantoin. Postnatal exposure to diphenylhydantoin results in *increased* [³H]diazepam binding to cortex	(Callager and Mallorga, 1980)
3. Rats exposed prenatally to THC are *supersensitive* to THC as adults. Postnatal exposure to THC results in adults who are *tolerant* to THC	(Fried, 1976)
4. Prepubertal treatment of rats with either beta-endorphin or naloxone (P1–21) resulted in a higher threshold for thermal stimulation (tail flick) at P90. This response does not occur following administration of either compound to adults.	(Moldow et al., 1981; Sandman et al., 1970)
5. Brains from rat pups nursed by mothers consuming alcohol show increased tyrosine hydroxylase (TOH) activity in caudate. Adults show reduced TOH activity in response to alcohol	(Branchey and Friedhoff, 1973)
6. Administration of methadone to infant rats alters synaptosomal uptake of catecholamines. Methadone given to adults does not alter synaptosomal uptake	(Slotkin et al., 1979)

be minimally teratogenic but markedly to potentiate the teratogenic effects of other cytotoxic agents. More work is needed in behavioral teratogenesis.

(8) Nicotine exposure, by mothers smoking during pregnancy, has been demonstrated to retard fetal growth and to produce long-lasting (11 years) hyperactivity with learning deficiencies. Similar results have been obtained with hypoxia per se, so one primary mechanism for damage may be via nicotine induced hypoxia. Postnatal exposure to nicotine changes catecholaminergic uptake mechanisms.

(9) Tricyclic antidepressants have been found to delay development and produce behavioral disturbances in animal studies. Offspring had altered sleep patterns, depressed exploratory activity, and deficient problem-solving ability. Environmental

Table 1.12. Sex of the animal may determine the consequence of perinatal drug exposure

1. Male rats, but not females, prenatally exposed to cannabinoids exhibited inferior learning behavior in a maze	(Fried, 1971; Gianutsos and Abbatiello, 1972)
2. Following prenatal exposure to methadone: Male rats responded fastest on a VI 40 schedule of reinforcement. Female rats, but not males, showed positive behavioral contrast on learning and S + S – discrimination. Also the females showed the greatest response suppression upon introduction of noncontingent shock	(Hutchings et al., 1979)
3. Following prepubertal treatment of rats with morphine, female offspring, but not males, responded to naloxone with an increase in plasma corticosterone. There were no signs of precipitated abstinence	(Zimmerman et al., 1974)
4. Prenatal exposure to alcohol in rats induces tolerance to alcohol, diazepam, and pentobarbital in female but not male offspring	(Abel et al., 1981)
5. The ontogeny of locomotion differs in male and female rats. So does the locomotor response following neonatal treatment with 6-hydroxydopamine	(Concannon and Schechter, 1981)

complexity is a determining factor in the expression of the drug-induced behavioral deficits.

(10) Neuroleptics have opposite effects following chronic exposure during prenatal development to those during postnatal development or in adults. Such offspring are impaired in the acquisition of conditioned avoidance responses, have reduced dopamine synthesis and utilization in limbic forebrain structures, and decreased dopamine receptor binding. Chronic postnatal exposure produces dopamine receptor supersensitivity, as in adults. Amphetamine treatment partially removes the behavioral deficits resulting from prenatal exposure, perhaps by its ability to stimulate catecholamine release.

(11) Diphenylhydantoin exposure during pregnancy causes fetal hydantoin syndrome, which includes abnormal morphology and reduced intellectual ability. Animal studies indicate delayed cerebellar maturation. Hydantoin-induced folic acid deficiency has been implicated in the drug damage.

(12) Aspirin has not been shown to induce physical malformations in humans, but in animals has been found to impair learning in otherwise healthy adults which had been exposed prenatally. One mechanism of drug damage may be via prostaglandin synthesis inhibition.

(13) Environmental influences modulate fetal development. Stress, hypoxia and malnutrition alter behavior in many ways that mimic drug exposure per se. These environmental factors have been found to exert an influence on brain growth rate, neurogenesis, synaptogenesis and neurotransmitter dynamics. Thus, it must be emphasized that developmental studies of drug effects should utilize an experimental design to distinguish these factors from actual pharmacological drug actions, e.g. with additional controls, pair-feeding, cross-fostering, and close match of rearing conditions.

(14) Various animal models have been suggested for studying childhood hyperactivity, also known as attention deficit disorder. To be a valuable animal model, three criteria should be met: (a) the behavior deficits produced should be replicate one or more of the cardinal features of the syndrome; (b) there should be a temporal correlation with the pathogenesis of the condition in humans; and (c) pharmacotherapy with stimulants must produce results consistent with those in humans. The models which best fulfill these criteria following perinatal treatment include 6-hydroxydopamine, neuroleptics, undernutrition and lead exposure. Other studies have considered perinatal drug influences, of, for example, opiates, marihuana, barbiturates, alcohol and amphetamine.

There are various other factors to consider, in addition to those discussed and summarized above: (1) Not all perinatal drug effects on behavior are negative (Table 1.10), for example, neonatal exposure to THC improved learning in the offspring. (2) Both acute and chronic responses are different in neonates and adults (Table 1.11). (3) Endocrinological influences on drug mechanisms have been implicated, since many studies show gender differences in several types of drug response (Table 1.12).

In conclusion, there is still much to be done in the field of development psychopharmacology. Mechanisms underlying drug-induced behavioral impairments are still being explored; the range of effectiveness of pharmacotherapy to rectify drug-induced neurological and behavioral impairments is still being investigated. Because neurological and behavioral damage are intimately related, and because behavioral teratology may indicate neural deficits without accompanying morphological damage, behavioral analysis should accompany, wherever possible, studies aimed at defining perinatal drug influences on developing brain mechanisms.

References

Abel, E.L. (1979) Behavioral teratology of marihuana extract in rats. Neurobehav. Toxicol. 1, 285–287.

Abel, E.L. (1980a) Procedural considerations in evaluating prenatal effects of alcohol in animals. Neurobehav. Toxicol. 2, 167–174.

Abel, E.L. (1980b) Prenatal exposure to cannabis: a critical review of effects on growth, development, and behavior. Behav. Neural Biol. 29, 137–156.

Abel, E.L., Bush, R. and Dintcheff, B.A. (1981) Exposure of rats to alcohol in utero alters drug sensitivity in adulthood. Science 212, 1531–1533.

Abel, E.L., Bush, R., Dintcheff, B.A. and Ernst, C.A.S. (1981) Critical periods of marihuana-induced intrauterine growth retardation in the rat. Neurobehav. Toxicol. 3, 351–354.

Abel, E.L., Dintcheff, B.A. and Day, N. (1980) Effects of marihuana on pregnant rats and their offspring. Psychopharmacology 71, 71–74.

Ahlenius, S., Brown, R., Engel, J. and Lundborg, P. (1973) Learning deficits in 4 week old offspring of the nursing mothers treated with the neuroleptic drug penfluridol. Naunyn-Schmiedeberg's Arch. Pharmacol. 279, 31–37.

Ahlenius, S., Engel, J., Hard, E., Larsson, K., Lundborg, P. and Sinnerstedt, P. (1977) Open field behavior and gross motor development in offspring of nursing rat mothers given penfluridol. Pharmacol. Biochem. Behav. 6, 343–347.

Ahlenius, S., Engel, J. and Lundborg, P. (1975) Antagonism by d-amphetamine of learning deficits in rats induced by exposure to antipsychotic drugs during early postnatal life. Naunyn-Schmiedeberg's Arch. Pharmacol. 288, 185–193.

Altman, J. and Sudarshan, K. (1975) Postnatal development of locomotion in the laboratory rat. Anim. Behav. 23, 896–920.

American Psychiatric Association: Diagnostic and Statistical Manual of Mental Disorders (1980) 3rd edn. Am. Psychiat. Assoc., Washington, D.C.

Annegers, J.F., Elveback, L.R., Hauser, W.A. and Kurland, L.T. (1974) Do anticonvulsants have a teratogenic effect? Arch. Neurol. 31, 364–373.

Armanda, J.V., Gorman, W., Bergsteinsson, H. and Gunn, T. (1977) Efficacy of caffeine in treatment of apnea in the low-birth-weight infant, J. Pediat. 90, 467–472.

Baker, P.C. and Hoff, K.M. (1975) The effects of LSD upon brain indoleamine maturation in the brain of the mouse. Gen. Pharmacol. 6, 19–22.

Barnes D. and Altman, J. (1973) Effects of two levels of gestational-lactational undernutrition on postweaning growth of the rat cerebellum. Exp. Neurol. 38, 420–428.

Barnes, C. and Fried, P.A. (1974) Tolerance to delta-9-THC in adult rats with differential delta-9-THC exposure when immature or during early adulthood. Psychopharmacologia 34, 181–190.

Barlow, S.M., Knight, A.F. and Sullivan, F.M. (1978) Delay in postnatal growth and development of offspring produced by maternal restraint stress during pregnancy in the rat. Teratology 18, 211–218.

Barlow, S.M., Knight, A.F. and Sullivan, F.M. (1979) Prevention by diazepam of adverse effects of maternal restraint stress on postnatal development and learning in the rat. Teratology 19, 105–110.

Beeley, L. (1981) Drugs and breast feeding. Clin. Obstet. Gynaecol. 8, 291–295.

Bergman, A., Rossellki-Austin, L., Yedwab, G. and Yanai, J. (1980) Neuronal deficits in mice following phenobarbital exposure during various periods in fetal development. Acta Anat. 108, 370–373.

Bergman, A. and Yanai, J. (1981) Neuronal deficits after neonatal exposure to phenobarbital. Exp. Neurol. 73, 199–208.

Bleyer, W.A. and Marshall, R.E. (1972) Barbiturate withdrawal in a passively addicted infant. J. Am. Med. Assoc. 221, 185–186.

Bolles, R.C. and Woods, P.J. (1964) The ontogeney of behavior in the albino rat. Anim. Behav. 12, 427–441.

Bond, N.W. and DiGusto, E.L. (1976) Effects of prenatal alcohol consumption on open-field behaviour and alcohol preference in rats. Psychopharmacology 46, 163–165.

Borgen, L.A., Davis, W.M. and Pace, H.B. (1973) Effects of prenatal delta-9-tetrahydrocannabinol on the development of rat offspring. Pharmcol. Biochem. Behav. 1, 203–206.

Branchey, L. and Friedhoff, A.J. (1973) The influence of ethanol administered to pregnant rats on tyrosine hydroxylase activity of their offspring. Psychopharmacology 32, 151–156.

Briggs, G.G., Samson, J.H. and Crawford, D.J. (1975) Lack of abnormalities in a newborn exposed to amphetamine during gestation. Am. J. Dis. Child. 129, 249–250.

Broitman, S.T. and Donoso, A.O. (1978) Effects of chronic imipramine and clomipramine oral administration on maternal behavior and litter development. Psychopharmacology 56, 93–101.

Butcher, R.E., Vorhees, C.V. and Kimmel, C.A. (1972) Learning impairment from maternal salicylate treatment in rats. Nat. (New Biol.) 236, 211–213.

Butler, N.R. and Goldstein, H. (1973) Smoking in pregnancy and subsequent child development. Brit. Med. J. 4, 573–574.

Butler, S.R. and Schanberg, S.M. (1975) Effect of maternal morphine administration on neonatal rat brain ornithine decarboxylase (ODC). Biochem. Pharmacol. 24, 1915–1918.

Butler, S.R. and Schanberg, S.M. (1977) Effect of maternal deprivation on polyamine metabolism in pre-weanling rat brain and heart. Life Sci. 21, 877–884.

Campbell, B.A., Lytle, L.D. and Fibiger, H.C. (1969) Ontogeny of adrenergic arousal and cholinergic inhibitory mechanisms in the rat. Science 166, 635–637.

Carakushansky, G., Neu, R.L. and Gardner, L.I. (1969) Lysergide and cannabis as possible teratogens in man. Lancet i, 150–151.

Carlsson, A. (1978) Mechanism of action of neuroleptic drugs. In: Psychopharmacology: A Generation of Progress (Lipton, M.A., MiMascio, A. and Killam, K.F. eds.) Raven Press, New York, pp. 1057–1070.

Clarren, S.K. and Smith D.W. (1978) The fetal alcohol syndrome, New Engl. J. Med. 298, 1063–1067.

Clemens, L.G., Popham, T.V. and Ruppert, P.H. (1979) Neonatal treatment of hamsters with barbiturate alters adult sexual behavior. Dev. Psychobiol. 12, 49–59.

Cole, P.V., Hawkins, L.H. and Roberts, D. (1972) Smoking during pregnancy and its effect on the fetus. J. Obstet. Gynecol. Brit. Commonw. 79, 782–787.

Concannon, J.T. and Schechter, M.D. (1981) Hyperactivity in developing rats: sex differences in 6-hydroxy-dopamine and amphetamine effects. Pharmacol. Biochem. Behav. 14, 5–10.

Cooper, J.R. (ed.) (1978) Sedative-hypnotic drugs: risks and benefits. DHEW Publication No. (ADM) 81–592.

Coyle, I.R. (1975) Changes in developing behavior following prenatal administration of imipramine. Pharmacol. Biochem. Behav. 3, 799–807.

Coyle, I.R. and Singer, G. (1975a) The interaction of post-weaning housing conditions and prenatal drug effects on behaviour. Psychopharmacology 41, 237–244.

Coyle, I.R. and Singer, G. (1975b) The interactive effects of prenatal imipramine exposure and postnatal rearing conditions on behavior and histology. Psychopharmacology 44, 253–256.

Coyle, I., Wayner, M.J. and Singer, G. (1976) Behavioral teratogenesis: a critical evalution. Pharmacol. Biochem. Behav. 4, 191–200.

46

Cragg, B.G. (1972) The development of cortical synapses during starvation in the rat. Brain 95, 143–150.

Da Silva, V.A., Ribeiro, M.J. and Masur, J. (1980) Developmental, behavioral and pharmacological characteristics of rat offspring from mothers receiving ethanol during gestation or lactation. Dev. Psychobiol. 13, 653–660.

Dalterio, S.L. (1980) Perinatal or adult exposure to cannabinoids alters male reproductive functions in mice. Pharmacol. Biochem. Behav. 12, 143–153.

Dalterio, S. and Bartke, A. (1979) Perinatal exposure to cannabinoids alters male reproductive function in mice. Science 205, 1420–1422.

Dalterio, S., Blum, K., Dalallo, L., Sweeney, C., Briggs, A. and Bartke, A. (1980) Perinatal exposure to Delta-^{9}-THC in mice: altered enkephalin and norpinephrine sensitivity in vas deferens. Substance, Alcohol Actions/Misuse 1, 467–478.

Davis, W.M. and Lin, C.H. (1972) Prenatal morphine effects on survival and behavior of rat offspring. Res. Commun. Chem. Pathol. Pharmacol. 3, 205–214.

Davison, A.N. (1977) The biochemistry of brain development and mental retardation. Brit. J. Psychiat. 131, 565–574.

Desmomd, M.M., Schwanecke, R.P., G.S. Yasunaga, S. and Burgdorff, I. (1972) Maternal barbiturate utilization and neonatal withdrawal symptomology. J. Pediatr. 80, 190–197.

Diaz, J. and Samson, H.H. (1980) Impaired brain growth in neonatal rats exposed to ethanol. Science 208, 751–753.

Diaz, J., Schain, R.J. and Bailey, B.G. (1977) Phenobarbital-induced brain growth retardation in artifically reared rat pups. Biol. Neonate 32, 77–82.

Dobbing, J. and Sands, J. (1971) Vulnerability of developing brain. IX. The effect of nutritional growth retardation on the timing of the brain growth-spurt. Biol. Neonate 19, 363–378.

Dobbing, J., Hopewell, J.W. and Lynch, A. (1971) Vulnerability of developing brain: VII. Permanent deficit of neurons in cerebral and cerebellar cortex following early mild undernutrition. Exp. Neurol. 32, 439–447.

Dow, T.G.B., Rooney, P.J. and Spence, M. (1975) Does anemia increase the risks to the fetus caused by smoking in pregnancy. Brit. Med. J. 4, 253–254.

Elmazar, M.M.A. and Sullivan, F.M. (1981) Effect of prenatal phenytoin administration on postnatal development of the rat: a behavioral teratology study. Teratology 24, 115–124.

Ellison, G., Eison, M.S., Huberman, H.S. and Daniel, F. (1978) Long-term changes in dopaminergic innervation of caudate nucleus after continuous amphetamine administration. Science 201, 276–278.

Engel, J. and Lundborg, P. (1974) Regional changes in monoamine levels and in the rate of tyrosine and tryptophan hydroxylation in 4 week old offspring of nursing mothers treated with the neuroleptic drug penfluridol. Naunyn-Schmiedeberg's Arch. Pharmacol. 282, 327–334.

Engel, J. and Lundborg, P. (1976) Reduced turnover in mesolimbic dopamine neurons in 4 week old offspring of nursing mothers treated with penfluridol. Brain Res. 110, 407–412.

Engel, J. and Lunborg, P. (1979) Increased mesolimbic ^{3}H-spiroperidol binding in 4-week old offspring of nursing rat mothers treated with penfluridol. Eur. J. Pharmacol. 60, 393–395.

Eriksson, M., Larsson, G. and Zetterstrom, R (1979) Abuse of alcohol, drugs and tobacco during pregnancy – consequences for the child. Paediatrician 8, 228–242.

Eriksson, M., Larsson, G., Winbladh, B. and Zetterstrom, R. (1978) The influence of amphetamine addiction on pregnancy and the newborn infant. Acta Paediatr. Scand. 67, 95–99.

Erinoff, L., Macphail, R.C., Heller, A. and Seiden, L.S. (1979) Age-dependent effects of 6-hydroxydopamine on locomotor activity in the rat. Brain Res. 164, 195–205.

Ernst, A.M. (1967) Mode of action of apomorphine and dexamphetamine on gnawing compulsion in rats. Psychopharmacology 10, 316–323.

Ewart, F.G. and Cutler, M.G. (1979) Effects of ethyl alcohol on development and social behavior in the offspring of laboratory mice. Psychopharmacology 62, 247–251.

Ferreira, S.H (1979) Site of analgesic action of aspirin-like drugs and opioids. In: Mechanism of Pain and Analgesic Compounds (Beers Jr. R.F. and Bassett, E.G. eds.) Raven Press, New York pp. 309–32.

Finnell, R.H. (1981) Phenytoin-induced teratogenesis: a mouse model. Science 211, 483–484.

Finnegan, L.P. (1979) Drug dependence in pregnancy: clinical management of mother and child. NIDA Services Research Monograph Series, DHEW Publication No. (ADM) 79–678.

Fish, I. and Winick, M. (1969) Effect of malnutrition on regional growth of the developing rat brain. Exp. Neurol. 25, 534–540.

Fishburne, P.M. and Cisin, L. (1980) National survey on drug abuse: main findings. National Institute on Drug Abuse, DHHS Publication No. (ADM) 80–976.

Fishman, R.H.B. and Yanai, J. (1983) Long-lasting effects of early barbiturates on the CNS and behavior. Neurosci. Biobehav. Rev. In press.

Fishman, R.H.B., Gaathon, A. and Yanai, Y. (1982) Early phenobarbital suppresses circulating thyroxine in mice. Dev. Brain Res. 5, 202–204.

Fishman, R.H.B., Ornoy, A. and Yanai, J. (1983) Neuronal degeneration after early phenobarbital exposure in mice. Exp. Neurol. 79, 212–222.

Fleischman, R.W., Hayden, D.W., Rosenkratz, H. and Braude, M.C. (1975) Teratologic evaluation of delta-9-tetrahydrocannabinol in mice, including a review of the literature. Teratology 12, 47–50.

Ford, D.H. and Rhines, R.K. (1979) Prenatal exposure to methadone HCl in relationship to body and brain growth in the rat. Acta Neurol. Scand. 59, 248–262.

Freedman, L.S., Samuels, S., Fish, I., Schwartz, S.A., Lange, B., Katz, M. and Morgano, L. (1980) Sparing of the brain in neonatal undernutrition: amino acid transport and incorporation into brain and muscle. Science 207, 902–904.

Fried, P.A. (1976) Cross-tolerance between inhaled cannabis and intraperitoneal injections of delta-9-THC. Pharmacol. Biochem. Behav. 4, 635–638.

Fried, P.A. (1976) Short and long-term effects of pre-natal cannabis inhalation upon rat offspring. Psychopharmacology 50, 285–291.

Fried, P.A. (1980) Marihuana use by pregnant women: neurobehavioral effects in neonates. Drug Alcohol Depend. 6, 415–424.

Fried, P.A. and Charlebois, A.T. (1979) Cannabis administered during pregnancy: first- and second-generation effects in rats. Physiol. Psychol. 7, 307–310.

Fuller, G.N. and Wiggens, R.C. (1981) A possible effect of the methylxanthines caffeine, theophylline and aminophylline on postnatal myelination of the rat brain. Brain Res. 213, 476–480.

Gallager, D.W. and Mallorga, P. (1980) Diphenylhydantoin: pre- and postnatal administration alters diazepam binding in developing rat cerebral cortex. Science 208, 64–66.

Gianutsos, G. and Abbatiello, E.R. (1972) The effect of pre-natal cannabis sativa on maze learning ability in the rat. Psychopharmacology 27, 117–122.

Giulian, D., McEwen, B.S. and Pohorecky, L.A. (1974) Altered development of the rat brain serotonergic system after disruptive neonatal experience. Proc. Natl. Acad. Sci. USA 71, 4106–4110.

Goldstein, A., Aronow, L. and Kalman, S.M. (1974) Principles of Drug Action: The Basis of Pharmacology, 2nd edn. Wiley, New York, Chapt. 10: Chemical Mutagenesis, pp. 623–666.

Golter, M. and Michaelson, I.A. (1975) Growth, behavior, and brain catecholamines in lead-exposed neonatal rats: a reappraisal. Science 187, 359–361.

Golub, M.S., Sassenrath, E.N. and Chapman, L.F. (1981) Regulation of visual attention in offspring of female monkeys treated chronically with delta 9-tetrahydrocannabinol. Dev. Psychobiol. 14, 507–512.

Goodrich, C. A., Hoff, K.M. and Baker, P.C. (1974) The maturational effects of LSD upon brain weight and behavior in the mouse. Comp. Gen. Pharmacol. 5, 153–155.

Goodwin, D.W., Schulsinger, F., Hermansen, L., Guze, S.B. and Winokur, G. (1975) Alcoholism and the hyperactive child syndrome. J. Nerv. Ment. Dis. 160, 349–353.

Gross, M.D. (1976) Growth of hyperkinetic children taking methylphenidate, dextroamphetamine, or imipramine/desipramine. Pediatrics 58, 423–431.

Gupta, C., Sonawane, B.R. and Yaffe, S.J. (1980) Phenobarbital exposure in utero: alterations in female reproductive function in rats. Science 208, 508–510.

48

Gupta, C., Yaffe, S.J. and Shapiro, B.H. (1982) Prenatal exposure to phenobarbital permanently decreases testosterone and causes reproductive dysfunction. Science 216, 640–642.

Hanson, J., Jones, K.L and Smith, D.W (1976) Fetal alcohol syndrome. J. Am. Med. Assoc. 235, 1458–1460.

Hanson, J.W., Myrianthopoulos, N.C., Harvey, M.A.S. and Smith, D.W. (1975) Risks to the offspring of women treated with hydantoin anticonvulsants, with emphasis on the fetal hydantoin syndrome. J. Pediat. 89, 662–668.

Harclerode, J., Nyquist, S.E., Nazar, B. and Lowe, D. (1979) Effects of cannabis on sex hormones and testicular enzymes on the rodent. In: Marihuana: Biological Effects (Nahas, G.G. and Paton, W.D.M., eds.) Permagon Press, New York, pp. 395–405.

Hecht, F., Beals, R., Lees, M., Jolly, H. and Roberts, P. (1968) Lysergic-acid-diethylamide and cannabis as possible teratogens in man. Lancet ii, 1087–1088.

Hedner, T., Lundborg, P. and Engel, J. (1979) Brain biochemical and behavioral changes in 4 week old rats after neonatal oxygen deprivation. Pharmacol. Biochem. Behav. 10, 647–650.

Heinonen, O.P., Slone, D. and Shapiro, S. (1977) Birth defects and drugs in pregnancy. Publishing Sciences Group, Inc. Littleton, MA.

Hembree III, W.C., Nahas, G.G., Zeidenberg, P. and Huang, H.F.S. (1979) Changes in human spermatozoa associated with high dose marihuana smoking. In: Marihuana: Biological Effects (Nahas, G.G. and Paton, W.D.M. eds.), Pergamon Press, New York, pp. 429–439.

Hill, R.M. (1973) Drugs ingested by pregnant women. Clin. Pharmacol. Ther. 14, 654–659.

Hill, R.M. and Stern, L. (1979) Drugs in pregnancy: effects on the fetus and newborn. Drugs 17, 182–197.

Hitzeman, B.A., Hitzemann, R.J., Brase, D.A. and Loh, H.H. (1976) Influence of prenatal d-amphetamine administration on development and behavior of rats. Life Sci. 18, 605–612.

Hubel, D.H. (1979) The visual cortex of normal and deprived monkeys. Am. Sci. 67, 532–543.

Hubel, D.H. and Wiesel, T.N. (1970) The period of susceptibility to the physiological effects of unilateral eye closure in kittens. J. Physiol. 206, 419–436.

Hutchings, D.E. and Gibbon, J. (1970) Preliminary study of behavioral and teratogenic effects of two 'stress' procedures administered during different periods of gestation in the rat. Psychol. Rep. 20, 239–246.

Hutchings, D.E., Towey, J.P., Gorinson, H.S. and Hunt, H.F. (1979) Methadone during pregnancy: assessment of behavioral effects in the rat offspring, J. Pharmacol. Exp. Ther. 208, 106–112.

Jonsson, G. and Hallman, H. (1980). Effects of neonatal nicotine administration on the postnatal development of central noradrenaline neurons. Acta Physiol Scand. Suppl. 479, 25–26.

Jonsson, G. and Hallman, H. (1982) Substance P counteracts neurotoxin damage on norepinephrine neurons in rat brain during ontogeny. Science 215, 75–77.

Jones, D.G. and Dyson, S.E. (1976) Synaptic junctions in undernourished rat brain—an ultrastructural investigation. Exp. Neurol. 51, 529–535.

Jones, K.L., Smith, D.W., Ulleland, C.N. and Streissguth, A.P. (1973) Pattern of malformation in offspring of chronic alcoholic mothers. Lancet i, 1267–1271.

Kasamatsu, T. and Pettigrew, J.D. (1976) Depletion of brain catecholamines: failure of ocular dominance shift after molecular occlusion in kittens. Science 194, 206–209.

Kastin, A.J., Kostrzewa, R.M., Schally, A.V. and Coy, D.H. (1980) Neonatal administration of met-enkephalin facilitates maze performance of adult rats. Pharmacol. Biochem. Behav. 13, 883–886.

Keller, E.A., Munaro, N.I. and Orsingher, O.A. (1982) Perinatal undernutrition reduces alpha and beta adrenergic receptor binding in adult rat brain. Science 215, 1269–1270.

Kernis, M.M., Pashayan, H.M. and Pruzansky, S (1973) Dilantin-induced teratogenicity and folic acid deficiency. Teratology 7, A19.

Kimmel, C.A., Butcher, R.E., Vorhees, C.V. and Schumacher, H.J. (1974) Metal-salt potentiation of salicylate-induced teratogenesis and behavioral changes in rats. Teratology 10, 293–300.

Kolansky, H. and Moore, W.T. (1972) Toxic effects of chronic marihuana use. J. Am. Med. Assoc. 222, 35–41.

Kornetsky, C. (1970) Psychoactive drugs in the immature organism. Psychopharmacologia 17, 105–136.

Koshakji, R.P. and Schulert, A.R. (1973) Biochemical mechanisms of salicylate teratology in the rat. Biochem. Pharmacol. 22, 407–416.

Kraus, H.F., Campbell, G.A., Fowler, M.W., Carton, A.C. and Farber, J.P. (1981) Maternal nicotine administration and fetal brain stem damage: a rat model with implications for sudden infant death syndrome. Am. J. Obstet. Gynecol. 140, 743–746.

Krsiak, M., Elis, J., Poschlova, N. and Masek, K. (1977) Increased aggressiveness and lower brain serotonin levels in offspring of mice given alcohol during gestation. J. Stud. Alcohol. 38, 1696–1704.

Lasky, D.I., Zagon, I.S. and McLaughlin, P.J. (1977) Effect of maternally administered heroin on the motor activity of rat offspring. Pharmacol. Biochem. Behav. 7, 281–284.

Lau, C., Bartolome, M. and Slotkin, T.A. (1977) Development of central and peripheral catecholaminergic systems in rats addicted perinatally to methadone. Neuropharmacology 16, 473–478.

Lauder, J.M. and Mugnaini, E. (1977) Early hyperthyroidism alters the distribution of mossy fibers in the rat hippocampus. Nature 268, 335–337.

Leahy, J.P., Stern, W.C., Resnick, O. and Morgane, P.J. (1978) A neuropharmacological analysis of central nervous system catecholamine systems in developmental protein malnutrition. Dev. Psychobiol. 111, 361–370.

Leathwood, P., Bush, M., Berent, C. and Mauron, J (1974) Effects of early malnutrition on Swiss white mice: avoidance learning after rearing in large litters. Life Sci. 14, 157–162.

LeMoal, M., Stinus, L., Simon, H., Tassin, J.P., Thierry, A.M., Blanc, G., Glowinski, J. and Cardo, B. (1977) Behavioral effects of a lesion in the ventral mesencephalic tegmentum: evidence for involvement of A10 dopaminergic neurons. Adv. Biochem. Psychopharmacol. 16, 237–245.

Loch, R.K., Rafales, L.S., Michaelson, I.A. and Bornschein, R.L. (1978) The role of undernutrition in animal models of hyperactivity. Life Sci. 22, 1963–1970.

Long, S.Y. (1972) Does LSD induce chromosomal damage and malformations? A review of the literature. Teratology 6, 75–90.

Longo, L.O. (1977) The biological effects of carbon monoxide on the pregnant woman, fetus, and newborn infant. Am. J. Obstet, Gynecol. 129, 69–103.

Lucchi, M.M., Spano, P.F. and Trabucchi, M. (1981) Dose-dependent and reversible effects of lead on rat dopaminergic system. Life Sci. 28, 795–799.

Lundborg, P. (1972) Abnormal ontogeny in young rabbits after chronic administration of haloperidol to the nursing mothers. Brain Res. 44, 684–687.

Lundborg, P. and Ross, B.E. (1974) Increased concentration of homovanillic acid in the brains of infant rabbits after administration of haloperidol to their nursing mothers. J. Pharm. Pharmacol. 26, 816–818.

McCall, M.A., Tieman, D.G. and Hirsch, H.V.B. (1979) Chronic intraventricular administration of LSD affects the sensitivity of cortical cells to monocular deprivation. Neurosci. Abstr. 5, 631.

McCullough, M.L. and Blackman, D.E. (1976) The behavioral effects of prenatal hypoxia in the rat. Dev. Psychobiol. 9, 335–342.

McGinty, J.F. and Ford, D.H. (1980) Effects of prenatal methadone on rat brain catecholamines. Dev. Neurosci. 3, 224–234.

McNutt, B.A., Boileau, R.A. and Cohen, M.N. (1977) The effects of long-term stimulant medication on the growth and body composition of hyperactive children. Psychopharmacol. Bull. 13, 36–38.

Manning, F.J., McDonough Jr., J.H., Elsmore, T.F., Saller, C. and Sodetz, F.J. (1971) Inhibition of normal growth by chronic administration of delta-9-tetrahydrocannabinol. Science 174, 424–426.

Manning, F., Wyn Pugh, E. and Boddy, K. (1975) Effect of cigarette smoking on fetal breathing movements in normal pregnancies. Brit. Med. J. 1, 552–553.

Marichich, E.S., Molina, V.A. and Orsingher, O.A. (1979) Persistent changes in central catecholaminergic system after recovery of perinatally undernourished rats. J. Nutr. 109, 1045–1050.

Marsh, L. and Fraser, F.C. (1973) Studies on dilantin-induced cleft palate in mice. Teratology 7, A23.

Martin, J.C. (1975) Effects on offspring of chronic maternal methamphetamine exposure. Dev. Psychobiol. 8, 397–404.

Martin, J.C. and Becker, R.F. (1970) The effects of nicotine administration in utero upon activity in the rat. Psychon. Sci. 19, 59–60.

Martin, J.C. and Becker, R.F. (1971) The effects of maternal nicotine absorption or hypoxic episodes upon appetitive bahavior of rat offspring. Dev. Psychobiol. 4, 133–147.

Martin, J.C. and Martin, D.C. (1981) Voluntary activity in the aging rat as a function of maternal drug exposure. Neurobehav. Toxicol. Teratol. 3, 261–264.

Martin, J.C., Martin, D.D., Radow, B. and Day, H.E. (1979) Life span and pathology in offspring following nicotine and methamphetamine exposure. Exp. Aging Res. 5, 509–522.

Martin, J.C., Martin, D.C., Radow, B. and Sigman, G. (1976) Growth, development and activity in rat offspring following maternal drug exposure. Exp. Aging Res. 2, 235–251.

Martin, J.C., Martin, D.C., Sigman, G. and Radow, B. (1978) Maternal ethanol consumption and hyperactivity in cross-fostered offspring. Physiol Psychol. 6, 362–365.

Meyer, M.B., Tonascia, J.A. and Buck, C. (1974) The interrelationship of maternal smoking and increased perinatal mortality with other risk factors. Further analysis of the Ontario Perinatal Mortality Study, 1960–1961. Am. J. Epidemiol. 100, 443–452.

Middaugh, L.D., Santos, III, C.A. and Zemp, J.W. (1975) Phenobarbital during pregnancy alters operant behavior of offspring in C57BL/6J mice. Pharmacol. Biochem. Behav. 3, 1137–1139.

Miller, F.E., Heffner, T.G., Kotake, C. and Seiden, L.S. (1981) Magnitude and duration of hyperactivity following neonatal 6-hydroxydopamine is related to the extent of brain dopamine depletion. Brain Res. 229, 123–132.

Miller, J.D. and Cisin, I.H. (Printed 1980) Highlights from the National Survey on Drug Abuse: 1979, DHHS Publication No. (ADM) 80–1032.

Millicovsky, G. and Johnston, M.C. (1981) Maternal hyperoxia greatly reduces the incidence of phenytoin-induced cleft lip and palate in A/J mice. Science 212, 671–672.

Mirmiran, M., Van DePoll, N.E., Corner, M.A., Van Oyen, H.G. and Bour, H.L. (1981) Suppression of active sleep by chronic treatment with chlorimipramine during early postnatal development: effects upon adult sleep and behavior in the rat. Brain Res. 204, 129–146.

Moldow, R.L., Kastin, A.J., Hollander, C.S., Coy, D.H. and Sandman, C.A. (1981) Brain beta-endorphin-like immunoreactivity in adult rats given beta-endorphin neonatally. Brain Res. Bull. 7, 683–686.

Monson, R.R., Rosenberg, L., Hartz, S.C., Shapiro, S., Heinonen, O.P. and Slone, D. (1973) Diphenylhydantoin and selected congenital malformations. N. Engl. J. Med. 289, 1049–1052.

Naeye, R.L. (1978) Effects of maternal cigarette smoking on the fetus and placenta. Brit. J. Obstet. Gynaecol. 85, 732–737.

Nair, V. (1974) Prenatal exposure to drugs: effect on the development of brain monoamine systems. In: Drugs and the Developing Brain (Vernadakis, A. and Weiner, N., eds.) Plenum Press. New York, pp. 171–197.

Nasello, A.G., Astrada, C.A. and Ramirez, O.A. (1974) Effects on the acquistion of conditioned avoidance responses and seizure threshold in the offspring of amphetamine treated gravid rats. Psychopharmacology 40, 25–31.

Nasello, A.G. and Ramirez, O.A. (1978) Brain catecholamines metabolism in offspring of amphetamine treated rats. Pharmarcol. Biochem. Behav. 9, 17–20.

Netzloff, M.L., Frias, J.L. and Rennert, O.M.(1977) Respiratory changes in 9-methyl PGA teratogenesis. Life Sci. 20, 1233–1238.

Netzloff, M.L., Streiff, R.R., Frias, J.L. and Rennert, O.M. (1979) Folate antagonism following teratogenic exposure to diphenylhydantoin. Teratology 19, 45–50.

Newman, R. (1974) Pregnancies of methadone patients. NY State J. Med., Part 1, 52–54.

Nolen, G.A. (1981) The effect of brewed and instant coffee on reproduction and teratogenesis in the rat. Toxicol. Appl. Pharmacol. 58, 171–183.

O'Callaghan, J.P. and Holtzman, S.G. (1976) Prenatal administration of morphine to the rat: tolerance to the analgesic effect of morphine in the offspring. J. Pharmacol. Exp. Ther. 197, 533–544.

Origuchi, Y., Nonaka, I., Uneo, T. and Usuku, G. (1975) Ultrastuctural changes in the cerebellum of young rats having received diphenylhydantoin during the embryonal stage. Kumamoto Med. J. 28, 84–93.

Ouelette, E.M., Rosett, H.L., Rosman, N.P. and Weiner, L. (1977) Adverse effects on offspring of maternal alcohol abuse during pregnancy. New Engl. J. Med. 297, 528–530.

Quigley, M.E., Sheehan, K.L., Wilkes, M.M. and Yen, S.S.C. (1979) Effects of maternal smoking on circulating catecholamine levels and fetal heart rates. Am. J. Obstet. Gynecol. 133, 685–690.

Radouco-Thomas, S., Magnan, F., Grove, R.N., Singh, P., Garcin, F. and Radouco-Thomas, C. (1976) Effect of chronic administration of delta-tetrahydrocannabinol on learning and memory in developing mice. In: The Pharmacolgy of Marihuana (Braude, M., and Szara, S., eds.) Raven Press, New York, pp. 487–489.

Ramer, C.M. and Lodge A. (1975) Clinical and developmental characteristics of infants of mothers on methadone maintenance. Add. Diseases 2, 227–234.

Rapoport, J.L., Jensvold, M., Elkins, R., Buchsbaum, M., Weingartner, H., Ludlow, C., Zahn. T., Berg, C. and Neims, A. (1981) Behavioral and cognitive effects of caffeine in boys and adult males. J. Nerv. Mental. Dis. 169, 726–732.

Rawat, A.K. (1977) Developmental changes in the brain levels of neurotransmitters as influenced by maternal ethanol consumption in the rat. J. Neurochem. 28, 1175–1182.

Rawat, A.K. (1980) Development of histaminergic pathways in brain as influenced by maternal alcoholism. Research Commun. Chem. Pathol. Pharmacol. 27, 91–103.

Richard, L.G. (Ed.) (1981) Demographic trends and drug abuse. 1980–1995. NIDA Research Monograph No. 35. DHHS publication number ADM (81–1069).

Riley, E.P., Lochry, E.A. and Shapiro, N.R. (1979a) Lack of response inhibition in rats prenatally exposed to alcohol. Psychopharmacology 62, 47–52.

Riley, E.P., Lochry, E.A., Shapiro, N.R. and Baldwin, J. (1979b) Response perseveration in rats exposed to alcohol prenatally. Pharmacol. Biochem. Behav. 10, 255–259.

Ritter, E.J., Scott, W.J., Wilson, J.G. Mathinos, P.R. and Randall, J.L. (1982) Potentiative interactions between caffeine and various teratogenic agents. Teratology 25, 95–100.

Roche, A.F., Lipman, R.S., Overall, J.E. and Wellington, H. (1979) The effects of stimulant medication on the growth of hyperkinetic children. Pediatrics 63, 847–850.

Rodier, P.M. (1977) Correlations between prenatally-induced alterations in CNS cell populations and postnatal function. Teratology 16, 235–246.

Rodier, P.M., Reynolds, S.S. and Roberts, W.N. (1979) Behavioral consequences of interference with CNS development in the early fetal period. Teratology 19, 327–336.

Rosengarten, H. and Friedhoff, A.J. (1979) Enduring changes in dopamine receptor cells of pups from drug administration to pregnant and nursing rats. Science 203, 1133–1135.

Rosenzweig, M.R., Bennett, E.L. and Diamond, M.C. (1972) Brain changes in response to experience. Sci. Am. 226, 22–30.

Safer, D., Allen, R. and Barr, E. (1972) Depression of growth in hyperactive children on stimulant drugs. New Engl. J. Med. 287, 217–220.

Sandman, C.A., McGivern, R.F., Berka, C., Walker, J.M., Coy, D.H. and Kastin, A.J. (1979) Neonatal administration of β-endorphin produces 'chronic' insensitivity to thermal stimuli. Life Sci. 25, 1755–1760.

Schain, R.J. and Watanabe, K. (1975) Effect of chronic phenobarbital administration upon brain growth of the infant rat. Exp. Neurol. 47, 509–515.

Schechter, M.D. and Concannon, J.T. (1982) Haloperidol-induced hyperactivity in neonatal rats: effect of lithium and stimulants. Pharmacol. Biochem. Behav. 16, 1–5.

Seiden, L.S. and Dykstra, L.A. (1977) Psychopharmacology: A Behavioral and Biochemical Approach. Van Nostrand Reinhold, Co., New York, Vol. 5, pp. 117–171.

Shalaby, I.A. and Spear, L.P. (1980) Chronic administration of haloperidol during development: later psychopharmacological responses to apomorphine and arecoline. Pharmacol. Biochem. Behav. 13, 685–690.

52

Shaywitz, B.A., Klopper, J.H., Jager, R.D. and Gordon, J.W. (1976b) Paradoxical response to amphetamine in developing rats treated with 6-hydroxydopamine. Nature 261, 153–155.

Shaywitz, B.A. and Pearson, D.A. (1978) Effects of phenobarbital on activity and learning in 6-hydroxy-
dopamine treated rat pups. Pharmacol. Biochem. Behav. 9, 173–179.

Shaywitz, B.A., Yager, R.D. and Klopper, J.H. (1976a) Selective brain dopamine depletion in developing
rats: an experimental model of minimal brain dysfunction. Science 191, 305–308.

Shoemaker, W.J. and Wurtman, R.J. (1971) Perinatal undernutrition: accumulation of catecholamines in
rat brain. Science 171, 1017–1019.

Shoemaker, W.J. and Wurtman, R.J. (1973) Effect of perinatal undernutrition on the metabolism of catecholamines in the rat brain. J. Nutr. 103, 1537–1547.

Silbergeld, E.K. and Goldberg, A.M. (1974) Lead-induced behavioral dysfunction: an animal model of
hyperactivity. Exp. Neurol. 42, 146–157.

Silbergeld, E.K. and Goldberg, A.M. (1975) Pharmacological and neurochemical investigations of lead-
induced hyperactivity. Neuropharmacology 14, 431–444.

Slotkin, T.A. (1979) Ornithine decarboxylase as a tool in developmental neurobiology. Life Sci. 24,
1623–1630.

Slotkin, T.A., Lau, C. and Bartolome, M. (1976) Effects of neonatal or maternal methadone administration
on ornithine decarboxylase activity in brain and heart of developing rats. J. Pharmacol. Exp. Ther.
199, 141–148.

Slotkin, T.A., Schanberg, S.M. and Kuhn, C.M. (1980) Synaptic development in brains of rats exposed
perinatally to ethanol. Experientia 36, 1005–1006.

Slotkin, T.A. and Thadani, P.V. (1980) Neurochemical teratology of drugs of abuse. In: Advances in the
Study of Birth Defects, Vol. 4: Neural and Behavioral Teratology (Persaud, T.V.N., ed.), MTP
Press, Lancaster, UK, pp. 199–234.

Slotkin, T.A., Whitmore, W.L., Salvaggio, M., and Seidler, F.J. (1979) Perinatal methadone addiction of
biogenic amine systems in the rat. Life Sci. 24, 1223–1230.

Smart, J.L., Dobbing, J., Adlard, B.P.F., Lynch, A. and Sands, J. (1973) Vulnerability of developing brain:
relative effects of growth restriction during the fetal and suckling periods on behavior and brain composition of adult rats. J. Nutr. 103, 1327–1338.

Snyder, S.H., Banerjee, S.P., Yamamura, H.I. and Greenberg, D. (1974) Drugs, neurotransmitters, and
schizophrenia. Science 184, 1243–1253.

Sobrian, S.K. (1977) Prenatal morphine administration alters behavioral development in the rat. Pharmacol. Biochem. Behav. 7, 285–288.

Sonawane, B.R. (1982) Effects of prenatal nicotine exposure on reproductive function of rat offspring. Teratology 25, 77A.

Sonderegger, T. and Zimmermann, E. (1978) Adult behavior and adrenocortical function following neonatal morphine treatment in rats. Psychopharmacology 56, 103–109.

Spear, L.P., Shalaby, I.A. and Brick, J. (1980) Chronic administration of haloperidol during development:
behavioral and psychopharmacological effects. Psychopharmacology 70, 47–58.

Speidel, B.D. and Meadow, S.R. (1972) Maternal epilepsy and abnormalities of the fetus and newborn.
Lancet ii, 839–843.

Spyker, J.M. (1975) Assessing the impact of low level chemicals on development: behavioral and latent effects. Fed. Proc. 34, 1835–1844.

Stoof, J.C., Dijkstra, H. and Hillegers, J.P.M. (1978) Changes in the behavioral response to a novel environment following lesioning of the central dopaminergic system in rat pups. Psychopharmacology 57,
163–166.

Strauss, M.E., Starr, R.H., Ostrea, E.M., Chavez, C.J. and Stryker, J.C. (1976) Behavioral concomitants
of prenatal addiction to narcotics. J. Pediatr. 89, 842–846.

Streissguth, A.P., Landesman-Dwyer, S., Martin, J.C. and Smith, D.W. (1980) Teratogenic effects of alcohol in humans and laboratory animals. Science 209, 353–361.

Strombom, U. (1975) On the functional role of pre- and postsynaptic catecholamine receptors in brain. Acta Physiol. Scand. Suppl. 431, 1–43.

Sullivan, F.M. and McElhatton, P.R. (1975) Teratogenic activity of the antiepileptic drugs phenobarbital, phenytoin, and primidone in mice. Toxicol. Appl. Pharmacol. 34, 271–282.

Thadani, P.V., Lau, C., Slotkin, T.A. and Schanberg, S.M. (1977a) Effects of maternal ethanol ingestion on amine uptake into synaptosomes of fetal and neonatal rat brain. J. Pharmacol. Exp. Ther. 200, 292–297.

Thadani, P.V., Slotkin, T.A. and Schanberg, S.M. (1977b) Effects of late prenatal or early postnatal ethanol exposure on ornithine decarboxylase activity in brain and heart of developing rats. Neuropharmacology 16, 298–293.

Thieme, R.E., Dijkstra, H. and Stoof, J.C. (1980) An evaluation of the young dopamine-lesioned rat as an animal model for minimal brain dysfunction (MBD). Psychopharmacology 67, 165–169.

Tonge, S.R. (1973a) Permanent alterations in catecholamine concentrations in discrete areas of brain in the offspring of rats treated with methylamphetamine and chlorpromazine. Brit. J. Pharmacol. 47, 425–427.

Tonge, S.R. (1973b) Permanent alterations in 5-hydroxyindole concentrations in discrete areas of rat brain produced by the pre- and neonatal administration of methylamphetamine and chlorpromazine. J. Neurochem. 20, 625–627.

Trulson, M.E. and Jacobs, B.L. (1979) Chronic amphetamine administration to cats: behavioral and neurochemical evidence for decreased central serotonergic function. J. Pharmacol. Exp. Ther. 211, 375–384.

Vardaris, R.M., Weisz, D.J., Fazel, A. and Rawitch, A.B. (1976) Chronic administration of delta-9-tetrahydrocannabinol to pregnant rats: studies of pup behavior and placental transfer. Pharmacol. Biochem. Behav. 4, 249–254.

Wagner, G.C., Ricaurte, G.A., Seiden, L.S., Schuster, C.R., Miller, J.J. and Wistley, J. (1980) Long-lasting depletions of striatal dopamine and loss of dopamine uptake sites following repeated administration of methamphetamine. Brain Res. 181, 151–160.

West, G.L., Sobotka, T.J., Brodie, R.E. and Beier, J.M. (1982) Physical and behavioral development of F1 albino rats after prenatal caffeine. Teratology 25, 81A.

West, J.R., Hodges, C.A. and Black, Jr., A.C. (1981) Prenatal exposure to ethanol alters the organization of hippocampal mossy fibers in rats. Science 211, 957–959.

Whatson, T.S. and Smart, J.L. (1978) Social behaviour of rats following pre- and early postnatal undernutrition. Physiol. Behav. 20, 749–753.

Wilson, G.S., Desmond, M.M. and Verniaud, W.M. (1973) Early development of infants of heroin-addicted mothers. Am. J. Dis. Child. 126, 457–462.

Wright, P.L., Smith, S.H., Keplinger, M.L., Calandra, J.C. and Braude, M.C. (1976) Reproductive and teratologic studies with delta-9-tetrahydrocannabinol and crude marijuana extract. Toxicol. Appl. Pharmacol. 38, 223–235.

Yanai, J. and Ginsburg, B.E. (1979) The relative contribution of pre- and neonatal ethanol administration to changes in mice behavior. Arch. Int. Pharmacodyn. 241, 235–244.

Yanai, J., Rosselli-Austin, L. and Tabakoff, B. (1979) Neuronal deficits in mice following prenatal exposure to phenobarbital. Exp. Neurol. 64, 237–244.

Yanai, J. and Tabakoff, B. (1980) Altered sensitivity to ethanol following prenatal exposure to barbiturates. Psychopharmacology 68, 301–303.

Yanai, J., Bergman, A., Shafer, R., Yedwab, J. and Tabakoff, B. (1981) Audiogenic seizures and neuronal deficits following early exposure to barbiturate. Dev. Neurosci. 4, 345–350.

Yanai, J., Fishman, R.H.B. and Feigenbaum, J.J. (1982) Lessened sensitivity to apomorphine induced-climbing behavior in mice following neonatal exposure to phenobarbital. Neurobehav. Toxicol. Teratol. 4, 535–538.

Zagon, I.S. and McLaughlin, P.J. (1977a) Effect of chronic maternal methadone exposure on perinatal development. Biol. Neonate 31, 271–282.

54

Zagon, I.S. and McLaughlin, P.J. (1977b) The effects of different schedules of methadone treatment on rat brain development. Exp. Neurol. 56, 538–552.

Zagon, I.S. and McLaughlin, P.J. (1977c) Methadone and brain development. Experientia 33, 1486.

Zagon, I.S. and McLaughlin, P.J. (1978) Perinatal methadone exposure and its influence on the behavioral ontogeny of rats. Pharmacol. Biochem. Behav. 9, 665–672.

Zagon, I.S. and McLaughlin, P.J. (1978) Perinatal methadone exposure and brain development: a biochemical study. J. Neurochem. 31, 49–54.

Zagon, I.S. and McLaughlin, P.J. (1979) Motor activity and learning ability in rats perinatally exposed to methadone. NIDA Res. Monogr. 27, 121–127.

Zagon, I.S., McLaughlin, P.J. and Thompson, C.I. (1979) Learning ability in adult female rats perinatally exposed to methadone. Pharmacol. Biochem. Behav. 10, 889–894.

Zelson, C., Lee, S.J. and Casalino, M. (1973) Neonatal narcotic addiction. N. Engl. J. Med. 289, 1216–1220.

Zelson, C., Sook, J.L. and Casalino, M. (1973) Neonatal narcotic addiction: comparative effects of maternal intake of heroin and methadone. N. Engl. J. Med. 287, 1216–1220.

Zemp, J.W. and Middaugh, L.D. (1975) Some effects of prenatal exposure to d-amphetamine sulfate and phenobarbital on developmental neurochemistry and on behavior. Addic. Dis. 2, 307–331.

Zimmerman, E., Branch, B., Taylor, A.N., Young, J. and Pang, C.N. (1974) Long-lasting effects of prepuberal administration of morphine in adult rats. In: Narcotics and the Hypothalamus (Zimmerman, E. and George, R., eds.) Raven Press, New York, pp. 183–194.

Neurobehavioral Teratology
edited by Joseph Yanai
© Elsevier Science Publishers BV 1984

2

POSSIBLE MECHANISMS UNDERLYING THE TERATOGENIC EFFECTS OF MEDICINES ON THE DEVELOPING BRAIN

Dick F. Swaab and Majid Mirmiran

Netherlands Institute for Brain Research, IJdijk 28, 1095 KJ Amsterdam, The Netherlands

DESPITE the fact that various clinically employed drugs present a serious threat to fetal brain development, the use of medication during pregnancy is reaching previously unheard of levels. A retrospective survey in Belgium showed that an average of 4.4 different drugs had been taken by expectant mothers (Meire et al., 1979), and this type of survey only traced 30% of the medicines actually used (Bodendorfer et al., 1979). A prospective survey disclosed that, in the United States, women take on the average eleven different drugs in the course of pregnancy (Doering and Stewart, 1978). Many of these preparations in fact contain a mixture of pharmaceutical compounds, and most of them are of the type that easily cross the placenta. Subsequently they readily reach the foetal brain, since the blood-brain barrier at this stage of development is not capable of preventing their passage. Probably because of the dramatic evidence furnished by the thalidomide tragedy, our awareness of the dangers of drug ingestion has cautioned us against the indiscriminate use of medicine only during the *initial* stages of pregnancy. However, even medicines that do not cause any gross physical malformations can cause microscopic defects (such as the vaginal tumors in children of mothers treated with diethylstilboestrol during gestation: Herbst, 1981) or alter the intricate structure or chemical composition of fetal brain tissue to such an extent that permanent behavioral deviations later develop. The latter field, which is known as 'behavioral teratology' is the subject of this chapter.

55

Substances affecting brain development

Those chemical compounds which are of importance for adult brain function appear in general to be involved in brain development as well (Swaab, 1980). At the present time this is best established for *sex hormones, corticosteroids, thyroid hormones*, and *neurotransmitters*. Substances which alter the balance of any of these compounds during ontogeny are therefore capable of altering the course of brain development in a permanent way.

Sex hormones in the rat, acting during the perinatal period, affect the maturation of the brain (both structurally and functionally) in a different way in the two sexes. For example, a light macroscopically evident sexual dimorphism occurs in the size of the nucleus preopticus medialis, which is determined by the levels of testosterone present around the time of birth (Gorski et al., 1978; Jacobson et al., 1980). There are relatively subtle effects such as those that undoubtedly constitute the biological basis for sex-related brain differences in animals as well as in humans. These differences include not only such obvious phenomena as sexual behavior patterns and the size of related brain structures, but also the performance in a variety of learning situations (Van de Poll et al., 1978). It is therefore a matter of considerable concern that progestatives, estrogens and/or combinations thereof have frequently been prescribed to pregnant women (Reinisch and Karow, 1977), in the mistaken belief that they prevent impending miscarriages. In the United States between one and 4.5 million pregnant women used diethylstilboestrol (DES) from 1945 until 1971. It was taken off the market only due to a probable carcinogenic effect on the cervix and vagina in female offspring (Herbst et al., 1981). It is worth mentioning that DES recently appeared to be supplied by Dutch mail order as a sex stimulating compound. Not only are these drugs ineffective in sustaining pregnancy, but their use entails a real possibility of inducing personality disorders in the offspring. Thus estrogen-exposed children have been found between 4 and 21 years of age to be generally less self-confident, less sensitive, and more dependent and group oriented than normal children (Reinisch and Karow, 1977). In addition, an increased percentage of infertility and interference with sexual function was found following intrauterine exposure to injected estrogens (Stenchever et al., 1981; Beral and Colwell, 1981). Prenatal administration of oestrogen and progesterone in boys has been reported to influence certain aspects of postnatal psychosexual development most noticeably (i.e. 'masculinity', 'aggressiveness' and athletic abilities) (Yalom et al., 1973).

Corticosteroids are used during pregnancy, for example in cases of allergic reactions, and to promote lung development in the child in cases of imminent parturition (as recommended by Liggins and Howie, 1972). In quite a number of patients this treatment does not seem to have the expected effect (Gariete et al., 1981). In addition, animal experiments indicate that exposure to corticosteroids can retard brain development and affect behavior in later life (Balazs et al., 1975; Taeusch, 1975; Dahlof et al., 1980; Sobel, 1978, Johnson et al., 1981). It has been demonstrated that corticosteroids also affect glial cell proliferation in rat brain (Howard and Benjamins, 1975). Marton et al. (1979) found a slowing of psychomotor development, which persisted at least up to 2 years of life in prematurely born children who had been exposed to corticosteroids.

Thyroid hormones have been injected directly into the amniotic fluid in order to enhance fetal lung maturation (Mashiach et al., 1978). No follow-up investigation of these children has been carried out to our knowledge, although it is known from animal experiments that such treatment may hamper brain development (Balazs, 1979).

Recent research indicates also that *neurotransmitters* – which can be subdivided into the following groups: acetylcholine, biogenic amines, amino acids and peptides – are essential for normal brain development.

(1) *Acetylcholine.* Pyridostigmine (an acetylcholinesterase inhibitor), when administered to neonatal rats, induces premature puberty and increased male sexuality in both sexes of the offspring (Hinz et al., 1978). Nicotine (an acetylcholine receptor agonist) enhances cell death in the rat foetal brain stem (Kraus et al., 1981) while neonatal administration of chlorisodamine (a nicotine-receptor blocker) prevented the normal postnatal increase in volume and cell number of the mouse superior cervical ganglion (Black and Geen, 1974).

(2) *Biogenic amines.* Apart from the serotonin-reuptake blocker (chlorimipramine) and the a-adrenergic agonist (clonidine), see below, there are many examples of medicines which, if used during pregnancy, impair normal brain development by upsetting the balance of the monoamines and/or influencing the sensitivity of the receptors. In animal experiments, reserpine (used as an antihypertensive as well as a tranquilizer) decreases the monoamine levels in the brain and has been shown to induce permanent brain and behavioral changes in the offspring (Thornburg and Moore, 1976; Hutchings, 1978; Patel et al., 1981; Barlow and Sullivan, 1975). These include reduced formation of neurons, hyperactivity, and increased susceptibility to audiogenic seizures. Amphetamine, which increases the release of catecholamines in the brain, is commonly used as a dieting aid but is also given to children in cases of enuresis nocturna or minimal brain dysfunction (Huygen, 1979; Hitzemann et al., 1976; Nasello and Ramirez, 1978; Gross and Wilson, 1974). Offspring of pregnant rats treated with such drugs show behavioral changes, most notably an inability in adulthood to adapt to new surroundings (Hutchings, 1978; Hitzemann et al., 1976). a-Methyl-dopa (a false transmitter precursor for noradrenaline) and propanolol (a β-adrenergic blocker), when taken by the pregnant mother, result in a reduced head circumference in the neonate (Moar et al., 1978; Pruyn et al., 1979). The use of neuroleptics such as chlorpromazine (a dopamine antagonist) during pregnancy has been reported to result in extrapyramidal disturbances in the newborn child (Hill et al., 1966), while in animal experiments it impaired learning ability (reviewed in Barlow and Sullivan, 1975). Barbiturates, which also stimulate dopamine receptors (Yanai and Feigenbaum, 1981), are commonly used as hypnotics, sedatives, anticonvulsives and for preventing neonatal jaundice. They may induce a long-term withdrawal syndrome lasting as much as 3 months

58

(Thornburg and Moore, 1976). In animal studies, barbiturates have been shown to impair reproductive function and maze-learning ability of the offspring despite the absence of obvious CNS deformities (Clemens et al., 1979; Gupta et al., 1980; Middaugh et al., 1975).

(3) *The amino acids.* Our present knowledge of the possible effects on brain development of drugs acting upon this group of transmitters is disappointingly small, even though amino acidic preparations are used in neonatology. It is important to emphasize that almost any disturbance in amino acid metabolism goes together with mental retardation (Lee, 1980). Prenatal or early postnatal treatment of rats with the often used transquilizer diazepam (which acts upon GABA receptors: Kruck and Pycock, 1979) produces long-lasting effects on brain enzymes, thereby resulting in behavioral disturbances such as hyperactivity and lack of acoustic startle reflexes (Fonseca et al., 1976; Kellog et al., 1980; Jakoubek, 1978). Diazepam administration during pregnancy in humans results in low Apgar scores, depressed respiration and impaired suckling (Cree et al., 1973; Patrick et al., 1972). Long-term follow-ups of such children are lacking.

(4) *Peptides.* Little is known about the possible long-term effects on brain development of this recently discovered group of neurotransmitters that were originally thought to be simply hormones produced by the hypothalamus, e.g. vasopressin, oxytocin, LHRH, TRH and somatostatin, but which later appeared to have important central effects as well (for review, see Swaab, 1982).

Oxytocin is routinely used in obstetrics and may cause fetal distress, including a rise in core temperature and possibly retarded motor and speech development. Preliminary observations in the rat revealed a permanent effect on water metabolism following administration of oxytocin to the developing rat (for references see Boer and Swaab, in press). It will probably take gynecologists some time to get used to the idea that even oxytocin can be considered as a neurotransmitter, and thus as a 'psychotropic drug' that may be detrimental to the child via a direct action on the developing brain. Vasopressin, which can permanently alter osmoregulation following perinatal administration (Boer and Swaab, 1983), and its analogues have been given to mentally retarded children (J. Eisenberg, pers. comm.; Waggoner et al., 1978; Anderson et al., 1979).

Naloxone, an opiate antagonist, is administered clinically in order to normalize fetal heart rate (Goodlin, 1981). Animal experiments have implicated naloxone as the cause of a permanent impairment of sensitivity to thermal stimuli (Sandman et al., 1979) and of maze-learning ability (Vorhees, 1981). β-Endorphin, used during delivery as an analgesic (Oyama et al., 1980), induces similar disturbances in the rat (Sandman et al., 1979).

Mechanisms of action of medicines on the developing brain

Drugs taken by the pregnant mother may impair the developing child's brain in different ways.

(1) This action may be *indirect,* as in the case of aspirin which, when taken by the pregnant mother, makes the fetus more susceptible to the stress of labor, thus resulting in a higher incidence of intracranial bleeding and perinatal mortality (Rumack et al., 1981; Collins, 1981).

(2) Drugs may affect brain development by interacting directly with the formation of the neuronal and glial network, e.g. by affecting cell division, cell death, cell migration, or the formation of neurites, synapses and receptors. Most, if not all, medicines in fact appear to affect several of these processes simultaneously.

Cell division is reported to be slowed down by a number of medicines, both in vivo and in vitro (Patel et al., 1981). Barbiturates were found e.g. to cause a 30% reduction in the number of cerebellar Purkinje cells and a 15% reduction in hippocampal pyramidal cells (Hutchings, 1978; Ornoy and Yanai, 1980; Culver and Vernadakis, 1979; Diaz and Schain, 1978). Other compounds which have similar deleterious effects include corticosteroids (De Lemos and Moore, 1976), chlorpromazine (Patel et al., 1980), alcohol (Barnes and Walker, 1981), reserpine (Patel et al., 1981), thyroid hormone (Balazs, 1979) and sex hormones (Gorski et al., 1978; Jacobson et al., 1980). Indirect evidence for decreased brain cell division is provided by the smaller head circumferences which have been found at birth following treatment with sex hormones (H.J. Huisjes, pers. comm.); with α-methyl-dopa or propanolol (Moar et al., 1978; Pruyn et al., 1979), and hydantoin (Hanson and Smith, 1976; Hanson, 1978; Hilesma et al., 1981), or by the use of alcohol (Iosub et al., 1981; Ouelette and Rosett, 1976) during human pregnancy.

Cell death is augmented by nicotine (Kraus et al., 1981) and accelerated by alcohol exposure prior to birth (Yanai, 1981).

Cell migration is disturbed by alcohol (Jones et al., 1976), while the *formation of neurites and synapses* is known to be affected by sex hormones (Arai et al., 1978; Greenough et al., 1977; Salaman, 1974; Toran-Allerand, 1976), by corticosteroids (Howard and Benjamin, 1975), by morphine/methadone (Hutchings, 1978; Slotkin et al., 1979); Strauss et al., 1979; Kreek, 1979; Kaltenbach et al., 1979), by anticonvulsive agents (Culver and Vernadakis, 1979) and by alcohol (Hammer and Scheibel, 1981; West et al., 1981).

Another direct effect of drugs is upon non-neuronal elements in the brain, e.g. the glia cells. There is strong evidence, for instance, that neuroleptic drugs inhibit glial adenylate cyclase activity (Henn, 1982), while corticosteroids probably affect glial cell proliferation (Howard and Benjamin, 1975). Clonidine interacts with glial cells to decrease the level of their cyclic AMP (Henn, 1982).

(3) The third mechanism involves effects of medicines on the *interaction of brain and behavior during development.* This has come to light in a study at our institute in which

the long-term effect of REM sleep ('active' sleep: AS) deprivation on brain and behavior development was studied. In man and other mammals AS occupies a large proportion of time in utero and in the early postnatal period, which is the period of brain development. This led to the question whether or not AS plays an important role in brain maturation.. Experimental suppression of AS during early postnatal life by means of clomipramine, clonidine, or instrumental deprivation in rats, revealed a clearcut reduction of cortical size, higher level of open field activity, deficient masculine sexual behavior, and disturbed sleep patterns in adulthood (Mirmiran et al., 1981; Mirmiran et al., 1983a). These results, and those of others using different pharmacological as well as non-pharmacological approaches, argue in favor of AS per se as a causal factor in normal brain maturation (Juvancs and Nowaczyk, 1975; Mitler, 1971; Saucier and Astic, 1975).

The specific reduction of cortical weight, together with decreased protein content, in the absence of any significant change in cell number, was highly reminiscent of the picture seen in rats reared under sensorially impoverished conditions (Rosenzweig and Bennett, 1978). This similarity suggested that the developmental effects of rearing in 'enriched' environments may entail an interaction between AS and experimental 'traces' laid down earlier during periods of wakefulness. This hypothesis is rendered still more credible by the demonstration that the amount of AS increases during enrichment rearing (Mirmiran et al., 1982). Furthermore, concomitant AS deprivation by means of clonidine neutralizes the effect that environmental enrichment normally exerts upon cortical growth (Mirmiran and Uylings, submitted). Another intriguing finding is that prolonged AS deprivation by means of clonidine even *prior to* the period of enrichment rearing interferes with the expected extra brain growth (Mirmiran et al., 1983b). Apparently, cortical mechanisms underlying 'plasticity' in later life can be adversely affected by the absence of AS and/or NA disturbances in early development. Such a phenomenon may implicate abnormal sleep patterns as a potential contributory factor to learning deficiences in humans as well.

A higher level of activity in the open-field test was found in adulthood in rats that were neonatally deprived of AS. This test is believed to measure the level of 'emotionality', i.e. 'fearfulness' (Aulich, 1976; Russel, 1973). Hyperactivity and emotional lability have also been described in children (e.g. in minimal brain dysfunction; Gross and Wilson, 1974). Although its etiology is largely unknown, prenatal complications are believed to increase the chance that such abnormalities will occur. It might not be premature, therefore, to express a word of caution about exposure of infants to drugs or situations affecting sleep (particularly AS) which, from animal experiments, are known to cause a comparable syndrome.

The drugs used in the AS-deprivation studies, viz. clomipramine (Anafranil®) and clonidine (Catapresan®) are also used in clinical practice (for treating depression, hypertension, migraine, nocturnal enuresis, sleep apnea, opiate withdrawal, minimal brain dysfunction, etc.). The potential seriousness of such exposure has been emphasized by Dr. N. Monod of the University of Paris, who discontinued clomipramine treatment in infants up to 3 months of age suffering from sleep apnea (pers. comm.), after learning about these animal experimental results (Mirmiran et al., 1980).

Clinical awareness required

A wide variety of chemical compounds having comparable effects upon monoamine systems and/or AS are currently in clinical use. It is both surprising and a source of concern that practically no follow-up studies appear to have been carried out on the possible long-lasting functional consequences of such treatments in man. Table 2.1 lists the most commonly used drugs during the prenatal and early postnatal periods. Some of these substances have demonstrable teratogenic effects, and almost all of them tend to suppress AS.

It is important to point out that almost all drugs used during gestation easily cross the placenta, and their level in the fetus (especially in the brain) is even higher than in the maternal circulation (Mirkin and Singh, 1976). In addition, humans are often more sensitive than animals to teratogenicity of drugs (Council on Environmental Quality, 1981). The offspring of many drug-addicted mothers exhibit withdrawal symptoms (Hill and Stern, 1979). The possibility of fetal sleep disturbances during gestation as well as during the withdrawal period has been ignored so far. However, one report does demonstrate a prolonged disturbance of sleep in babies born from heroin-addicted mothers (David and Glass, 1980). A similar mechanism might be responsible for the smaller head circumferences in boys, up to 4 years of age, born to mothers treated with a-methyl-dopa during late gestation (Moar et al., 1978; Ounsted et al., 1980).

The direct and indirect effects of a variety of clinically used drugs upon the development of the brain have been reviewed here. Taken together, the literature on this subject points to a potential health hazard not only during the first trimester of pregnancy (as is now generally accepted) but also throughout the entire period of gestation, and even during lactation. Obstetricians and pediatricians should therefore be aware of the fact that the immediate beneficial effects of many drugs may be offset by the induction of permanent behavioral and psychological defects within the children's developing brains. This is an especially relevant consideration in cases involving children suffering from minimal brain dysfunction who are often subjected to extremely high doses of imipramine- or amphetamine-like drugs (for review, see Gross and Wilson, 1974) despite the fact that improvement often occurs eventually even in the absence of any medication whatsoever. The same point can be made, of course, for the treatment of nocturnal enuresis by means of antidepressants. It is an unfortunate commentary at the present time that the mothers themselves are often more aware of the potential dangers inherent in the use of medicines during pregnancy than are the physicians who prescribe them. We suggest that the investigation of the link between experimental and clinical medicine in this area, viz. the question of behavioral teratological sequelae of medications administered during early development, ought to be encouraged.

Table 2.1. Sequelae of chronic drug exposure during gestation, labor, lactation and childhood in man and other mammals

Drugs	Brain and behavioral teratogenicity in man	Brain and behavioral teratogenicity in animals	AS-deprivation effect
Antihypertensiva			
α-Methyl-dopa	Questionable neurological status, smaller head circumference (Moar et al., 1978)	Hyperanxiety and delayed motor coordination (Saucier and Astic, 1975)	Saucier and Astic, 1975 Valatx and Nowaczyk, 1977
	Delayed visual motor performance, smaller head circumference (Ounsted et al., 1980)	Hyperactivity (Juvancs and Nowaczyk, 1975)	
Propanolol	Light for dates, smaller head circumference, bradycardia (Pruyn et al., 1979)	No data available	Lanfumey and Adrien, 1981
	Prolonged labor, neonatal respiratory depression, bradycardia (Habib and McCarthy, 1977)		
Reserpine	Anorexia, lethargy (Yaffe and Stern, 1976)	Reduced brain cell proliferation (Patel et al., 1981)	Hoffman and Domino, 1969
Clonidine (also used for migraine, in opiate withdrawal and for depression)	No data available	Increased anxiety, reduced masculine sexual behavior smaller brain (Mirmiran et al., 1983a)	Autret et al., 1977 Putkonen et al., 1977 Kleinlogel et al., 1975 Miettinen, 1981
Anticonvulsants and hypnosedatives			
Barbiturates	'Barbiturate withdrawal syndrome': hyperactivity, restlessness, disturbed sleep, excessive crying, tremors, hyperreflexia (Bleyer and Marshall, 1972) Reduced responsiveness to sensory stimuli (Brazelton, 1970)	Increased activity in novel environment, smaller brain, reduced brain DNA (Diaz and Schain, 1978) Reduced masculine sexual behavior (Clemens et al., 1979) Increased locomotion in openfield, decreased acquisition in passive avoidance, less response to environmental stimuli (Middaugh et al., 1975) Reduced brain weight; destroys already formed neurons; impairement of learning (Yanai, 1980)	Oswald et al., 1963 Stotsky et al., 1971 Hartmann, 1978

Hydantoin	Low IQ scores (Hanson and Smith, 1975) Microcephaly, mental retardation (Hanson, 1978) Smaller head circumference, mental deficiency (IQ < 85) (Hanson et al., 1976) 2–3 times higher rate of mental retardation (Amer. Acad. Pediat.; Committee on Drugs, 1979) Smaller head circumference (Hilesma et al., 1981; Ogawa et al., 1982; for review see Bossi, 1982)	No data available	Cohen et al., 1968
ACTH	Apathy, drowsiness, pseudodementia (Langenstein et al., 1979)	Accelerates the onset of eye opening and motor behavior (Swaab and Martin, 1981)	Gillin et al., 1974
Tranquillizers Diazepam	Low Apgar scores, reluctance to eat (Cree et al., 1973)	Increased locomotion and decreased defecation in males; lower performance in maze learning (Fonseca et al., 1976)	Kales and Scharf, 1973
	Lethargy, impaired suckling (Patrick et al., 1972) Depressed reflexes (McCarthy et al., 1973)	Lack of acoustic startle reflexes (Kellog et al., 1980)	
Alcohol (It has also been used to prevent premature labor (Fuchs, 1965))	Microcephaly, mental retardation, hyperactivity, speech and language problems (Iosub et al., 1981)	Sexual behavior deficiency (Cicero and Badger, 1977)	Williams and Salamy, 1972
	Poor suckling, smaller head circumference (Oullette et al., 1976)	Smaller cortical pyramidal cells with less extensive dendritic branching (Hammer and Sheibel, 1981)	
	Low Apgar and high incidence of respiratory distress (Zervoudakis, 1980)	Destroys already formed neurons; depression of aggressive behavior; impairment of learning (Yanai, 1981)	
Amphetamine	Withdrawal symptoms (Hill and Stern, 1979)	Marked reduction in ability to habituate to new surroundings (Nasello and Ramirez, 1978)	Rechtschaffen and Maron, 1964

Enhancement of fetal lung maturation			
Corticosteroids (in addition used in pregnant women for infertility and subsequent maintenance of pregnancy)	Light for dates, Delayed psychomotor development (Marton et al., 1979)	Smaller brain (Johnson et al., 1981) Reduced masculine sexual behavior (Dörner, 1979; Dählof et al., 1980) Reduction in brain weight and DNA content (De Lemos and Moore, 1976) Reduction in brain weight and lipids (Romano et al., 1977)	Gillin et al., 1972
Thyroxine (Mashiach et al., 1978; Wu et al., 1973)	No data available	Cell proliferation ceases prematurely throughout the brain (Balazs, 1979)	Dunleavy et al., 1974
Antidepressants			
Imipramine-like compounds	Poor suckling, irritability urinary retention, breathlessness, tachypnoea, cyanosis (Hill and Stern, 1979)	Increased emotionality, decreased masculine sexual behavior, smaller brain and cortical size (Mirmiran et al., 1983a)	Shimizu and Himwich, 1969 Mirmiran et al., 1981 Dunleavy et al., 1972 Khazan and Sulman, 1966 Ritvo et al., 1967
Neuroleptics			
Chlorpromazine	Extrapyraidal dysfunction (e.g. tremor, hypertonus, etc.) (Hill et al., 1966)	Reduction in brain DNA content (Patel et al., 1980; Vertes et al., 1980) Impairment of maze learning and reduction of exploratory behavior (Hoffelt and Webster, 1965) Increased locomotion and impaired maze learning (Fonseca et al., 1976)	Khazan et al., 1967 Hartman, 1978 Lewis and Evans, 1969
Prevention of abortion			
Estrogen	Decrease independency, sensitivity, self-assurance (Reinisch, 1977) Decrease 'masculinity', aggressiveness and athletic ability (Yalow et al., 1973) Lower proportion of marriage (Beral and Colwell, 1981) Smaller head circumference H.J. Huisjes, pers.comm.)	Effects upon various behaviors depending upon the dosage used and the sex of the animals	Branchey et al., 1971

References

American Academy of Pediatrics, Committee on Drugs. Anticonvulsants and Pregnancy (1979) pp. 331–333.

Anderson, L.T., David, R., Bennet, K. and Dancis, J. (1979) Passive avoidance learning in Lesch-Nyhan disease: effect of 1-desamino-8-arginine vasopressin. Life Sci. 24, 905–910.

Arai, Y., Matsumoto, A. and Nishizuka, M. (1978) Synaptogenic action of estrogen on the hypothalamic arcuate nucleus (ARCN) of the developing brain and of the deafferented adult brain in female rats. In: Hormones and Brain Development (Dorner, G. and Kawakami M., eds.), Elsevier, Amsterdam, pp. 43–48.

Aulich, D. (1976) Escape versus exploratory activity: an interpretation of rat's behavior in the open-field and light-preference test. Behav. Process 1, 153–164.

Autret, A. (1977) Effects of clonidine on sleep pattern in man. Eur. J. Clin. Pharmacol. 12, 319–322.

Balazs, R. (1979) Cerebellum: certain features of its development and biochemistry. In: Development and Chemical Specificity of Neurons, Progress in Brain Research, Vol. 51 (Cuenod, M., Kreutzberg, G.W. and Bloom, F.E., eds.), Elsevier/North-Holland Biomedical Press, Amsterdam, pp. 357–372.

Balazs, R., Patel, A.J. and Hajos, F. (1975) Factors affecting the biochemical maturation of the brain: effects of hormones during early life. Psychoneuroendocrinology 1, 25–36.

Barlow, S.M. and Sullivan, F.M. (1975) Behavioural teratology. In: Teratology, Trends and Applications (Berry, C.L. and Poswillo, D.E., eds.), Springer-Verlag, New York, pp. 103–120.

Barnes, D.E. and Walker, D.W (1981) Prenatal ethanol exposure permanently reduces the number of pyramidal neurons in rat hippocampus. Dev. Brain Res. 1, 333–340.

Beral, V. and Colwell, L. (1981) Randomised trial of high doses of stilboestrol and ethisterone therapy in pregnancy: long-term follow-up of the children. J. Epid. Comm. Health 35, 155–160.

Black, I.B. and Geen, S.C. (1974) Inhibition of the biochemical and morphological maturation of adrenergic neurons by nicotinic reporter blockade. J. Neurochem. 22, 301–306.

Bleyer, W.A. and Marshall, R.E (1972) Barbiturate withdrawal syndrome in a passively addicted infant. J. Am. Med. Assoc. 221, 185.

Bodendorfer, T.W., Briggs, G.G. and Gunning, J.E. (1979) Obtaining drug exposure histories during pregnancy. Am. J. Obstet. Gynecol. 135, 490–494.

Boer, G.J. and Swaab, D.F. (1983) Longterm effects on brain and behavior of early treatments with neuropeptides. In: Application of Behavioral Pharmacology in Toxicology (Zbinden, G., Cuomo, V., Racagni, G. and Weiss, B., eds.) Raven Press, New York, pp. 251–263.

Bossi, L. (1982) Neonatal period including drug disposition in newborns: review of the literature. In: Epilepsy, Pregnancy and the Child (Janz, D., Dam, M., Richens A., Bossi, J., Helge, H. and Schmidt, D., eds.), Raven Press, New York, pp. 327–341.

Branchey, M. (1971) Effects of estrogen and progesterone on sleep patterns of female rats. Physiol. Behav. 6, 743–746.

Brazelton, T.B. (1970) Effects of prenatal drugs on the behavior of the rat. Am. J. Psychiat. 126, 1261–1266.

Cicero, T.J. and Badger, T.M. (1977) Effects of alcohol on the hypothalamo-pituitary gonadal axis in the male rat. J. Pharmacol. Exp. Ther. 201, 427–433.

Clemens, L.G., Popham, T.V. and Rupport, P.H. (1979) Neonatal treatment of hamsters with barbiturates alters adult sexual behavior. Dev. Psychobiol. 12, 49–59.

Cohen, H.B., Duncan, F. and Dement, W.C. (1968) The effects of diphenylhydantoin on sleep in the cat. Clin. Neurophysiol. 24, 401–408.

Collins, E. (1981) Maternal and fetal effects of acetaminophen and salicylates in pregnancy. Obstet. Gynecol. 58, Suppl. 57S–62S.

Council on environmental quality, Chemical hazards to human reproduction. Prepared by Clement Associates, Inc. for the Council on Environmental Quality, January 1981, Government Printing Office, USA.

66

Cree, J.E., Meyer, S. and Hailey, D.M. (1973) Diazepam in labour: its metabolism and effect on the clinical condition and thermogenesis of the newborn. Brit. Med. J. 4, 251–255.

Culver, B. and Vernadakis, A. (1979) Effects of anticonvulsant drugs on chick embryonic neurons and glia in cell culture. Dev. Neurosci. 2, 74–85.

Dahlof, L.G., Larsson, K. and Hard, E. (1980) Sexual differentiation and adult sexual behavior of male offspring of mothers treated with corticosteroids during pregnancy. Neurosci. Lett. Suppl. 5, 128.

Davis, M.M. and Glass, P. (1980) Fetal exposure to narcotics: neonatal sleep as a measure of nervous system disturbances. Science 209, 619–621.

De Lemos, R.A. and Moore, (Eds.) (1976) Lung maturation and the prevention of hyaline membrane disease. Report of the 70th Ross Conf. on Pediatric Research, Columbus, Ohio, pp. 77–80.

Diaz, J., and Schain, R. (1979) Phenobarbital: effects of longterm administration on behavior and brain of artificially reared rats. Science 199, pp. 90–91.

Doering, P.L. and Stewart, R.B. (1978) The extent and character of drug consumption during pregnancy. J. Am. Med. Assoc. 239, 843–846.

Dörner, G. (1979) Psychoneuroendocrine aspects of brain development and reproduction. In: Psychoneuroendocrinology in Reproduction, An Interdisciplinary Approach (Zichella, L. and Pancheri, P., eds.) Elsevier, Amsterdam, pp. 43–54.

Dunleavy, D.L.F., Brezinova, V., Oswald, I., Maclean, A.W. and Tinker, M. (1972) Changes during weeks in effects of tricyclic drugs on the human sleeping brain. Brit. J. Psychiat. 120, 663–672.

Dunleavy, D.L.F., Oswald, I., Brown and Strong, J.A. (1974) Hyperthyroidism, sleep and growth hormone. Electroenceph. Clin. Neurophysiol. 36, 259–263.

Erskine, M.S., Geller, E. and Yuwiler, A. (1979) Effects of neonatal hydrocortisone treatment on pituitary and adrenocortical response to stress in young rats. Neuroendocrinology 29, 191–199.

Fonseca, N.M., Sell. A.B. and Carlini, E.A. (1976) Differential behavioral responses of male and female adult rats treated with five psychotropic drugs in the neonatal state. Psychopharmacology 46, 263–268.

Frank, L. and Roberts, R.J. (1979) Effects of low-dose prenatal corticosteroid administration on the premature rat. Biol. Neonate 36, 1–9.

Fuchs, F. (1965) Treatment of threatened premature labour with alcohol. J. Obstet. Gynaecol. Brit. Commonw. 72, 1011–1013.

Gariete, T.J., Freeman, R.K., Linzey, E.M., Braly, P.S. and Dorchester, W.L. (1981) Perspective randomised study of corticosteroids in the management of premature rupture of the membranes and the premature gestation. Am. J. Obstet, Gynecol. 141, 508–515.

Gillin, R., Jacobs, L.S., Fram, D.H. and Snyder, F. (1972) Acute effect of a glucocorticoid on natural human sleep. Nature 237, 398–399.

Gillin, J.C., Jacobs, L.S., Snyder, F. and Henkin, R.I. (1974) Effects of ACTH on the sleep of normal subjects and patients with Adison's disease. Neuroendocrinology 15, 21–31.

Goodlin, R. (1981) Naloxone and its possible relationship to fetal endorphin levels and fetal distress. Am. J. Obstet. Gynecol. 136, 16–19.

Gorski, R.A., Gordon, J.H., Shryne, J.E. and Southam, A.M. (1978) Evidence for a morphological sex difference within the medial preoptic area of the rat brain. Brain Res. 148, 333–346.

Greenough, W.T., Carter, C.S., Steerman, C. and Devoogd, T.J. (1977) Sex differences in dendritic patterns in hamster preoptic area. Brain Res. 126, 63–72.

Greer, G. (1972) The Female Eunuch, p. 99, Paladin (pocket), London.

Gross, M.B. and Wilson, W.C. (Eds.) (1974) Minimal brain dysfunction, Brunner/Mazel, New York.

Gupta, C., Sonawane, B.R., Yaffe, S.J. and Shapiro, B.H. (1980) Phenobarbital exposure in utero: alternations in female reproductive function in rats. Science 208, 508–510.

Habib, A. and McCarthy, J.S. (1977) Effects on the neonate of propranolol administered during pregnancy. J. Pediat. 9, 808–811.

Hammer, R.P. and Scheibel, A.B. (1981) Morphological evidence for a delay of neuronal maturation in fetal alcohol exposure. Exp. Neurol. 74, 587–596.

Hanson, J.W. and Smith, D.W. (1975) The fetal hydantoin syndrome. J. Pediat. 87, 285–290.

Hanson, J.W., Myrianthopoulos, N.C., Harvey, M.A.S. and Smith, D.W. (1976) Risks to the offspring of women treated with hydantoin anticonvulsants, with emphasis on the fetal hydantoin syndrome. J. Pediat. 89, 662–668.

Hanson, J.W. (1978) Fetal hydantoin syndrome. Teratology 13, 185–188.

Haram, K. and Bakke, O.M. (1980) Diazepam as an induction agent for Caesarean section. A clinical and pharmacokinetic study of fetal drug exposure. Brit. J. Obstet. Gynaecol. 87, 506–512.

Henn, F. (1983) Neurotransmitters and astroglia lead to neuromodulation. In: Chemical Transmission in the Brain (Buijs, R.M., Pevet, P. and Swaab, D.F., eds.), Progress in Brain Research, Vol. 55, Elsevier, Amsterdam, pp. 241–252.

Herbst, A.L. (1981) Diethylstilbestrol and other sex hormones during pregnancy. Obstet. Gynec. 58, Suppl. 35S–40S.

Herbst, A.L., Hubby, M.M., Azizi, F. and Makii, M.M. (1981) Reproductive and gynecologic surgical experience in diethystillbestrol-exposed daughters. Am. J. Obstet. Gynecol. 141, 1019–1028.

Hillesmaa, V.K., Teramo, K., Granstrom, M.-L. and Bardy, A.H. (1981) Fetal head growth retardation associated with maternal antiepileptic drugs. Lancet ii, 165–167.

Hill, R.M. (1973) Drugs ingested by pregnant women. Clin. Pharmacol. Ther. 14, 654–659.

Hill, R.M. and Stern, L. (1979) Drugs in pregnancy: effects on the fetus and newborns. Drugs 17, 182–197.

Hill, R.M., Desmond, M.M. and Kay, J.I. (1966) Extrapyramidal dysfunction in an infant of a schizophrenic mother. J. Pediat. 69, 589–595.

Hinz, G., Docke, F. and Dorner, G. (1978) Long-term changes of sexual functions in rats treated neonatally with psychotropic drugs. In: Hormones and Brain Development (Dorner, G. and Kawakami, M., eds.) Elsevier, Amsterdam, pp. 121–127.

Hitzemann, B.A., Hitzemann, R.J., Brase, D.A. and Loh, H.H. (1976) Influence of prenatal d-amphetamine administration on development and behavior of rats. Life Sci. 18, 603–612.

Hoffelt, D.R. and Webster, R.L. (1965) Effects of injection of tranquillizing drugs during pregnancy on offspring. Nature 205, 1070–1072.

Hoffman, J.S. and Domino, E.F. (1969) Comparative effects of reserpine on the sleep cycles of man and cat. Pharmacol. Exp. Ther. 170, 190–198.

Howard, E. and Benjamin, J.A. (1975) DNA, ganglioside and sulfatide in brains of rats given corticosterone in infancy, with an estimate of cell loss during development. Brain Res. 92, 73–87.

Huisjes, H.J., Rijksuniversiteit Groningen, Personal Communication.

Hutchings, D.E. (1978) Behavioral teratology: embryopathic and behavioral effects of drugs during pregnancy. In: Early Influences, Studies on the Development of Behavior and the Nervous System (Gottlieb, G., Ed.) Academic Press, New York, pp. 7–34.

Huygen, F.J.A. (1979) De behandeling van enuresis nocturna. Ned. T. Geneesk. 123, 748–752.

Iosub, S., Fuchs, M., Bingol, N. and Gromisch, D.S. (1981) Fetal alcohol syndrome revisited. Pediatrics 68, 475–479.

Jacobson, C.D., Shryne, J.E., Shapiro, F. and Gorski, R.A. (1980) Ontogeny of the sexually dimorphic nucleus of the preoptic area. J. Comp. Neurol. 193, 541–548.

Jakoubek, B. (1978) The effect of ACTH and/or tranquillizers on the development of brain macromolecular metabolism. In: Hormones and Brain Development (Dorner, G. and Kawakami, M., eds.) Elsevier/North-Holland Biomedical Press, Amsterdam, pp. 259–264.

Johnson, J.W.C., Mitzner, W., Beck, J.C., London, W.T., Sly, D.L., Lee, P.A., Khouzami, V.A. and Calvalieri, R.L. (1981) Long-term effects of betamethasone on fetal development. Am. J. Obstet. Gynecol. 141, 1053–1064.

Jones, G.E.S. (1973) Luteal phase insufficiency. Clin. Obstet. Gynecol. 16, 255–273.

Jones, K.L., Smith, D.W. and Hanson, J.W. (1976) The fetal alcohol syndrome: clinical delineation. Ann. NY Acad. Sci. 273, 130–137.

Juvancs, P. and Nowaczyk, T. (1975) Effects of early postnatal a-methyl-Dopa treatment on behavior in the rat. Psycopharmacologia (Berl.) 42, 95–97.

Kales, A. and Scharf, M.B. (1973) Sleep laboratory and clinical studies of the effects of benzodiazepine on sleep: flurazepam, diazepam, chlordiazepoxide. In: The Benzodiazepines (Grattini, S., Mussini, E. and Randall, L.O., eds.) Raven Press, New York, pp. 577–598.

Kaltenbach, K., Graziani, L.J. and Finnegan, L.P. (1979) Methadone exposure in utero: developmental status at one and two years of age. Pharmacol. Biochem. Behav. 11, Suppl. 15–17.

Kellog, C., Tervo, D., Ison, J., Parisi, T. and Miller, R.K. (1980) Prenatal exposure to diazepam alters behavioral development in rats. Science 207, 205–207.

Khazan, N. and Sulman, F.G. (1966) Effects of imipramine on paradoxical sleep in animals with reference to dreaming and enuresis. Psychopharmacology 10, 89–95.

Khazan, N., Bar, R. and Sulman, F.G. (1967) The effects of cholinergic drugs on paradoxical sleep in the rat. Int. J. Neuropharmacol. 6, 279–282.

Kleinlogel, H., Scholtysik, C. and Sayers, A.C. (1975) Effects of clonidine and BS 100-141 on the EEG sleep pattern in the rat. Eur. J. Pharmacol. 33, 159–163.

Kreek, M.J. (1979) Methadone disposition during the perinatal period in humans. Pharmacol. Biochem. Behav. 11, 7–13.

Kraus, H.F., Campbell, G.A., Fowler, M.W., Catron, A.C. and Farber, J.P. (1981) Maternal nicotine administration and fetal brain stem damage: a rat model with implications for sudden infant death syndrome. Am. J. Obstet. Gynecol. 140, 743–746.

Kruck, Z.L. and Pycock, C.J. (1979) Neurotransmitters and drugs. Croom Helm Biology in Medicine Series, Croom Helm, London.

Lagenstein, I., Willig, R.P. and Kuhne, D. (1979) Cranial computed tomography (CCT) findings in children treated with ACTH and dexamethasone: first results. Neuropaediatrie 10, 370–384.

Lanfumey, L. and Adrien, J. (1981) Effects of a noradrenergic agonist on sleep in the rat. Sleep 1980 (Koella, W.P., ed.) Karger, Basel, pp. 290–291.

Lee, M.-L. (1980) Aminoacidopathy and mental retardation. In: Prevention of Mental Retardation and Other Developmental Disabilities (McCormack, M.K., ed.), Marcel Dekker, New York, pp. 135–150.

Lewis, P.D., Patel, A.J., Bendek, G. and Balazs, R. (1977) Effect of reserpine on cell proliferation in the developing rat brain: a quantitative histological study. Brain Res. 129, 299–308.

Lewis, S.A. and Evans, J.I. (1969) Some effects of chlropromazine on human sleep. Psychopharmacology 14, 342–348.

Liggins, G.C. and Howie, R.N. (1972) A controlled trial of antepartum glucocorticoid treatment for prevention of the respiratory distress syndrome in premature infants. Pediatrics 50, 515–525.

Marton, I.S., Gati, I., Nemenyi, M. and Szøndy, M. (1979) Psychomotor development and cord endocrine parameters of premature newborns exposed to steroid in utero. An interdisciplinary approach. In: Psychoneuroendocrinology in Reproduction (Zichella, L. and Pancheri, P., eds.) Elsevier, Amsterdam, pp. 509–514.

Mashiach, S., Barkai, G., Sack, J., Stern, E., Goldman, B., Brisk, M. and Serr, D.M. (1978) Enhancement of fetal lung maturity by intra-amniotic administration of thyroid hormone. Am. J. Obstet. Gynecol. 130, 289–293.

McCarthy, G.T., O'Connell, B. and Robinson, A.E. (1973) Blood levels of diazepam in infants of two mothers given large doses of diazepam during labour. J. Obstet. Gynecol. 70, 349–352.

Meire, F., Vuylsteek, K., Buylaert, W. and Bogaert, M. (1979) Geneesmiddelengebruik tijdens de zwangerschap. Ned. T. Geneesk. 123, 703–706.

Middaugh, L.D., Santos, C.A. and Zemp, J.W. (1975) Effects of phenobarbital given to pregnant mice on behavior of mature offspring. Dev. Psychobiol. 8, 305–313.

Miettinen, M.V.J. (1981) a-Adrenergic function and sleep in kittens. In: Sleep 1980 (Koella, W.P., ed.) Karger, Basel, pp. 287–289.

Mirkin, B.L. and Singh, S. (1976) Placental transfer of pharmacologically active molecules. In: Perinatal Pharmacology and Therapeutics (Mirkin, B.L., ed.), Academic Press, New York, pp. 1–69.

Mirmiran, M., Van de Poll, N., Corner, M., Boer, G. and Van Oyen, H. (1980) Lasting sequelae of chronic treatment with chlorimipramine during early postnatal development in the rat. IRCS Med. Sci. 8, 200–202.

Mirmiran, M., Van de Poll, N., Corner, M., Van Oyen, H. and Bour, H. (1981) Suppression of active sleep by chronic treatment with chlorimipramine during postnatal development: effects upon adult sleep and behavior in the rat. Brain Res. 204, 129–146.

Mirmiran, M., Van den Dungen, H. and Uylings, H.B.M. (1982) Sleep patterns during rearing under different environmental conditions in juvenile rats. Brain Res. 233, 287–298.

Mirmiran, M., Scholtens, J., Van de Poll, N.E., Uylings, H.B.M., Van der Gugten, J. and Boer, G.J. (1983a) Effects of experimental suppression of active (REM) sleep during early development upon adult brain and behavior. Dev. Brain Res., 7, 277–286.

Mirmiran, M. and Uylings, H.B.M. (1983) The environmental enrichment effect upon cortical growth is neutralized by concomitant pharmacological suppression of active sleep in female rats. Brain Res. 261, 331–334.

Mirmiran, M., Uylings, H.B.M. and Corner, M.A. (1983b) Pharmacological suppression of REM sleep prior to weaning counteracts the effectiveness of subsequent environmental enrichment on cortical growth in rats. Dev. Brain Res. 7, 102–105.

Mitler, M. (1971) Some developmental observations on the effects of prolonged deprivation of low voltage fast wave sleep in the deer mouse. Dev. Psychobiol. 4, 293–311.

Moar, V.A., Jefferies, M.A., Mutch, L.M.M., Ounsted, M.K. and Redman, C.W.G. (1978) Neonatal head circumference and the treatment of maternal hypertension. Brit. J. Obstet. Gynaecol. 85, 933–937.

Nahas, G. and Goujard, J. (1979) Phenothiazines, benzodiazepines, and the fetus. In: Reviews in Perinatal Medicine, Vol. 3 (Scarpelli, E.M. and Cosmi, E.V., eds.) Raven Press, New York, pp. 243–280.

Nasello, A.G. and Ramirez, O.A. (1978) Brain catecholamines metabolism in offspring of amphetamine-treated rats. Pharmacol. Biochem. Behav. 9, 17–20.

Ogawa, Y., Nomura, Y., Kaneko, S., Suzuki, K. and Sato, T. (1982) Insidious effect of antiepileptic drugs in the perinatal period. In: Epilepsy, Pregnancy, and the Child (Janez, D., Dam, M., Richens, A., Bossi, L., Helge, H. and Schmidt, D., eds.) Raven Press, New York, pp. 197–202.

Ornoy, A. and Yanai, J. (1980) Central nervous system teratogenicity: experimental models for human problems. In: Advances in the Study of Birth Defects, Neural and Behavioural Teratology (Vol. 4 Persaud, T.V.N., ed.) MTP Press Ltd., pp. 1–21.

Oswald, I., Berger, R.J., Jaramillo, B.A., Ketidie, K.M.G., Olley, P.C. and Plunkett, G.B. (1963) Melancholia and barbiturates: a controlled EEG, body and eye movement study of sleep. Brit. J. Psychiat. 109, 66–78.

Ouelette, E.M. and Rosett, H.L. (1976) A pilot study of the fetal alcohol syndrome at the Boston City Hospital. Part II: The Infants. Ann. NY Acad. Sci. 273, 123–129.

Ounsted, M.K., Moar, V.A., Good, F.J. and Redman, C.W.G. (1980) Hypertension during pregnancy with and without specific treatment: the development of the children at the age of four years. Brit. J. Obstet. Gynaecol. 87, 19–24.

Oyama, T., Matsuki, A., Taneichi, T., Ling, N. and Guillemin, R. (1980) β-Endorphin in obstetric analgesia. Am. J. Obstet. Gynaecol. 137, 613–616.

Patel, A.J., Vertes, Zs., Lewis, P.D. and Lai, M. (1980) Effect of chlorpromazine on cell prolifetration in the developing rat brain. A combined biochemical and morphological study. Brain Res. 202, 415–428.

Patel, A.J., Barochovsky, O. and Lewis, P.D. (1981) Psychotropic drugs and brain development: effects on cell replication in vivo and in vitro. Neuropharmacology 20, 1243–1249.

Patrick, M.J., Tilstone, W.J., Reavey, P. (1972) Diazepam and breast feeding. Lancet i, 542.

Pruyn, S.C., Phelan, J.P. and Buchanan, G.C. (1979) Long-term propanolol therapy in pregnancy: maternal and fetal outcome. Am. J. Obstet. Gynecol. 135, 485–489.

Putkonen, P.T.S., Leppavuori, A. and Stenberg, D. (1977) Paradoxical sleep inhibition by central α-adrenoreceptor stimulant (clonidine) antagonized by alpha-receptor blocker yohimbine. Life Sci. 21, 1059–1066.

Rechtschaffen, A. and Maron, L. (1964) The effect of amphetamine on the sleep cycle. Neurophysiology 16, 438–445.

Reinisch, J.M. (1981) Prenatal exposure to synthetic progestins increases potential for aggression in humans. Science 211, 1171–1173.

Reinisch, J.M. and Karow, W.G. (1977) Prenatal exposure to synthetic progestins and estrogens: effects on human development. Arch. Sex. Behav. 6, 257–288.

Ritvo, E., Ornitz, E., La Franchi, S. and Walter, R. (1967) Effects of imipramine on the sleep-dream cycle: an EEG study in boys. Electroenceph. Clin. Neurophysiol. 22, 465–468.

Roman, M.C. (1977) Prednisone effects on postnatal brain development of rats following maternal therapy. Pediat. Res. 11, 1042–1045.

Rosenzweig, M.R. and Bennett, E.L. (1978) Experimental influences in brain anatomy and brain chemistry in rodents. In: Studies on the Development of Behavior and the Nervous System, Vol. 4: Early Influences (Gottlieb, G., ed.) Academic Press, New York, pp. 289–327.

Rumack, C.M., Guggenheim, M.A., Rumack, B.H., Peterson, R.G., Johnson, M.L. and Braithwaite, W.R. (1981) Neonatal intracranial hemorrhage and maternal use of aspirin. Obstet. Gynecol. 58, Suppl. 52S–56S.

Russel, P.A. (1973) Relationship between exploratory behavior and fear: a review, Brit. J. Psychol. 64, 417–433.

Salaman, D.F. (1974) The role of DNA, RNA, and protein synthesis in sexual differentiation of the brain. In: Integrative Hypothalamic Activity Progress in Brain Research, Vol. 41, (Swaab, D.F. and Schade, J.P., eds.) Elsevier, Amsterdam, pp. 349–362.

Sandman, C.A., McGivern, R.F., Berka, C., Walker, M., Coy, D.H. and Kastin, A.J. (1979) Neonatal administration of β-endorphin produces 'chronic' insensitivity to thermal stimuli. Life Sci. 25, 1755–1760.

Saucier, D. and Astic L. (1975) Effets de l'alpha-methyl-Dopa sur le sommeil du chat nouveau-ne. Evolution comportementale au cours du 1er mois postnatal. Psychopharmacologia 42, 299–303.

Shimizu, A. and Himwich, H.E. (1969) Effects of psychotropic drugs on the sleep-wakefulness cycle of the developing kittens. Dev. Psychobiol. 2, 161–167.

Slotkin, T.A., Whitmore, W.L., Salvaggio, M. and Seidler, F.J. (1979) Perinatal methadone addiction affects brain synaptic development of biogenic amine systems in the rat. Life Sci. 24, 1223–1230.

Sobel, E.H. (1978) Effects of neonatal stunting on the development of rats: early and late effects of neonatal cortisone on physical growth and skeletal maturation. Pediat. Res. 12, 945–947.

Stenchever, M.A., Williamson, R.A., Leonard, J., Karp, L.E., Ley, B., Shy, K. and Smith, D. (1981) Possible relationship between in utero diethylstilbestrol exposure and male fertility. Am. J. Obstet. Gynecol. 140, 186–193.

Strauss, M.E., Lessen-Firestone, J.K., Chavez, C.J. and Stryker, J.C. (1979) Children of methadone-treated women at five years of age. Pharmacol. Biochem. Behav. 11, Suppl. 3–6.

Strotzky, B.A., Cole, J.O., Tang, Y.T. and Gahm, I.G. (1971) Sodium butabarbital (Butisol Sodium) as a hypnotic agent for aged psychiatric patients with sleep disorders. J. Am. Geriat. Soc. 19, 860–870.

Swaab, D.F. (1980) Neuropeptides and brain development – a working hypothesis. In: A Multidisciplinary Approach to Brain Development, Proc. Internat. Meeting, Selva di Fasano, Italy, April 18–20 (Di Benedetta, C., Balazs, R., Gombos, G. and Porcellati, P., eds.) Elsevier/North-Holland Biomedical Press, Amsterdam, pp. 181–196.

Swaab, D.F. and Martin, J.T. (1981) Functions of β-melanotropin and other opiomelanocortin peptides in labour, intrauterine growth and brain development. In: Peptides of the Pars Intermedia, Ciba Foundation Symp. 81 (Evered, D. and Lawrenson, G., eds.), Pitman, London, pp. 196–217.

Swaab, D.F. (1982) Neuropeptides. Their distribution and function in the brain. In: Chemical Transmission in the Brain, Progress in Brain Research, Vol. 55 (Buijs, R.M., Pevet, P. and Swaab, D.F., eds.), Elsevier, Amsterdam, pp. 97–122.

Taeusch, H.W. (1975) Glucocorticoid prophylaxis for respiratory distress syndrome: a review of potential toxicity. J. Pediat. 87, 617–623.

Thornburg, J.E. and Moore, K.E. (1976) Pharmacologically induced modifications of behavioral and neurochemical development. In: Perinatal Pharmacology and Therapeutics (Mirkin, B.L., ed.), Academic Press, New York, pp. 269–354.

Tonjes, R., Hecht, K., Hinz, G., Docke, F. and Dorner, G. (1981) Effects of neonatal pyridostigmine treatment on sexual maturation and adult behaviour in female rats subjected to maternal deprivation. Endokrinologie 78, 1–11.

Toran-Allerand, C.D. (1976) Sex steroids and the development of the newborn mouse hypothalamus and preoptic area in vitro: implications for sexual differentiation. Brain Res. 106, 407–412.

Valatx, J.L. and Nowaczyk, (1977) Essai de suppression pharmacologique du sommeil paradoxal chez le rat nouveau-ne. Rev. EEG Neurophysiol. 7, 269–277.

Van de Poll, N.E., De Bruin, J.P.C. Van Dis, H. and Van Oyen, H.G. (1978) Gonadal hormones and the differentiation of sexual and agressive behavior and learning in the rat. In: Maturation of the Nervous System. Progress in Brain Research, Vol 48, (Corner, M.A., Baker, R.E., van de Poll, N.E., Swaab, D.F. and Uylings, H.B.M., eds.), Elsevier, Amsterdam, pp. 309–325.

Vertes, Z., Vertes, M. and Kovacs, S. (1980) Further study of maternal chlorpromazine effect on the DNA synthesis in the rat brain. Neurosci. Lett. Suppl. 5, S 407.

Vorhees C.V. (1981) Effects of prenatal naloxone exposure on postnatal behavioral development of rats. Neurobehav. Toxicol. Teratol. 3, 295–301.

Waggoner, R.W., Slonim, A.E. and Armstrong, S.H. (1978) Improved psychological status of children under dDAVP therapy for central diabetes insipidus. Am. J. Psychiat. 135, 361–362.

West, J.R., Hodges, C.A. and Black, A.C. (1981) Prenatal exposure to ethanol alters the organization of hippocampal mossy fibers in the rat. Science 211, 957–959.

Williams, H.L. and Salamy, A. (1972) Alcohol and Sleep. In: The Biology of Alcoholism (Kissin, B. and Begleiter, H., eds.), Plenum Press, New York, pp. 435–483.

Wu, B. (1973) The effect of thyroxine on the maturation of fetal rabbit lungs. Biol. Neonate 22, 161–168.

Yaffe, S.J. and Stern, L. (1976) Clinical implications of perinatal pharmacology. In: Perinatal Pharmacology and Therapeutics (Mirkin, B.L., ed.), Academic Press, New York, pp. 355–429.

Yalom, I.D., Green, R. and Fisk, N. (1973) Prenatal exposure to female hormones. Effect on psychosexual development in boys. Arch. Gen. Psychiat. 28, 554–561.

Yanai, J. (1981) Comparison of early barbiturate and ethanol effects on the CNS. Substance Alcohol Actions Misuse 2, 79–91.

Yanai, J. and Feigenbaum, J.J. (1981) Lessened sensitivity to apomorphine induced hypothermia following prenatal exposure to phenobarbital. IRCS Med. Sci. 9, 965.

Zervoudakis, I.A., Krauss, A., Fuchs, F. and Wilson, K.H. (1980) Infants of mothers treated with ethanol for premature labor. Am. J. Obstet. Gynecol. 137, 713–718.

Neurobehavioral Teratology
edited by Joseph Yanai
© Elsevier Science Publishers BV 1984

3

THE ETIOLOGY OF
CENTRAL NERVOUS SYSTEM DEFECTS

Marcus A. Klingberg[1], Howard S. Cuckle[1,2], Cheri M. Papier[1] and Juan Chemke[3]

[1] Department of Preventive and Social Medicine, Sackler School of Medicine, Tel Aviv University, Tel Aviv, Israel, [2] Nuffield Department of Clinical Medicine, Cancer Studies, University of Oxford, Radcliffe Infirmary, Oxford, England and [3] Department of Clinical Genetics, Kaplan Hospital (affiliated with the Hebrew University and the Hadassah Medical School), Rehovot, Israel

THE guiding principle of epidemiology is derived from the ancients' 'man is the measure of all things'. Thus, according to this principle, unless a phenomenon related to the health of humans can be demonstrated in human rather than in animal populations, it should be considered as unproven. However, although theoretically sound, practical considerations often lead us to ignore this principle and to draw conclusions on the basis of experimental work alone, or on the basis of only weak corroborative epidemiological support. For example, consider the widespread use of antiemetics in pregnancy; while there is ample justification from animal experiments to suggest an etiological role in birth defects, there is insufficient epidemiological evidence to support this hypothesis in humans. Given the fact that alternative non-pharmacological means of treating nausea in pregnancy are available (e.g. eating crackers), it seems prudent to limit the use of antiemetics. However, care must be exercised to avoid jumping to hasty conclusions: that is, not to conclude that a causal relationship exists just because we agree that the drug is contraindicated; nor to exclude the possibility of a causal relationship just because of insufficient epidemiological support. While human harm is the final arbiter of 'proof', we cannot afford to wait until that harm is done. One could argue, in that case, that practical decisions should be based on experimental work and that justification – or vilification – of the decision should be left to epidemiologists looking at the situation retrospectively. However, we would thus eliminate the vast majority of foodstuffs, medicines and household chemicals (including petroleum) which are an integral part of our lives. The answer, it seems, lies in balancing risks and gains. Balance is required so that a modest risk may be considered acceptable if substantial benefit is derived.

The function of epidemiology in the area of teratology ('teratoepidemiology') is to quantify these risks in human subjects and to estimate the statistical variability of the risk (i.e. to determine the minimal and maximal values of the risk on the basis of human data). However, although epidemiology can be used as a safety net to detect large risks to humans, intermediate risks are likely to go unnoticed by epidemiological monitoring, and small risks may not emerge until considerable numbers of individuals have been exposed and many harmed. It is worthwhile considering why epidemiology is so poor at establishing a small risk. This arises mainly from human variability; genetically, environmentally, and habitually; it also arises from our inability to measure these factors precisely. Even if we are interested in studying the relationship between a simple, well-defined etiological agent, such as a newly-prescribed pharmacological preparation, and a gross, easily diagnosable outcome such as anencephalus (although such an association has in fact not been found), and the risk is low, natural variability and the imprecision of the investigator may prevent discovery of the connection. Anencephalus is not a new disorder which emerged concurrently with the introduction of this hypothetical new drug; its etiology is multifactorial, being influenced apparently by race, parity, diet, family history and other factors. Our study must measure these factors as well. In addition, while the drug is manufactured under quality control procedures, its use is likely to be variable and subject to imprecise measurement. Did the patient always comply with the regimen? Is its use potentiated by ingestion of certain foods? Does its effect depend on body weight? Is the mother exaggerating her use of it in order to 'blame' the birth of her malformed baby on some exogenous factor? Is she underestimating her use out of guilt? Again, anencephalus is problematic. Most cases abort spontaneously early in pregnancy and are never diagnosed, and an increasing proportion are being therapeutically aborted in mid-pregnancy following antenatal diagnoses. In countries which do not legally require registration of pregnancy outcome in therapeutic abortions, this could be an important factor in preventing the drug/malformation risk from being detected.

If such difficulties exist in studying the relationships between well-defined agents and adverse pregnancy outcomes, then it can readily be seen that questions involving behavioral outcomes, such as whether smoking in pregnancy causes moderate intellectual impairment in the offspring, are extremely difficult to study epidemiologically. Hence it is to be expected that the epidemiology of neurobehavioral outcomes would be sparse and raise difficulties of interpretation. The main endpoints are, after all, small developmental changes subject to imprecision of measurement and established, for the most part, only years after the exposure.

Human neurobehavioral teratology

Behavioral teratology is an attempt to integrate the domains of teratology and experimental psychology. Its principal concern is the study of neurobehavioral changes resulting from pre- or early postnatal exposure to various environmental disturbances or events with the intent of understanding the embryopathic mechanisms by which these changes are produced.

A possible scheme for the elucidation of neurobehavioral effects could be considered as parallel to that of teratogenic effects with structural outcomes. According to Wilson (1973), teratogenic agents initiate a series of pathogenic effects starting at the level of the cell. They may interfere with some physiologic function such as protein synthesis or enzyme activity, resulting in either cell death or improper cellular function. He hypothesizes that the various types of pathogenesis "may converge into a relatively narrow channel of abnormal development, for example, one that would lead ultimately to insufficient cells or cell products to carry out morphogenesis or to carry on function at the site of the final defect" (Wilson, 1973, p. 25). The final defect in the impaired developmental sequence could be death, malformation, growth retardation, or neurobehavioral malfunction. Although Wilson's paradigm has been used specifically for elucidating teratogenic mechanisms leading to gross structural malformations, the same type of model could apply to mechanisms of agents which may result in developmental retardation, neurobehavioral impairment and perhaps even death, but not gross structural malformations. Some drugs such as heroin, methadone, some tranquilizers, stimulants and hypnotics may interfere directly in the neurochemical processes of the developing fetal brain rather than by selectively killing embryonic cells.

Among the more well-studied agents which are known from epidemiological evidence to produce syndromes of both structural malformations and neurobehavioral deficits are alcohol (Smith, 1980; Clarren and Smith, 1978; Streissguth et al, 1978), the hydantoin anticonvulsants (Bergsma, 1979; Hanson and Smith, 1976), and methyl mercury (Matsumoto et al, 1965; Takeuchi and Matsumoto, 1969; Harada, 1978). The characteristic defects produced by chronic maternal alcoholism include growth deficiency (on average, infants experience 65% of normal postnatal linear growth rate and 40% of normal rate of weight gain), mental retardation (on average, an IQ of 63), dysmorphic craniofacial features, microcephaly, variable joint anomalies, cardiac defects (especially ventricular septal defect) and poor fine motor coordination (Bergsma, 1979; Smith, 1980). As this pattern of defects seems to be characteristic of children born to chronic alcoholic mothers, it is thought that alcohol (ethanol) is the agent responsible. However, one of its metabolic breakdown components, such as acetaldehyde, could also possibly be the etiologic factor. Other hypotheses for causes of 'fetal alcohol syndrome' include general maternal malnutrition or a deficiency of a particular vitamin or nutrient, perhaps folic acid.

Fetal hydantoin syndrome, in which prenatal exposure to hydantoin anticonvulsants (diphenylhydantoin, mephenytoin, ethotoin) occurs, is also characterized by both structural and functional neurobehavioral defects. These may include pre- and postnatal growth deficiency, microcephalus and performance shortcomings, such as developmental delays or mental retardation. Dysmorphic craniofacial features and hand anomalies are also common in this syndrome (Bergsma, 1979). It is estimated that 10–30% of hydantoin-exposed fetuses exhibit features of this syndrome (Bergsma, 1979; Hanson and Smith, 1976).

Congenital Minamata disease, a neurological disorder of the newborn caused by maternal ingestion of fish contaminated by methyl mercury compounds in Japan, resulted in numerous children born with neurological symptoms similar to cerebral palsy. Severe cases often exhibited structural malformations such as microcephalus, limb defects, muscle hypotony and strabismus, as well as various neurological, growth, mental and nutritional dysfunctions (Matsumoto et al, 1965; Takeuchi and Matsumoto, 1969; Harada, 1978).

Other agents, such as heroin, methadone and cigarette smoking, for which little epidemiological evidence exists linking them to structural malformations, apparently do lead to neurobehavioral impairments. With regard to prenatal exposure to heroin and methadone, there is an initial neonatal withdrawal syndrome, consisting of tremors, irritability, hyperreflexia, sleep disturbances, and prolonged high-pitched crying. Later on, long-term neurobehavioral disorders, such as hyperactivity and short attention span, occur (Wilson et al, 1973). These long-term effects have not been revealed so much through epidemiologic studies as through follow-up surveys of cases with severe neonatal symptoms in order to determine possible subsequent sequelae.

Maternal cigarette smoking, aside from the well-known and consistently found relationship with low birthweight (average of 200 g less than babies of nonsmoking mothers), also has been shown to increase the risk of spontaneous abortion by 30–70% (Kline et al, 1977), but as yet has not been found to cause structural malformation. Regarding neurobehavioral effects, studies have reported such long-term sequelae as impaired neurological and intellectual development including minimal brain dysfunction and abnormal ECGs (Dunn et al., 1977), growth retardation, measurable emotional, behavioral and intellectual deficits (USDHEW, 1979), abnormal infant behavior patterns (Saxton, 1978), hyperkinesis (Denson, 1975), and stunted growth at least until age 11 (Butler and Goldstein, 1973).

Other agents, such as hormones taken by pregnant women, have also been reported in association with behavioral and personality disorders (Yalom et al., 1973; Reinisch, 1977).

However, despite the growing literature in the field of human behavioral teratology, the fact remains that it is very difficult to reveal causal associations between prenatal exposures and postnatal behavioral abnormalities. The specific reasons, in addition to the general difficulties of studying small risk, discussed above, are mainly twofold: human behavior spans an enormous range of so-called 'normal' behaviors; and the intervening events and variables between the time of exposure and the time of evaluation of effects only serve to confound potential associations (Bornschein, 1980).

Even establishing the causal relationship between thalidomide and the gross limb-reduction deformities was not an easy task; therefore prenatal insults resulting in slight behavioral inpairments diagnosed well after birth are all the more difficult to reveal using current epidemiological techniques.

Some of the difficulties encountered in the follow-up of infants of 30 heroin-addicted mothers (Wilson et al., 1973), for example, are summarized as follows:

(1) The infants were not necessarily representative of infants of heroin addicts. They were under special observation because of their withdrawal symptoms, not because of volunteered information.

(2) It was difficult to obtain an adequate history of drug taking (not only for heroin, but other drugs as well); the purity of illegally acquired drugs was similarly impossible to determine.

(3) Drug addicts tend to have poor diets, high infection rates, and generally poor health; factors that in and of themselves could lead to a high risk of adverse developmental sequelae in infants.

(4) There was no adequate comparison group.

(5) It was difficult to obtain permission for long-term follow-up, either from the mothers, their relatives, or from foster parents.

It is not far-fetched to presume, though, that many, if not most, teratogenic agents which cause malformations of the central nervous system might also result in some neurobehavioral deficits. The degree of structural, functional, or behavioral anomaly might depend upon a number of factors, such as amount (or dosage), length, and time of exposure as well as individual susceptibility.

If such a presumption is made, it would be theoretically feasible to conduct a prospective epidemiological investigation starting with exposed and unexposed pregnant women (exposed to a drug, for example, suspected of causing CNS malformations, and using a variable protocol for dose, timing and length of administration); then one could follow up the children born for possible neurobehavioral dysfunctions. Such data are not available.

Looking in the other direction (that is, beginning with childhood neurobehavioral disorders) is even more problematic from a methodological point of view. Even if physicians or psychologists dealing with these children were to consider the possibility of a prenatal cause of the disorders (a highly unlikely possibility, even more unlikely if our assumption is incorrect; i.e. if the neurobehavioral manifestations do not occur in conjunction with structural defects), trying to trace maternal exposures retrospectively is fraught with difficulties.

Behavioral lesions?

As hinted at in the previous section, it does not follow ipso facto that if intrauterine exposure to a specific agent produces a behavioral effect, then it also must be associated

78

with a CNS lesion. Deformities such as clubfoot can lead to psychological and behavioral problems especially in childhood while as yet there is no suggestion of an associated CNS lesion. Even abnormal behavior with a known neurological basis does not necessarily indicate the presence of a CNS lesion. An inborn error of metabolism, for example, may affect neural processes but be determined by genetically controlled biochemical factors only.

Conversely, it is not known for sure whether a teratological agent responsible for a CNS lesion could also produce behavioral problems. In other words, there is no dose-response 'rule' by which all doses produce a certain CNS lesion; that is, higher doses leading to a congenital CNS malformation and lower doses to behavioral problems. However, while there is no such rule, that kind of mechanism is likely to play some part. When a causal relationship is established, the mechanism is often unknown, so that such a dose-response rule cannot easily be excluded. It may therefore be useful to accept as a working hypothesis that whatever causes CNS malformations may potentially, at a lower level of exposure, result in behavioral faults. Consequently, a knowledge of the epidemiology of CNS malformations may be a useful asset in studying neurobehavioral teratology.

Classification of CNS defects

The CNS defects form a broad group of distinct malformations. The major components are the neural tube defects (anencephalus and spina bifida), hydrocephalus and microcephalus, but also included, for example, are brain damage, CNS teratomas and macrocephalus. From the anatomical point of view this is a well-defined classification scheme; all anomalies of neurological tissue or conditions strongly associated with such anomalies are included; other defects, such as spina bifida oculta, which have some similarities to the included defects are not. From an etiological point of view this scheme may not be ideal: i.e. all defects that are etiologically similar are not necessarily included and those that are etiologically dissimilar are not necessarily excluded. Although acknowledging this as a problem, the fact remains that some kind of classification scheme is needed, or else we would be reduced to studying individual malformations with small numbers of cases. In the following review of the epidemiological literature relating to CNS malformations, consideration has been given to the separate subtypes wherever possible. In the presentation of our own findings on CNS malformations in Israel, small numbers of cases preclude such a breakdown.

Epidemiology of CNS defects

The major epidemiologic features of CNS defects will be presented in this section, based on both descriptive and analytical studies. Anencephalus and spina bifida (sometimes referred to as the neural tube defects or NTDs) will be discussed together, for the most part, as their characteristic features seem to be similar; where appropriate, hydrocephalus and microcephalus will also be discussed.

The neural tube defects are among the most frequently occurring and severe malformations worldwide. Rates, at birth, vary tremendously among the studied populations, although they may not reflect the true incidence of the conditions. This is due, in part, to the fact that the majority of embryos with NTDs miscarry. In Japan, for example, where NTD rates at birth are very low (about 0.9/1000) (Neel, 1958), those for late-embryo and early-fetal abortuses are about 6.2/1000 (Nishimura, 1975). In Londen, the respective figures are 3.0/1000 in total births (Carter and Evans, 1973a) and 30/1000 in abortuses (Creasy and Alberman, 1976).

Given a general population miscarriage rate of 15%, for example, the proportion of Japanese abortuses with NTDs would be 88%, while that for London, 64% (Leck, 1977). In addition, recent developments in prenatal diagnosis, such as alpha fetoprotein screening and ultrasound have made it possible to prevent the birth of fetuses with neural tube defects, by mid-pregnancy termination.

Taking these factors into consideration, then, as well as the usual difficulties in making international comparisons (such as differential diagnostic criteria, differential ascertainment procedures, and 'fashionable' or 'trendy' diagnoses), we shall present a few 'gross' geographic figures for very high and very low areas which may well represent real differences in incidence. According to a multinational survey by Stevenson et al. (1966), rates for anencephalus vary 40-fold from highs in Belfast, Ireland and Alexandria, Egypt to lows in Bogota, Colombia and Ljubljana, Yugoslavia. In Ireland, rates of NTDs combined reached 8.7/1000 (Stevenson et al., 1966). One of the highest rates for total CNS defects is found in S. Wales (8.1/1000).

With regard to ethnic groups, studies of different groups residing in the same geographic area reveal high rates of NTDs among the Sikhs of India (Searle, 1959), and low rates among Ashkenazi (European-origin) Jews (Naggan and MacMahon, 1967; Naggan, 1971). Lower rates have also been found among blacks living in the United States and England originating from West Africa than among whites living in the same areas (Alter, 1963; Leck, 1972; Erickson, 1976). Interestingly enough, however, studies of black populations in West Africa and Kenya have not shown such low rates (Gupta, 1969; Khan, 1965). One of the lowest reported rates of anencephalus among Caucasoid populations was reported in Finland during the period 1965–1973 with a rate of 0.32/1000 births (Granroth, 1978).

In most populations, the common CNS defects occur more frequently among females than males (Biggar et al., 1976; Laurence et al., 1968; Record and McKeown, 1949), in particular anencephalus (Coffey and Jessop, 1957; Czeizel and Révész, 1970; Hay, 1971). The sex ratio is less marked in populations exhibiting low anencephalus rates, such as American blacks (Gittelsohn and Milham, 1965) and Ashkenazi Jews (Naggan, 1971).

The question of 'nature versus nurture' invariably arises in the search for etiologic factors in such conditions. It is a difficult question as different lines of evidence suggest, but do not provide conclusive proof of either one or the other. The truth most probably lies somewhere in between and the most appropriate 'catch-all' hypothesis is that CNS defects are 'multifactorial' in origin, being influenced both by genetic and environmental factors.

A look at studies of migrant populations should be helpful in this regard. One such study compared rates of spina bifida among Japanese living in Japan with those of descendents of Japanese migrants living in Hawaii. The tendency was for a shift in rates from those of the original home country to those of the new area. In other words, the rates among descendents of Japanese migrants living in Hawaii were higher than those for Japan, but lower than those for the Caucasoids of Hawaii (Morton et al., 1967). Another study, comparing rates of NTDs in Ireland with those of Irish migrants to Boston, revealed the same tendency for rates to shift towards those of the new area; a more marked change in rates was found for migrants' grandchildren than for their children (Naggan and MacMahon, 1967; Naggan, 1971). These studies tend to implicate environmental rather than genetic factors, although an interaction between the two cannot be excluded.

A report attempting to delineate the role of environmental versus genetic factors in NTD etiology, revealed that in a low-prevalence area (Los Angeles County, California) environmental factors played a less important role than genetic factors. This was tested by comparing the epidemiologic features of NTDs in Los Angeles County with those of high-prevalence areas. The characteristics indicative of genetic factors differed considerably in the low versus high-prevalence areas, while the environmental factors did not (Sever, 1982).

A look at recurrence rates of NTDs in families should offer some insight into the nature-nurture question: following the birth of a child with either anencephalus or spina bifida in the United Kingdom, there is a 5% chance of recurrence in another child (Carter et al, 1968); following the birth of two children with NTDs, the risk of another rises to 13% (Masterson, 1962). This is in comparison to an approximate 0.5% risk in the general population. However, though these represent tremendously increased familial risks, it cannot be stated definitively that genetic factors are in operation. According to Yen and MacMahon (1968), "The recurrence of these anomalies in siblings is as likely to be due to persistence or recurrence of environmental factors as to a common genetic inheritance". Reports of the offspring of parents with CNS defects, although scanty, indicate an approximate 3–4% increase in risk of being affected (Carter and Evans, 1973b: Tünte, 1971).

Studies of twins are similarly ambiguous and difficult to interpret. In general, concordance rates (i.e. rates in which both individuals are affected) are higher in monozygous than in dizygous twin pairs (De Haan, 1966). However, the majority of monozygous twin pairs are not concordant for NTDs (Yen and MacMahon, 1968). As monozygous twins have indentical genetic make-ups, anything less than 100% concordance rates lends credence to an environmental interaction theory.

Other avenues of exploration of a possible genetic role in the NTDs include analyses of chromosomal, blood group and consanguinity data. Chromosomal abnormalities have been found, for example, in the parents of affected index children and their siblings (de Grouchy et al., 1964; Ellis and Penrose, 1961) and in anencephalic births (Arias-Bernal and Jones, 1967); other reports of anencephalic fetuses and their parents, however, do not show unusual karyotypes (Frézal et al., 1964; Masterson, 1962; Harnden et al., 1959). Similarly, no differences were found in series of anencephalic and control births for ABO or Rhesus blood groups (Smithells et al., 1964).

With regard to consanguinity, a World Health Organization study (1970) showed a significant association between CNS malformations and parental consanguinity in Egypt and India. Similarly, in Israel, an initial report based on the first 7 years of a congenital malformations survey at Kaplan Hospital (upon which our present analysis is based) also showed significant differences in CNS rates between consanguineous versus non-consanguineous parents (at the second-cousin level or closer) independent of ethnic group (Chemke et al., 1973). However, among parents of spina bifida and hydrocephalic children in Japan, there was no increase in consanguineous mariages (at the first cousin level) over the general population (Imaizumi, 1977a, b).

If genetics cannot account for the majority of NTDs, what other factors can? A look at time trends in incidence shows that although no consistent seasonal trend has been noted, a very marked long-term secular trend was found in both Boston, Massachusetts, and Providence, Rhode Island over the years 1920–1949, with 1930 being the peak year (MacMahon and Yen, 1971), suggestive of an epidemic hypothesis. A second peak was found in Providence, but not Boston, in the early 1940s. Another study by Naggan (1969), predating the other, analyzed NTD frequency from 1930 to 1965 in Boston which also showed a clear decline over that period. In examination of fathers' occupational class (which corresponds to Warner's well-known social class gradient), he noted the intriguing finding of a peak for the lowest occupational class in the early 1940s, similar to that later found by MacMahon and Yen in Providence. All of the classes showed the 1930 peak. These findings may be interpreted to indicate that while all social classes experienced some factor which led to the 1930 peak, the later peak resulted from something which most seriously affected the lower socioeconomic classes. Correspondingly, it was subsequently reported that the Providence data were derived from the Providence Lying-in Hospital, a hospital serving primarily a lower-class segment of the population compared to the Boston Lying-in Hospital. Other social class gradients have been noted in Scotland for anencephaly (Edwards, 1958) and in Rotterdam for NTDs (Hamersma, 1966).

A variety of indicators of social class (or socioeconomic status) have been used, such as paternal occupation, location and type of home, income, type of hospital accommodation at birth, and others. NTDs, in general, seem to be less frequent among those of higher socioeconomic status, according to these indicators (Coffey and Jessop, 1957; Edwards, 1958; Butler et al., 1969; Wilson, 1971). The prevalence of NTDs by paternal occupation, ranked on a scale similar to the five social classes in the UK (Office of Population Censuses and Surveys, 1970), varies from study to study. In England, a four-fold increase was found over the five categories in some areas (Wilson, 1971) and smaller gradients in others (Leck, 1974). No such increases were observed in Hungary (Czeizel and Révész, 1970) or among Jews in Israel or the United States (Naggan and MacMahon, 1967; Naggan, 1971). Only recently has the idea of maternal and/or paternal exposures at the workplace as possible teratogenic agents come into being; therefore, variations in the prevalence of NTDs or other malformations by occupation may not be reflecting social class differences as much as differences in chemical, radiation, or other exposures.

A number of maternal features have been investigated in relation to the frequency of NTDs, such as age, parity, previous abortions, and chronic diseases. In general, age and parity are difficult to separate, as younger women usually exhibit lower parity. Anencephalus, for example, occurs most frequently among young, primiparous women and women over 40 (Record and McKeown, 1949; Masterson, 1962). In Hungary, the prevalence of NTDs among first births remained higher than the other birth ranks over all maternal ages (Czeizel and Révész, 1970). Among the Jewish population of Israel, one study showed peak prevalence for birth ranks 1 and 4 at ages 30–34 years, with parity 4+ generally higher over all ages (Naggan, 1971). In a review of the literature on maternal age and anencephaly by Fedrick (1970a), the majority of studies showed a U-shaped pattern; i.e. higher risks for younger and older mothers with a trough occurring in the middle, around ages 25–29 years. Paternal age, which has been considered as a risk factor in Down syndrome (Stene et al., 1977; Matsunaga et al., 1978; Hook et al., 1981; Klingberg et al., 1982), has not been closely examined for its role, if any, in neural tube defects. In general, it is difficult methodologically to separate out a possible paternal from a maternal age effect, due to the fact that older women tend to have older husbands.

A multivariate study by Elwood et al. (1978) which controlled for place, year, season of birth and maternal ethnic origin, showed that death rates for anencephaly were no longer found to be associated with maternal age, but rather with previous stillbirths and infant deaths.

Prior and subsequent abortion and stillbirths have been shown to be more frequent in mothers of anancephalics (Stevenson and Warnock, 1959; Masterson, 1962), and in mothers of children with CNS defects in general (Granroth et al., 1978).

The following are among the environmental agents which have been considered as possibly associated with CNS defects:

(1) Infectious agents such as rubella related to microcephalus; cytomegalovirus related to mental and motor retardation in about 10% of affected infants, sometimes accompanied by microcephalus; herpes simplex virus, associated with microcephalus and mental retardation; toxoplasmosis, related to microcephalus and hydrocephalus and in severe neonatal illness, often resulting in neurological sequelae, such as mental retardation and seizures; syphilis, in which the central nervous system may be involved; and influenza, with contradictory reports, some claiming an association with

anencephalus and other congenital malformations, but this has not been confirmed (Sever et al., 1976).

(2) Chemicals such as methylmercury related to microcephalus in congenital Minamata disease (Takeuchi and Matsumoto, 1969); and organic solvents associated with CNS defects in general (Holmberg et al., 1979).

(3) Radiation, including X- and gamma-radiation during pregnancy in relation to microcephalus, growth and mental retardation (Brent, 1979); and exposure of women to the atomic blast at Hiroshima in relation to microcephalus (Miller, 1956; Brent, 1979). Possible behavioral effects of intrauterine radiation in humans are extremely difficult to evaluate because: they may be related to postnatal environmental influences; animal tests for behavioral outcomes are not necessarily applicable to humans; reports are often contradictory and not dose-related; and it is impossible to correlate behavioral effects with neuroanatomical changes (Brent, 1979).

(4) Nutritional factors such as tea consumption (Fedrick, 1974); canned peas and cured meat, have been suggested to be due to the magnesium salts in the peas and the nitrates or nitrites in the meat (Knox, 1972); and soft water found in England and Wales (Fedrick, 1970b; Lowe et al., 1971) and in Holland (Verstege, 1971), due to the low calcium or trace mineral levels. A recent study suggests that lowered rates of anencephalus in the Fylde peninsula (UK) may have been mitigated by a change in water hardness from soft to slightly hard, maybe by the addition of a trace mineral (Bound et al., 1981). Vitamin deficiencies, in particular folic acid, may confer added risk of neural tube defects (Smithells et al., 1976); clinical trials in the United Kingdom of periconceptional vitamin supplementation are currently underway in an attempt to reduce the recurrence rate of NTDs and initial reports have been encouraging (Smithells et al., 1980).

(5) Physical factors such as hyperthermia of the mother during pregnancy have been incriminated in higher rates of CNS defects (Miller et al., 1978; Halperin and Wilroy, 1978); however, whether caused by febrile illness or sauna bathing, these findings are tenuous indeed. Hyperthermia caused by sauna bathing seems almost incredible as a risk factor in CNS defects, as Finland, where sauna bathing is a part of everyday life, exhibits one of the lowest rates in the world (0.32/1000 births) (Granroth, 1978).

A survey of birth defects

In order to select the important etiological features from this maze of possible causation, we will relate some of the putative risk factors to the actual associations we have found in a consecutive series of 35 546 births at Kaplan Hospital (Rehovot, Israel) during the period 1966–1976.

As birth certificates in Israel do not include malformation information, it was essential to compile a special questionnaire for recording all births. The data recorded on

Table 3.1. Births with CNS malformations at the Kaplan Hospital, Israel (1966–76)

	All births	Births with CNS malformations
Live births		
Singletons	34455	65
Twins	701	0
Triplets	15	0
Stillbirths		
Singletons	341	30
Twins	31	2
Triplets	3	0
Total	35546	97

the questionnaire included demographic information as well as family history, genetic factors, details of the delivery and parental health, with special emphasis on chronic diseases.

Examination of all newborns was performed by a single neonatologist. In case of suspected malformation, the clinical geneticist was consulted and when necessary, other specialists (e.g. orthopedic surgeons, neurologists, ophthalmologists) were called in. The information obtained from each gravida was recorded on the questionnaire by the pediatrician, obstetrician and social worker. All neonates, whether suspected of having an abnormality or not, were examined twice during their stay in the hospital; within the first 24 hours of birth and before discharge from hospital, usually on the fourth day of life. Postmortem examinations were performed on all stillbirths, and on infants who died during their stay in the newborn nursery. The diagnosis thus

Table 3.2. Maternal factors

	All pregnancies	CNS malformations	
		Pregnancies	Prevalence/1000
Age (year)			
Under 20	1535	2	1.30
20–24	12484	31	2.48
25–29	11474	33	2.88
30–34	5966	19	3.18
35 or more	3709	11	2.96
Previous pregnancies			
0	9543	26	2.72
1	8193	24	2.93
2	5860	16	2.73
3	3934	6	1.52
4+	7638	24	3.14

Table 3.3. Oral contraceptive use

	All pregnancies	CNS malformations	
		Pregnancies	Prevalence/1000
Oral contraceptive use			
Yes	4536	10	2.20
No	30632	86	2.81

obtained was recorded on a precoded checklist of congenital malformations included in the questionnaire.

The survey was designed to study all malformations either occurring alone or in combination with others (up to six malformations could be recorded for each infant). Some results have previously been published (Klingberg et al., 1971a, b; Chen et al., 1970; Chemke et al., 1973). In this presentation, only infants with a CNS malformation (whether it was the primary or an associated defect) will be discussed.

Results of the survey
During the period of study a total of 35546 infants were born; 97 had CNS malformations (see Table 3.1). The percentage of multiple births among those affected (2 out of 97; 2%) was the same as the overall figure (750 out of 35546; 2%). Although the numbers are too small for any conclusions, it is of interest that the two affected twins were from the same pregnancy. Tables 3.2–5 relate to pregnancies rather than births. There were 96 affected pregnancies in a total of 35168 giving a birth prevalence of 2.73/1000. The tables show the results of maternal factors (age and previous pregnancies); oral contraceptive use; maternal diabetes; socioeconomic factors (paternal education and paternal occupation); and familial factors (ethnic origin and consanguinity).

Maternal factors (Table 3.2). Neither of the factors studied show a strong effect. The increased risk is in the direction expected from the literature, but of little magnitude. Moreover, neither the number of previous pregnancies nor maternal age account for many cases of CNS malformation.

Table 3.4. Diabetes mellitus

	All pregnancies	CNS malformations	
		Pregnancies	Prevalence/1000
Diabetes mellitus *			
Yes	156	4	25.64
No	35012	92	2.63

* $t = 5.58$, $P \ll 0.00001$.

86

Table 3.5. Socioeconomic factors

	All pregnancies	CNS malformations	
		Pregnancies	Prevalence/1000
Paternal education			
≤ 11 years or unknown	22 738	66	2.90
12 years	6 638	15	2.26
13 years or more	5 792	15	2.59
Paternal occupation			
Administrators, academics and professionals	9 505	26	2.74
Clerks, salespersons and skilled workers	11 404	34	2.98
Service, agricultural and unskilled workers	8 263	25	3.03
Army	3 382	5	1.48
Unemployed or unknown	2 614	6	2.30

Oral contraceptive use (Table 3.3). In this population, previous oral contraceptive use does not appear to be associated with increased risk of CNS defects. This negative finding is in accordance with other published results (Heinonen et al., 1977; Bracken et al., 1978; Robinson, 1971; Royal College of General Practitioners, 1976; Vessey et al., 1979; Cuckle and Wald, 1982).

Diabetes mellitus (Table 3.4). Looking at maternal (non-gestational) diabetes, a clear risk is found. The four CNS cases in 156 diabetic pregnancies (25.64/1000) represent a statistically significant excess over that found for non-diabetics (92 cases in 35 012 pregnancies, or 2.63/1000). We do not know the extent to which diabetic con-

Table 3.6. Familial factors

	All pregnancies	CNS malformations	
		Pregnancies	Prevalence/1000
*Ethnic origin**			
Asian	9 615	29	3.02
African	10 288	28	2.72
Ashkenazi (or Western)	15 444	36	2.33
Other	179	3	16.75
Consanguinity			
Unrelated or unknown	32 637	78	2.39
Second cousins	1 232	3	2.44
First cousins	1 213	15	12.37
Uncle-niece/aunt-nephew	86	0	–

* Based on the country of birth of the maternal grandmother.

trol in pregnancy had been achieved. Although the risk factor is clearly operating, it cannot account for many cases since diabetes was a rare condition in our study.

Although diabetes has often been reported in association with congenital malformations in general (Pederson, 1964; Kučera, 1971; Day and Insley, 1976) only a few studies have noted a slightly increased risk of this disease with CNS defects (Malins, 1978; Granroth, 1978).

Socioeconomic factors (Table 3.5). As mentioned in the review, social class is an associated factor, an indirect measure of diet, housing conditions, cleanliness or some other underlying feature. Since the underlying feature is unknown, an indirect approach is necessary. In our survey, education and occupation were used as indicators of social class. The occupations have been arranged according to income based on the published earnings of Israelis during the study period. Army personnel and the unemployed have been entered separately, as they were difficult to categorize according to income level. The justification for grouping years of education as we have done is that 12 years are required in Israel for the attainment of certain skills and 13 or more for advanced education.

Although no clear pattern emerges, there is a tendency for those with less education and less skilled jobs to have a higher prevalence, as expected, but as with maternal factors, the magnitude is not great.

Familial factors (Table 3.6). Regarding the role of genetic factors in the etiology of CNS malformations, the present consensus is that a genetic predisposition exists, but that one or more environmental triggers are needed to activate it. Such a mechanism is difficult to study epidemiologically; some studies mentioned in the previous epidemiological review which were originally conducted in order to reveal a genetic component could just as well be considered indicative of a common or unchanging environment. Rather than using the term 'genetic factors' then, we have looked at 'familial factors', which imply a genetic component to a greater or lesser extent. We have studied two such factors, ethnic origin and consanguinity. Ethnic origin was determined by the maternal grandmother's place of birth in order to avoid a large Israeli-born category; this would have been unavoidable using maternal place of birth. The results do show a reasonably large excess of births in those of Asian origin; the 'other' group, mainly Arab and Israeli-born, is too small to place confidence in the result.

Our most striking finding is the high risk in first-cousin marriages. This is a five-fold relative risk compared to those less closely related. To put it in another way, over 15% of pregnancies associated with CNS malformations are the result of first cousin or closer marriages in comparison to about 3.5% in the total population; therefore about 12% of CNS malformations are attributable to this factor. It is interesting to note that no 'intermediate-level risk' was demonstrated in second-cousin marriages. Their risk was the same as those unrelated.

Conclusion

From what we know of the epidemiology of CNS malformations, it is clear that no single environmental agent can be shown to account for a substantial proportion of the birth prevalence. Also, among the agents suspected of involvement, none stands up to epidemiological investigation. What then are the implications for behavioral teratology? If well-defined conditions like CNS defects are intractable to this method, how can behavioral effects be determined epidemiologically? Certainly the idea of checking for behavioral effects of agents involved in CNS lesions is not presently effective. Nonetheless, the argument is still tenable, and it therefore would be reasonable to check any proven CNS teratogens which emerge in the future for possible neurobehavioral outcomes.

Acknowledgment

This analysis has been made possible by a grant from the Sapir Memorial Fund of Mifal Hapayis, Tel Aviv.

References

Alter, M. (1963) Anencephalic births in a northern and a southern community. Am. J. Dis. Child. 106, 536–544.

Arias-Bernal, L. and Jones Jr., H.W. (1967) An anencephalic male with XX sex chromosome complement. Am. J. Obstet. Gynecol. 99, 877–878.

Bergsma, D. (ed.) (1979) Birth Defects Compendium, 2nd edn., Alan R. Liss, New York.

Biggar, R.J., Mortimer Jr. E.A. and Haughie, G.E. (1976) Descriptive epidemiology of neural tube defects, Rochester, New York, 1918–1938. Am. J. Epidemiol. 104, 22–27.

Bornschein, R.L. (1980) The role of behavioral assessment in standard in vivo teratogenicity testing. In: Proceedings of Workshop on Methodology for Assessing Reproductive Hazards in the Workplace (Infante, P.F. and Legator, M.S., eds.) NIOSH Pub. No. 81–100, Bethesda, MD, pp. 227–245.

Bound, J.P., Harvey, P.W., Brookes, D.M. and Sayers, B. McA. (1981) The incidence of anencephalus in the Fylde peninsula 1956–76 and changes in water hardness. J. Epidemiol. Community Health 35, 102–105.

Bracken, M.B., Holford, T., White, C. and Kelsey, J. (1978) Role of oral contraception in congenital malformation of offspring. Int. J. Epidemiol. 7, 309–317.

Brent, R.L. (1979) Effects of ionizing radiation on growth and development. In: Epidemiologic Methods for Detection of Teratogens (Klingberg, M.A., Weatherall, J.A.C. and Papier, C., eds.) Karger, Basel, pp. 147–183.

Butler, N.R., Alberman, E.D. and Schutt, W.H. (1969) The congenital malformations. In: Perinatal Problems (Second Report of the British Perinatal Mortality Survey) (Butler, N.R. and Alberman, E.D., eds.) Livingstone, Edinburgh, pp. 283–320.

Butler, N.R. and Goldstein, H. (1973) Smoking in pregnancy and subsequent child development. Brit. Med. J. iv, 573–575.

Carter, C.O., David, P.A. and Laurence, K.M. (1968) A family study of major central nervous system malformations in South Wales. J. Med. Genet. 5, 81–106.

Carter, C.O. and Evans, K. (1973a) Spina bifida and anencephalus in Greater London. J. Med. Genet. 10, 209–234.

Carter, C.O. and Evans, K. (1973b) Children of adult survivors with spina bifida cystica. Lancet ii, 924–926.

Chemke, J., Chen, R., Klingberg, M.A. and Levin, S. (1973) Some indications for genetic factors in congenital malformations. Israel J. Med. Sci. 9, 1400–1403.

Chen, R., Weissman, S.L., Salama, R. and Klingberg, M.A. (1970) Congenital dislocation of the hip (CDH) and seasonality: The gestational age of vulnerability to some seasonal factor. Am. J. Epidemiol. 92, 287–293.

Clarren, S.K. and Smith, D.W. (1978) The fetal alcohol syndrome. New Engl. J. Med. 298, 1063–1067.

Coffey, V.P. and Jessop, W.J.E. (1957) A study of 137 cases of anencephaly. Brit. J. Prev. Soc. Med. 11, 174–180.

Creasy, M.R. and Alberman, E.D. (1976) Congenital malformations of the central nervous system in spontaneous abortions. J. Med. Genet. 13, 9–16.

Cuckle, H.S. and Wald, N.J. (1982) Evidence against oral contraceptives as a cause of neural-tube defects. Brit. J. Obstet. Gynaecol. 89, 547–549.

Czeizel, A. and Révész, C. (1970) Major malformations of the central nervous system in Hungary. Brit. J. Prev. Soc. Med. 24, 205–222.

Day, R.E. and Insley, J. (1976) Maternal diabetes mellitus and congenital malformation. Arch. Dis. Child. 51, 935–938.

Denson, R., Nanson, J.L. and McWatters, M.A. (1975) Hyperkinesis and maternal smoking. Can. Psychiatr. Assoc. J. 20, 183–187.

Dunn, H.G., McBurney, A.K., Ingram, S. and Hunter, C.M. (1977) Maternal cigarette smoking during pregnancy and the child's subsequent development. II. Neurological and intellectual maturation to the age of $6\frac{1}{2}$ years. Can. J. Public Health 68, 43–50.

Edwards, J.H. (1958) Congenital malformations of the central nervous system in Scotland. Br. J. Prev. Soc. Med. 12, 115–130.

Ellis, J.R. and Penrose, L.S. (1961) Enlarged satellites and multiple malformations in the same pedigree. Ann. Hum. Genet. 25, 159.

Elwood, J.M., Raman, S. and Mousseau, G. (1978) Reproductive history in the mothers of anencephalics. J. Chron. Dis. 31, 473–481.

Erickson, J.D. (1976) Racial variations in the incidence of congenital malformations. Ann. Hum. Genet. 39, 315–320.

Fedrick, J. (1970a) Anencephalus: Variation with maternal age, parity, social class and region in England, Scotland and Wales. Ann. Hum. Genet. 34, 31–38.

Fedrick, J. (1970b) Anencephalus and the local water supply. Nature 227, 176–177.

Fedrick, J. (1974) Anencephalus and maternal tea drinking: Evidence for a possible association. Proc. R. Soc. Med. 67, 356–360.

Frézal, J., Kelley, J., Guillemot, M.L. and Lamy, M. (1964) Anencephaly in France, Am. J. Hum. Genet. 16, 336–350.

Giroud, P. and Giroud, A. (1964) Anencéphalie et rickettsioses maladies in apparentes. Bull. Acad. Nat. Méd. 621, 1964.

Gittelsohn, A.M. and Milham, S. (1965) Total records of congenital malformations in New York State. In: Genetics and the Epidemiology of Chronic Diseases (Neel, J.V., Shaw, M.S. and Schull, W.J., eds.) U.S.P.H.S. Publication No. 1163, Washington.

Granroth, G. (1978) Risk indicators for defects of the central nervous system. Dissertation, University of Helsinki, Helsinki.

Granroth, G., Haapakoski, J. and Hakama, M. (1978) Defects of the central nervous system in Finland. II. Birth order, outcome of previous pregnancies and family history. Teratology 17, 213–222.

de Grouchy, J., Brissaud, M.E., Repessé, G. and Lamy, M. (1964) Anencéphalie familiale et remaniement de deux chromosomes 13–15. C. R. Acad. Sci. (Paris) 258, 691.

Gupta, B. (1969) Incidence of congenital malformations in Nigerian children. W. Afr. Med. J. 18, 22–27.

De Haan, Q.C. (1966) Monozygotic anencephalic twins. Report of a case. Obstet. Gynecol. 28, 559–560.

Halperin, L.R. and Wilroy Jr., R.S. (1978) Maternal hyperthermia and neural-tube defects. Lancet i, 212–213.

Hamersma, K. (1966) Anencephalie en Spina Bifida. Drukkerij Romijn, Apeldoorn, The Netherlands.

Hanson, J.W. and Smith, D.W. (1976) Fetal hydantoin syndrome. Lancet i, 692.

Harada, M. (1978) Congenital Minamata disease: Intrauterine methylmercury poisoning. Teratology 18, 285–288.

Harnden, D.G., Briggs, J.H. and Stewart, J.S.S. (1959) Nuclear chromatin of anencephalic foetuses. Lancet ii, 126–127.

Hay, S. (1971) Sex differences in the incidence of certain congenital malformations. A review of the literature and some new data. Teratology 4, 277.

Heinonen, O.P., Slone, D. and Shapiro, S. (1977) Birth Defects and Drugs in Pregnancy. PSG Publishing, Littleton, MA.

Holmberg, P.C. (1979) Central-nervous-system defects in children born to mothers exposed to organic solvents during pregnancy. Lancet ii, 177–179.

Hook, E.B., Cross, P.K., Lamson, S.H., Regal, R.R., Baird, P.A. and Uh, S.H. (1981) Paternal age and Down syndrome in British Columbia. Am. J. Hum. Genet. 33, 123–128.

Imaizumi, Y. (1977a) Incidence of spina bifida and parental consanguinity in Japan. Congenital Anomalies 17, 471–478.

Imaizumi, Y. (1977b) Consanguinity among parents of congenital hydrocephalus in Japan. Congenital Anomalies 17, 479–486.

Khan, A.A. (1965) Congenital malformations in African neonates in Nairobi. J. Trop. Med. Hyg. 68, 272–274.

Kline, J., Stein, Z.A., Susser, M. and Warburton, D. (1977) Smoking: A risk factor for spontaneous abortion. New Engl. J. Med. 297, 793–796.

Klingberg, M.A., Chemke, J., Chen, R. and Levin, S. (1971a) A survey of congenital malformations in Israel. The effect of some factors associated with ethnic origin. Israel J. Med. Sci. 7, 1529–1534.

Klingberg, M.A., Chen, R., Chemke, J. and Levin, S. (1971b) An epidemiologic study of congenital malformations among different ethnic and social groups in Israel. Dev. Med. Child. Neurol. 13, 735–745.

Klingberg, M.A., Chen, R., Papier, C.M., Chemke, J. and Amizur, G. (1982) Paternal age and Down syndrome. Congenital Anomalies 22, 1–6.

Knox, E.G. (1972) Anencephalus and dietary intakes. Brit. J. Prev. Soc. Med. 26, 219–223.

Kučera, J. (1971) Rate and type of congenital anomalies among offspring of diabetic women. J. Reprod. Med. 7, 73–82.

Laurence, K.M., Carter, C.O. and David, P.A. (1968) Major central nervous system malformations in South Wales. II. Pregnancy factors, seasonal variation and social class effects. Brit. J. Prev. Soc. Med. 22, 212–222.

Leck, I. (1972) The etiology of human malformations: Insights from epidemiology. Teratology 5, 303–314.

Leck, I. (1974) Paediatric aspects of epidemiology – insights into the causation of disorders of early life. In: Scientific Foundations of Paediatrics (Davis, J.A., and Dobbing, J., eds.) Heinemann, London, pp. 727–757.

Leck, I. (1977) Correlations of malformation frequency with environmental and genetic attributes in man. In: Handbook of Teratology, Vol. III, (Wilson, J.G. and Fraser, F.C., eds.) Plenum, New York, pp. 243–324.

Lowe, C.R., Roberts, C.L. and Lloyd, S. (1971) Malformations of the central nervous system and softness of local water supplies. Brit. Med. J. 2, 357–361.

MacMahon, B. and Yen, S. (1971) Unrecognized epidemic of anencephaly and spina bifida. Lancet i, 31–33.

Malins, J.M. (1978) Congenital malformations and fetal mortality in diabetic pregnancy. J. R. Soc. Med. 71, 205–207.

Masterson, J.G. (1962) Empiric, genetic counseling and preventive measures in anencephaly. Acta Genet. 12, 219.

Matsumoto, H.G., Koya, G. and Takeuchi, T. (1965) Fetal Minamata disease. A neuropathological study of two cases of intrauterine intoxication by a methylmercury compound. J. Neuropathol. Exp. Neurol. 24, 563–574.

Matsunaga, E., Tonomura, A., Oishi, H. and Kikuchi, Y. (1978) Reexamination of paternal age effect in Down's syndrome. Hum. Genet. 40, 259–268.

Miller, R.W. (1956) Delayed effects occurring within the first decade after exposure of young individuals to the Hiroshima atomic bomb. Pediatrics 18, 1–18.

Miller, P., Smith, D.W. and Shepard, T.H. (1978) Maternal hyperthermia as a possible cause of anencephaly. Lancet i, 519–521.

de Morsier, G. and Bammater, F. (1960) Études sur les dysraphies cranio-cérébrales. Rev. Neurol. 103, 513.

Morton, N.E., Chung, C.S. and Mi, M.-P. (1967) Genetics of Inter-racial Crosses in Hawaii. Monographs on Human Genetics, Vol. 3, Karger, Basel.

Naggan, L. (1969) The recent decline in prevalence of anencephaly and spina bifida. Am. J. Epidemiol. 89, 154–160.

Naggan, L. (1971) Anencephaly and spina bifida in Israel. Pediatrics 47, 577–586.

Naggan, L. and MacMahon, B. (1967) Ethnic differences in the prevalence of anencephaly and spina bifida in Boston, Massachusetts. New Engl. J. Med. 277, 1119–1123.

Neel, J.V. (1958) A study of major congenital defects in Japanese infants. Am. J. Hum. Genet. 10, 398–445.

Nishimura, H. (1975) Prenatal versus postnatal malformations based on the Japanese experience on induced abortions in the human being. In: Aging Gametes: Their Biology and Pathology, (Blandau, R.J., ed.) Karger, Basel, pp. 349–368.

Office of Population Censuses and Surveys (1970) Classification of Occupations 1970. Her Majesty's Stationery Office, London.

Pedersen, L.M., Tygstrup, I. and Pedersen, J. (1964) Congenital malformations in newborn infants of diabetic women. Lancet i, 1124–1126.

Record, R.G. and McKeown, T. (1949) Congenital malformations of the central nervous system. I. A survey of 930 cases. Brit. J. Prev. Soc. Med. 4, 183.

Reinisch, J. (1977) Prenatal exposure of human foetuses to synthetic progestin and oestrogen affects personality. Nature 266, 561.

Robinson, S.C. (1971) Pregnancy outcome following oral contraceptives. Am. J. Obstet. Gynecol. 109, 354–358.

Royal College of General Practitioners Oral Contraceptive Study (1976) The outcome of pregnancy in former oral contraceptive users. Brit. J. Obstet. Gynaecol. 83, 608–616.

Saxton, D.W. (1978) The behaviour of infants whose mothers smoke in pregnancy. Early Hum. Dev. 24, 363–369.

Searle, A.G. (1959) The incidence of anencephaly in a polytypic population. Ann. Hum. Genet. 23, 279–288.

Sever, J.L., Fuccillo, D.A. and Bowes Jr., W.A. (1976) Environmental factors: Infection and immunization. In: Prevention of Embryonic, Fetal, and Perinatal Disease (Brent, R.L. and Harris, M.I., eds.) DHEW Publication No. (NIH) 76–853, Bethesda, MD, pp. 199–209.

Sever, L.E. (1982) An epidemiologic study of neural tube defects in Los Angeles County. II. Etiologic factors in an area with low prevalence at birth. Teratology 25, 323–334.

Smith, D.W. (1980) Alcohol effects on the fetus. In: Drug and Chemical Risks to the Fetus and Newborn (Schwarz, R.H. and Yaffe, S.J., eds.) Alan R. Liss, New York, pp. 73–82.

Smithells, R.W., Chinn, E.R. and Franklin, D. (1964) Anencephaly in Liverpool. Dev. Med. Child Neurol. 6, 231–240.

Smithells, R.W., Sheppard, S. and Schorah, C.J. (1976) Vitamin deficiencies and neural tube defects. Arch. Dis. Child. 51, 944–950.

Smithells, R.W., Sheppard, S., Schorah, C.J., Seller, M.J., Nevin, N.C., Harris, R., Read, A.P. and Fielding, D.W. (1980) Possible prevention of neural tube defects by periconceptional vitamin supplementation. Lancet i, 399–400.

92

Stene, J., Fischer, G. and Stene, E. (1977) Paternal age effect in Down's syndrome. Ann. Hum. Genet. 40, 299–306.

Stevenson, A.C., Johnston, H.A., Stewart, M.I.P. and Golding, D.R. (1966) Congenital malformations. A report of a study of a series of consecutive births in 24 centers. Bull. WHO 34, Suppl.

Stevenson, A.C. and Warnock, H.A. (1959) Observations on the results of pregnancies in women resident in Belfast. I. Data relating to all pregnancies ending in 1957. Ann. Hum. Genet. 23, 382.

Streissguth, A.P., Herman, C.S. and Smith, D.W. (1978) Intelligence, behavior and dysmorphogenesis in the fetal alcohol syndrome: A report on 20 patients. J. Pediatr. 92, 363–367.

Takeuchi, T. and Matsumoto, H. (1969) Minamata disease of human fetuses. In: Methods for Teratological Studies in Experimental Animals and Man (Nishimura, H. and Miller, R.W., eds.) Igaku Shoin, Tokyo.

Tünte, W. (1971) Fortpflanzungsfähigkeit, Heiratshäufigkeit und Zahl und Beschaffenheit der Nachkommen bei Patienten mit Spina bifida aperta. Humangenetik 13, 43.

USDHEW (1979) Smoking and Health: A Report of the Surgeon General. USDHEW No. 79–50066.

Verstege, J.C.W. (1971) Anencephalie in Nederland 1951–1968. Centraal Bureau voor de Statistiek, Staatsuitgeverij, The Hague.

Vessey, M., Meisler, L., Flavel, R. and Yeates, D. (1979) Outcome of pregnancy in women using different methods of contraception. Brit. J. Obstet. Gynaecol. 86, 548–556.

Wilson, T.S. (1971) A study of congenital malformations of the central nervous system among Glasgow births 1964–1968. Health Bull. 29, 79–87.

Wilson, J.G. (1973) Environment and Birth Defects. Academic Press, New York.

Wilson, G.S., Desmond, M.M. and Verniaud, W.M. (1973) Early development of infants of heroin-addicted mothers. Am. J. Dis. Child. 126, 457–462.

World Health Organization (1970) Genetic factors in congenital malformations. WHO Tech. Rep. Ser. 438.

Yalom, I.D., Green, R. and Fisk, M. (1973) Prenatal exposure to female hormones: Effect on psychosexual development in boys. Arch. Gen. Psychiat. 28, 554–561.

Yen, S. and MacMahon, B. (1968) Genetics of anencephaly and spina bifida? Lancet ii, 623–626.

Neurobehavioral Teratology
edited by Joseph Yanai
© Elsevier Science Publishers BV 1984

4

IN VITRO EMBRYO CULTURES AS A METHOD FOR THE STUDY OF CENTRAL NERVOUS SYSTEM MALFORMATIONS

Asher Ornoy and Igor Zusman

Laboratory of Teratology, Department of Anatomy and Embryology, Hebrew University, Jerusalem, Israel

CENTRAL nervous system anomalies constitute a widespread group of defects, all impairing the integrity and function of the nervous system. The etiology of these different anomalies is usually poorly understood. These anomalies are also considered to be the most difficult defects for treatment in humans, because even in cases where surgery might be effective (such as hydrocephaly and meningomyelocele) there is a certain degree of damage already done that is not curable. Moreover, many expressions of slight, minor CNS anomalies are behavioral and cognitive deficits, which can be detected only with fine quantitative techniques. One can understand the wide range and high incidence of these various anomalies while considering the complexity of embryonic development of the central nervous system. The brain is therefore susceptible to many different factors throughout pregnancy, many of which are yet undefined. This applies to man as well as experimental animals.

Concomitantly with the investigation of the normal pattern of CNS development, many studies were made to assess possible teratogenic effects on the CNS. These in vivo studies were performed in different animal species. However, with the introduction of even one major environmental change (e.g. administration of a drug during pregnancy, hypoxia) many factors come into play due to different metabolic pathways being affected. Therefore, any conclusions drawn from one animal species and applied

93

to another and especially to man, must be drawn with much caution. In vitro experiments on whole embryo culture are, however, free of metabolic changes caused by the maternal metabolism, and may therefore be more suitable for teratogenic studies. However, such embryos can only be held in culture for a limited period, which is too short in terms of brain development for the study of the whole array of possible teratogenic effects on the CNS.

Development of the central nervous system

The CNS is the first system to develop and to differentiate, and one of the last to be completed. The neural plate, the first sign of the future CNS, can be first observed at days 7.5–8 in the mouse and rabbit, and at days 9–9.5 in the rat (Edwards, 1968; Rugh, 1968). Some major developmental events of the CNS are very rapid so that by day 14, for example, the mouse has a typical mammalian brain. On the other hand, various parts of the CNS develop at different rates in the same animal. For instance, the cerebellum in not entirely differentiated at birth in many animals. In the mouse the neural tube is closed in part at 8 days, by which time neural crest cells have spread ventrolaterally and cranial ganglia V–X are apparent. At 8.5–9.5 days the anterior and posterior neuropores close. At that stage, the three primary brain vesicles form, as well as the brain flexures. Different structures, such as the optic cup, the otic vesicle, Rathke's pocket and the roof of the rhombencephalon can be observed at the same developmental stage. At 10 days the telencephalic vesicles as well as the other brain vesicles are clearly evident. The same developmental rate of the brain is found in rabbits, but in rats all these changes are one day later. At 10.5 days in the mouse or at 11.5 days in rats more structures are defined, such as the lamina terminalis, infundibulum, various cranial nerves, including ganglia of the trigeminal nerve (V), facial (VII) and acoustic nerves (VIII). The metameric cervical spinal ganglia are also formed. At 11 days in the mouse and at 12 days in the rat, the infundibulum begins to pinch off from the diencephalon and the roof of the fourth ventricle thins out, concomitant with the formation of the choroid plexus. In the lateral view the diencephalon can be identified, with its optic chiasma and infundibulum being obscured in part by the enlarging mesencephalon. The cerebellar plates arise from the metencephalon forming a transverse fold posterior to the mesencephalon. Just posterior to the center of the metencephalon is the triangular and lucid thin roof of the myelencephalon, which tapers rapidly into the spinal cord. During day 12 in the mouse and day 13 in the rat the cerebellum is much thickened, the posterior choroid plexus is apparent in the roof of the myelencephalon, the pontine flexure is present, the telencephalic vesicles are enlarging, and the spinal ganglia are visible to about the level of somite 40. During the next day of development the cerebral hemispheres partly cover the diencephalon, the anterior choroid plexus projects into the lateral and third ventricles, close to which the corpora striata, thalamus and hypothalamus appear. During the future development of the brain all these parts will enlarge and develop, but the basic relationships remain unchanged. Migration of neuroblasts from the deeper ventricular zones will form the cortical plate which appears in the mouse and in the rat at slightly different development stages (Ornoy and Yanai, 1980). In man, the primary developmental events of the neural tube follow a similar pattern to that of rodents. The earliest evidence of neural plate formation is the appearance of the neural epithelium 15–17 days after fertilization (stage 7) by which time the notochordal process starts to form. The neural folds begin to fuse during the 22nd day (stage 10), after the first 6–7 pairs of somites have been formed. The anterior neuropore closes at day 24 (stage 11), by which time the three brain vesicles can already be identified. Formation of the neural tube is completed by day 26 (stage 12) with the closure of the posterior neuropore. However, the telencephalic (cerebral) vesicles first appear at days 32–33, at the time when the right and left cerebellar plates can also be identified (Lemire et al., 1975; O'Rahilly and Gardner, 1971, 1977). The cortical plate appears quite late during development, at 7.5–8 weeks after conception. In man, too, the cerebellar cortex develops mainly during the second half of gestation, and is completed at term or shortly after birth. Similarly, maturation of the cerebral cortex also extends into the postnatal period (O'Rahilly and Gardner, 1977; Dobbing and Sands, 1973).

Organ culture of mammalian embryos

The method of in vitro cultivation of whole early somite mammalian embryos is now used widely in the main branches of teratology (clinical, behavioral, experimental) for the study of some mechanisms of abnormal development. Short-term 'organism culture' (Mintz, 1967) of early stages in the mammalian development has become a practical reality. As a result, more and more in vitro experiments under controlled conditions can be anticipated. Novel techniques have already been introduced for the manipulation of development in vitro, and some problems of fundamental theoretical as well as practical significance can be studied with the use of these methods (for review, see Kaufman, 1981).

It is possible to divide the in vitro culture methods into two main parts: culture of preimplantation embryos and culture of early somite embryos. In vitro studies of preimplantation embryos allow studies of some problems of fertilization in vitro (Bavister, 1980; Stewart, 1981; Trotnow et al., 1981; Kuehl and Dukelow, 1982), the development of early cleavage stages (Brinster, 1963; Hsu et al., 1974; Spindle, 1980) or differentiation of the early blastocyst stage (Hsu, 1971, 1972, 1973; Rottmann and Lampeter, 1981; Wu et al., 1981a, b). Many reasons have increased interest of investigators in studying the development of preimplantation embryos in in vitro culture systems, in particular because this method allows the study of some problems in the genetic control of differentiation, both normal and abnormal. But for the study of normal and abnormal development of the brain the in vitro culture method of early somite

96

embryos is more suitable. The first successful attempts to culture rat embryos in vitro were performed about 50 years ago (Nicholas and Rudnick, 1934, 1938; Jolly and Lieure, 1938), but the modern history of whole embryo culture of mammalian embryos during early organogenesis began only when D.A.T. New published his first articles in this field (New and Stein, 1964; New, 1966). The method has been improved by New himself (New et al., 1973; New, 1978) and by other investigators (Rizzino and Sherman, 1979; Sadler, 1979; Tam and Snow, 1980), and is now used in many laboratories for the culture of rat and mouse embryos.

In the rat, using this tehnique, it is possible to achieve normal development of embryos at late primitive streak and head-fold stages (Figs. 4.1–4). Later developmental stages, up to 13.5 days of gestation, can be kept in culture for somewhat shorter periods (Cockroft, 1976; Buckley et al., 1978). For the mouse, good growth and development of early somite embryos in vitro were achieved for periods of up to 48 h (Sadler, 1979). This modified culture technique has been used to maintain 10.5 day rabbit embryos (stages of early organogenesis) in vitro for up to 24 h (Stokes et al., 1981).

It is possible to study with this method normal development of early embryos of different species or the same species during their early organogenesis, including the study of abnormal differentiation of the separate parts of embryos and their correla-

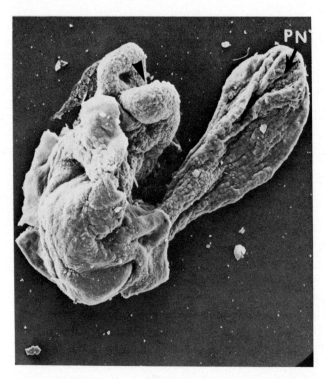

Fig. 4.1. A scanning electron (SE) macrograph of a 10½ day old rat embryo cultured for 24 h in vitro in the rat serum. Note the cranial neural folds (arrows) and the posterior neuropore (PN). × 86.

tions (Hsu, 1979; Copp, 1980, 1981; Spielmann et al., 1980; Papaioannou, 1982). It has been found that the development of early mouse and rat embryos in vitro depends on conditions during incubation (Wordinger and Kell, 1978; Naeslund, 1979; Sellens and Sherman, 1980). It has been shown that normal in vitro development of rat embryos at 9.5 days of gestation, before organogenesis, depends on the method of preparation of the serum for culture (Steele and New, 1974). Serum prepared from blood centrifuged after clotting causes the formation of double hearts in embryos with retarded growth, in contrast to the embryos cultured in serum prepared from blood centrifuged before clotting; these develop normally.

It was found in other experiments that 8 day old mouse embryos can successfully develop through early somite stages and begin differentiation of the central nervous system in rat serum at the same rate as in human cord serum (Wu et al., 1981b).

It has been shown repeatedly that the development of rat or mouse embryos in an in vitro culture system under optimal conditions is no different from that in vivo. Rat embryos explanted at early head-fold stage and grown in vitro over a period of 48 h show very similar rates of growth and differentiation to embryos of the same period of gestation developed in vivo (New et al., 1976). Mouse embryos from the beginning of neuralation (head-fold stage) to the closure of the neural tube and formation of the

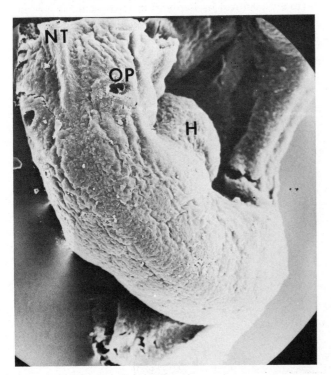

Fig. 4.2. An SE macrograph of the posterior view of an 11½ day old rat embryo cultured for 48 h in vitro. Note the heart (H), otic placode (OP) and the closed neural tube (NT). × 86.

limb buds, when cultured in vitro, grow and develop in a similar way to age-matched embryos in vivo (Sadler and New, 1981). There were no significant differences in the development of the body (number of somites), central nervous system, circulatory system and protein content.

Moreover, in vitro developmental stages which mimic the in vivo conditions were also described for earlier developmental stages. Development of mouse embryos cultured in vitro from the early preimplantation stage (2–4 cell stage embryos) to blastocyst formation is obtained within 2–3 days, similar to the in vivo situation. Similarly, mouse embryos can be cultured in vitro from the blastocyst to early somite stage, undergoing the same developmental stages as in vivo although at a somewhat lower developmental rate (Libbus and Hsu, 1980). After 7 days of incubation these embryos exhibit development of somites, neural folds and heart, reaching stage 14 of mouse development. On the eighth day of culture, further differentiation to stage 15 occurs. In vitro recapitulation of in vivo developmental stages can be considered as a prerequisite for any teratogenic studies performed in this culture system, if conclusions are to be drawn for the in vivo situation.

In vitro culture techniques are important not only for the study of embryonic development but for the development of fetal membranes too. For example, both at 9.5 and 11.5 days, rat embryos were virtually identical in vivo and in vitro as far as volume density and surface density of the vascular system in the yolk sac endoderm were concerned (Gupta et al., 1981).

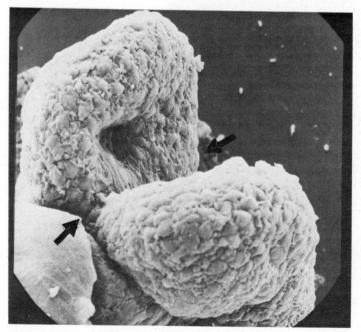

Fig. 4.3. An SE micrograph of the dorsal aspect of the cranial neural folds of the same embryo that is in Fig. 4.1. Note the open anterior neuropore (arrows). × 360.

The apparently normal development through early organogenesis supports the use of cultured embryos as a model system for investigations on the regulation of embryonic development and differentiation. It is therefore not surprising that various teratogenic agents have been tested in this system. Trypan blue, for instance (a well known teratogen in rodents), at concentrations of 150, 300 or 450 μg/ml, is more teratogenic during the first 24 hours of culture of rat embryos at 9.5 days of gestation than when administered to embryos cultured at 10.5 days (Gupta et al., 1981; Gulamhusein, 1981). These data confirm the observations by other investigators that the teratogenic activity of trypan blue at the above mentioned concentrations decreases after 10.5 days of gestation in vivo (Beck and Lloyd, 1966; Berry, 1970). It seems, therefore, that with respect to early organogenesis stages, extrapolation from the in vitro system to the whole animal in vivo can be justified.

Description of the method

Two points are to be emphasised in the description of this method: dissection of the embryos and preparation of the medium for culture (for details, see New, 1978).

At 8–10 days of gestation, pregnant animals (rats or mice) are killed, the uterine horns with embryos are cut out and placed in sterile saline solution and then the conceptuses are removed. These are transfered to fresh saline solution, and the outermost membranous layer, Reichert's membrane, with attached trophoblast and parietal

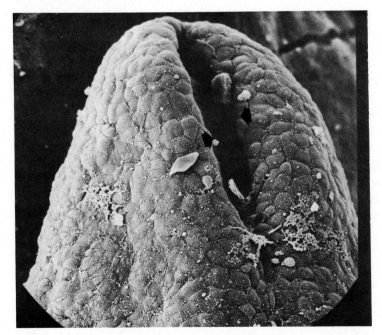

Fig. 4.4. An SE micrograph of the dorsal aspect of the caudal neural folds of the same embryo that is in Fig. 4.1. Note the open posterior neuropore (arrows). × 480.

entoderm is opened and removed, but the visceral yolk sac, amnion and ectoplacental cone are left intact and explanted with the embryo.

Various culture media have been used for the cultivation of mammalian embryos during organogenesis. It has been found that successful results can be obtained using immediately centrifuged rat serum (Steele and New, 1974; Buckley et al., 1978). Blood in sterile conditions is immediately centrifuged (10 min at 3000 revs./min). After 30 min the fibrin clot is formed and the plasma is then recentrifuged. The supernatant serum is stored frozen in sterile tubes. In order to prevent bacterial growth in this highly nutritive medium an antibiotic mixture is added to the serum (penicilin 100 IU/ml and streptomycin 100 μg/ml serum). The serum is inactivated (30 min at 56°C) before use.

The procedure of culture technique is relatively simple. The explanted conceptuses are transfered into sterile glass bottles containing inactivated serum prewarmed at 37°C. One ml of serum is used for each embryo. Between 2 and 6 conceptuses are placed in each culture bottle and are cultured at 37°C for 48 h in a roller incubator chamber (New et al., 1973). The following gassing procedure is used in the Department of Anatomy (Professor F. Beck), University of Leicester, England, and recently in our own laboratory of teratology. The cultures of rat embryos are gassed for 2 min with: beginning of culture; 5% O_2, 5% CO_2, 90% N_2: after 24 h; 20% O_2, 5% CO_2, 75% N_2: after 42 h; 40% O_2, 5% CO_2, 55% N_2. This gassing procedure is vital to the survival and normal growth and differentiation of the rat embryos in culture. The mouse embryos of the same age are cultured during the first 24 h in a gas phase of 5% O_2, 5% CO_2, 90% N_2 and during the second day in a new atmosphere of 20% O_2, 5% CO_2 and 75% N_2 (Sadler, 1979). After two days of culture the embryos are removed from the medium and investigated by morphological or biochemical methods. In order to obtain the maximal benefit of whole-embryo culture techniques, definitive parameters have been developed for the quantitative estimation of embryonic growth and development (Brown and Fabro, 1981). An objective scoring system has been devised which provides a precise measure of morphological development, and several parameters are examined as estimates of embryonic growth.

The use of this morphological scoring system in embryo culture experiments provides a precise index of embryonic development and allows a quantitative comparison of development and growth. Moreover, as the developing nervous system is easily seen at these early stages from the dorsal surface of the embryos (Figs. 4.1–4), one can study the development of different parts of the brain (brain vesicles formation, anterior and posterior neuropore closure, development of the optic system, etc.) by relatively simple macroscopic observations, with the assistance of magnifying lenses. It is therefore not surprising that the embryo culture system became a relatively popular way for the study of CNS malformations, much more than for the study of developmental defects of other organs.

The morphological studies can obviously be accompanied by biochemical studies. A good parameter of embryonic growth and development is the determination of protein content in whole embryos (Gulamhusein, 1981; Sadler and New, 1981; Green-away, et al., 1982). Determination of protein synthesis in different parts of the embryo, as well as the rate of DNA and RNA synthesis under normal conditions and following exposure to teratogens are also of significant value (LaMarca and Wassarman, 1979; Sherman, 1979).

The study of CNS malformations in embryo culture systems
The above described method enables the study of the direct effects of different terato-genic agents on various embryonic organs, including the brain, with subsequent extra-polation of in vitro obtained data to the in vivo situation (Morris and Steele, 1974, 1977; Bruckner et al., 1981; Eto et al., 1981; Sheth et al., 1981; Huxham et al., 1982).

Organ culture systems have also been used for comparison of in vivo and in vitro abnormal neural tube development. In particular, the development of a genetically induced CNS malformation in a mutant, curly tail, mouse has been studied (Copp et al., 1982). In vivo, the majority of non-mutant embryos undergo posterior neuro-pore closure between the 30 and 34 somite stage, whereas approximately 50% of mu-tant (curly tail) embryos show delayed closure, and around 20% maintain an open posterior neuropore even at advanced stages of development. A similar result has been found for embryos developing in vitro from the headfold stage. Later in development, 50–60% of mutant embryos in vivo develop tail flexion defects, and 15–20% lumbo-sacral myeloschisis. This supports the view that delayed posterior neuropore closure is the main developmental lesion leading to the appearance of caudal neural tube de-fects in these mutant mice.

The role of microfilaments and proteoglycans during neuroepithelial morphogene-sis has been studied by using the whole embryo culture method (Morriss-Kay, 1981). It has been shown that microfilament contraction is essential for the development and maintenance of the concave curvature of the neural epithelium. It has also been sug-gested that microfilament contraction is only of morphogenetic significance in the transverse plane at the midbrain/hindbrain regions, whereas in the forebrain it is prob-ably important in all planes. Short-term interruption of microfilament contraction does not necessarily result in open neural tube defects, but has an effect on the size and shape of the neural tube and other embryonic structures. Proteoglycans are also important for growth and specific developmental patterns during the period of cranial neurulation in rat embryos. Chondroitin sulphate proteoglycans probably have a role in relation to neuroepithelial cell shape and cell proliferation, while heparan sulphate proteoglycans may be involved in cell adhesion.

Many articles have been devoted to the in vitro study of the effects of different tera-togenic factors on the development and differentiation of the CNS in order to under-stand the mechanism of their in vivo action (Fraser and Hansen, 1981; Gulamhusein, 1981; Mirkes and Greenaway, 1981a; Schmid et al., 1981; Sim et al., 1981; Walsh et al., 1981). It has been shown, for instance, that cyclophosphamide in doses of 25 μg/ml has teratogenic effects on day 10 rat embryos cultured in vitro (Mirkes and Greenaway, 1981b). Rat embryos exposed to cyclophosphamide (25 mg/kg) in vivo on day 10 of gestation demonstrated the same malformations as the embryos treated with cyclophosphamide (25 μg/ml) in vitro (Greenaway et al., 1982). The most characteristic defects in in vivo and in vitro studies included hypoplasia of the prosencephalon leading to ventrolateral protusions (hammerhead) in the area of the future telencephalon. Histologically, embryos showed a significant reduction in mean mitotic number fron 4.8 to 2.7 mitotic figures per neural tube cross section.

A combination of maternal treatment with in vitro culture has often been used to evaluate the effect of teratogens on embryonic development in the rat. Using this method, specific teratogenic actions of some drugs (thiadiazole, cadmium sulfate, dinoseb, trypan blue, etc.) was shown on 9 and 10 day old rat embryos. (Beaudoin and Fisher, 1981). Each chemical administered at day 9 of pregnancy induced a significant delay in neural tube closure in the cultured embryos, and after 42 h of culture there were still many embryos with open neural tubes. Treatment at day 10 was less inhibitory than treatment at day 9, but thiadiazole, dinoseb and trypan blue significantly reduced the incidence of neural tube closure at 24 h.

It is known that some antibiotics in high doses cause different malformations in embryos when given to pregnant animals. The same results have been observed in in vitro culture systems. For example, rifampicin at concentrations from 12.5 to 50 μg/ml was teratogenic for day 10 rat embryos cultivated in vitro (Greenaway et al., 1981). The anterior neuropore failed to close. Cells along the neural tube lumen were rounded up and often apparently free from the rest of the neural ectoderm. These histological changes were different from those observed in the open neural tube following cytochalasin exposure. It is possible to suggest that although the ultimate defect may be the same, exencephaly, the mechanism of its development varies.

The whole embryo culture technique is particularly suitable for the study of embryos during neurulation, since during this period the embryo and yolk sac are directly exposed to the culture medium or to the gas atmosphere, and substances added to the medium have free access to the embryonic cells. It has been shown that in a gas phase of 5% CO_2 and 20% O_2 a high proportion of cultured rat embryos developed with abnormal or unclosed neural tubes during the first day of culture (days 9.5 to 10.5 of gestation). This was overcome by using a gas phase containing only 5% O_2 during the period of neurulation, although 20% O_2 was found to support normal development for the subsequent 24 h (New et al., 1976a, b).

Some mechanisms of this phenomenon have been studied using transmission electron microscopy (Morriss and New, 1979). In embryos developing in vivo and in vitro with a 5% O_2 gas phase during neurulation, the mitochondria of neuroblasts have few cristae and therefore suggest anaerobic metabolism. In embryos cultured in a 20% O_2 gas phase, the mitochondria had an appearance typical of those in cells with aerobic metabolism. A direct correlation was therefore demonstrated in vitro between aerobic metabolism and abnormal development of the cranial neural tube. It seems that anaerobic metabolism is necessary for normal cranial neural tube development

(Morriss-Kay, 1981). It is possible to explain this correlation knowing the normal in vivo process of neurulation which occurs when the growing rat embryo becomes partially separated from the maternal oxygen source by the enveloping yolk sac.

Another advantage of the in vitro culture method is also the possibility of studying more exactly the teratogenic effect of some factors which have no demonstrable pathological effect in vivo. Cytochalasin D, for instance, in doses of 400 μg/kg, exhibits minimal teratogenicity in rats in vivo, leading in one study to two excencephalic fetuses among the 111 fetuses delivered (Fantel et al., 1981). This low in vivo teratogenicity is contrasted with the very high teratogenic potency of cytochalasin D in rat embryos cultured in vitro. Embryos exposed to cytochalasin D in concentrations at or above 0.31 μg/kg on day 10 showed significant frequencies of neural tube abnormalities, decreased protein content, low somite counts and reduced crown–rump length.

It is known that neural tube defects in man have an overall high frequency with marked geographical variations (for review, see Kaufman, 1981). Their etiology is not well understood but it is accepted that both genetic and environmental factors have a place in this phenomenon. Among the latest environmental factors to be found is vitamin A, which has in experimental animals a significant role in causing neural tube defects.

Morriss (1980) has found genetic differences in the sensitivity of early mouse embryos to the vitamin A effect: administration of vitamin A in relatively low doses (5 and 10 mg/kg) to pregnant mice on day 9 of gestation resulted in significant differences in the rate of malformations between fetuses of mutant (curly tail) and normal (control) strains. While in a regular control strain the malformation rate was 54%, it was only 33–36% in the fetuses of the curly tail strain.

In experiments with in vitro culture methods vitamin A in concentrations over 0.5 μg/ml inhibited the overall growth and differentiation of rat embryos at the primitive streak stage (Morriss and Steele, 1974). Embryos cultured in vitro at the neural plate stage (day 9) in serum containing retinol or retinoic acid at a concentration of 0.5 μg/ml demonstrated multiple malformations, mainly abnormal differentiation of the head and failure of closure of the neural tube (Morris and Steele, 1977). All these abnormalities were in a manner similar to those previously seen in vivo (Morriss, 1972).

Abnormal development of the CNS has been found in experiments with chemically induced diabetes in pregnant animals. Serum from rats made diabetic by the intraperitoneal administration of streptozotocin caused CNS malformations among early somite-stage mouse embryos cultured in vitro (Sadler, 1980a). A high percentage of embryos grown in this serum exhibited inhibition of neural tube closure (exencephaly) which was dose- and age related: a higher incidence of malformations occured among younger (2–3 versus 4–6 somite) embryos and among embryos exposed to serum from severely diabetic animals. Neural folds in the exencephalic embryos were usually wide spaced and were open in the fore, mid or hindbrain regions, or in all three areas simultaneously. A large amount of pyknotic cellular debris (cell death) was found in the neuroepithelium and neural crest cells of embryos cultured for 48 h in serum from severely diabetic animals.

Several factors, including hyperinsulinism, altered glucose levels and ketone bodies, have been suggested as agents responsible for producing abnormalities among diabetic offspring (Landauer, 1972; Cockroft and Coppola, 1977; Horton and Sadler, 1981). Problems arise, however, in trying to evaluate teratogenic effects of these factors in vivo, and in vitro culture methods seems to be more appropriate for achieving this goal. Early somite mouse embryos were therefore cultured in excess glucose, (6.2–9.2 mg/ml versus 1.2 mg/ml in control) and exhibited a high frequency of neural tube defects which were age- and dose related (Sadler, 1980b). More older embryos were affected at the higher concentration of glucose, and younger embryos were affected more often than older embryos. The malformations were characterized by inhibition of cranial neural fold closure involving primary mid and hindbrain regions. In some instances, neural folds were wide-spaced and the lack of fusion extended from the prosencephalon through the rhombencephalon.

Similarly, the ketone β-hydroxybutyrate, was found to produce neural tube malformations in early somite (2–3 somites) mouse embryos, and its effects on embryos cultured at 4 mg/ml displayed inhibition of neural fold closure in cranial (exencephaly) and/or caudal (spina bifida) regions. None of the 5–6 somite embryos were affected at any dose of β-hydroxybutyrate (Horton and Sadler, 1981).

The results obtained in the embryo culture system are similar to those obtained in vivo with induced diabetes in mice and rats (Watanable and Ingalls, 1969; Ornoy and Cohen, 1980), where the high incidence of congenital malformations amongst the offspring was mainly due to CNS malformations. In contrast, the offspring of diabetic women have an increased rate of malformations of various organs, i.e. cardiovascular, skeletal and CNS (Gabbe, 1977).

Conclusions

There are indeed many advantages to the use of the in vitro organ culture system of early somite embryos for the study of teratogenic effects on the developing CNS. However, in spite of these advantages there are specific limitations which make this system only of partial help. The embryos can be kept in culture for a limited period, covering only the initial steps of brain development. Many of the teratogenic effects are not distinct at early developmental stages, but exert their effect during later embryonic development. It is also known that many of the brain developmental defects are minute and have mainly functional significance without evident morphological defects (Ornoy and Yanai, 1980). Such defects will obviously not be observed in the organ culture system. This is even more significant when one considers the whole array of possible behavioral changes caused by teratogenic agents. All these described limitations have been considered against the main advantage of the organ culture system, which offers, apart from relative comfort of the experimental set up, a possibility to detect the direct effect of teratogens on the embryo without maternal or placental modifications. It is apparently best for the assessment of teratogenic potential of different agents to combine both in vitro and in vivo studies.

References

Bavister, B.D. (1980) Recent progress in the study of early events in mammalian fertilization. Dev. Growth Diff. 22, 385–402.

Beadoin, A.R. and Fisher, D.L. (1981) An in vivo/in vitro evaluation of teratogenic action. Teratology 23, 57–61.

Beck, F. and Lloyd, J.B. (1966) The teratogenic effects of azo dyes. In: Advances in Teratology, Vol. 1 (Woollam, D.H.M., ed.) Academic Press, London, pp. 131–193.

Berry, C.L. (1970) The effect of trypan blue on the growth of the rat embryo in vivo. J. Embryol. Exp. Morphol. 23, 213–218.

Brinster, R.L. (1963) Method for in vitro cultivation of mouse ova from two-cell to blastocyst. Exp. Cell Res. 32, 205–208.

Brown, N.A. and Fabro, S. (1981) Quantitation of rat embryonic development in vitro: A morphological scoring system. Teratology 24, 65–98.

Bruckner, A., Henneberry, R. and Freese, F. (1981) Teratogenic effects of valproic acids and phenyloin on mouse embryos in vitro. Teratology 23, 30A.

Buckley, S.K.L., Steele, C.E. and New, D.A.T. (1978) In vitro development of early postimplantation rat embryos. Dev. Biol. 65, 396–403.

Cockroft, D.L. (1976) Comparison of in vitro and in vivo development of rat fetuses. Dev. Biol. 48, 163–172.

Cockroft, D.L. and Coppola, P.T. (1977) Teratogenic effects of excess glucose on head-fold rat embryos in culture. Teratology 16, 141–146.

Copp, A.J. (1980) The development of field vole (*Microtus agrestis*) and mouse blastocysts in vitro: A study of trophoblast cell migration. Placenta I, 47–60.

Copp, A.J. (1981) The mechanism of mouse egg cylinder morphogenesis in vitro. J. Embryol. Exp. Morphol. 61, 277–278.

Copp, A.J., Seller, M.J. and Polani, P.E. (1982) Neural tube development in mutant (curly tail) and normal mouse embryos: The timing of posterior neuropore closure in vivo and in vitro. J. Embryol. Exp. Morphol. 69, 151–167.

Dobbing, J. and Sands, J. (1973) Quantitative growth and development of human brains. Arch. Dis. Child. 48, 757–764.

Edwards, J.A. (1968) The external development of the rabbit and rat embryos. In: Advances in Teratology, Vol. 3 (Woollam, D.H.M., ed.) Logo Press, London, pp. 239–263.

Eto, K., Figueroa, A., Tamura, G. and Pratt, R.M. (1981) Induction of cleft lip in cultured rat embryos by localized administration of tunicamycin. J. Embryol. Exp. Morphol. 64, 1–9.

Fantel, A.G., Greenaway, J.C., Shepard, T.H., Juchau, M.R. and Selleck, S.B. (1981) The teratogenecity of cytochalasin D and its inhibition by drug metabolism. Teratology 23, 223–231.

Fraser, F.C. and Hausen, C. (1981) Increase in neural tube defects in sibs of probands with other kinds of malformation. Teratology 23, 35A.

Gabbe, S.G. (1977) Congenital malformations in infants of diabetic mothers. Obstet. Gynecol. Surv. 32, 125–132.

Greenaway, J.C., Fantel, A.G. and Shepard, T.H. (1981) In vitro metabolic activation of rifampicin teratogenecity. Teratology 23, 37A.

Greenaway, J.C., Fantel, A.G., Shepard, T.H. and Juchau, M.R. (1982) The in vitro teratogenecity of cyclophosphamide in rat embryos. Teratology 25, 335–343.

Gulamhusein, A.P. (1981) Trypan blue teratogenesis in the rat in vitro. In: Culture Technique (Neubert, D. and Merker, H.J., eds.) Walter de Grysler, Berlin, pp. 43–56.

Gupta, M., Gulamhusein, A.P., Beck, F. and Moore, W.J. (1981) The extrapolation of action of a teratogen from the in vitro to the in vivo situation. Teratology 24, 41A–42A.

Horton Jr., W.E. and Sadler, T.W. (1981) The effect of the ketone body, β-hydroxybutyrate on cultured mouse embryos. Teratology 23, 54A.

Hsu, Y.C. (1971) Post-blastocyst differentiation in vitro. Nature 231, 100–102.

Hsu, Y.C. (1972) Differentiation in vitro mouse embryos beyond the implantation stage. Nature 239, 200–202.

Hsu, Y.C. (1973) Differentiation in vitro of mouse embryos to the stage of early somite. Dev. Biol. 33, 403–411.

Hsu, Y.C. (1979) In vitro development of individually cultured whole mouse embryos from blastocyst to early somite stage. Dev. Biol. 68, 453–461.

Hsu, Y.C., Baskar, J., Stevens, L.C. and Rash, J.E. (1974) Development in vitro of mouse embryos from the two-cell stage to the early somite stage. J. Embryol. Exp. Morphol. 31, 235–245.

Huxham, I.M., Gupta, M., Azoubel, R. and Beck, F. (1982) Dose-dependent induction on embryonic abnormalities in vitro by tissue homogenates of placenta and decidua. Brit. J. Exp. Pathol. 63, 95–102.

Jolly, J. and Lieure, C. (1938) Recherches sur la culture des oeufs des mammiferes. Arch. d'Anat. Microsc. Morphol. Exp. 34, 307–374.

Kaufman, M.H. (1981) The role of embryology in teratological research, with reference to the development of the neural tube and heart. J. Reprod. Fert. 62, 607–623.

Kuehl, T.J. and Dukelov, W.R. (1982) Time relations of squirrel monkey (Saimiri sciureus) sperm capacitation and ovum maturation in an in vitro fertilization system. J. Reprod. Fert. 64, 135–137.

LaMarca, M.J. and Wassarman, P.M. (1979) Program of early development in the mammal: changes in absolute rates of syntheses of ribosomal proteins during oogenesis and early embryogenesis in the mouse. Dev. Biol. 73, 103–109.

Landauer, W. (1972) Is insulin a teratogen? Teratology 5, 129–136.

Lemire, R.J., Loeser, J.D., Leech, R.W. and Olvard, E.C. (1975) Normal and Abnormal Development in the Human Nervous System. Harper Low, New York.

Libbus, B.L. and Hsu, Y.C. (1980) Sequential development and tissue organization in whole mouse embryos cultured from blastocyst to early somite stage. Anat. Rec. 197, 317–329.

Mintz, B. (1967) Mammalian embryo culture. In: Methods in Developmental Biology (Wilt, F.M. and Wessells, N.K., eds.) Crowell, New York, pp. 379–400.

Mirkes, P.E. and Greenaway, J.C. (1981a) Teratogenecity of chlorambucil in rat embryos cultured in vitro. Teratology 23, 53A.

Mirkes, P.E. and Greenaway, J.C. (1981b) Teratogenecity of cyclophosphamide teratogenecity in rat embryos cultured in vitro. Teratology 23, 53A.

Morriss, G.M. (1972) Morphogenesis of the malformations induced in rat embryos by maternal hypervitaminosis A. J. Anat. 113, 241–250.

Morriss, G.M. (1980) Neural tube defects: towards prevention and understanding. Nature 284, 121–122.

Morriss-Kay, G.M. (1981) Growth and development of pattern in the cranial neural epithelium of rat embryos during neurulation. J. Embryol. Exp. Morphol. 65, 225–241.

Morriss, G.M. and New, D.A.T. (1979) Effect of oxygen concentration on morphogenesis of cranial neural folds and neural crest in cultured rat embryos. J. Embryol. Exp. Morphol. 54, 17–35.

Morriss, G.M. and Steele, C.E. (1974) The effect of excess vitamin A on the development of rat embryos in culture. J. Embryol. Exp. Morphol. 32, 505–514.

Morriss, G.M. and Steele, C.E. (1977) Comparison of the effects of retinol and retinoic acid on postimplantation rat embryos in vitro. Teratology 15, 109–120.

Naeslund, G. (1979) The effect of glucose-, arginine-, and leucine-deprivation on mouse blastocyst outgrowth in vitro. Upsala J. Med. Sci. 84, 9–20.

New, D.A.T. (1966) Development of rat embryos cultured in blood sera. J. Reprod. Fertil. 12, 509–524.

New, D.A.T. (1978) Whole-embryo culture and the study of mammalian embryos during organogenesis. Biol. Rev. 53, 81–122.

New, D.A.T., Coppola, P.T. and Cockroft, D.L. (1976a) Improved development of headfold rat embryos in culture resulting from low oxygen and modifications of the culture serum. J. Reprod. Fertil. 48,. 219–222.

New, D.A.T., Coppola, P.T. and Cockroft, D.L. (1976b) Comparison of growth in vitro and in vivo of post-implantation rat embryos. J. Embryol. Exp. Morphol. 36, 133–144.

New, D.A.T., Coppola, P.T. and Terry, S. (1973) Culture of explanted rat embryos in rotating tubes. J. Reprod. Fertil. 35, 135–138.

New, D.A.T. and Stein, K.F. (1964) Cultivation of post-implantation mouse and rat embryos on plasma clots. J. Embryol. Exp. Morphol. 12, 101–110.

Nicholas, J.S. and Rudnick, D. (1934) The development of rat embryos in tissue culture. Proc. Natl. Acad. Sci. USA 20, 656–658.

Nicholas, J.S. and Rudnick, D. (1938) Development of rat embryos cylinder to head fold stages in plasma cultures. J. Exp. Zool. 78, 205–232.

O'Rahilly, R. and Gardner, E. (1971) The timing and sequence of events in the development of the human nervous system during the embryonic period proper. Z. Anat. Entwicklungsgesch. 134, 1–17.

O'Rahilly, R. and Gardner, E. (1977) The developmental anatomy and histology of the human central nervous system. In: Handbook of Clinical Neurology, Vol. 30, Pt 1, (Vinken, P.J. and Bruyn, G.W., eds.) North-Holland, Amsterdam, pp. 15–40.

Ornoy, A. and Cohen, A.M. (1980) Teratogenic effects of sucrose diet in diabetic and nondiabetic rats. Isr. J. Med. Sci. 16, 789–791.

Ornoy, A. and Yanai, J. (1981) Central nervous system teratogenicity: experimental model for human problems. In: Advances in the Study of Birth Defects. Vol. 4, Neural and Behavioral Teratology (Persamd, T.V.N., ed.) MTP Press Lancaster, pp. 1–21.

Papaioannou, V.E. (1982) Lineage analysis of inner cell mass and trophoectoderm using microsurgically reconstituted mouse blastocyst. J. Embryol. Exp. Morphol. 68, 199–209.

Rizzino, A. and Sherman, M.I. (1979) Development and differentiation of mouse blastocysts in serum-free medium. Exp. Cell Res. 121, 221–233.

Rottmann, O.J. and Lampeter, W.W. (1981) Development of early mouse and rabbit embryos without zona pellucida. J. Reprod. Fertil. 61, 303–306.

Rugh, R. (1968) The Mouse. Its Reproduction and Development. Burgess Minneapolis, MN, pp. 237–242.

Sadler, T.W. (1979) Culture of early somite mouse embryos during organogenesis. J. Embryol. Exp. Morphol. 49, 17–25.

Sadler, T.W. (1980a) Effects of maternal diabetes on early embryogenesis. I: The teratogenic potential of diabetic serum. Teratology 21, 339–347.

Sadler, T.W. (1980b) Effects of maternal diabetes on early embryogenesis. II: Hyperglycemia induced exencephaly. Teratology 21, 349–356.

Sadler, T.W. and New, D.A.T. (1981) Culture of mouse embryos during neurulation. J. Embryol. Exp. Morphol. 66, 109–116.

Schmid, B.P., Kao, J., Goulding, E.H. and Fabro, S. (1981) Assesment of in vitro teratogenecity of postimplantation mouse embryos treated with cadmium and valproate. Teratology 24, 47A–49A.

Sellens, M.H. and Sherman, M.I. (1980) Effects of culture conditions on the developmental programme of mouse blastocysts. J. Embryol. Exp. Morphol. 56, 1–22.

Sherman, M.I. (1979) Developmental biochemistry of preimplantation mammalian embryos. Annu. Rev. Biochem. 48, 443–470.

Sheth, K., Koszalka, T.R. and Brent, R.L. (1981) The uptake of steroids by rat embryo explants. Teratology 23, 61A–62A.

Sim, F.R.P., Matsumoto, N., Goulding, E.H., Denny, K.H. and Pratt, R.M. (1981) Specific development defects induced by jervine in cultured rodent embryos. Teratology 23, 62A.

Spielmann, H., Jacob-Muller, J. and Beckord, W. (1980) Immunosurgical studies on inner cell mass development in rat and mouse blastocyst before and during implantation in vitro. J. Embryol. Exp. Morphol. 60, 255–269.

Spindle, A. (1980) A improved culture medium for mouse blastocysts. In Vitro 16, 669–674.

Steele, C.E. and New, D.A.T. (1974) Serum variants causing the formation of double hearts and other abnormalities in explanted rat embryos. J. Embryol. Exp. Morphol. 31, 707–719.

Stewart, J. McD. (1981) In vitro fertilization and embryo rescue. Environm. Exp. Bot. 21, 301–315.

Stokes, P.A., Vardy, P.H. and McBride W.G. (1981) Advances in rabbit embryo culture during organogenesis. Dev. Growth Diff. 23, 623–627.

Tam, P.P.L. and Snow, M.H.L. (1980) The in vitro culture of primitive-streak-stage mouse embryos. J. Embryol. Exp. Morphol. 55, 131–143.

Trotnow, S., Al-Hasani, S. and Sadler, M. (1981) Experience with in vitro fertilization of follicular rabbit oocytes and embryos transfer. Arch. Gynecol. 231, 41–50.

Walsh, D.A., McEwen, S.E., Webster, W.S. and Lipson, A.H. (1981) Effects of acute ethanol exposure using in vitro rat embryo cultures. Teratology 23, 68A.

Watanable, G. and Ingalls, T.H. (1969) Congenital malformations in the offspring of alloxan-diabetic mice. Diabetis 12, 66–72.

Wordinger, R.J. and Kell, J.A. (1978) The influence of different simple tissue culture media on the in vitro development of the past blastocyst mouse embryo. IRCS Med. Sci. Biomed. Technol. 6, 12–15.

Wu, T.-C., Wan, Y.-J. and Damjanov, I. (1981a) Positioning of inner cell mass determines the development of mouse blastocysts in vitro. J. Embryol. Exp. Morphol. 65, 105–117.

Wu. T.-C., Wan, Y.-J. and Damjanov, I. (1981b) Rat serum promotes the in vitro development of mouse blastocysts during early somite stages of embryogenesis. J. Exp. Zool. 217, 451–453.

Section II
DRUGS OF USE AND ABUSE
A. BARBITURATES AND OTHER ANTICONVULSANTS,
BENZODIAZEPINES AND ALCOHOL

Neurobehavioral Teratology
edited by Joseph Yanai
© Elsevier Science Publishers BV 1984

5

AN ANIMAL MODEL FOR THE EFFECT OF BARBITURATE ON THE DEVELOPMENT OF THE CENTRAL NERVOUS SYSTEM

Joseph Yanai

Department of Anatomy and Embryology, The Hebrew University–Hadassah Medical School, Box 1172, 91010 Jerusalem, Israel

T HE study of the central nervous system and the behavioral outcome of early (pre- and neotatal) exposure to barbiturate, and the establishment of an animal model of these effects, are pertinent since barbiturate use and abuse is fairly common. According to the U.S. Senate Investigating Committee, in the early seventies there were 500 000 to 1 million barbiturate addicts in the United States alone, and many others using barbiturates in smaller doses for medical purposes. Among pregnant women, 24–32% use sedatives including barbiturates (Forfar and Nelson, 1973; Hill, 1973). Barbiturate indication in pregnant women varies from prophylaxis of neonatal hyperbilirubinemia when administered late in pregnancy (Thomas, 1976; Trolle, 1968), through its antiepileptic effect when given to epileptic pregnant women during the entire pregnancy (Char et al., 1979), to a drug given routinely to manage preeclampsia (Speroff, 1973). In addition, phenobarbital is given during early childhood for the prevention of seizure (Wallace, 1980). Some information is available on the short- and long term consequences of prenatal and neonatal exposure to barbiturates in humans, including changes in CNS and behavior. These investigations are not discussed here and the reader is referred to papers which discuss this subject extensively (Myers and Myers, 1979; Fishman and Yanai, 1983; Wallace, Chapter 6). In general evidence has accumulated indicating that early barbiturate exposure may cause gross malformations (Bethenod and Frederich, 1975) as well as long-lasting behavioral disabilities (Wolf and Forsythe, 1978). The data led to the defining of the 'fetal barbiturate syndrome' (Smith, 1977).

Despite extensive exposure to barbiturates during early development, studies on an animal model for the long-term effect on CNS of early chronic exposure to barbiturates are relatively scarce. By comparison, extensive studies have been conducted on the effects of early administration of another sedative hypnotic, ethanol, on the CNS, and an animal model for the fetal alcohol syndrome is well established (Abel, 1981). The animal studies into the long-term effects on CNS of early exposure to barbiturates have been recently reviewed and compared to similar studies on exposure to ethanol (Yanai, 1981; Fishman and Yanai, 1983). These studies will therefore not be discussed here. Briefly, however, the studies into the effects of early exposure to barbiturates on animal CNS and behavior started 30 years ago with the pioneering work of Armitage (1952), who demonstrated various behavioral changes in adult rats prenatally exposed to phenobarbital. These changes also included learning deficits. No major new data were generated during the subsequent two decades, but one important study which should be mentioned was that of Murai (1966), who also showed learning deficits as well as other behavioral changes in rats prenatally exposed to barbiturates. However, only since the mid-seventies has there been a significant acceleration in the interest and research effort devoted to the study of the effect of early exposure to barbiturates on animal CNS and behavior. A few research groups have provided most of the available data: Middaugh, Zemp and associates (Middaugh et al., 1975; 1981) studied behavioral and neurochemical changes in mice after prenatal exposure to phenobarbital; Schain, Diaz and associates (Schain and Watanabe, 1975; Diaz et al., 1977) studied mainly changes in rat brain weight, but also some behavioral and biochemical changes after neonatal exposure to phenobarbital. Gupta and associates (Gupta et al., 1980a, b) conducted studies on the reproductive physiology of rats after prenatal exposure to phenobarbital; Yanai and associates studied long-lasting behavioral, neurochemical, neuromorphological and metabolic changes in mice of inbred and outbred strains after prenatal and/or neonatal exposure to phenobarbital; these studies are the subject of this chapter.

Methods of administration, the resulting barbiturate levels, and the strains used

In our studies, adult mice used as parents were housed in mating groups of 1 male and 4 females and maintained under standard laboratory conditions. Their offspring (the subjects of the experiments) received phenobarbital prenatally via the placenta, or neonatally via daily injections.

Prenatal administration   The method has been described before (Yanai et al., 1979). Briefly, female parent mice were checked daily at 08.00 h and those that conceived, as evidenced by the existence of a vaginal plug, were separated from the males and housed with other pregnant females. On gestation day 9 (GD 9; the day in which the plug was found is considered GD 1), the females were housed in individual cages. Treated females then received milled mouse food containing 3 g/kg phenobarbital in acid form (their only food source) and water, both available ad libitum. Control females received milled food and water. Drug administration continued until GD 18 when the phenobarbital and control diets were replaced with regular mouse pellets. Appropriate cross-fostering was carried out after delivery as previously described (Yanai et al., 1979), in order to control for the possible carry-over effect of phenobarbital on maternal milk production or behavior. Following delivery and cross-fostering, the barbiturate-exposed offspring and control offspring were maintained with their mothers under standard laboratory conditions and received no further drug treatment.

Neonatal administration   See Yanai and Bergman 1981. In this group, parent females were not checked for vaginal plugs. Instead, female mice were left with the males until pregnancy became apparent, at which time they were moved to individual cages. After delivery, the pups in each litter were divided into control (C) and barbiturate-treated groups. Toe cuttings were used for identification. Treated pups received a daily subcutaneous injection of 50 mg/kg sodium phenobarbital in sterilized water (10 ml vehicle/kg mouse) on days 2–21 (delivery day = 1). Control pups received vehicle injections. After day 21 all of the pups were maintained with their mothers under standard laboratory conditions with no further drug treatment. Although many investigators have administered various drugs to the pups via the mother's milk (by feeding the drug to the mother), we chose the more laborious method of direct administration to the pups in order to avoid the possible indirect effects of the barbiturate known to induce changes in maternal milk production and behavior.

    Phenobarbital concentrations in the treated mother, their fetuses and treated neonates have been described (Yanai et al., 1979; Yanai and Bergman, 1981). Briefly, blood phenobarbital concentration in the pregnant mice averaged 113 ± 12 μg/ml (mean $\pm$ SEM) during most of the phenobarbital feeding period. The phenobarbital levels of the fetuses were similar to the mothers. Treated neonates had at day 2 brain phenobarbital levels of about 45 μg/g, which remained almost unchanged throughout the 24 h postinjection period. Clearance was accelerated on day 10 so that no phenobarbital remained at 24 h postinjection. At 20 days, brain phenobarbital concentration rose only to about a third of the peak concentration of days 2 and 10 and disappeared rapidly so that virtually no phenobarbital remained in the brain after 4 h.

    Unless otherwise specified, experiments employed HS/Ibg (HS) mice. This strain was derived through crosses of eight inbred strains and was deliberately maintained genetically heterogeneous(McClearn et al., 1970). A few studies also employed the heterogeneous albino Sabra strain. Inbred C57BL/10 (C57) and DBA/1 (DBA) were employed in a neuromorphological study (see below). Genetically heterogeneous mice are very prolific and maintain their pregnancy and pups under drug treatment far better than inbred strains. Because of the large gene pool possessed by heterogeneous populations, a case could be made for the general applicability of the effects found. Furthermore, these animals are likely to exhibit effects which inbred strains may not show because of possible specific genetic peculiarities. On the other hand, inbred strains offer uniform, replicable genetic material and may enable demonstration of genotype-environment interaction in studies of early drug effects, as described below.

Neuromorphological deficits

Early studies showing a reduction in brain weight after neonatal exposure to pheno-barbital prompted us to explore whether this change indicated long-lasting fine neuro-morphological deficits after prenatal or neonatal exposure to phenobarbital. In the early studies (Schain and Watanabe, 1975), 30 or 60 mg/kg per day phenobarbital were administered to rat pups via injections on postnatal days 3 to 21. On day 21 the brains of the animals treated with 60 mg/kg phenobarbital weighed 12% less than control brains. Treatment with 30 mg/kg phenobarbital had no effect on brain weight. In subsequent investigations, rat pups were raised artificially, using gastric cannulas on postnatal days 5 to 18 and were given daily injections of 60 mg/kg phenobarbital (Diaz et al., 1977). This method offers a powerful control for undernutrition which may result from changes in suckling behavior as well as any potential change in moth-er-pup interaction stemming from the possible inability of the treated pups to display the cues which will elicit the proper maternal behavior. The 12% reduction in brain weight was again demonstrated in the treated pups suggesting that the effect of barbi-turates on brain morphology is direct and not mediated through undernutrition or changes in maternal care.

In our studies the brains of prenatally and neonatally treated HS mice offspring were removed at age 50 days and prepared for histological studies using the standard haematoxylin/eosin staining technique. Prenatal administration (Yanai et al., 1979) and neonatal administration (Yanai and Bergman, 1981) of phenobarbital caused 8% and 12% reductions in brain weight respectively. These results demonstrated that the reduction in brain weight caused by neonatal phenobarbital administration (Schain and Watanabe, 1975) was considered long lasting, as it persisted into adulthood, and that similar long-lasting changes in brain weight occurred after prenatal phenobarbi-tal exposure. Prenatal exposure to barbiturate resulted in a 30% deficit in the number of the prenatally forming cerebellar Purkinje cells and 15% in the number of the hip-pocampal pyramidal cells. The deficits of these macroneurons did not affect the subse-quent appearance of the neonatally forming granule cells. The area of the cerebellar and hippocampal layers and the neurons of the cerebral cortex were also unaffected by prenatal barbiturate administration (Yanai et al., 1979).

In a subsequent study (Bergman et al., 1980) phenobarbital was given at various periods between gestation days 9 to 18. Similar deficits in the number of Purkinje and pyramidal neurons occurred after all periods of phenobarbital administration, without correlation to the time of origin of the cells. This suggested that phenobarbital can destroy even newly formed neurons.

As expected, the number of neonatally forming granule cells was reduced in the cerebellum and hippocampus by 22–33% following neonatal exposure to phenobarbital (Yanai and Bergman, 1980). However, neonatal administration of phenobarbital also caused a 35% deficit in the number of already formed Purkinje and pyramidal cells. Furthermore, unlike the consequences of prenatal phenobarbital administration, neonatal exposure resulted in a decrease of the area of the hippocampal and cerebellar layers (although only in the higher 50 mg/kg dose and not in the lower 40 mg/kg dose). The cerebral cortex, which was unaffected by prenatal phenobarbital administration, also showed deficits in area and in cell number following neonatal phenobarbital administration. The Purkinje cell losses were later confirmed in rats (Hannah et al., 1982).

The findings presented above suggest that phenobarbital is not as mild a drug as has often been presumed. Many relatively mild insults destroy only proliferating migrating and differentiating brain cells. Examples of these effects are low levels of X-irradiation (Altman, 1975), 5-azacytidine (Rodier, 1977) and undernutrition (Clos et al., 1977). However, phenobarbital destroyed even already formed neurons. In this respect it possesses a similar neurotoxicity to another sedative hypnotic, ethanol. Thus, adult rats neonatally treated with ethanol had a brain weight of approximately 12% lower than those in the control group, and had a reduction in the area of the cerebellar layers and a deficit of about 20% in the number of the granule and Purkinje cells (Bauer-Moffet and Altman, 1977).

Further studies were carried out to assess the dendritic architecture of the surviving neurons, employing the Purkinje cells and using the Golgi staining technique (Yanai and Iser, 1981). Prenatally treated Sabra animals were studied at age 50 days; neonatally treated animals were studied at both ages 14 and 50 days. Several alternative outcomes could have been expected: (1) that deficits would occur in the dendritic tree of the cells which survived after early exposure to phenobarbital, (2) that these cells would actually have a more developed dendritic tree as a compensating mechanism for the lost neurons, and (3) that no early phenobarbital-induced changes would be found. The results showed that neither prenatal nor neonatal exposure affected the area of the two-dimensional Purkinje cell dendritic tree. The number of branches at the various levels in the dendritic tree was not affected by early phenobarbital exposure. The numer of dendritic spines per mm in the prenatally exposed animals was normal, but the neonatally exposed animals had both short- (day 14) and long-lasting deficits in the number of dendritic spines. The deficits were relatively small, but it should be noted that they added to the already existing deficits in the number of Purkinje cells. In general, however, it may be concluded that the deficits in the dendritic tree architecture induced by early administration of phenobarbital were minimal. This was in contrast to the extensive damage to the dendritic tree induced by milder insults such as undernutrition (Pysh. et al., 1979). One possible explanation is that postnatal undernutrition, which destroyed the cerebellar granule cells but spared the Purkinje cells, markedly decreased the ratio of granule cells to Purkinje cells. On the other hand, neonatal phenobarbital administration, which destroyed both types of neurons, did not have a significant effect on the ratio of granule cells to Purkinje cells. Thus it is possible that degeneration would occur in the Purkinje dendritic tree if it did not have enough granule cells to which to synapse.

A detailed study was conducted on the ultrastructure of the cerebellar cortex at the area of the pyramis vermis. The long-term effect of phenobarbital was studied at age 50 days in prenatally and neonatally treated mice. In addition, short-term effects were studied in neonatally treated mice on day 14 (Fishman et al., 1983). In all groups studied, extensive degenerative processes and abnormalities were found, including mitochondrial degeneration, which ranged from swelling, collapse of cristae and vacuolization, to total granularization. Severly degenerated mitochondria ended up clustered. Lamellar bodies were found throughout the cytoplasm and cell processes. In addition, there was myelin sheath degeneration throughout, including scattered swelling, collapse and twisting of the coat and electron dense inclusions. Many examples of the degeneration appeared to have occurred relatively shortly before the brain was removed. Thus, outcomes of phenobarbital were unique since, despite the rapid clearance of the drug, not only was the degeneration it induced long lasting, but apparently even the *degenerative processes* themselves were long lasting. It would be interesting further to study the mechanisms of the degenerative processes still present in adult animals 50 days after the drug has cleared. Because of the extensive neural damage induced by early phenobarbital administration, it became pertinent to assess the effects of phenytoin, one of the preferred phenobarbital substitutes in the treatment of seizures. Since the two drugs are often indicated in combination, we have studied the cerebellar ultrastructure in mice after neonatal exposure to 50 mg/kg phenobarbital (as described above), 50 mg/kg phenytoin, or a phenobarbital-phenytoin combination of 25 mg/kg each (Fishman et al., 1982a). As in the previous experiments, phenobarbital induced long-lasting ultrastructural degeneration. Both phenytoin and the phenytoin-phenobarbital combination induced extensive ultrastructural deficits. The deficits from the two drugs combined would have probably been the most severe; however, the effect of this treatment was exceedingly toxic and many of the pups died, possibly allowing a selection against the most affected individuals to take place. A triad of neuronal abnormalities was found: mitochondrial degeneration, myelin breakdown and lamellar-forming bodies. These were not equally distributed in all treatment groups. Phenobarbital exposure was strongly associated with myelin deficits and marked mitochondrial degeneration at days 14 and 50. In the phenobarbital-phenytoin group similar mitochondrial degeneration appeared, mainly at age 14 days.

The response of the CNS to input of various agents, including drugs, may be dependent in its extent on genetic factors. This phenomenon, well known as genotype-environment interaction (Holdane, 1946), was studied extensively and reviewed by Broadhurst (1978), and it is the central theme of the scientific field 'psychopharmacogenetics' (Eleftheriou, 1975). A similar phenomenon during prenatal development was well established in behavior-genetic analysis (Thompson and Olian, 1961; DeFries, 1964). It was expected that similar genotype-environment interaction would occur when drugs were used as the environmental variable. Indeed, the extent of the fetal alcohol syndrome in humans is determined in part by genetic factors (Christoffel and Salafs-key, 1975). Consequently, an animal model was established for the assessment of the possible heritable components in the neuronal sensitivity to phenobarbital (Yanai et al., 1983). Pups of the strains HS/Ibg (HS), C57BL/10 (C57) and DBA/1 (DBA) were injected with phenobarbital neonatally, as described above. In order to control for the possible genetic effect on maternal behavior or milk production, all pups were fostered by lactating HS dams. The cerebellar histology of the neonatally treated animals was studied at adulthood. Some of the phenobarbital-induced deficits previously seen in HS mice were again demonstrated in all three strains to a similar extent. The deficits included a reduction in brain weight and in the number of Purkinje cells. However, the area of the cerebellar layers was reduced significantly in HS and C57 strains but not in the DBA strain, clearly suggesting genotype-environment interaction. Although strain differences in CNS morphology were previously shown (Roderick et al., 1973; Wimer et al., 1980), it is still noteworthy that the strains markedly differed in almost every component of the cerebellar morphology. Thus, control C57 had smaller cere-bellar layers than HS, and DBA had smaller cerebellar layers than both HS and C57. The strain differences in the number of Purkinje cells did not correspond to the differ-ences in the cerebellar layers, for while both C57 and DBA had fewer Purkinje cells than HS, they did not differ from each other in this variable. In addition to the demonstration of genotype-environment interaction, the study provided other infor-mation:

(1) Inbreeding depression may occur in brain morphology, since the cerebellum was quantitatively less developed in inbred strains compared to the heterogeneous stocks.

(2) The inbreeding depression did not include the neurosensitivity to early pheno-barbital administration. On the contrary, the inbred DBA strain suffered less neuro-morphological damage than either HS or C57. This may be explained by the fact that the DBA strain possesses relatively great CNS resistance to barbiturate upon initial exposure (Sieman and Chan, 1976) despite its relatively slow rate of barbiturate meta-bolism. The fact that inbred strains were not necessarily more neurosensitive to barbi-turate during development than outbred stocks may represent a general phenomenon in drug teratology, and, in fact, in a study on ethanol teratogenicity (Giknis et al., 1980) the outbred strains did not generally exhibit a greater resistance to ethanol than the inbred strains.

An autoradiographic study provided more insight into the process of neuronal losses following prenatal exposure to phenobarbital. Control and phenobarbital-treated pregnant mice were given a single [³H]-thymidine injection on gestation day 13, 15 or 17. The number of labelled cells was counted at age 50 days (Yanai et al., 1982a). A marked reduction in the number of labelled cells occurred among the treated animals in the prenatally formed neurons of the cerebellum, hippocampus and cerebral cortex. Thus barbiturate apparently decreased the number of nerve cells added to the brain (reduction of cell 'birthdays'). This could occur via several mechanisms, including a reduction in the number of cell divisions or via a prolongation of the phases of cell division. In the absence of a compensatory addition of cells, as no shift in the labelling curve could be demonstrated, the final number of cells would have to be smaller and, indeed, was smaller in adult animals (Yanai et al., 1979). It is also possible that part of the reduction in labelling represents a destruction by phenobarbital of labelled cells, since phenobarbital could destroy even already formed neurons (Yanai and Bergman, 1981). The decrease in labelling was much larger than the final decrease in the number of cells (Yanai et al., 1979). Moreover, extensive reduction in labelling was shown even in the cortex, where no deficit in the final number of cells could be demonstrated before. (Yanai et al., 1979). Although it is likely that autoradiography is a more sensitive method for the detection of neural changes than the conventional methods of cell counting, only the existence of some recovery of cell number can explain the discrepancy between the results of the two methods. Recovery does not necessarily require compensatory addition of new cells. Rather, it may be mediated by a compensatory reduction of normal cell death (Cowan, 1973).

Early exposure to phenobarbital affects the levels and metabolism of sex hormones (Gupta et al., 1980a,b; Weidenfeld et al., in press; see below for further discussion) and, potentially, the sex-related area of the brain. Thus, it became pertinent to study the effect of prenatal exposure to phenobarbital on the sexually dimorphic medial preoptic area (MPOA). Autoradiographic study was conducted on the MOPA using a design similar to that of the experiment described above. In general, females had a greater packing density (cells/mm^2) than males. This sex difference disappeared in animals prenatally exposed to phenobarbital, possibly due to a marked early phenobarbital-induced decrease in cell 'birthdays' (labelling) in females but not in males (Yanai et al., 1982b). The greatest reduction of labelled cells occurred in the most sexually dimorphic areas of the MPOA.

Sensitivity and tolerance to barbiturate and ethanol

Repeated exposure to barbiturates or various other psychotrophic drugs results in reduced sensitivity to the drugs upon further exposure. This phenomenon, referred to as tolerance, is transient (Kalant et al., 1971; Tabakoff et al., 1978a). On the other hand, when the barbiturate is administered during early development, the changes in brain response to the drug last longer (Yanai and Tabokoff, 1979). Thus, 50 day old male offspring prenatally exposed to the drug and control animals received a daily injection of 50 mg/kg pentobarbital ip. Sleep time and temperature loss were monitored. The injection was repeated for three consecutive days. Both barbiturate and control offspring developed functional (CNS) tolerance following the repeated pento-barbital administration, demonstrated by their shorter sleep time and their higher brain pentobarbital levels upon awakening. However, barbiturate-treated offspring had shorter sleep time with higher brain pentobarbital levels than controls upon awakening, as well as less temperature loss. The greatest differences occurred on the second injection day. This suggests that the effect was not only on brain sensitivity to barbiturate, but possibly also on the rate of development of tolerance. These findings have been confirmed on rats. The rat mothers received barbital in their drinking water during pregnancy and lactation. The offspring had a shorter sleep time following a single pentobarbital injection. Since brain levels were not monitored, it is not yet known whether the shortened sleep time resulted from functional or metabolic changes (Harris and Case, 1979). More recently, the possible generality of this phenomenon to other sedative hypnotics was demonstrated with ethanol (Abel et al., 1981).

Cross-functional tolerance between barbiturate and ethanol is a well established phenomenon (Wahlstrom, 1971; Frankel et al., 1977) which, like other types of tolerance, is expected to be transient. Yet adult mice who were prenatally exposed to phenobarbital had a shorter sleep time than controls following a single injection of 3.5 g/kg ethanol. This lessened sensitivity was due to factors residing within the CNS, as the barbiturate-derived offspring had higher brain ethanol levels upon awakening. The rate of ethanol metabolism was not affected by prenatal barbiturate exposure (Yanai and Tabakoff, 1980). This phenomenon also seemed true for rats. In Harris and Case's study (1979) offspring born to rats had a shorter sleep time following 3 g/kg ethanol than control offspring. It is not known if this change was functional or metabolic as ethanol levels were not monitored.

The results demonstrate the new phenomenon of prenatally induced long-term tolerance and cross tolerance. This phenomenon is of potential significance since if tolerance is related to the addictive process, adults whose mother consumed barbiturate during pregnancy may be more liable to addiction to barbiturate or alcohol upon subsequent exposure. More recent studies have been conducted to elucidate the possible mechanisms mediating the prenatally induced long-term tolerance. Research results demonstrating changes in sensitivity of the post-synaptic dopamine receptors are promising, and are discussed below with other biochemical changes.

Susceptibility to audiogenic seizures

Mice display convulsive seizures as part of the withdrawal syndrome after chronic barbiturate consumption at adulthood (Freund, 1971; Belknap et al., 1973). These symptoms start when a great proportion of the drug has already cleared, and they disappear shortly after complete clearance.

In our studies, HS mice prenatally or neonatally exposed to phenobarbital were tested for susceptibility to audiogenic seizures at age 28 days (Yanai et al., 1981). While animals with prenatal exposure to phenobarbital did not differ from controls in seizure susceptibility, animals exposed to phenobarbital at age 2–21 days had a three-fold increase over control levels in susceptibility to audiogenic seizure, thus suggesting that the neonatal period is the sensitive period for the induction of susceptibility to audiogenic seizures. In previous studies, Murai (1966) injected rats with daily doses of 5 mg/kg phenobarbital on gestation days 5–8 or 17–20. The offspring were tested at adulthood for electroshock seizure. As in the mouse experiment discussed above, administration of barbiturate late in pregnancy did not affect seizure. However, rat offspring whose mothers received barbiturate during early pregnancy were less susceptible to electroshock seizures than controls. Electroshock seizures and audiogenic seizures do not necessarily share a common etiology, and the two experiments described differed in the species of the test animals and the time during pregnancy of the drug administration. Yet the data seem to suggest that prenatal administration of barbiturate does not enhance seizure susceptibility. The neonatal period was the more sensitive in the effect of barbiturate on seizure.

The increased susceptibility to audiogenic seizures appears as a general phenomenon after early administration of various agents. It seems to represent a general hyperexcitability of the CNS rather than prolonged withdrawal, since it may result from both addictive and non-addictive substances, which do not cause withdrawal. Accordingly, early ethanol administration induces the susceptibility to audiogenic seizure where the sensitive period was the neonatal one (Yanai and Ginsberg, 1979). However, prenatal administration of methylmercury (Menashi et al., 1982) or bacterial endotoxin (Hazart, 1982) also induced a long-term increase in susceptibility to audiogenic seizures.

Changes in hippocampal behaviors: spontaneous alternations and performance in an eight-arm maze

Relatively few studies have attempted to demonstrate a causal relationship between behavioral changes and early induced neuromorphological and neurochemical deficits. One apparent reason is that early insults affect the morphology of extensive regions of the brain, thus making it difficult to correlate specific neuromorphological damage with particular functional (behavioral) changes. It may be possible, however, to ascertain the correlation if 'region-specific behaviors' are studied. Obviously, no behavior can be attributed entirely to one specific brain region. However, certain behaviors have been correlated mainly with a specific brain region. The hippocampus is a region which has been investigated very extensively in structure, biochemistry and function (O'Keefe and Nadel, 1978; Olton, 1977; Storm-Mathison, 1977). The behavior in a radial maze (Olton and Samuelson, 1976) was correlated electrophysiologically with the hippocampus (Olton et al., 1978), and the integrity of the hippocampus and its afferents and efferents is necessary for the normal expression of this behavior (Olton and Papas, 1979). Similarly, spontaneous alternation (Dennis and Sollenberger, 1934) is commonly regarded as a 'hippocampal' behavior (Roberts et al., 1962). Indeed, in our studies, we have demonstrated that early barbiturate administration which impaired the hippocampus (among other structures) also caused extensive deficiencies in radial maze behavior and spontaneous alternation. Thus, mice prenatally or neonatally exposed to phenobarbital were tested for spontaneous alternation at ages 22, 28, 35 and 42 days (Pick and Yanai, 1982). Neonatally treated animals had significantly fewer alternations than controls on all testing days. The differences in alternation between controls and animals prenatally treated with phenobarbital were small and did not reach statistical significance. The more sensitive test, delayed spontaneous alternation (30 s), was subsequently applied to an additional group of prenatally treated animals at age 42 days. This test demonstrated markedly less alternation in treated animals than in controls. It should be noted that the greater behavioral deficits induced by neonatal as compared to prenatal phenobarbital exposure corresponded to the greater neuronal deficits that occurred after treatment in this period. Yet, this association between the behavioral and the neuromorphological events should be considered only indicative of a possible correlation. Further extensive studies are required in order to establish adequately the causal relationship between changes in hippocampal morphology induced by early phenobarbital treatment and changes in spontaneous alternations.

In another 'hippocampal' behavior, performance in the radial eight-arm maze (Pick and Yanai, 1982), control mice had 7.9 correct entries out of a maximum possible 8.0, after the fifth test day. However, mice prenatally or neonatally exposed to phenobarbital needed an average of 25% more entries to reach the water reward in all eight arms during the five test days. The number of phenobarbital exposed mice attaining the maximum score was one third that of controls.

Long-lasting induction of a microsomal drug-oxidizing system

Changes in the activity of the hepatic enzymes that metabolize drugs have consequences on behavior since they mediate response to the drugs (metabolic tolerance) and affect hormonal levels. It is known that following phenobarbital administration to pregnant female rodents, the fetuses and the neonates may demonstrate the activity of a microsomal drug-oxidizing system similar to that found in adults (Hart et al., 1962). The studies demonstrated only short-term effects, and the possibility that the metabolic changes were long-lasting was not investigated, perhaps because enzyme induction in adults is mostly transient. This fact is particularly true for the induction of a microsomal drug-oxidizing system (Conney, 1967).

The activity of a microsomal drug-oxidizing system was studied in 45 day old HS mice prenatally exposed to phenobarbital (Yanai, 1979). The barbiturate-exposed offspring had a 32% higher in vitro activity of microsomal enzymes. The significance of this finding is the demonstration that, in contrast to induction at adulthood, induction of the microsomal drug-oxidizing system during the prenatal period, when the liver is still developing, is long term. This unique long-term enzyme induction could have significant consequences, even on behavior, since microsomal enzymes metabolize steroids, including sex hormones (Conney and Klutch, 1963). Indeed, the offspring with the induced microsomal enzyme activity also had a smaller seminal vesicle size than controls (Yanai, 1979), probably indicating low testosterone levels (Hershberger et al., 1953). Recently, Gupta et al. (1980b;1982) directly demonstrated a reduction in testosterone and reproductive function in male rats after prenatal exposure to phenobarbital. Our studies suggested that mice neonatally exposed to phenobarbital showed less in vitro enzymatic aromatization of brain [1,2-^{3}H]testosterone to estradiol than controls (Weidenfeld et al., in press). Unlike the changes in hepatic enzymes and steroid hormones caused by prenatal phenobarbital exposure, the changes in testosterone aromatization induced by *neonatal* phenobarbital administration were short term. However, the potential ensuing behavioral changes could be long lasting.

The phenomenon of long-term enzyme induction by prenatal substrate administration is not restricted to barbiturate; it was also demonstrated with ethanol (Sze et al., 1976). Yet it is entirely different from what appears as a long-term microsomal drug induction by TCDD and similar substances (Lucier et al., 1975) as this substance and other compounds with a similar action are metabolized very slowly. Thus, unlike barbiturate and ethanol, which are metabolized immediately, these compounds are still present in the body at adulthood so that the enzyme induction they produce is actually short term.

Changes in thyroid hormone levels

Many of the neural and behavioral changes induced by early barbiturate administration resembled the changes induced by manipulating the thyroid hormone system either during development or at adulthood. Among the changes were brain cell proliferation and ultrastrucural degeneration (Lauder, 1977), sensitivity to narcosis induced by barbiturate (Breese et al., 1975) or ethanol (Breese et al., 1974), susceptibility to audiogenic seizures (Seyfried et al., 1979) and changes in the catecholamine neurotransmitters (Safaei and Timiras, 1982), including sensitivity of postsynaptic dopamine receptors (Atterwille, 1981). Consequently, it became pertinent to study changes in thyroid hormone levels induced by early exposure to phenobarbital as a possible mediator of some of the phenobarbital-induced neural and behavioral changes. Normally, serum thyroxine levels (T_4) peak sharply at the end of the second postnatal week in mice. However, treating neonatal mice with phenobarbital completely eliminated this marked T_4 peak (Fishman et al., 1982b). This particular effect was transient, although its possible neural and behavioral consequences could be long lasting.

Changes in neurotransmitter systems

It appears particularly relevant to study changes induced by early phenobarbital administration in the dopaminergic system. This is due to the known relationship between the state of arousal of the dopaminergic system and behavioral and biochemical processes affected by early phenobarbital administration. For example, prenatal exposure to barbiturates resulted in long-term deficits in various measures related to learning (Armitage, 1952; Harris and Case, 1979; Middaugh et al., 1975; Murai, 1966; Pick and Yanai, 1982). These behaviors were implicated in many studies as being affected by the state of the dopaminergic synapse (Shayweitz et al., 1978). Locomotor activity which can be induced by stimulating the post-synaptic dopaminergic receptors (Kelly et al., 1975) was also affected in some of these studies by prenatal exposure to barbiturates. The susceptibility to audiogenic seizures is also altered by manipulating the dopaminergic system (Anlezark et al., 1978) and seizure incidence was enhanced by neonatal phenobarbital exposure (Yanai et al., 1981). Similarly, the relationship between thyroid hormones and the sensitivity of the postsynaptic dopamine receptors is well established (Atterwille, 1981), and phenobarbital has been shown to eliminate the thyroid hormone peak which normally appears during development (Fishman et al., 1982b). Mice prenatally exposed to phenobarbital had long-lasting reduction in brain sensitivity to barbiturate and ethanol (Yanai and Tabakoff, 1979; 1980) and an accelerated acquisition of functional (CNS) tolerance to barbiturate (Yanai and Tabakoff, 1979). The relationship between the dopaminergic system and CNS response to barbiturate has not been clearly established. Only a few attempts have been made to study the sensitivity of the dopamine receptors in adult animals that became tolerant to barbiturate as a result of chronic exposure. The results were inconsistent (Tarsy and Badessarini, 1974; Seeber and Kuschensky, 1975). In studies with a related sedative hypnotic, ethanol, results were equivocal as some studies showed the dopamine receptors' supersensitivity (Engel and Liljequist, 1976; Lai et al., 1980), while others demonstrated subsensitivity following chronic ethanol exposure (Hoffman and Tabakoff, 1977; Rabin et al., 1980; Tabakoff et al., 1978b). Using the opposite experimental approach, dopaminergic receptor supersensitivity was induced in mice via the well established methods of chronic exposure to haloperidol or via icv injection of 6-hydroxydopamine (6-OHDA) preceded by desipramine (DMI) treatment (Yanai and Feigenbaum, 1982). The treated animals had a lower CNS sensitivity to barbiturate and ethanol narcosis than controls. On the other hand, when the dopamine receptors of rats were rendered subsensitive via prenatal exposure to haloperidol, the animals had an increased CNS sensitivity to barbiturate narcosis (Yanai and Fishman, 1983). The results suggest that resistance to barbiturate and ethanol may be mediated by supersensitivity of the post-synaptic dopaminergic receptors. It follows that the offspring of barbiturate-consuming mothers that possess CNS resistance to ethanol and barbiturate should also have supersensitive dopamine receptors. In order to test this hypothesis, adult mice prenatally exposed to phenobarbital were tested for apomorphine-induced hypothermia (Yanai and Feigenbaum, 1981). Treated offspring were more resistant to apomorphine hypothermia than controls. Apomorphine is a dopamine agonist which induces hypothermia apparently by acting on the dopamine receptors in the rostral hypothalamus (Sweatman and Jell, 1977) or the mesolimbic system (Grabowska and Ander, 1976). Accordingly, one may assume that prenatal exposure to phenobarbital induces subsensitivity of the dopamine receptors. To verify this assumption prenatally treated mice were tested for apomorphine-induced locomotor activity. This behavior is considered an indication of the sensitivity of dopamine receptors, primarily in the nucleus accumbens (Kelly et al., 1975). Prenatal exposure to phenobarbital increased apomorphine-induced locomotor activity by as much as 32% ($p < .001$, Yanai, 1983). There is an apparent contradiction between the two consequences of apomorphine administration, hypothermia and locomotor activity. Therefore, studies were conducted in our laboratory on the etiology of apomorphine-induced hypothermia (Feigenbaum and Yanai, 1982). Supersensitivity of the dopamine receptors was induced in adult mice via DMI, 6-OHDA treatment. As expected the treatment accentuated apomorphine-induced locomotor activity. However, the treated animals were more resistant than controls to the hypothermic effect of apomorphine, demonstrating that resistance to apomorphine hypothermia is an indication of dopamine receptor supersensitivity. It may be concluded that prenatal exposure to phenobarbital induces long-term supersensitivity of the postsynaptic dopamine receptors, as demonstrated by both the increase in locomotor activity and the decrease in hypothermia after apomorphine injection.

Apomorphine induces stereotyped 'climbing behavior' in mice, presumed to be mediated by stimulation of striatal and possibly nucleus accumbens-located dopamine receptors (Costall et al., 1980; Protais et al., 1976). Neonatal exposure to phenobarbital caused short-term reduction in climbing behavior (Yanai et al., 1982c), suggesting striatal receptor subsensitivity. These results do not necessarily contradict the findings of the effect of prenatal phenobarbital on apomorphine-induced locomotor activity and hypothermia because (a) this experiment differed from the aforementioned research in chosen time of phenobarbital administration (prenatal vs. neonatal), and (b) the changes demonstrated in climbing behavior were short term, disappearing at adulthood when the animals were rendered resistant to barbiturate and ethanol narcosis. However, the issue of the relationships between outcomes of different apomorphine-induced behaviors in animals with early phenobarbital administration, requires further study involving direct assessment with binding assays. At the time of writing, we are conducting such an investigation.

The catecholaminergic system was further investigated, since presynaptic events in the dopaminergic system could effect the sensitivity of the postsynaptic dopamine (DA) receptors and because there is a known relationship between tolerance and the noradrenergic (NE) system (Tabakoff et al., 1978a). Striatal and hypothalamic NE and DA were assayed after prenatal or neonatal exposure to phenobarbital. The levels of both neurotransmitters were found to be below control levels (Yanai, 1983). The turnover of these neurotransmitters is under study. These findings are in agreement with those of Middaugh et al. (1981), who showed a reduction in whole brain NE and DA levels after prenatal exposure to barbiturate. In addition, treated offspring had a greater uptake of DA, NE, serotonin and γ-aminobutyric acid than controls.

The serotonergic system mediates some of the behaviors which are known to be affected by early phenobarbital exposure. Among them is the development of barbiturate tolerance (Kahanna et al., 1980). Consequently, tryptophan hydroxylase (TPH) activity was studied after prenatal and neonatal exposure to phenobarbital as an indicator of the serotonergic system. There were only small and not statistically significant differences between treated and control offspring for TPH activity, suggesting a more central role of the catecholaminergic systems rather than the serotonergic system in mediating the early phenobarbital-induced changes in behavior, particularly changes in sensitivity and tolerance to barbiturate and ethanol (Yanai, 1983).

Methodological considerations

A central methodological issue in the early administration of barbiturate, as well as in many other insults, is the question of direct effect versus non-specific, indirect effect. Within this issue a major problem is undernutrition, since sedated pregnant females may not be able to consume normal amounts of food, and sedated pups may not be able to suckle enough milk. Possible undernutrition or malnutrition is particularly relevant in studies on early ethanol administration, since ethanol may replace more nutritious food. It appears that undernutrition does not mediate the effect of early barbiturate administration for the following reasons.

(1) Unlike ethanol, barbiturates have no caloric value and under the conditions in my laboratory did not decrease food intake. In fact, barbiturates are known to enhance food intake (Opitz and Akinlaja, 1966). (2) Prenatally treated adult offspring achieved normal body weight (Yanai et al., 1979). Among neonatally treated mice only males had a small reduction in body weight from control levels (Yanai and Bergman, 1981), yet both females and males had neural and behavioral deficits. (3) Rat neonates raised artificially, under conditions that completely controlled for undernutrition, still had deficits in brain weight similar to those found in our experiment (Diaz et al., 1977). (4) Similarly, administration of phenobarbital to a fetal mouse spinal cord culture induced morphological and biochemical deficits (Bergey et al., 1981). (5) Many of the deficits occurring after early phenobarbital administration did not resemble those induced by undernutrition. For example, phenobarbital destroyed neurons which were already formed (Yanai and Bergman, 1981), while undernutrition destroyed only proliferating cells (Clos et al., 1977). On the other hand, undernutrition caused extensive dendritic aberrations (Griffin et al., 1977; Pysh et al., 1979), while phenobarbital did not affect the dendritic branches but caused specific deficits in the dendritic spines (Yanai and Iser, 1981). Furthermore, (6) the result of prenatal pheno-

barbital administration was opposite to that of undernutrition; while undernutrition is known to potentiate the effects of ethanol and barbiturate, prenatal ethanol administration acted specifically to decrease sensitivity to barbiturate and ethanol (Yanai and Tabakoff, 1979; 1980).

Other possible indirect effects of barbiturate should be taken into account. Among them is the hypothermic effect occurring in high doses, which alone is teratogenic. The fact that barbiturate impairs maternal behavior and milk production necessitated its direct administration to the pups, but even this condition does not offer complete control for indirect effects, since impaired pups may have a suckling disability or an inability to display the cues necessary to elicit the proper maternal care.

There are, of course, countless other indirect ways in which barbiturates can act. For example, phenobarbital depresses uterine contraction. All these possibilities should be taken into account when evaluating outcomes of early barbiturate administration.

Summary: mechanisms mediating phenobarbital effect

The findings presented in this chapter are summarized below in a heuristic manner designed to suggest mechanisms possibly mediating the effects of early phenobarbital administration on behavior; however, studies of these mechanisms are still in their earliest stages. Several possible mechanisms may be proposed, but only tentatively, since there remain alternative hypotheses which have not yet been ruled out. Our studies demonstrated that early exposure to phenobarbital affected several behaviors, including susceptibility to audiogenic seizures (Yanai et al., 1981), CNS sensitivity to barbiturate and ethanol and accelerated acquisition of barbiturate functional tolerance (Yanai and Tabakoff, 1979; 1980), spontaneous alternations and performance in the eight-arm maze (Pick and Yanai, 1982), and various apomorphine-induced behaviors (Yanai and Feigenbaum, 1981; 1982; Yanai et al., 1982c). Studies conducted in other laboratories demonstrated changes in certain other behaviors; among them were learning (e.g. Armitage, 1952; Middaugh.et al., 1975), activity (Murai, 1966; Middaugh et al., 1981), and sexual function (Gupta et al., 1980a; 1982), as discussed earlier in this chapter.

Early administration of phenobarbital induced changes in the thyroid hormone system (Fishman et al., 1982b) either via the induction of a microsomal drug-oxidizing system (Yanai, 1979) or via more direct pathways. It is possible that thyroid hormone could change behavior via its effect on CNS morphology (Lauder, 1977). The relationship between neuromorphological alterations and the behaviors which are affected by early phenobarbital exposure was best demonstrated in the case of audiogenic seizures (Ginsburg, 1967), although most other behaviors are probably affected by the neuromorphological alterations. Another mode of action for thyroid hormone is through its known effect on catecholamines and dopamine receptors (Alterwill, 1981). Here the behaviors most likely to be affected are barbiturate and ethanol sleep time (Yanai and Tabakoff, 1979; 1980) and apomorphine-induced behaviors (Yanai and Feigenbaum, 1981; 1982; Yanai et al., 1982c).

Early phenobarbital administration altered sex hormones (Gupta et al., 1980b; Weidenfeld et al., in press), either directly or via the induction of a microsomal drug-oxidizing system (Yanai, 1979). The alteration in sex hormone was the most probable cause of a decrease in sexual function (Gupta et al., 1980b; 1982). In addition, estrogen could have acted on behaviors by altering dopamine receptors (Bedard et al., 1978; Gordon et al., 1980), as in the thyroxine effect on dopamine receptors. The most likely behaviors to have been affected this way were sensitivity to drugs and the apomorphine-induced behaviors cited above. Changes in steroid hormones are also a possible cause for the elimination of sexual dimorphism in brain structure (Yanai et al., 1982b) and the resulting sexual differences in behavior.

As discussed above, phenobarbital effects on behavior could have taken place via pathways which include the hepatic microsomal drug-oxidizing system, thyroid hormone and sex hormones. On the other hand, phenobarbital could have acted directly by means of other, as yet uninvestigated, routes to alter CNS morphology or chemistry. In future investigations, attention could well be given to pathways where the relationship between the neural and the behavioral events is already established. In our system the study of the possible mediation of phenobarbital-induced changes in audiogenic seizures (Yanai et al., 1981), performance in the eight-arm maze and spontaneous alternations (Pick and Yanai, 1982) by alteration in the hippocampal morphology (Yanai and Bergman, 1981) appears most promising. Also promising would be research into possible mediations of phenobarbital-induced changes in sensitivity to drugs (Yanai and Tabakoff, 1979; 1980) and apomorphine-induced behaviors (Yanai and Feigenbaum, 1981; 1982; Yanai et al., 1982c) by studying changes in the sensitivity of the postsynaptic dopamine receptors.

Acknowledgment

This work was supported by USPHS grant DA 2365.

References

Abel, E.L., (Ed.) (1981) Fetal Alcohol Syndrome. Vol. I. An Annotated and Comprehensive Bibliography, CRC Press, Boca Raton.

Abel, E.L., Bush, R. and Dintcheff, B.A. (1981) Exposure of rats to alcohol in utero alters drug sensitivity in adulthood. Science 212, 1531–1533.

Altman, J. (1975) Effect of interference with cerebellar maturation on the development of locomotion. An experimental model. In: Brain Mechanism in Mental Retardation (Buchwald, N.A. and Brazier, A.B., eds.) Academic Press, New York, pp. 41–91.

128

Anlezark, G.M., Horton, R.W. and Meldrum, B.S. (1978) Dopamine agonists and reflex epilepsy. Adv. Biochem. Psychopharmacol. 19, 383–388.

Armitage, S.G. (1952) The effects of barbiturates on the behavior of rat offspring as measured in learning and reasoning situations. J. Comp. Physiol. Psychol. 45, 146–152.

Atterwill, C.K. (1981) Effect of acute and chronic T₃ to rats on central 5-HT and DA mediated behavior and brain biochemistry. Neuropharmacology 20, 131–134.

Bauer-Moffet, C. and Altman, J. (1977) The effect of ethanol chronically administered to preweanling rats on cerebellar development: a morphological study, Brain Res. 119, 249–268.

Bedard, P., Dankova, J., Boucher, R. and Langelier, P. (1978) Effect of estrogens on apomorphine-induced circling behavior in the rat. Can J. Physiol. Pharmacol. 56, 538–541.

Belknap, J.K., Waddingham, S. and Ondrusek, G. (1973) Barbiturate dependence in mice induced by a simple short-term oral procedure. Physiol. Psychol. 1, 394–396.

Bergey, G.K., Swaiman, K.F., Schrier, B.K., Fitzgerald, S. and Nelson, P.G. (1981) Adverse effect of phenobarbital on morphological and biochemical development of fetal mouse spinal cord neurons in culture. Ann. Neurol. 9, 584–589.

Bergman, A., Rosselli-Austin, L., Yedwab, G. and Yanai, J. (1980) Neuronal deficits in mice following phenobarbital exposure during various periods in fetal development. Acta. Anat. 108, 370–373.

Bethenod, M. and Frederich, A. (1975) Les enfants des antiepileptiques, Pediatrie 30, 227–248.

Breese, G.R., Cott, J.M., Cooper, B.R., Prange, A.J. and Lipton, M.A. (1974) Antagonism of ethanol narcosis by thyrotropin releasing hormone. Life Sci. 14, 1053–1063.

Breese, G.R., Cott, J.M., Cooper, B.R., Prange, A.P., Lipton, M.A. and Plotnikoff, N.P. (1975) Effects of thyrotropin-releasing hormone (TRH) on the actions of pentobarbital and other centrally acting drugs. J. Pharmacol. Exp. Ther. 193, 11–22.

Bradhurst, P.L. (1978) Drugs and the Inheritance of Behavior. Plenum Press, New York.

Char, F., Hearty, J.B. and Dungan, W.T. (1979) Problems in counseling the epileptic mother. Birth Defects (original article series) XV (SE) 261–266.

Christoffel, K.K. and Salafsky, I. (1975) Fetal alcohol syndrome in dizygotic twins, J. Pediatr. 87, 963–967.

Clos, J., Favre, C., Selme-Matrat, M. and Legrand, J. (1977) Effect of undernutrition on cell formation in the rat brain and specially on cellular composition of the cerebellum. Brain Res. 123, 13–26.

Conney, A.H. and Klutch (1963) Increased activity of androgen hydroxylase in liver microsomes of rats pretreated with phenobarbital and other drugs. J. Biol. Chem. 238, 1611–1617.

Conney, A.H. (1967) Pharmacological implications of microsomal enzyme induction. Pharmacol. Rev. 19, 317–366.

Costal, B., Naylor, R.J. and Dohria, V. (1980) On the importance of mesolimbic mechanisms for the control of apomorphine induced climbing behavior in the mouse, Brit. J. Pharmacol. 68, 175P–176P.

Cowan, W.M. (1973) Neuronal death as a regulative mechanism in the control of cell number in the nervous system. In: Development and Aging of the Nervous System (Rockstein, M., ed.) Academic Press, New York, pp. 19–41.

DeFries, J.C. (1964) Prenatal maternal stress in mice: differential effect on behavior. J. Hered. 55, 289–295.

Dennis, W.J. and Sollenberger, R.T. (1934) Negative adaptation in the maze exploration of albino rats. J. Comp. Psychol. 18, 197–206.

Diaz, T., Schain, R.J. and Bailey, B.G. (1977) Phenobarbital-induced brain growth retardation in artificially reared rat pups. Biol. Neonate. 32, 77–82.

Eleftheriou, B.E. (ed.) (1975) Psychopharmacogenetics, Plenum Press, New York.

Engel, J. and Liljequist, S. (1976) The effect of long-term ethanol treatment on the sensitivity of dopamine receptors in the nucleus accumbens. Psychopharmacology 49, 253–257.

Feigenbaum, J.J. and Yanai, J. (1982) Lessened sensitivity to apomorphine hypothermia is associated with postsynaptic dopaminergic receptor supersensitivity, Proceedings of the 13th CINP Congress, p. 211.

Fishman, R.H.B. and Yanai, J. (1983) Long-lasting effects of early barbiturates in central nervous system and behavior. Neurosci. Biobehav. Rev., 7, 19–28.

Fishman, R.H.B., Ornoy, A. and Yanai, J. (1982a) Ultrastructural evidence of cerebellar degeneration after early exposure to phenytoin and/or phenobarbital (PhB) in mice, Proceedings of the 9th European Teratology Society Meeting.

Fishman, R.H.B., Gaaton, A. and Yanai (1982b) Barbiturate treatment eliminates thyroxin peak in neonatal mice. Dev. Brain Res. 5, 202–205.

Fishman, R.H.B., Ornoy, A. and Yanai, J. (1983) Ultrastructural evidence of long-lasting cerebellar degeneration following early exposure to phenobarbital in mice, Exp. Neurol., 79, 212–222.

Forfar, J.O. and Nelson, M.N. (1973) Epidemiology of drugs taken by pregnant women: drugs that may effect the fetus adversly. Clin. Pharmacarol. Ther. 14, 632–642.

Frankel, D., Khanna, J.M., LeBlanc, A.E. and Kalant, H. (1977) Effect of p-chlorophenylalanine on development of cross-tolerance between pentobarbital and ethanol. Can J. Physiol. Pharmacol. 55, 954–957.

Freund, G. (1971) Alcohol, barbiturate, and bromide withdrawal syndrome in mice. In: Recent Advances in Studies of Alcoholism (Mendelson, J.H. and Mello, N.K., eds.) U.S. Govt. Printing Office, Washington, D.C., pp. 453–471.

Garbowska, M. and Anden, N-E. (1976) Apomorphine in the rat nucleus accumbens: effect on the synthesis of 5-Hydroxytryptamine and noradrenaline, the motor activity and body temperature. J. Neural Trans. 38, 1–8.

Giknis, M.L.A., Damjanov, I. and Rubin, E. (1980) The differential transplacental effect of ethanol in four mouse strains. Neurobehav. Toxicol. 2, 235–237.

Ginsburg, B.G. (1967) Genetic parameters in behavioral research. In: Behavior-Genetics Analysis (Hirsh, J., ed.) McGraw-Hill, New York, pp. 135–153.

Gordon, J.H., Gorski, R.A., Borison, R.L. and Diamond, B.I. (1980) Postsynaptic efficency of dopamine: possible suppression by estrogen. Pharmacol. Biochem. Behav. 12, 515–518.

Griffin, W.S.T., Woodward, D.J. and Chanda, R. (1977) Malnutrition-induced alterations of developing Purkinje cells. Exp. Neurol. 56, 298–311.

Gupta, G., Shapiro, B.H. and Yaffe, S.J. (1980a) Reproductive dysfunction in male rats following prenatal exposure to phenobarbital. Pediatr. Pharmacol. 1, 55–62.

Gupta, G., Sonawane, B.R., Yaffe, S.J. and Shapiro, B.H. (1980b) Phenobarbital exposure in utero: alterations in female reproductive function in rats. Science 208, 508–510.

Gupta, C., Yaffe, S.J. and Shapiro, B.H. (1982) Prenatal exposure to phenobarbital permanently decreases testosterone and causes reproductive dysfunction. Science 216, 640–641.

Haesaert, B., (1982) Transplacental effect of endoxin on the development of mice embryos. MSc Dissertation, Dept. Anatomy Embryology, The Hebrew University, Jerusalem, Israel.

Haldane, J.B.S. (1946) The interaction of nature and nurture. Ann. Eugen. 13, 197–205.

Hannah, R.S., Roth, S.H. and Spira, A.W. (1982) The effect of chloropromazine and phenobarbital on cerebellar Purkinje cells. Teratology 26, 21–25.

Harris, R.A. and Case, J. (1979) Effects of maternal consumption of ethanol, barbital, or chlordiazepoxide on the behavior of the offspring. Behav. Neurol. Biol. 26, 234–247.

Hart, L.G., Adamson, R.H., Dixon, R.L. and Fouts, J.R. (1962) Stimulation of hepatic microsomal drug metabolism in the newborn and fetal rabbit. J. Pharmacol. Exp. Ther. 137, 103–106.

Hershberger, L.G., Shipley, E.G. and Meyer, R.K. (1953) Myotrophic activity of 19-nortestosterone and other steroids determined by modified levator ani muscle method. Proc. Soc. Biol. Med. 83, 175.

Hill, R.M. (1973) Drugs ingested by pregnant women. Clin. Pharmacol. Ther. 14, 654–659.

Hoffman, P.L. and Tabakoff, B. (1977) Alterations in dopamine receptor sensitivity by chronic ethanol treatment. Nature 268, 551–553.

Kalant, H., LeBlanc, A.E. and Gibbons, R.J. (1971) Tolerance to, and dependence on, some non-opiate psychotropic drugs. Pharmacol. Rev. 23, 135–180.

Kelly, P.H., Seviour, P.W. and Iversen, S.D. (1975) Amphetamine and apomorphine responses in the rat following 6-OHDA lesions of the nucleus accumbens septi and corpus striatum. Brain Res. 94, 507–522.

130

Khanna, J.M., Kalant, H., Le, A.D., Mayer, J. and LeBlanc, A.E. (1980) Effect of *p*-chlorophenylalanine on the acquisition of tolerance to the hypnotic effect of pentobarbital, barbital and ethanol. Can. J. Physiol. Pharmacol. 58, 1031–1041.

Lai, H., Carino, M.A. and Houta, A. (1980) Effect of ethanol on central dopamine functions. Life Sci. 27, 299–304.

Lauder, J.M. (1977) Effects of thyroid state on development of rat cerebellar cortex. In: Thyroid Hormones and Brain Development (Grave, G.D., ed.) Raven Press, New York, pp. 235–254.

Lucier, G.W., Sonawane, B.R., McDaniel, O.S. and Hook, G.E.R. (1975) Postnatal stimulation of hepatic microsomal enzymes following administration of TCDD to pregnant rats. Chem.-Biol. Interact. 11, 15–26.

McClearn, G.E., Wilson, J.R. and Meredith, W. (1970) The use of isogenic and heterogenic mouse stocks in behavioral research. In: Contributions to Behavior-Genetic Analysis: The Mouse as a Prototype (Lindzey, G. and Thiessen, D.D., eds.) Appleton-Century-Crofts, New York, pp. 3–22.

Menashi, M., Ornoy, A. and Yanai, J. (1982) Transplacental effects of methymercury chloride in mice with specific emphasis on the audiogenic seizure response. Dev. Neurosci. 5, 216–221.

Middaugh, L.D., Santos III, C.A. and Zemp, J.W. (1975) Effects of phenobarbital given to pregnant mice on behavior of mature offspring. Dev. Psychobiol. 8(4), 305–313.

Middaugh, L.D., Thomas, T.N., Simpson, L.W. and Zemp, J.W. (1981) Effect of prenatal maternal injections of phenobarbital on brain neurotransmitters and behavior of young C57 mice. Neurobehav. Toxicol. Teratol. 3, 271–275.

Murai, N. (1966) Effect of maternal medication during pregnancy upon behavioral development of offspring. Tohuku J. Exp. Med. 89, 265–272.

Myers, R.E. and Myers, S.E. (1979) Use of sedative analgestic, and anesthetic drugs during labor and delivery: bane or boon? Am. J. Obstet. Gynecol. 133, 83–104.

O'Keefe, J. and Nadel, L. (1978) The Hippocampus as a Cognitive Map. Clarendon Press, Oxford.

Olton, D.S. (1977) Spatial memory. Sci. Am. 236, 82–98.

Olton, D.S. and Papas, B.C. (1979) Spatial memory and hippocampal function, Neuropsychology 17, 669–682.

Olton, D.S. and Samuelson, R.J. (1976) Remembrance of places passed: spatial memory in rats. J. Exp. Psychol. Anim. Behav. Processes 2, 97–116.

Olton, D.S., Branch, M. and Best, P.J. (1978) Spatial correlates of hyppocampal unit activity. Exp. Neurol. 58, 587–409.

Opitz, K. and Akinlaja, A. (1966) Zur Beeinflusung der Nahrungsaufnahme durch Psychopharmaka. Psychopharmacologia 9, 307–319.

Pick, C.G. and Yanai, J. (1982) Changes in hippocampal behaviors after early exposure to phenobarbital in mice, Proc. Int. Soc. Dev. Neurosci. p. 182.

Protais, P., Consentin, J. and Schwartz, J.C. (1976) Climbing behavior induced by apomorphine in mice: a simple test for the study of dopamine receptors in striatum. Psychopharmacologia 50, 1–6.

Pysh, J.J., Perkins, R.E. and Singer Beck, L. (1979) The effect of postnatal undernutrition on the development of the mouse Purkinje cell dendritic tree. Brain Res. 163, 165–170.

Rabin, R.A., Wolfe, B.B., Dibner, M.D., Zahniser, N.R., Melchior, C.L. and Milinoff, P.B. (1980) Effect of ethanol administration and withdrawal on neurotransmitter receptor systems in C57 mice. J. Pharmacol. Exp. Ther. 213, 491–496.

Roberts, W.W., Dember, W.N. and Brodwick, M. (1962) Alternation and exploration in rats with hippocampal lesions. J. Comp. Physiol. Psychol. 55, 695–700.

Roderick, T.H., Wimer, R.E., Wimer, C.C. and Schwartzkroin, P.A. (1973) Genetic and phenotypic variation in weight of brain and spinal cord between inbred strains of mice. Brain Res. 64, 345–353.

Rodier, P.M. (1977) Correlations between prenatally-induced alterations in CNS cell populations and postnatal function. Teratology 16, 235–246.

Safaei, R. and Timiras (1982) Hormone induction and catecholamine enzyme induction in neural tissue by thyroid hormones. Program and Abstracts, 3rd Int. Meet. Soc. Dev. Neurosci., p. 193.

Schain, R.J. and Watanabe, K. (1975) Effects of chronic phenobarbital administration upon brain growth of the infant rat. Exp. Neurol. 47, 509–515.

Seeber, V. and Kuschensky, K. (1976) Dopamine-sensitive adenylate cyclase in homogenates of rat striata during ethanol and barbiturate withdrawal. Arch. Toxicol. 35, 247–253.

Seyfried, T.N., Glaser, G.H. and Yu, R.K. (1979) Thyroid hormone influence on the susceptibility of mice to audiogenic seizures. Science 205, 598–600.

Shaywitz, S.E., Cohen, D.J. and Shaywitz, B.E. (1978) Biochemical basis of minimal brain dysfunction. J. Pediatr. 92, 179–187.

Siemens, A.J. and Chan, A.W.K. (1976) Differential effects of phenobarbital and ethanol in mice. Life Sci. 19, 581–590.

Smith, D.W. (1977) Teratogenicity of anticonvulsive medications. J. Dis. Child. 131, 1337–1339.

Speroff, L. (1973) Toxemia of pregnancy – mechanism and therapeutic management. Am. J. Cardiol. 32, 582–591.

Storm-Mathisen, J. (1977) Localization of transmitter candidates in the brain: the hippocampal formation as a model. Prog. Neurobiol. 8, 119–181.

Sweatman, P. and Jell, R.M. (1977) Dopamine and histamine sensitivity of rostral hypothalamic neurons in the cat: possible involvement in thermoregulation. Brain Res. 127, 173–178.

Sze, P.Y., Yanai, J. and Ginsburg (1976) Effects of early ethanol input on the activities of ethanol metabolizing enzymes in mice. Biochem. Pharmacol. 25, 215–217.

Tabakoff, B., Yanai, J. and Ritzmann, R.F. (1978a) Brain noradrenergic systems as a prerequisite for developing tolerance to barbiturates. Science 200, 449–451.

Tabakoff, B., Hoffman, P.L. and Ritzmann, R.F. (1978b) Dopamine receptor function after chronic injection of ethanol. Life Sci. 23, 643–648.

Tarsy, D. and Baldessarini, R.J. (1974) Behavioral supersensitivity to apomorphine following chronic treatment with drugs which interfere with synaptic function of catecholamines. Neuropharmacology 13, 927–940.

Thomas, C.R. (1976) Routine phenobarbital for prevention of neonatal hyperbilirubinemia. Obstet. Gynecol. 47, 304–308.

Thompson, V.C. and Olian, S. (1961) Some effects on offspring behavior of maternal adrenalin injections during pregnancy in three inbred mouse strains. Psychol. Rep. 8, 87–90.

Trolle, D. (1968) Phenobarbitone in neonatal icteruf. Lancet i, 251–252.

Wahlstrom, G. (1971) Changes in a hexobarbital anaesthesia threshold in rats induced by repeated long term treatment with barbital or ethanol, Psychopharmacology 19, 366–380.

Wallace, S.J. (1980) Successful prophylaxis against fibrile convulsions with valproic acid or phenobarbitone. Brit. Med. J. 280, 353–354.

Weidenfeld, J. Schiller and Yanai, J. Effect of early exposure to phenobarbital on in vitro aromatization of testosterone by neonatal male mouse brain. Neuroendocrinol. Lett. in press.

Wimer, R.E., Wimer, C.C., Chernow, C.R. and Balvanz, B.A. (1980) The genetic organization of neuron number in the pyramidal cell layer of hippocampal regio superior in house mice. Brain Res. 196, 59–77.

Wolf, S.M. and Forsythe, A. (1978) Behavioral disturbance, phenobarbital and febrile seizures. Pediatrics 61, 728–731.

Yanai, J. (1979) Long term induction of microsomal drug oxidizing system in mice following prenatal exposure to barbiturate. Biochem. Pharmacacol. 28, 1429–1430.

Yanai, J. (1981) Comparison of early barbiturate and ethanol effects on the CNS. Substance and Alcohol Actions/Misuse 2, 79–91.

Yanai, J. (1983) Possible dopaminergic involvement in early phenobarbital induced changes in sensitivity to barbiturate. Teratology, 27, 86A.

Yanai, J. and Bergman, A. (1981) Neuronal deficits in mice after neonatal exposure to phenobarbital. Exp. Neurol. 73, 199–208.

132

Yanai, J. and Feigenbaum, J.J. (1981) Lessened sensitivity to apomorphine induced hypothermia following prenatal exposure to phenobarbital. IRCS Med. Sci. 9, 965.

Yanai, J. and Feigenbaum J.J. (1982) Early exposure to phenobarbital, dopamine receptors sensitivity and tolerance. Proc. 3rd Meet. Int. Soc. Dev. Neurosci. p. 231.

Yanai, J. and Fishman, R.H.B. (1983) Sensitivity to barbiturate is changed by developmental alteration of dopamine receptor sensitivity. Dev. Neurosci., in press.

Yanai, J. and Ginsburg, B.E. (1979) The relative contribution of pre and neonatal administration of changes in mice behavior. Arch. Int. Pharmacodyn. Ther. 241, 235–245.

Yanai, J. and Iser, C. (1981) Stereologic study on Purkinje cells in mice following early exposure to phenobarbital. Exp. Neurol. 74, 707–716.

Yanai, J. and Tabakoff, B. (1979) Increased tolerance in mice following prenatal exposure to barbiturate. Psychopharmacology 64, 325–327.

Yanai, J. and Tabakoff, B. (1980) Altered sensitivity to ethanol following prenatal exposure to barbiturate. Psychopharmacology 68, 301–303.

Yanai, J., Rosselli-Austin, L. and Tabakoff, B. (1979) Neuronal deficits in mice following prenatal exposure to phenobarbital. Exp. Neurol. 64, 237–244.

Yanai, J., Bergman, A., Shafer, R., Yedwab, J. and Tabakoff, B. (1981) Audiogenic seizures and neuronal deficits following early exposure to barbiturate. Dev. Neurosci. 4, 345–350.

Yanai, J., Wolf, M. and Feigenbaum, J.J. (1982a) Autoradiographic study of phenobarbital's effect on development of the central nervous system. Exp. Neurol. 78, 437–449.

Yanai, J. Wolf, M. and Feigenbaum, J.J. (1982b) Morphological alterations in the medial preoptic area after prenatal administration of phenobarbital. Acta Anat. 114, 347–354.

Yanai, J., Feigenbaum, J.J. and Fishman, R.H.B. (1982c) Lessened sensitivity to apomorphine induced climbing behavior in mice following neonatal exposure to phenobarbital. Neurobehav. Toxicol. Teratol. 4, 535–538.

Yanai, J., Bergman, A. and Feigenbaum, J.J. (1983) Genetic factors influencing neurosensitivity to early phenobarbital administration in mice. Acta Anat. 115, 40–46.

Neurobehavioral Teratology
edited by Joseph Yanai
© Elsevier Science Publishers BV 1984

6

STUDIES ON THE EFFECTS OF ANTICONVULSANT DRUGS ON THE DEVELOPING HUMAN BRAIN

Sheila J. Wallace

University Hospital of Wales, Heath Park, Cardiff CF4 4XW, UK

WHEN considering possible neurobehavioural teratological effects of anticonvulsant drugs on the human brain it is essential to relate the timing of drug administration to the stage of anatomical and physiological development of the brain.

In this chapter a short statement on the phases of human brain growth is followed by a brief general consideration of possible ways drugs might interact with the central nervous system. For phenobarbital, primidone, phenytoin, carbamazepine, valproate and ethosuximide there is consideration of the chemistry, mode of action, possible direct effects on neurobehavioural development and possible secondary effects on the brain due to alteration in endocrine function. In particular, attention is given to studies which might indicate the clinical importance of neurological, cognitive and behavioural changes induced in children by the ingestion of drugs used over long periods in the treatment of epilepsies.

The maturing brain

Growth of the total mass of the brain is very rapid from 4 to 5 months gestation until the end of the first postnatal year, moderately fast during the second year and gradually becomes almost imperceptible after the fifth year. Measurement of human brain weight shows that it increases until at least the age of 8 years. (Dobbing and Sands, 1973). The occipitofrontal circumference of the head continues to increase until about 16 to 18 years of age and it may be presumed that the mass of the brain does likewise.

The periods of most rapid alteration in brain state are comprehensively described by Volpe (1981a, b). In the normal central nervous system dorsal and ventral induction are completed by 6 weeks of gestation. Neuronal proliferation occurs from 2 to 4 months gestation, migration from 3 to 5 months gestation, organisation, which includes development of synapses, from 6 months to several years postnatally and myelination from 9 months gestation to several years postnatally (Volpe, 1981 a). Not all parts of the brain undergo the same sort of development at the same time. In particular the neuronal development of the forebrain occurs between 2 to 4 months gestation, but that of the cerebellum at about 8 months gestation to 1 to 2 months postnatally. In order for development to occur in an ideal manner a normal pool of amino acids must be available and the hormonal status appropriate. (Balazs, 1976).

In recognition that brain development proceeds throughout childhood, possible teratological actions of anticonvulsant drugs on the nervous system will be considered by examining studies performed on children up to the age of 16 years.

Interactions between drugs and the developing nervous system

In theory, drugs might affect the energy metabolism of neurones, the excitability of neuronal membranes, the vascular supply to the brain, the supporting glial cells and/ or transmitter metabolism or post-synaptic receptors. In practice, anticonvulsant drugs are effective because of their abilities to reduce the excitability of neuronal membranes and their effects on either neurotransmitter metabolism or post-synaptic receptors. Most drugs affecting behaviour probably act by altering the availability or effectiveness of neurotransmitters and it has been suggested that such drugs have the greatest potential for selectively affecting brain function. In a discussion of the concept of negative feedback and neurotransmitter metabolism, the dependency of normal development of synaptic connections on neurotransmitter metabolism has been explored (Weiner, 1974). It is considered that modification of neurotransmitter metabolism during maturation may have important effects on ultimate central nervous system development and on behaviour. Hinwich (1974) has examined amino acid metabolism in the context of brain development. He comments that during rapid cerebral growth the free amino acid pool in the brain serves as a source of building material for brain proteins and that some members of this pool, for example, γ-aminobutyric acid (GABA) serves as a neurotransmitter. GABA is known to be of importance in inhibition of seizure discharges and its brain level to be influenced by the use of at least some of the commonly used anticonvulsant drugs. It is possible that a disturbance of balance amongst free amino acids could affect reactions necessary for the normal development of the brain. Experiments in animals have shown that 'blood-brain' and 'blood-cerebrospinal fluid' barrier systems alter with maturation. As a result of decreasing permeability of cerebral capillaries and volume of glial cells and the growth of neuronal processes, decreasing permeability of the ependymal lining and increasing production and flow of cerebrospinal fluid and increasing transport across the choroid plexus, substances which tend to cross from the blood to the brain in young animals pass more readily into the cerebrospinal fluid than the brain in older animals. Comparable details are not available for human infants and young children, but it is well known that their responses to sedatives, in particular barbiturates, are different from those of adults. It might be justifiable to postulate that alteration in anticonvulsant drug access to the brain could be a factor in considering possible neurobehavioural teratology.

In any study of the effects of drugs on the central nervous system, it is essential to recognise that age, specific brain structure studied and the selected neurological concept being examined may influence the result.

Effects of unspecified anticonvulsant drugs on brain development

A few reports are available where specific effects of separate anticonvulsant drugs have not been sought.

47 infants who were exposed to various anticonvulsants in utero were studied by Jager-Roman et al. (1982). One fifth of the babies had birth weights less than the tenth centile for gestational age. 42 of the infants were followed to 6 months of age, when 21 of them were considered to have minor neurological abnormalities, but of 23 seen at 24 months only 3 were considered abnormal. Slight psychomotor retardation was noted in 7 of 42 at 6 months, 10 of 35 at 12 months and 3 of 23 of those seen at 24 months. The authors conclude that initial neurodevelopmental problems may exist in children exposed prenatally to anticonvulsants, but that these abnormalities resolve with time. Of the 23 examined at 24 months, the number of the 21 children thought to be abnormal at 6 months is not stated, making the authors' conclusions of doubtful validity. Granstrom (1982) examined 93 children of epileptic mothers. The 66 of these children whose mothers received antiepileptic therapy during pregnancy are compared with 66 control infants who were healthy and born in the same obstetric unit. No difference in neurological development was found between the two groups. A further study of 19 infants of mothers with epilepsy reports that 4 of the 19 had minor abnormalities at birth (Latis, 1982). Only 1 of the 4 was permanently disadvantaged, having been apathetic at birth and having a persistent right hemisyndrome and reduced overall abilities.

Thus where anticonvulsant drugs are looked at as a group rather than individually, it appears that there is little evidence that they affect prenatal brain development.

Phenobarbital

Phenobarbital is a weak acid which is protein bound. With a half-life of 53 to 140 h, 3 weeks may be needed before there is constancy of the serum level. The latter is in equilibrium with the brain level and is stable over long periods under continuous therapy.The mechanisms of action of phenobarbital have been reviewed by Prichard (1982). Phenobarbital increases the threshold to electrical and chemical stimuli, prolongs inhibitory potentials in isolated cerebral cortex, depresses physiological excitations and enhances inhibitions. Interactions with GABA are involved in the enhancing mechanisms. It can also reduce calcium uptake by depolarised nerve terminals. A rise in total brain 5-hydroxytryptophan may occur. Evidence that phenobarbital may be more active against abnormal than physiological electrical activity is given by Prichard (1982), who reports that local acidosis, such as may happen in a focal seizure discharge, leads to a change of stable phenobarbital into a more active form. Morrell et al. (1959) showed that in rabbits phenobarbital inhibited the spread of abnormal activity from chronic cortical freeze foci to adjacent cortex and the diencephalon and suppressed firing of the foci themselves. Kindling experiments may be very relevant models of childhood seizure disorders. In such models in cats and baboons, phenobarbital was found to retard the kindling process (Wada, 1977). In addition to other activities, phenobarbital may lead to primary depression of energy metabolism. Prichard concluded his review by stating that a combination of actions in some critical proportion may be more relevant in the antiepileptic effect of phenobarbital than attempts to attribute the latter to one chemical or pharmacological property. Although the above studies emphasise the relatively minor effects of phenobarbital on normal electrophysiological processes, there is evidence from the electroencephalograph (EEG) that it must cause electrical alterations even if their clinical importance is not immediately obvious. The 20–30 Hz activity seen on the EEG of people receiving phenobarbital is said to be due to its action on the mesencephalic reticular formation.

There has been some investigation of the effects of phenobarbital on hormonal secretion. Masala et al. (1980) reported that there was an impaired response of prolactin to thyrotropin-releasing hormones in children who received phenobarbital for between 10 and 20 months. No effect was noted if the duration of treatment was less than 10 months. Increased removal of thyroxine (T_4) from the blood of children on phenobarbital is countered by increased T_4 production, and individuals remain euthyroid. Phenobarbital was found to have no effect on growth hormone secretion.

Thus on theoretical grounds, from the cerebral electrical viewpoint, since phenobarbital preferentially inhibits abnormal or unusual discharges it might, in the developing brain, inhibit the formation of new synaptic connections, restricting potential intracerebral paths of communication. From the hormonal viewpoint prenatally administered phenobarbital might cause reduction in brain cell numbers, with defective myelinisation being a consequence of its use peri- and postnatally.

Neurological effects

When phenobarbital has been taken during pregnancy the infants may suffer with-drawal symptoms and signs. Desmond et al. (1972) reported that tremors may persist for days to months after delivery. The anatomical correlate of the tremors has not been postulated. Although phenobarbital was given on a large scale in the late 1960s and early 1970s to newborn babies with jaundice, the possible long-term neurological ef-fects of its use in this age group were not explored. Ataxia and nystagmus which may appear at any age just after starting phenobarbital medication are adapted to unless toxic levels persist in the serum. In a study of childred aged 6 months to 5 years, of whom 26 received continuous phenobarbital over a 2-year period, and a further 34 phenobarbital at some stage over the same time, no child became ataxic. (Wallace, unpublished data). Those who received phenobarbital for 2 years were specifically tested for cerebellar dysfunction at 3-monthly intervals, with negative results. There is no report in the literature of a systematic study of the long-term neurological effects of phenobarbital which might be related to permanent alteration in brain structure or function.

Cognitive effects

No study has looked at the cognitive effects of the pre-, peri- or immediate postnatal use of phenobarbital. Several authors have considered possible effects when phenobar-bital is given in the prophylaxis of febrile convulsions. The age range is usually 6 months to 3 years, but may extend to 5 years, thus brain systems which might be vul-nerable are organisation, including synaptic development, and myelination. Camfield et al. (1979) tested children at 8 months and 12 months after they had started on phe-nobarbital. No pre-test scores were available. They found no difference in IQ scores between placebo and phenobarbital-treated groups and no difference between the five Binet subcategories. There was possibly a slight difference in short-term memory favouring the placebo group, but since the Binet subscales are not meant to be used as independent parameters, this finding may be spurious. Hellstrom and Barlach-Christoffersen (1980) also report that there is no deterioration in intelligence if pheno-barbital is given to pre-school children for 12 months, but these children were not tested prior to commencing therapy. Aldridge Smith and Wallace (1982) tested 16 children before starting phenobarbital and at intervals during 24 months of continuous treatment during which no further convulsions occurred. The mean Griffiths Develop-mental Quotient was 103.9 (SD 20.7) before phenobarbital was commenced and 106.1 (SD 21.5) 24 months later. These findings were not significantly different from those of 21 children who had had no drugs and no seizures over the same time period. Wolf et al. (1981) tested 21 children treated for febrile convulsions with phenobarbital for a mean of 35 months. The drug was withdrawn and the children retested. The results were comparable whether or not phenobarbital was being given. In addition, they were not significantly different from those for 25 children who had had febrile convul-sions, but who had not received phenobarbital.

In children of school age, Holdsworth and Whitmore (1974) noted that those with epilepsy who were attending schools for normal pupils tended to do better if they were on phenobarbital than if they were on no therapy. Trimble and Corbett (1980), whose study is restricted to children with severe epilepsy, report a fall-off of intelligence where chronic therapy includes phenobarbital, but their study fails to consider the effects of the seizure disorder. Wapner et al. (1962) gave phenobarbital 1.2–3.7 mg/kg per day to 36 epileptic children aged 8 to 10 years. Effects on learning ability were studied in comparison with controls matched for sex, race and IQ. The tests were administered over a 6-week period and included the multiple T stylus maze and the Full-Range Picture Vocabulary Test of Ammons and Ammons. Acquisition of vocabulary was equivalent in the children with epilepsy and the controls. The initial performance on the maze was slightly, but not significantly better in the controls, but the net gain in skill was comparable over the 6-week period in the two groups. Wapner et al. concluded that in this time period the rate of learning was not impaired by phenobarbital. Hutt et al. (1968) reported subclinical deficits in adaptive capacity which became more obvious the higher the serum phenobarbital level. They found further that the rate of speech production in open-ended conversation increased. In general, they concluded that phenobarbital had no effect on tasks which are brief or simple, but might reduce the efficiency with which those requiring sustained attention were performed. Hutt et al. worked in strictly controlled surroundings and the importance of their findings in day-to-day learning was not explored. The early optimism of Barnes and Fetterman (1938), Somerfeld-Ziskind and Ziskind (1940) and Lennox (1942), who all reported either improved intellect, lack of deleterious effects or improved mentation after phenobarbital was given to their patients, appears to have been justified. However, despite the availability and very widespread use of phenobarbital over a period of 70 years, a properly conducted study of its effects on cognitive function in school children of normal intelligence remains to be performed. On present evidence it seems unlikely that phenobarbital causes important permanent changes in cerebral structure of function if given after the neonatal period.

Behavioural effects

Babies born to mothers who have received phenobarbital during pregnancy may be irritable and over-excitable for months later (Desmond et al., 1972). This is presumably due to withdrawal of sedative effects, but the anatomical and physiological substrates have not been postulated.

In early childhood excitement, irritability, tearfulness and aggression appear to be specific effects of barbiturates since they are not seen with other anticonvulsants (Stores, 1975). Such behavioural changes may be secondary to actions of the phenobarbital on neurotransmitter systems or might occur in young children more readily than adults because of differences in blood-brain barrier mechanisms. Mattson and Cramer (1982) suggest that the behavioural changes may have a secondary effect on learning, but this hypothesis has not been further explored. The incidence of behavioural intolerance to barbiturates given to pre-school children for prophylaxis of febrile convulsions is at least 19%.Thorn (1975) reported this problem in 34 of 174 children. Wolf and Forsythe (1978) found that 46 of 109 (42%) children developed a behaviour disturbance when given phenobarbital. Treatment was discontinued in 20%. The problems began soon after commencing therapy and were not related to serum phenobarbital levels. Abnormal behaviour prior to therapy increased the risk of an adverse response. The behavioural changes were all reversible on discontinuance of phenobarbital. In a personal study where a behavioural profile was obtained before commencing phenobarbital the parents of 20 of 41 children reported deterioration in at least one aspect of behaviour 2–3 weeks after starting treatment. Improvement in at least one aspect of behaviour was reported in 5 of the 41. Of 18 children given no drugs over the same period 3 were stated to have deterioration and 4 improvement in at least one aspect of behaviour. The differences between phenobarbital and no treatment are significant for deterioration ($p < 0.02$) (Wallace, unpublished data). In the same study, withdrawal of phenobarbital after 24 months from 16 children produced no behavioural change in 6, improvement in at least 3 aspects of behaviour in 4, deterioration in at least 3 aspects in one and a change in one or two aspects, largely improvements, in 5. Since it is usual to discontinue phenobarbital if adverse behaviour occurs, the possible teratological effects in children who react unfavourably have not been considered.

No prospective study of the behavioural effects of phenobarbital on school-age children has been reported. Holdsworth and Whitmore (1974) found that children with epilepsy who were in normal schools and who had no behaviour disturbance were significantly more likely to be receiving phenobarbital than those with a behaviour disturbance ($p < 0.01$). On the other hand, children in a special school because of severe epilepsy who were being treated with phenobarbital were significantly more likely to have a conduct disorder than those receiving carbamazepine (Trimble and Corbett, 1979).

Conclusions
Possible neurological, cognitive and behavioural effects of phenobarbital which might lead to permanent alteration in brain structure or function are virtually unexplored. Such studies as exist suggest that, at least after the first few months of life, important, irreversible changes are unlikely.

Primidone

Primidone is a combination of phenobarbital and phenylethylmalonamide. After absorption it is broken down into these two major components. Thus many properties of primidone are identical to those of phenobarbital. There is controversy about the pharmacological actions of the phenylethylmalonamide, but it is felt that this sub-

140

stance possesses an epileptic effect in its own right. The mechanism of this effect is unknown.

Neurological effects

An acute idiosyncratic reaction consisting of ataxia, nystagmus and nausea occurring within 1–2 h of ingestion would lead to immediate cessation of treatment with primidone. Otherwise adverse neurological findings appear related to toxicity (Booker, 1972). No prospective study investigating possible long-term neurological effects in infancy or childhood has been conducted.

Cognitive and behavioural effects

No prospective study of the cognitive or behavioural effects of primidone in early childhood has been reported. Nolte et al. (1980) have shown that the mean performance quotient of the Wechsler Intelligence Scale for Children (WISC) was higher in 4 children 6 months after they had discontinued primidone than when they were on treatment.

Conclusions

Studies on phenobarbital are relevant to the use of primidone. No prospective examination of possible neuro-behavioural teratological effects of primidone has been undertaken.

Phenytoin

Phenytoin is a weak organic acid which is protein bound. It is absorbed slowly from the intestinal tract. The half-life is about 22 h in adults, but may be as long as 42 h in the human newborn. The total phenytoin concentration has been estimated to be between one and three times that in plasma, with the free concentration in the brain being six to ten times higher than the plasma level. The many actions of phenytoin have been very comprehensively reviewed by Woodbury (1982). Multiple effects on neurotransmitters are recorded, but it is believed that the major action of phenytoin is on movements of sodium and calcium ions across cellular or subcellular membranes. In excitable tissues the main effect is a reduction in sodium influx which leads to a fall in intracellular sodium and calcium ions with consequent blockage of neurotransmitter release. The phospholipid-calcium interactions in the cell membrane are affected. This may influence active transport of sodium and potassium ions across synaptic membranes, particularly where the sodium-potassium transport system is compromised as in an epileptic focus. Under such circumstances both release of the neurotransmitter from the nerve ending and its active re-uptake are affected. Between convulsions phenytoin given in dosage appropriate for suppression of seizures does not affect brain respiration (i.e. metabolism) and in therapeutic dosage there is no effect on the EEG. Thus when considering potential effects of phenytoin on the developing brain, organisation and the maturation of neurotransmitter systems might be the most vulnerable to teratogenic effects.

In addition to direct action of phenytoin on the brain, secondary abnormalities might, in theory, be caused by abnormal endocrine function. Dam (1982) has reviewed studies of alterations in measurements of endocrine function induced by treatment with phenytoin. In summary, there is an increase in the metabolism of corticosteroids, enhanced peripheral conversion of T_4 to T_3, inhibition of glucose-induced insulin release and increased plasma concentration of sex hormone-binding globulin in females. The clinical importance of the endocrine findings is not immediately apparent, but since the developing brain is known to be vulnerable to defective corticosteroid and thyroid output, these actions of phenytoin should not be completely ignored.

Fetal hydantoin syndrome
Hanson and Smith (1975) described craniofacial malformations in infants of mothers given phenytoin in pregnancy. Neurological or behavioural correlates were not noted initially, but Hoyte and Billson (1978) subsequently suggested that optic nerve hypoplasia could be an additional feature of this syndrome. More recently, Janz (1982) has argued that the findings in this condition, which are attributed to phenytoin, had been described in infants of mothers with epilepsy before phenytoin became available.

Neurological effects
Much has been made of neurological changes occurring in association with phenytoin therapy, but it is now recognised that these are mainly due to chronic overdosage. No permanent neurological sequelae have been convincingly correlated with fetal exposure to phenytoin. Theoretical dangers of damage to the rapidly developing cerebellum if phenytoin is given in the early neonatal period have never been confirmed on pathological material. 'Diphenylhydantoin encephalopathy' presenting with ataxia, dysarthria, nystagmus and vertigo is considered by Dam (1982) to be reversible. Dam further suggests that there is no convincing evidence that phenytoin ever causes permanent pathological changes in the cerebellum in man. Systematic studies of the clinical neurological effects of phenytoin have not been reported in childhood. There is, however, no reason to suppose that the impairment of motor function observed by Chadwick et al. (1976) and Dodrill (1975) in adults would not also occur in children. Such impaired motor function could, in theory, lead to secondary visuospatial learning difficulties, but studies exploring this possibility have yet to be performed.

Cognitive effects
There is no evidence that prenatal exposure to phenytoin leads to permanent cognitive deficits. There is a total absence of studies of possible cognitive effects of phenytoin in preschool children.

Stores and Hart (1976) reported that children with epilepsy who were attending

142

normal schools had significantly lower reading skills if they had received phenytoin for at least 2 years, as compared to other anticonvulsant therapy. Trimble and Corbett (1980) found a fall-off in intelligence in association with phenytoin in children with severe epilepsy attending a special school, but the findings are not correlated with seizure frequency. Conversely, Nolte et al. (1980) recorded that the mean test scores on the WISC improved after treatment with phenytoin, provided the serum phenytoin did not rise above 22 μg/ml, when there was a fall in the verbal quotient. The groups studied were very small and therefore unsuitable for statistical analysis. Nolte et al. also tested children initially while they were receiving phenytoin and retested them after discontinuance of therapy. The retest scores were higher than those obtained while the children were on phenytoin. The same authors (Nolte et al., 1982) have more recently performed a prospective controlled trial in which children received high dose or low dose phenytoin or no therapy, and were tested at 6-month intervals. High dose phenytoin was associated with a slight reduction in the verbal quotient. No significant difference was noted for concentration, visual memory, comprehension, and reproduction (Benton test), intellectual function (HAWK) and fine motor function, but there were trends towards better scores when children were off therapy rather than receiving phenytoin. From these studies there is at least a suspicion that cognitive function may be suboptimal while children of school age receive phenytoin, and that improvement may occur if the clinical state allows phenytoin to be discontinued. To date, information on pre-treatment and post-treatment abilities in a prospectively studied group of children is not available and possible permanent changes have not been identified.

Behavioural effects
The only study in which behavioural parameters are mentioned is that of Nolte et al. (1980). Children placed on low dose phenytoin were noted to improve in social adaptiveness to school tasks, which resulted in increased ability to concentrate on and benefit from education.

Conclusions
Considering the mechanisms of action of phenytoin, depression of synaptogenesis and of neurotransmitter systems might be predicted. However, although much has been written about possible adverse effects of phenytoin on neurobehavioural function, precise studies of these mechanisms on the developing brain are almost entirely lacking.

Carbamazepine

Carbamazepine is derived from iminostilbene. It is absorbed slowly from the gastrointestinal tract. The usual half-life of 6–8 h quoted for adults is probably longer than that for children, in whom more rapid turnover is likely. The exact mechanism of action of carbamazepine has not been defined, but it probably exerts its anticonvulsant activity via the noradrenergic and serotonergic pathways. There are effects on the thyroid hormone levels in the peripheral blood, but these are of doubtful clinical importance. In theory, carbamazepine might have neurobehavioural teratological effects either through direct action on developing neurotransmitter systems or by causing thyroid abnormalities which might secondarily affect either cellular numbers in the brain, or if occurring later, myelination.

Neurological effects

If the occipito-frontal circumference of the head can be meaningfully related to brain size, carbamazepine could be suspected of interference with the overall growth of the brain. Hiilesmaa et al. (1982) have reported reduction in the mean occipito-frontal circumference at birth in babies whose mothers received carbamazepine as their only antiepileptic drug during pregnancy. This finding did not appear to have any long-term clinical significance.

No study of the possible permanent neurological effects of carbamazepine given during childhood has been reported. Meinardi (1972) reviewed the neurologic side-effects of carbamazepine and recorded that nystagmus and difficulties with heel-toe walking and repetitive knee-bending were not dose-related, whereas the incidences of headache, disturbance of vision and dysarthria bore a linear relationship to the plasma carbamazepine level. There is no evidence that any neurological side-effect persists after reduction or discontinuance of carbamazepine dosage.

Cognitive effects

In the expectation that carbamazepine might lead to improved cognitive abilities a number of studies have been performed in both epileptic and non-epileptic populations. None relate to children of below school age. Therefore there is no information on possible permanent effects on cognition if carbamazepine is given at times of very rapid anatomical and physiological change in the brain.

Martin et al. (1965) reported better organisation, perceptive structuring and ability to use 'concrete experiments', but no improvement in visuographic structuring or drawing human figures when epileptic children of below average ability were treated with carbamazepine. Jacobides (1977) found that carbamazepine improved scholastic abilities and Hamster and Petruch (1977) recorded better intellectual performance, but the improvement was not statistically significant. Groh (1977) tested non-epileptic and epileptic children separately before and after giving carbamazepine. Compared with placebo the non-epileptic children were significantly more able to perform psychological tests when on carbamazepine. The same did not hold for children with epilepsy. Trimble and Corbett (1980) found no fall-off in intelligence in children with severe epilepsy being educated in a special school who had received long-term carbamazepine. Kalska (1976) could find no effect of carbamazepine on intellectual or memory quotients.

No prospective study gives cognitive abilities before and after long-term treatment with carbamazepine, but on the available evidence it seems unlikely that this drug would be deleterious.

Behavioural effects

There are no reports of studies of behaviour of infants or children exposed to carbamazepine prenatally, in infancy or early childhood. Transient drowsiness, anxiety or restlessness sometimes occurs at the commencement of therapy. Trimble and Corbett (1979), in their examination of children with severe epilepsy in a special school, found those receiving carbamazepine were significantly less likely to have a conduct disorder than those on phenorbarbital. Early suggestions that a positive psychotropic advantage accrued as a result of treatment with carbamazepine have not been fully explored. If such an advantage occurred, it might be relevant to look for withdrawal effects in children in whom carbamazepine had been used. No such study has been recorded.

Conclusions

There has been virtually no work designed to consider whether carbamazepine can be permanently harmful to the developing brain. The finding that infants exposed to carbamazepine in utero have small head circumferences requires further investigation. In particular it would be important to determine whether defects in higher nervous function become apparent in these children after school age.

Valproate

Valproate is usually administered as valproic acid or as sodium valproate. It is known to increase the whole brain content of the inhibitory neurotransmitter GABA, but this is felt not to be its basic anticonvulsant mechanism (Johnston and Salter, 1982). It is known further to cause hyperpolarisation of membrane potentials and to selectively augment post-synaptic GABA-mediated inhibition. Furthermore, inhibition of the glycine cleavage system may lead to hyperglycinaemia and hyperglycinuria (Mortensen et al, 1980). Secondary hyperammonemia can occur in patients with propionyl CoA carboxylase deficiency, with raised propionate levels (Coutter and Allen, 1980). Long-term treatment with valproate results in significant dose-dependent reduction in the plasma levels of protein-bound iodine, T_4 and T_3 (Fichsel and Knopfle, 1977). Thus valproate might have the potentiality to permanently affect brain development by interfering with new synapse formation, altering the amino acid pool necessary for structural development or by secondary effects associated with alterations in thyroid availability.

Neurological effects

There is no study relating possible permanent neurological disorder to the prenatal or immediate post-natal use of valproate. In 59 children aged 6 months to 5 years who

were given valproate for periods from 2 weeks to 2 years no alteration in clinical neurological status was noted despite careful monitoring (Wallace, unpublished data). In
particular, the 17 of the 59 children who received valproate continuously for 2 years
during which their motor ability was examined at 3-monthly intervals were completely
without signs that valproate affected fine or gross movement. Tremor is a recognised
feature of long-term treatment with valproate in older children and adults, but its nature and reversibility have not been systematically studied.

Cognitive effects

The possible prenatal and immediate post-natal effects of valproate on cognitive development have not been studied.

In 13 children treated with valproate in the prophylaxis of febrile convulsions, the
mean Griffiths Developmental Quotient was 113.8 (SD 13.3) prior to commencing
therapy and 115.9 (SD 14.2) 24 months later. (Aldridge Smith and Wallace, 1982).
These findings were not significantly different from those of 21 children of comparable
age and seizure status who had received no drugs over the same 24-month period.

No systematic study of the effects of valproate on older children has been performed.

Behavioural effects

No information is available on the possible behavioural effects on infants whose mothers have been given valproate during pregnancy. In a prospective study of such effects
in children aged 6 months to 5 years, mothers were asked to give a profile of their
child's behaviour pattern prior to commencing valproate. (Wallace and Aldridge
Smith, 1980). Two to three weeks after starting valproate the parents of 7 of 34 children reported deterioration in at least one aspect of behaviour. In comparable children
given no drug over the same period, the parents of 3 of 18 children reported deterioration in at least one aspect of behaviour. Improvement in at least one aspect was commented upon in 10 of 34 children given valproate and 4 of the 18 on no drugs. The
differences between the valproate and no treatment groups are not significant for
either deterioration or improvement. During this study, which continued for 2 years,
it was not necessary to withdraw valproate from any child on behavioural grounds.
Valproate was withdrawn after 2 years in 15 children (Wallace, unpublished data).
No behaviour change was noted in 7 of the 15. At least three aspects of behaviour
improved in only 1 child and deteriorated in 3. One or two aspects of behaviour deteriorated in a further 4. Children were apt to be more irritable, more active, sleep less
well, cry more and be less easy to manage after withdrawal of valproate. Within 3
months of stopping valproate all parents considered their children to be back to normal. Herranz et al. (1982) reported some behavioural side-effects in 56 of 88 children
on valproate monotherapy. 30 of the 56 had alterations in their sleep patterns, with
17 having longer and deeper sleep and 13 more superficial sleep. 17 of the 56 with
behaviour changes were more irritable after commencing valproate. The authors do

not consider possible long-term effects of alteration in sleep behaviour. In a further study of sleep patterns after taking valproate, it was found that in 10 normal young people no consistent alteration occurred as compared with placebo. (Harding et al., 1982). However, withdrawal of valproate affected rapid eye movement sleep. Excessive appetite was noted to be a complication of treatment with valproate soon after its introduction. Egger and Brett (1981) have reviewed this behavioural complication in detail, and emphasise the lack of understanding of its mechanism.

Conclusions

There is a paucity of studies on the effects of valproate given at periods of maximal brain growth and differentiation. The metabolic effects relating to alterations in behaviour, particularly those involving sleep disturbance and appetite, might in the long-term be of permanent disadvantage to the developing child, but further information is required on this aspect of valproate therapy.

Ethosuximide

Ethosuximide is used almost exclusively in absence seizures, when, in those patients who respond, there is clearance of the typical 3 Hz spike and wave activity on EEG within 48 h. No other effect on the EEG has been recorded. Ferrendelli and Klunk (1982) have reviewed the possible mechanisms of action of ethosuximide. It has an inhibitory effect which may be selective for $(Na^+ + K^+)$-ATPase existing in plasma membranes of nerve terminals, but this is thought not to explain its anticonvulsant effect. There is a possibility that it may enhance the influence of inhibitory neurotransmitters, but this is by no means proven. Thus the anticonvulsant properties of ethosuximide remain incompletely explained. In considering long-term effects on brain development it is therefore difficult to anticipate which features of maturation might be selectively affected.

Neurological effects

Since absence seizures are rare after puberty, it would be unusual for ethosuximide to be given in pregnancy. No reports of studies of infants of mothers given this drug have appeared in the literature. In older children neurological complications do not seem to have been studied prospectively. This is possibly because abnormal neurological signs have not been reported as a complication of treatment with ethosuximide.

Cognitive effects

All available studies refer to children of school age. Guey et al. (1967) reported intellectual deterioration manifested by memory disorders and speech disturbances in 25 children with various seizure types who received ethosuximide. However, the role of ethosuximide in the deterioration is uncertain, except that improvement occurred on its discontinuation. All 25 children were receiving other anti-epileptic drugs and 15 of them were known to be mentally retarded. When children received ethosuximide monotherapy for absence seizures no deterioration in abilities was found (Penry et al., 1972). 40 children were studied using the Halsted-Reitan neuropsychological battery and it was felt there might be some improvement in function. Such improvement is likely to be related, at least in part, to suppression of the abnormal EEG activity associated with the underlying condition. Improvement in intellectual function while taking ethosuximide was also reported by Smith et al. (1968). These authors treated children with learning disorders and 14–6 positive spikes on their EEGs with ethosuximide. The full scale and verbal quotients of the WISC increased significantly, though the performance quotient did not. The authors comment neither on whether improvement was maintained in the long term, nor on whether withdrawal led to regression.

Behavioural effects
Possible long-term behavioural effects of ethosuximide have not been studied. Drowsiness, fatigue and lethargy have been noted as side effects and are considered always to be dose related and reversible.

Conclusions
Ethosuximide is usually given in middle to late childhood when all aspects of brain growth are past their peak rates. In studies where it has been used as sole medication for either absence seizures or learning disorders some improvement in cognitive function has been observed. It is unlikely that ethosuximide has neurobehavioural teratological effects.

Comment

Most anticonvulsant drugs have been shown to be effective because of their ability to reduce excitation at neuronal membranes or alter neurotransmitter efficacy. Thus it might be anticipated that in infancy and childhood the development of new central nervous system pathways would be jeopardised by exposure to antiepileptic treatment. The study of this subject is still in its infancy. It is even uncertain whether any deleterious effects noted during treatment are permanent.

Extended follow-up studies of infants exposed to barbiturates in utero are required, and the neurological, cognitive and behavioural findings before, during and after treatment with phenobarbital in later childhood are still unquantified. Primidone has so much in common with phenobarbital that unless the phenylethylmalonamide component were examined separately effects of primidone itself would be difficult to ascertain. On theoretical grounds phenytoin might be expected to cause widespread interference with brain development, but no prospective study has explored this potentiality prior to school age. Studies on carbamazepine have started with the assumption

148

that it might benefit behaviour and cognitive function and have failed to comment on whether any improvement observed acutely is maintained, and on whether there is regression after the drug is discontinued. Effects of valproate on the normal fetal and epileptic childhood brain remain to be defined. Ethosuximide, because of its specific action in relation to absence seizures tends to be given only in middle to late childhood. Any neurobehavioural effect is likely to be associated with improvement through relief of absences.

Anticonvulsant drugs, excepting where a fetus receives them through passive transfer, are prescribed almost exclusively for infants and children with seizure disorders. In examining possible drug effects on the brain, it may be difficult to quantify neurobehavioural teratological effects of the seizures themselves.

Acknowledgment

Miss M. Chilcott has given secretarial assistance.

References

Aldridge Smith, J. and Wallace, S.J. (1982) Febrile convulsions: Intellectual progress related to recurrence of fits and to anticonvulsant therapy. Arch. Dis. Child. 57, 104–107.
Balazs, R. (1976) Hormones and brain development. Prog. Brain Res. 45, 139–159.
Barnes, M.R. and Fetterman, J.L. (1938) Mentality of dispensary epileptic patients. Arch. Neurol. 40, 903–910.
Booker, H.E. (1972) Primidone: Toxicity. In: Antiepileptic Drugs, Woodbury, D.M., Penry, J.K. and Schmidt, R.P., (eds.) Raven Press, New York, pp. 377–383.
Camfield, C.S., Chaplin, S., Doyle, A-B., Shapiro, S.H., Cummings, C. and Camfield, P.R. (1979) Side effects of phenobarbital in toddlers; behavioural and cognitive aspects. J. Pediat. 95, 361–365.
Chadwick, D., Reynolds, E.H. and Marsden, C.D. (1976) Anticonvulsant-induced dyskinesias: a comparison with dyskinesias induced by neuroleptics. J. Neurol. Neurosurg. Psychiat. 39, 1210–1218.
Coulter, D.L. and Allen, R.J. (1980) Secondary hyperammonemia: a possible mechanism for valproate encephalopathy. Lancet i, 1310–1311.
Dam, M. (1982) Phenytoin: Toxicity. In: Antiepileptic Drugs, Woodbury, D.M., Penry, J.K. and Pippenger, C.E., (eds.) Raven Press, New York, pp. 247–256.
Desmond, M.M., Schwanecke, R.P., Wilson, G.D., Yasunaga, S. and Burgdorff, I. (1972) Maternal barbiturate utilisation and neonatal withdrawal symptomatology. J. Pediatr. 80, 190–197.
Dobbing, J. and Sands, J. (1973) The quantitative growth and development of the human brain. Arch. Dis. Child. 48, 757–767.
Dodrill, C.B. (1975) Diphenylhydantoin serum levels, toxicity and neuropsychologial performance in patients with epilepsy. Epilepsia 16, 593–600.
Egger, J. and Brett, E.M. (1981) Effects of sodium valproate in 100 children with special reference to weight. Brit. Med. J. 283, 577–581.
Ferrendelli, J.A. and Klunk, W.E. (1982) Ethosuximide: Mechanisms of action. In: Antiepileptic Drugs. Woodbury, D.M., Penry, J.K. and Pippenger, C.E., (eds.) Raven Press, New York, pp. 655–661.
Fischel, H., Knopfle, G. (1978) Influence of anticonvulsive drugs on thyroid hormones in epileptic children.

In: Advances in Epileptology – 1977. Meinardi, H. and Rowan, A.J., (eds.) Swets and Zeitlinger, Amsterdam-Lisse, pp. 346–349.

Granstrom, M-L. (1982) Development of children of epileptic mothers: Preliminary results from the prospective Helsinki study. In: Epilepsy, Pregnancy and the Child. Janz, D., Dam, M., Richens, A., Bossi, L., Helge, H. and Schmidt, D., (eds.) Raven Press, New York, pp. 403–408.

Groh, C. (1978) Studies on the psychotropic effect of carbamazepine. In: Advances in Epileptology – 1977 Meinardi, H. and Rowan, A.J., (eds.) Swets and Zeitlinger, Amsterdam-Lisse, pp. 109–113.

Guey, J., Charles, C., Coquery, C., Roger, J. and Soulayrol, R. (1967) Study of the psychological effects of ethosuximide (Zarontin) in 25 children suffering from petit mal epilepsy. Epilepsia 8, 129–141.

Hamster, W. and Petruch, F. (1978) Psychometric studies in epileptics before therapy and under carbamazepine. In: Advances in Epileptology – 1977. Meinardi, H. and Rowan, A.J., (eds.) Swets and Zeitlinger, Amsterdam-Lisse, pp. 104–108.

Hanson, J.W. and Smith, D.W.(1975) The fetal hydantoin syndrome. J. Pediatr. 87, 285–290.

Harding, G.A., Alford, C.A. and Powell, T.E. (1982) Effect of sodium valproate on the sleep and performance of normal subjects. Paper persented at the 14th Epilepsy International Symposium, London.

Hellstrom, B. and Barlach-Christoffersen, M. (1980) Influence of phenobarbital on the psychomotor development and behaviour in pre-school children with convulsions. Neuropaediatrie 11, 151–160.

Herranz, J.L., Arteaga, R. and Armijo, J.A. (1982) Side-effects of sodium valproate in monotherapy controlled by plasma levels: a study in 88 pediatric patients. Epilepsia 23, 203–214.

Hiilesmaa, V.K., Teramo, K., Granstrom, M-L. and Bardy, A.H. (1982) Fetal growth and antiepileptic drugs: preliminary results of the prospective Helsinki study. In: Epilepsy, Pregnancy and the Child. Janz, D., Dam, M., Richens, A., Bossi, L., Helge, H. and Schmidt, D., (eds.) Raven Press, New York, pp. 203–205.

Himwich, W.A. and Davis, J.M. (1974) Free amino acids in the developing brain as affected by drugs. In: Drugs and the Developing Brain. Vernadakis, A. and Weinar, N., (eds.) Plenum Press, New York, pp. 231–242.

Holdsworth, L. and Whitmore, K. (1974) A study of children with epilepsy attending ordinary schools. I. Their seizure patterns, progress and behaviour in school. Dev. Med. Child Neurol. 16, 746–758.

Hoyte, C.S. and Billson, F.A. (1978) Maternal anticonvulsants and optic nerve hypoplasia. Brit. J. Ophthalmol. 62, 3–6.

Hutt, S.J., Jackson, P.M., Belsham, A. and Higgins, G. (1968) Perceptual motor behaviour in relation to blood phenobarbitone level: a preliminary report. Dev. Med. Child Neurol. 10, 626–632.

Jacobides, G.M. (1978) Alertness and scholastic achievement in young epileptic patients treated with carbamazepine. In: Advances in Epileptology – 1977 Meinardi, H. and Rowan, A.J., (eds.) Swets and Zeitlinger, Amsterdam-Lisse, pp. 114–119.

Jager-Roman, E., Rating, D., Koch, S., Gopfert-Geyer, I., Jacob, S. and Helge, H. (1982) Somatic parameters, diseases and psychomotor development in the offspring of epileptic parents. In: Epilepsy, Pregnancy and the Child. Janz, D., Dam, M., Richens, A., Bossi, L., Helge, H. and Schmidt, D., (eds.) Raven Press, New York, pp. 425–432.

Janz, D. (1982) On major malformations and minor abnormalities in the offspring of parents with epilepsy: review of the literature. In: Epilepsy, Pregnancy and the Child. Janz, D., Dam, M., Richens, A., Bossi, L., Helge, H. and Schmidt, D., (eds.) Raven Press, New York, pp. 211–222.

Johnston, D. and Slater, G.E. (1982) Valproate: Mechanisms of action. In: Antiepileptic Drugs. Woodbury, D.M., Penry, J.K. and Pippenger, C.E. (eds.) Raven Press, New York, pp. 611–616.

Kalska, H. (1976) The effects of some antiepileptic drugs on cognitive performance. In: Epileptology Janz, D., (ed.) Georg Thieme, Stuttgart, pp. 183–187.

Latis, G.O., Battino, D., Boldi, B., Breschi, F., Ferraris, G., Moise, A., Molteni, B. and Simionato, L. (1982) Preliminary data of a neuropediatric follow-up of infants born to epileptic mothers. In: Epilepsy, Pregnancy and the Child. Janz, D., Dam, M., Richens, A., Bossi, L., Helge, H. and Schmidt, D., (eds.) Raven Press, New York, pp. 419–423.

150

Lennox, W.G. (1942) Brain injury, drugs and environment as causes of mental decay in epilepsy. Am. J. Psychiat. 99, 174–180.

Martin, F., Movarrekhi, M. and Gisiger, M.G. (1965) Etude de quelques effets du Tegretol sur une population d'enfants epileptiques. Schweiz. Med. Wschr. 95, 982–989.

Massala, A., Meloni, T., Alagna, S., Rovasio, P.P., Mele, G. and France, V. (1980) Pituitary responsiveness to gonadotrophin-releasing and thyrotrophin-releasing hormones in children receiving phenobarbitone. Brit. Med. J. 281, 1175–1178.

Mattson, R.H. and Cramer, J.A. (1982) Phenobarbital: toxicity. In: Antiepileptic Drugs, Woodbury, D.M., Penry, J.K. and Pippinger, C.E., (eds.) Raven Press, New York, pp. 351–363.

Meinardi, H. (1972) Carbamazepine. In: Antiepileptic Drugs, Woodbury, D.M., Penry, J.K. and Schmidt, R.P., (eds.) Raven Press, New York, pp. 487–496.

Morrell, F., Bradley, W. and Ptashne, M. (1959) Effects of drugs on discharge characteristics of chronic epileptogenic lesions. Neurology 9, 492–498.

Mortensen, P.B., Kølvraa, S. and Christensen, E. (1980) Inhibition of the glycine cleavage system: Hyperglycinaemia and hyperglycinuria caused by valproic acid. Epilepsia 21, 563–569.

Nolte, R., Wetzel, B., Brugmann, G. and Brintzinger, I. (1980) Effects of phenytoin- and primidone-monotherapy on mental performance in children. In: Antiepileptic Therapy. Advances in Drug Monitoring. Johanessen, S.I., Morselli, P.L., Pippenger, C.E., Richens, A., Schmidt, D. and Meinardi, H., (eds.) Raven Press, New York, pp. 81–88.

Nolte, R., Wetzel, B., Brugmann, G. and Brintzinger, I. (1982) Phenytoin monotherapy in school children. A prospective study. Presented at the 14th Epilepsy International Symposium, London.

Penry, J.K., Porter, R.J. and Dreifuss, F.E. (1972) Ethosuximide: Relation of plasma levels to clinical control. In: Antiepileptic Drugs. Woodbury, D.M., Penry, J.K. and Schmidt, R.P., (eds.) Raven Press, New York, pp. 431–448.

Prichard, J.W. (1982) Phenobarbital: mechanisms of action. In: Antiepileptic Drugs. Woodbury, D.M., Penry, J.K. and Pippenger, C.E., (eds.) Raven Press, New York, pp. 365–376.

Smith, W.L., Philippus, M.J. and Guard, H.K. (1968) Psychometric study of children with learning problems and 14–6 positive spike EEG patterns treated with ethosuximide (Zarontin) and placebo. Arch. Dis. Child. 43, 616–619.

Somerfeld-Ziskind, E. and Ziskind, E. (1940) Effects of phenobarbital on mentality of epileptic patients. Arch. Neurol. 43, 70–79.

Stores, G. (1975) Behavioural effects of antiepileptic drugs. Dev. Med. Child. Neurol. 17, 647–658.

Stores, G. and Hart, J. (1976) Reading skills of children with generalised or focal epilepsy attending ordinary school. Dev. Med. Child Neurol. 18, 705–716.

Thorn, I. (1975) A controlled study of prophylactic long-term treatment of febrile convulsions with phenobarbital. Acta Neurol. Scand. (suppl. 75) 60, 67–73.

Trimble, M. and Corbett, J. (1979) Anticonvulsant drugs and behaviour – preliminary report. Presented to 11th Epilepsy International Symposium, Firenze.

Trimble, M. and Corbett, J. (1980) Anticonvulsant drugs and cognitive function. In: Advances in Epileptology: The Xth Epilepsy International Symposium. Wada, J.A. and Penry, J.K. (eds.) Raven Press, New York, pp. 113–120.

Volpe, J.J. (1981a) Neurology of the Newborn. Saunders, Philadelphia, pp. 3–27.

Volpe, J.J. (1981b) Neurology of the Newborn. Saunders, Philadelphia, pp. 28–59.

Wada, J.A. (1977) Pharmacological prophylaxis in the kindling model of epilepsy. Arch. Neurol. 34, 389–395.

Wallace, S.J. and Aldridge Smith, J. (1980) The effectiveness of dipropylacetate compared with phenobarbitone or no therapy in the prevention of convulsions with fever. In: Antiepileptic therapy: Advances in Drug Monitoring. Johanessen, S.I., Morselli, P.L., Pippenger, C.E., Richens, A., Schmidt, D. and Meinardi H. (eds.) Raven Press, New York, pp. 63–73.

Wapner, I., Thurston, D.L. and Holowach, J. (1962) Phenobarbital: Its effect on learning in epileptic children. J. Am. Med. Assoc. 182, 937.

Weiner, N. (1974) Neurotransmitter systems in the central nervous system. In: Drugs and the Developing Brain. Vernadakis, A. and Weiner N. (eds.) Plenum Press, New York, pp. 105–132.

Wolf, S.M. and Forsythe, A. (1978) Behaviour disturbance, phenobarbital and febrile seizures. Pediatrics 61, 728–731.

Wolf, S.M., Forsythe, A., Stunden, A.A., Friedman, R. and Diamond, H. (1981) Long-term effect of phenobarbital on cognitive function in childern with febrile convulsions. Pediatrics 68, 820–823.

Woodbury, D.M. (1982) Phenytoin: mechanisms of action. In: Antiepileptic Drugs. Woodbury, D.M., Penry, J.K. and Pippenger, C.E. (eds.) Raven Press, New York, pp. 269–281.

Neurobehavioral Teratology
edited by Joseph Yanai
© Elsevier Science Publishers BV 1984

7

A Review of Diazepam and Other Benzodiazepines in Pregnancy

Veronika E. Grimm

The Hebrew University of Jerusalem and The Weizmann Institute of Science, Rehovot, Israel

SINCE their introduction in 1960, the benzodiazepines (chlordiazepoxide, diazepam, fluorazepam, oxazepam etc.) have been used extensively to modify behavior in a wide variety of clinical problems. The usefulness of this family of drugs for seemingly diverse clinical conditions stems from at least four distinct behavioral effects, which include: anticonvulsant, muscle relaxant, anxiolytic and sedative-hypnotic properties (Tallman et al., 1980).

The use of benzodiazepines (BZDs) increased steadily throughout the 1970s. A conservative estimate indicates that in 1977 at least 8000 tons of these drugs were consumed in the United States (Tallman et al., 1980). Parallel with the increase in use in the general population, the use of diazepam (DZP) and other BZDs during pregnancy and labor increased throughout these years. In obstetric care they have been widely used to reduce anxiety, induce sedation or muscular relaxation, to reduce the average duration of normal larbor and in the treatment of eclampsia and preeclampsia (Bepko et al., 1965; Flowers et al., 1969; Friedman et al., 1969; Joyce and Kenyon, 1972; Lean et al., 1968; Sagen and Haram, 1973; Niswander, 1969).

Today, the use of drugs during the first trimester of pregnancy is not recommended. Since diazepam is one of the most commonly used drugs in the world, and became for many an easily available household remedy against psychological tensions, unpleasant moods or sleep disturbances, it is possible that a woman uses it without being aware of pregnancy in its early stages. Finally, diazepam is prescribed for psychiatric complications of pregnancy and is sometimes used to treat a threatened abortion (Ekkola et al., 1974).

In the 1960s clinical and research reports (Bepko et al., 1965; Joyce and Kenyon, 1972; Niswander, 1969; Berger, 1966; Toulouse and Maffei, 1965) considered the use of benzodiazepines in pregnancy and labor to be completely safe. Later studies increasingly drew attention to undesirable side effects and some even indicated that the administration of diazepam in early pregnancy was a possible teratogen in the formation of oral clefts (Saxen and Saxen, 1975; Aarskog, 1975; Safra and Oakley, 1975).

Drug disposition in mother, foetus and infant

After administration the BZDs are widely distributed in the body, but accumulate preferentially in lipid-containing areas, such as adipose tissue and brain. The pharmacologically active metabolites of BZDs are often long lived. Metabolism of BZDs is carried out primarily in the liver and their excretion by the kidneys. DZP, the most frequently used benzodiazepine, is metabolized by demethylation and hydroxylation to form demethyldiazepam and oxazepam, which, after conjugation, are excreted through the kidneys and bile and can be detected for the following 2 weeks in both urine and faeces. The half life of DZP is 24–48 h, that of demethyldiazepam is 42–96 h and that of oxazepam is 9–11 h. All three of these are biologically active (Gillberg, 1977).

DZP is a lipid-soluble drug with a small molecular weight so it crosses the placenta rapidly (Cavanagh and Condo, 1964) and is detectable in the fetal blood flow 5 min after maternal administration (Erkkola et al., 1973). De Silva et al. (1969) found a 1:1 ratio of distribution of diazepam between the maternal and fetal circulation at delivery, while Idänpään-Heikkilä et al. (1971) found that the concentration in fetal blood was consistently higher than that in maternal blood from 1 to 6 h after maternal administration in early pregnancy.

Mandelli et al. (1975), in a careful study, showed DZP to be present in fetal circulation in concentrations similar to those present in maternal plasma, 12 min after i.v. administration. With time, DZP plasma levels appear to be higher in the fetus than in the mother, and after repeated DZP administration both DZP and its metabolite N-demethylDZP show accumulation in the fetal unit.

The drug is not metabolized at all in the fetal liver or small intestine, and thus the fetus may be susceptible to its effects (Ananth, 1976). The newborn infant metabolizes DZP at a very low rate and only after 8–10 days of age do hydroxylated compounds appear in urine (Morselli et. al., 1973; 1974). Especially high levels of benzodiazepines were observed by Mandelli et al. (1975) in the heart, lungs and brain of foetus who received the drug and possibly also its metabolite from the mother through placental circulation (Mandelli et al., 1975).

The floppy infant syndrome

Exposure to DZP during the prenatal period resulted in significant hypothermia in the infants at birth, which lasted for at least 9 h (Owen et al., 1972). While the mechanism for the exaggerated fall in temperature is not clear, the authors point out the similarity of DZP-associated hypothermia to that seen in infants that suffered asphyxial incidents at birth. Alternatively they suggest that DZP may have a direct effect on the central regulation of temperature.

Doses larger than 30 mg given to the mother during labor were shown to result in low Apgar scores at birth, apnoeic spells, hypotonia, reluctance to feed and an impaired metabolic response to cold stress (Cree et al., 1973).

In the foetus, diazepam causes reduction of the beat-to-beat heart rate variability. This effect is visible on the heart rate tracing within minutes of maternal administration of the drug (Scher et al., 1972; van Geijn et al., 1980) and lasts through the first postnatal days. The duration of this reduction in heart rate variability depends on the dose of DZP, and may reflect a disturbance in neural regulation.

An increasing number of reports in the literature describe the 'floppy infant syndrome' in babies born to women treated chronically with DZP during pregnancy (Gillberg, 1977; Drury et al., 1977; Rowlatt, 1978; Spreight, 1977). This syndrome includes many or all of the following: failure to start breathing, shallow inadequate respiration, periodic cessation of respiration, floppiness, hypotonia, hyporeflexia, subnormal temperature and poor sucking. These effects last several days, during which significant plasma levels of diazepam and of its active metabolites can be detected.

In some infants withdrawal symptoms were described after prolonged intrauterine exposure to DZP. These included tremor, loose stools, vomiting, hyperactivity, irritability, hypertonicity, etc. The symptoms tended to appear a few hours after birth and last 10 days to 6 weeks in infants whose mothers received DZP therapy during 3–5 months of pregnancy (Rementeria and Bhatt, 1977).

In addition to passing the placenta, DZP and its active metabolites will pass from the mother's blood into breast milk. Measurable blood levels of these compounds then occur in breast-fed newborns. The infant metabolizes these substances more slowly than adults and an accumulation of them in the infant is therefore possible (Cole and Hailey, 1975; Brandt, 1976; Erkkola and Kanto, 1972).

Most of the conditions listed above are related to the amount of drug or its active metabolites present in the newborn. With the development of metabolic and eliminative mechanisms most of these symptoms lessen or disappear and the infants generally recover sufficiently to be released from hospital with no attempt being made to follow their long term development or to monitor later behavioral sequelae of the drug effects. There are two surveys reported in the literature attempting to assess the effects of chlordiazepoxide and another tranquilizing drug, meprobamate, on fetal and childhood development in a large sample of varied population. The results of the two reports contradict each other. One (Milkovich and van den Berg, 1974) found evidence for teratogenic effects for these drugs if taken early in pregnancy, while the other (Hartz et al., 1975) found no evidence for malformations nor any deleterious effects on motor development at 8 months of age, or at age 4 years on a general IQ measure. However, one might question the sensitivity of general IQ measures for the evaluation of the long term consequences of prenatal drug exposure, especially in the light of the increasing attention that is being drawn to the problems of children with learning disabilities. Many children who suffer from various forms of learning disabilities, attention deficit disorders, hyperkinetic problems and other conditions that are often diagnosed as having minimal brain dysfunction (MBD) show normal or even above average performance on general IQ measurements.

Animal studies

The early toxicological studies, similarly to the early human clinical reports, found negligible deleterious effects of BZDs in general or DZP, on reproduction and growth in the rat (Randall et al., 1961). Later studies on placental transfer have shown an accumulation of DZP in the liver and brain in the mouse, hamster and monkey fetus (Idänpään-Heikkilä et al., 1969). Dietary administration of any of six BZDs tranquilizers to mating pairs of mice resulted in reduced birth weight of the offspring and in significant decreases in postnatal survival (Guerriero and Fox, 1977). Relatively few reports focused on the effects of prenatal exposure of BZDs on behavioral development in the offspring. Among these, one investigation found somewhat superior performance for prenatally exposed male mice in a simple Y maze (Fox et al, 1977). However, reports from the same laboratory have shown reduction in litter size in BZD-treated mice, so the experimental group and the controls in this case may have come from extremely different intrauterine background, where the small number of surviving fetuses in the BZD group may have represented the most viable ones both in physical and behavioral terms, while the controls were selected from a wider distribution.

A low dose of DZP (1 mg/kg twice daily) given during pregnancy to rat dams undergoing severe restraint stress was shown to counteract effectively the long term negative influences of maternal stress on measures of behavioral development in the pups (Barlow et al., 1979). Orally adminstered DZP throughout pregnancy to non-stressed rats was shown to cause delayed sexual maturation and impaired acquisition of a conditional avoidance response (Ljubimov et al., 1974).

Prenatal exposure of rats to DZP in the third (final) week of gestation, a period when rapid cellular differentiation occurs in the central nervous system, was shown to interfere with the development of arousal processes in the offspring. The characteristic potentiation of locomotion responses and acoustic startle reflexes that normally appear in the third postnatal week were absent in these pups. The authors suggest that the loss of these behaviors reflects a long term effect that may result from changes in cellular development (Kellogg et al., 1980).

Similar long term effects were shown in my laboratory (Gai et al., 1982; Gai and Grimm, 1982; Frieder and Grimm, 1982). In a series of studies DZP (2.5, 5 or 10 mg/ kg) or an equivalent volume of vehicle was injected into pregnant Wistar dams for 16 days starting on day 4 of pregnancy. The resulting DZP offspring were compared to the vehicle-exposed ones with various measures of physical and behavioral development from birth up to 3 months of age. The results indicated that prenatal exposure to DZP (especially at the two larger doses) induces significant changes in some aspects of development and behavior. The early motor retardation, seen in feeble climbing on an inclined plane at 5 days of age, which may be due to the actual presence of the drug in the body, is not seen by 7 days of age. DZP had no effect on later motor development as tested by coordination, balance and running on a narrow elevated bar at 30 days of age. However, at about the same age, DZP offspring showed less rearing and longer latencies in an open field than the controls, possibly reflecting 'fearfulness' or 'reduced curiosity' (Barnett and Cowan, 1976). One of the most interesting behavioral results of this series of studies concerns the learning performance of DZP-exposed animals 2 or 3 months after the intrauterine drug exposure. At this age (i.e. 2–3 months) DZP and control animals learned two types of brightness-discrimination tasks. In the successive brightness-discrimination task, where the animal is presented only the rewarded stimulus (S+) or the nonrewarded stimulus (S–) on any given trial, but never the two together, DZP-exposed animals learned to run to S+ and not to run to S– just as fast as did the controls. When the reward contingencies were reversed in this task DZP and control rats reached criterion for reversal learning in the same number of trials. However, in a brightness-discrimination maze where S+ and S– are presented simultaneously at six choice points, the animal having to make six decisions on each trial in order to reach the goal, large and significant differences appeared both in running time and error measures between DZP and control animals. The prenatally DZP-exposed animals showed dose-dependent deficits both in acquisition and in the retention of this task 10 days after the learning. Prenatally DZP-exposed animals gave the impression of 'impulsivity', 'distractability', i.e. an inability to suppress incorrect responses.

Preliminary histological investigation of brain slices from these animals show extensive gliosis and perivascular cuffing in the cortex and some subcortical areas, but not in the cerebellum. Gliosis, the proliferation of small glia cells replacing neurons, the functioning nerve cells, is thought to be an indication of neuronal loss or degeneration. The cufflike thickness that was observed surrounding some blood vessels may indicate an allergic reaction to a foreign substance.

Mechanism of action

The benzodiazepines and more specifically diazepam given during pregnancy and labor are implicated in the occurrence of a wide variety of undesirable regulatory dysfunctions in the newborn and may exert long range deleterious influences, as some forms of learning disabilities or attention deficit disorders. The mechanisms by which the drug exerts these effects is not yet clarified. Some in vitro studies show a damaging effect of DZP in cell cultures. In an electron microscope study Breen and Stenchever (1970) noticed some alterations in a cell culture of human fibroblasts when DZP was added at different concentrations. A concentration of 1 g/ml of DZP was high enough to cause deformation in the membranous elements of the cells. It was also demonstrated that diazepam is capable of producing chromosome breakage in vitro and in vivo and that it is capable of retarding the growth rate of cells (Stenchever and Frankel, 1969; Stenchever et al., 1970). The histological finding of gliosis and perivascular cuffing (Frieder and Grimm, 1982) would support the idea of neuronal damage resulting from the early drug exposure.

The finding of chromosomal breakage is in disagreement with an earlier study by Staigen (1969), who found no deleterious effects for chlordiazepoxide nor diazepam on the chromosomes of diploid human fibroblasts. White et al. (1974) reported no increase in chromosomal aberration after single administration of 12–20 mg DZP i.v.

The benzodiazepines have saturable stereospecific and high affinity binding to synaptic plasma membranes obtained from mammalian brain (Mohler and Okada, 1977). A high correlation was found between the pharmacological and clinical effects of the BZPs and their affinities to these brain-specific benzodiazepine receptors. Studies on the ontogenetic development of these receptors found that they are detectable in the rat brain 8 days before birth, and that almost maximal concentration of receptors is achieved about 1 week after birth (Braestrup and Nielsen, 1978).

Available data on the neurochemical effects of benzodiazepines refer to current knowledge of brain neurotransmitters (Garattini et al., 1977). Accordingly, diazepam (and other BZDs investigated) does not interfere with steady state levels of brain monoamines, including dopamine (DA), noradrenaline (NE) and serotonin (5-HT) in the rodent brain (Taylor and Javerty, 1969). However, at high dose levels BZDs tend to decrease NE turnover in the thalamus, midbrain, cortex and cerebellum, DA turnover in the striatum and 5-HT turnover in the cortex of the rat (Lidbrink et al., 1974).

Diazepam was consistently found to increase the levels of acetylcholine (Ach) in the mouse whole brain (Consolo et al., 1972) and in the striatum and hippocampus of the rat (Consolo et al., 1975). The researchers investigating BZD effects on brain neurotransmitters used adult animals. There is no data as yet on the effects of prenatally administered BZD on these neurotransmitter systems in the developing fetus or young animals. Frieder and Grimm (1982) measured [³H]choline uptake to synaptosomes in 10 day old rat pups that were born to chronically DZP-treated dams (a treatment that resulted in specific learning disabilities in older animals, as was described above). The findings indicate a 46% reduction of [³H]choline uptake in comparison to vehicle-treated controls. At 20 days of age the reduction in [³H]choline uptake was somewhat milder but still significant, suggesting that prenatal exposure to DZP might interfere with the normal development of the cholinergic system.

It is by now generally accepted that BZDs exert most of their pharmacological effects by facilitating the action of GABA at the level of postsynaptic receptor sites in the central nervous system (Costa and Guidotti, 1979). Daily DZP treatment during pregnancy does not appear to change the number and affinity characteristics of [³H]diazepam binding in newborn rats. The same treatment also failed to change the binding characteristics of [³H]GABA. However, the capability of muscimol to increase [³H]diazepam binding was greatly reduced in the DZP-exposed animals, suggesting that daily administration of DZP during pregnancy may result in an alteration in the mechanism of coupling between GABA and benzodiazepine receptors (Braestrup et al., 1979; Massotti et al., 1980).

It is not yet known to what extent this alteration of the GABA-benzodiazepine receptor complex resulting from the prenatal exposure is involved in the various behavioral and developmental changes seen in the DZP exposed offspring.

Conclusion

The effects of prenatal exposure to BZPs are of two kinds: (a) the so called 'floppy infant syndrome' covering a variety of regulatory dysfunctions in the neonate, that are directly related to the presence of the drug or its active metabolites in its body; and (b) the long range consequences which can no longer be attributed to the presence of these compounds in the body and which include again a wide range of behavioral alterations from a reduced response output in open field, through flattened arousal, lowered inhibition of competing resonses in complex situations, and to impaired recall of learned tasks.

At the time of writing the nature of the physiological or molecular mechanisms responsible for the floppy infant syndrome are little known, and even less is known about mechanisms that mediate the long range behavioral consequences of prenatal exposure. Further research is needed in order to explore the effects of prenatal DZP exposure on those neurotransmitter systems that play important parts in mediating arousal, activity level, attention and memory processes.

The benzodiazepines have been shown to be effective tools in the management of severe anxiety conditions and useful adjuncts in the treatment of some convulsive disorders. The evidence presented in this review strongly cautions against the use of these drugs in pregnancy. However, very high anxiety levels or frequent convulsive attacks of the pregnant mother may in themselves pose a serious threat to the developing fetus. The respectivce dangers should be seriously weighed in each case before medication is prescribed during pregnancy.

References

Aarskog, D. (1975) Association between maternal intake of diazepam and oral clefts. Lancet ii, 921.

Barlow, S.M., Knight, A.F. and Sullivan, F.M. (1979) Prevention by diazepam of adverse effects of maternal restraint stress on postnatal development and learning in the rat. Teratology 19, 105–110.

Barnett, S.A. and Cowan, P.E. (1976) Activity, exploration, curiosity and fear: An ethological study. Interdiscip. Sci. Rev. 1, 43–63.

Bepko, F., Lowe, E. and Waxman, B. (1965) Relief of the emotional factor in labor with parentally administered diazepam. Obstet. Gynecol. 26, 852–857.

Berger, M. (1966) The use of Diazepam with 3000 parturients. Arzneim. Forsch. 16, 1110–1113.

Braestrup, C. and Nielsen, M. (1978) Ontogenic development of benzodiazepine receptors in the rat brain. Brain Res. 147, 170–173.

Braestrup, C., Nielsen, M. and Squires, R.F. (1979) No changes in rat benzodiazepine receptors after withdrawal from continuous treatment with lorazepam and diazepam. Life Sci. 24, 347–350.

Brandt, R. (1976) Passage of diazepam and desmethyldiazepam into breast milk. Drug Res. 26, 454–457.

Breen, P.C. and Stenchever, M.A. (1970) Some effects of diazepam on the fine structure of human fibroblasts in tissue culture. Am. J. Obstet. Gynecol. 108, 520–527.

Cavanagh, D. and Condo, C.S. (1964) Diazepam – a pilot study of drug concentrations in maternal blood, amniotic fluid and cord blood, Curr. Therap. Res. 6, 122–126.

Cole, A.P. and Hailey, D.M. (1975) Diazepam and active metabolite in breast milk and their transfer to the neonate. Arch. Dis. Child. 50, 741–742.

Consolo, S., Ladinsky, H., Peri, G. and Garattini, S. (1972) Effect of central stimulants and depressants on mouse brain acetylcholine and choline levels. Eur. J. Pharmacol. 18, 251–255.

Consolo, S., Garatinni, S. and Ladinsky, H. (1975) Action of the benzodiazepines on the cholinergic system. In: Mechanism of Action of Benzodiazepines (Costa, E. and Greengard, P., eds.) Raven Press, New York, pp. 45–61.

Cree, J.E., Meyer, J., Hailey, D.M. 1973, Diazepam in labour: Its metbolism and effect on the clinical condition and thermogenesis of the newborn. Brit. Med. J. 4, 251–255.

De Silva, J.A.F., D'Arconte, L. and Kaplan, J. (1964) The determination of blood levels and the placental transfer of diazepam in humans. Curr. Ther. Res. 6, 115–121.

Drury, K.A.D., Spalding, E., Donaldson, D. and Rutherford, D. (1977) Floppy infant syndrome: is oxazepam the answer? Lancet ii, 1126–1127.

Erkkola, R., Kangas, L. and Pekkarinen, A. (1973) The transfer of diazepam across the placenta during labor. Acta Obstet. Gynecol. Scand. 52, 167–170.

Erkkola, R. and Kanto, J. (1972) Diazepam and breast-feeding. Lancet i, 1235–1236.

Erkkola, R., Kanto, J. and Sellman, R. (1974) Diazepam in early human pregnancy. Acta Obstet. Gynecol. Scand. 53, 135–138.

Flowers, C.E., Rudolph, A.J. and Desmond, M.M. (1969) Diazepam (Valium) as an adjunct in obstetric analgesia. Obstet. Gynecol. 34, 68–81.

Fox, K.A., Abendschein, D.R. and Lahcen, R.B. (1977)Effects of benzodiazepam during gestation and infancy on Y-maze performance of mice. Pharmacol. Res. Comm. 9, 325–338.

Frieder, B. and Grimm, V.E. (1982) Prenatal exposure to diazepam: behavioral, neurochemical and histological findings. 4th ESN Meeting of the European Society for Neurochemistry, 398.

Friedman, E.A., Niswander, K.R. and Sachtleben, M.R. (1969) Effect of diazepam on labour. Obstet. Gynecol. 34, 82–86.

Gai, N. and Grimm, V.E. (1982) The effect of prenatal exposure to diazepam on aspects of postnatal development and behavior in rats. Psychopharmacology, 78, 225–229.

Gai, N., Jancourt, A., Assael, M. and Grimm, V.E. (1982) Development of rats after prenatal exposure to diazepam. 13th C.I.N.P. Congress.

Garattini, S., Marcucci, F. and Mussini, E. (1977) The metabolism and pharmacokinetics of selected benzo-diazepines. In: Psychotherapeutic Drugs, (Usdin, E. and Forrest, I. F., eds.), Marcel Dekker, New York, pp.1030–1087.

Gillberg, C. (1977) 'Floppy infant syndrome' and maternal diazepam. Lancet ii, 244.

Guerrero, F.J. and Fox, K.A. (1977) Benzodiazepines and development of Swiss-Webster mice. Pharmacol. Res. Comm. 9, 187–196.

Hartz, S.C., Heinonen, O.P., Shapiro, S., Siskind, V. and Slone, D. (1975) Antenatal exposure to meproba-mate and chlordiazepoxide in relation to malformations, mental development and childhood morta-lity. New. Engl. J. Med. 292, 726–728.

Idänpään-Heikkilä, J.E., Jouppila, P.I., Puolakka, J.O. and Vorne, M.S. (1971) Placental transfer and fetal metabolism of diazepam in early human pregnancy. Am. J. Obstet. Gynecol. 109, 1011–1016.

Idänpään-Heikkilä, J.E., Taska, R.J., Allen, H.A. and Schoolar, J.G. (1969) Placental transfer of diaze-pam-^{14}C in mice, hamsters and monkeys. J. Pharmacol. Exp. Ther. 176, 752–757.

Joyce, D.N. and Kenyon, V.G. (1972) The use of diazepam and hydrallazine in the treatment of severe pre-eclampsia. J. Obstet. Gynaecol. Brit. Commonw. 79, 250–254.

Kawathekar, P., Anusuya, S.R., Sriniwas, P. and Lagali, S. (1973) Diazepam (calmpose) in eclampsia: A preliminary report of 16 cases. Curr. Ther. Res. 15, 645–655.

Kellogg, C., Tervo, D., Ison, J., Parisi, T. and Miller, R.K. (1980) Prenatal exposure to diazepam alters behavioral development in rats. Science 207, 205–207.

Lean, T.H., Ratman, S.S. and Sivasamboo, R.R. (1968) Use of benzodiazepines in the management of eclampsia. J. Obstet. Gynaecol. Brit. Commonw. 75, 856–862.

Lidbrink, P., Corrodi, H. and Fuxe, K. (1974) Benzodiazepines and barbiturates. Turnover changes in cen-tral 5-hydroxytryptamine pathways. Eur. J. Pharmacol. 26, 35–40.

Ljubimov, B.I., Smolnikova, N.M. and Strekalova, S.N. (1974) Effect of diazepam on the development of the offspring. Bull. Exp. Biol. Med. 78, 1156–1158.

Mandelli, M., Morselli, P.L., Nordio, S., Pardi, G., Principi, N., Sereni, F. and Tognoni, G. (1975) Placen-tal transfer of diazepam and its disposition in the newborn. Clin. Pharmacol. Ther. 17, 564–572.

Massotti, M., Alleva, F.R., Balazs, T. and Guidotti, A. (1980) Gaba and the benzodiazepine receptors in the offspring of dams receiving diazepam: ontogenic studies. Neuropharmacology 19, 951–957.

Milkovich, L. and Van Den Berg, B. (1974) Effects of prenatal meprobamate and chlordiazepoxide hydro-chloride on human embryonic and fetal development. New. Engl. J. Med. 291, 1268–1271.

Mohler, H. and Okada, T. (1977) Benzodiazepine receptor: demonstration in the central nervous system. Science 198, 849–851.

Morselli, P.L., Mandelli, M., Tognoni, G., Principi, N., Pardi, G. and Sereni, F. (1974) Drug interactions in the human foetus and in the newborn infant. In: Drug Interactions, (Morselli, P.L., Garattini, S. and Cohen, S.N., eds.) New York, Raven Press, pp.259–270.

Morselli, P.L., Principi, N., Tognoni, G., Reali, E., Belvedere, G., Standen, S.M. and Sereni, F. (1973) Diazepam elimination in premature and full term infants, and children. J. Perinat. Med. 1, 133–141.

Niswander, K.R. (1969) Effects of diazepam on meperidine requirements in patients during labor. Obstet. Gynecol. 34, 62–67.

Owen, J.R., Irani, S.F. and Blair, A.W. (1972) Effect of diazepam administered to mothers during labour on temperature regulation of neonate. Arch. Dis. Child. 47, 107–110.

Randall, L.O., Heise, G.A., Schallek, W., Bagdon, R.E., Banziger, R., Boris, A., Moe, R.A. and Abrams, W.B. (1961) Pharmacological and clinical studies on valium: A new psychotherapeutic agent of the benzodiazepine class. Curr. Therap. Res. 3, 405–425.

Randall, L.O., Schallek, W., Heise, G.A., Keith, E.F. and Bagdon, R.F. (1960) The psychosedative proper-ties of methamino diazepoxide. J. Pharmacol. Exp. Ther. 129, 163–166.

Rementeria, J.L. and Bhatt, K. (1977) Withdrawal symptoms in neonates from intrauterine exposure to diazepam. J. Pediat. 90, 123–126.

Rowlat, R.J. (1978) Effect of maternal diazepam on the newborn. Brit. Med. J. 1, 985.

Safra, M.J. and Oakley, G.P. (1975) Association between cleft lip with or without cleft palate and prenatal exposure to diazepam. Lancet ii, 478.

Sagen, N. and Haram, K. (1973) Diazepam (valium) as an anaesthetic for operative vaginal delivery. Acta Obstet. Gynecol. Scand. 52, 153–156.

Saxen, I. and Saxen, L. (1975) Association between maternal intake of diazepam and oral cleft. Lancet ii, 496.

Scher, J., Hailey, D.M. and Beard, R.W. (1972) The effects of diazepam on the fetus. J. Obstet. Gynaecol. Brit. Commonw. 79, 635–638.

Speight, A.N.P. (1977) Floppy-infant syndrome and maternal diazepam and/-or nitrazepam. Lancet ii, 878.

Strenchever, M.A. and Frankel, R.B. (1969) Some effects of diazepam (on chromosomes of human leucocytes in vivo) in human cells in vitro. Am. J. Obstet. Gynecol. 103, 836–842.

Stenchever, M.A., Frankel, R.B. and Jarvis, J.A. (1970) Effect of diazepam on chromosomes of human leukocytes in vivo. Am. J. Obstet. Gynecol. 107, 456–460.

Tallman, J.F., Paul, S.M., Skolnick, P. and Gallager, D.W. (1980) Receptors for the age of anxiety: Pharmacology of the benzodiazepines. Science 207, 274–281.

Taylor, K.M. and Laverty, R. (1969) The effect of chlordiazepoxide, diazepam and intrazepam on catecholamine metabolism in regions of the rat brain. Eur. J. Pharmacol. 8, 296–301.

Toulouse, R. and Maffei, J.L. (1965) The utilization of valium in obstetrics. Rev. Franc. Gynecol. Obstet. 60, 263–270.

Van Geijn, H.P., Jongsma, H.W., Doesburg, W.H., Lemmens, W.A.J.G., de Haan, J. and Eskes, T.K.A.B. (1980) The effect of diazepam administration during pregnancy or labor on the heart rate variability of the newborn infant. Eur. J. Obstet. Gynecol. Reprod. Biol. 10, 187–201.

Yeh, S.Y., Paul, R.H., Cordero, L. and Hon, E.H. (1974) A study of diazepam during labor. Obstet. Gynecol. 43, 363–373.

Neurobehavioral Teratology
edited by Joseph Yanai
© Elsevier Science Publishers BV 1984

8

NEUROHISTOLOGICAL AND NEUROBIOLOGICAL ASPECTS OF FETAL ALCOHOL SYNDROME IN THE RAT

Benedikt Volk

Institute of Pathology, Department of Neuropathology, University of Freiburg, Albertstrasse 19, D-7800 Freiburg i.Br., FRG

THE toxicity of alcohol to the embryo and fetus was suspected in the last centuries (Ryan, 1837; Sullivan, 1899). However, it was only in 1968 that Lemoine et al., then later Ulleland et al. (1970), Jones et al. (1973) and Jones and Smith (1973, 1975) established the 'fetal alcohol syndrome' (FAS) as a nosological entity. The phenotype of the FAS shows a high variability. The main clinical features include intrauterine and postnatal growth retardation, microcephaly, facial characteristics (such as short palpebral fissures, hypoplastic philtrum, retrognathia etc.) and joint, limb and cardiac malformations (Clarren and Smith, 1978; Majewski, 1980). Dysfunction of the central nervous system such as mental retardation is one of the most common and most serious clinical symptoms in FAS (Majewski et al., 1976; Streissguth et al., 1980). There are few reports of autopsies of children with FAS. Jones and Smith (1975), and Peiffer et al. (1979) observed dysraphic disorders, porencephaly, agenesis of the corpus callosum and heterotopias in neuropathological investigations.

FAS is suspected to be one of the most common intrauterine lesions in the countries of the western world (Bierich et al., 1976; Clarren and Smith, 1978). In the United States Tenbrink and Buchin (1975) expected 4000–5000 births with FAS per year. According to Leiber (1977), in the Federal Republic of Germany 1500–3000 children a year show alcohol-induced birth defects and in France, Semaille-Viellette and Semaille (1977) reported an incidence of 3 ‰.

164

Placental transfer of alcohol

Ethyl alcohol is a short chain aliphatic hydrocarbon which easily passes biological membranes and the placental barrier. In experimental animals, Kesäniemi and Sippel (1975) observed that 20 min after alcohol administration to pregnant rats, blood alcohol levels in the fetal circulation were similar to the maternal values. On the other hand, alcohol metabolites such as acetaldehyde were only present in maternal blood and placental tissue, but not in the fetus. Sippel and Kesäniemi (1975) concluded that the placenta may have a barrier function protecting the fetus against products of alcohol oxidation. Mann et al. (1975) also noticed almost identical alcohol concentrations in the maternal and fetal circulation in pregnant sheep. In man, alcohol penetrates rather quickly through the placenta (Berlinkoff and Hall, 1950; Fetchko et al., 1951) and can be detected in the bloodstream of the newborn. However, differences in placental transfer of ethanol may be due to species variation (Waltman and Iniquez, 1972). Autoradiographic studies also show a fast passage of alcohol to the fetus (Åkesson, 1974) and regional differences within the fetal central nervous system (Ho et al., 1972). Ho and coworkers found in monkeys and hamsters a higher concentration of alcohol in cortical areas. Within the gray matter they found accumulation of activity in the cerebellum, putamen, visual cortex and hippocampus. They postulate that this pattern of distribution might explain the effect of alcohol on coordination and on the visual system.

The metabolism of alcohol

After oral intake of alcohol about 20% is resorbed by the stomach mucosa and about 80% by the intestines (Teschke and Lieber, 1978). The oxidation of alcohol by alcohol dehydrogenase (ADH) occurs mainly in the liver. Furthermore ADH is located in other organs such as kidney, lung, stomach, intestines and the brain (Isselbacher and Carter, 1973; Moser et al., 1969). Investigations of Raskin and Sokoloff (1968) and Rawat and Kuriyama (1972) have shown that after long term alcohol administration small amounts will be metabolized in the central nervous system. It is still under discussion as to whether ethanol oxidation in the brain may enhance the acute or chronic action of alcohol on the central nervous system. A further interesting but still hypothetical point is the possible interaction of biogenic aldehydes or acetaldehyde with catecholamines during alcohol metabolism forming morphine-like alkaloids (Cohen, 1977; Collins, 1977; Collins and Bigdeli, 1975; Deitrich and Erwin, 1975). These condensation products are neurotoxic and may induce neuronal degeneration in chronic alcoholism.

Besides ADH, the microsomal ethanol-oxidizing system (MEOS) located in the endoplasmic reticulum of hepatocytes plays an inportant role in ethanol metabolism in man and experimental animals. Lieber and DeCarli (1972) have shown that in the normal rat about 25% of ethanol metabolism is effected by the MEOS, which also metabolizes higher aliphatic alcohols such as propanol, butanol, etc. (Teschke et al., 1974). However, in contrast to ADH, the microsomal oxidation shows no coupling of oxidation to phosphorylation (Lieber, 1975). Therefore, a decrease in body weight after chronic alcohol consumption in man and experimental animals (Lieber et al., 1965) may be caused by the energy cost of wasteful pathways of alcohol metabolism (Pirola and Lieber, 1972). This may be an important point explaining the growth deficiency and developmental delay in the FAS. Majewski (1980) observed that in chronic drinkers there is a significant increase in children with FAS. Thus the intrauterine hypotrophy of these children may be induced or enhanced by the insufficient caloric utilization of the microsomal alcohol oxidation in their mother's metabolism.

After consumption and distribution of alcohol in the maternal body and after passing the placenta (Idanpään-Heikklä et al., 1972), alcohol can only be metabolized slowly by the fetal organism (Pikkarainen and Räiha, 1967; Räiha, et al., 1967; Sippel and Kesäniemi, 1975; Hollstedt and Rydberg, 1970). However, in young rats the ADH system develops rather quickly. In 3 week old animals, adult levels of this enzyme were observed by Räiha et al. (1967). There may be a similar situation in premature human infants. They are capable of oxidizing alcohol but not with the same capacity as their mothers (Gärtner and Ryden, 1972; Wagner et al., 1979).

Animal models

Teratogenetic effects of alcohol

In the early 20th century Stockard (1910) observed developmental abnormalities in the brain and the spinal cord of the fish *Fundulus heterolicus*, when its eggs were exposed to different alcohol concentrations. Sandor (1968) and Sandor and Elias (1968) reported malformations and prenatal death in the chick after alcohol treatment of the eggs. A direct toxic effect of alcohol on organogenesis was described by Kronick (1976). Pregnant mice (C57BL6J) were injected ip on different gestational days with a single dose of ethanol. Experimental animals which were treated on day 8, 9 or 10 displayed the highest number of malformations which were comparable in some way with the malformations of the human FAS described by Jones and Smith (1973) and Jones et al. (1973). After ethanol application to pregnant mice (5th to the 10th day of gestation) in a liquid diet fetuses displayed skeletal, heart and anomalies of the fore and hind limbs (Randall et al., 1977). Subsequent observations showed the direct teratogenicity in further mouse models. After ip injection of alcohol to pregnant mice (C57BL6J) at day 7 fetuses showed (7 days after application of ethanol) a reduction of brain size and craniofacial malformations (Sulik et al., 1981). Haddad and Dumas also (1982) reported midfacial hypoplasia and eye defects of mice fetuses of which the mothers received a single oral dose of alcohol during pregnancy. Furthermore, they observed that fetuses of C57BL6J mice were more sensitive to alcohol than fetuses of CBAJ mice. These experiments clearly show the teratogenicity of ethanol for various rodents. The observed malformations are comparable with some of the clinical features of the human FAS.

Prenatal and postnatal growth deficiency

Animal experiments have shown that prenatal alcohol application to maternal animals causes intrauterine and postnatal growth retardation in the offspring. After oral alcohol administration Papara-Nicholson and Telford (1957) observed a reduced birth weight in the offspring of guinea pigs. Similar effects were observed in beagles (Ellis and Pick, 1976), rats (Abel, 1978; Martin et al., 1977; Volk, 1977) and mice (Chernoff, 1977; Swanberg and Crumpacker, 1977; Yanai and Ginsburg, 1977; Randall and Taylor, 1979; Sulik, 1981). Although there has been an increasing interest in recent years in experimental work concerning FAS (Abel, 1980), only few neurohistological investigations have been reported. Volk (1977) and Kornguth et al. (1979) observed in the FAS of rats a reduced cerebellar mass and a retarded maturation of the cerebellar cortex. Barnes and Walker (1981) have shown that after prenatal alcohol exposure in the rat, experimental animals displayed a reduction of hippocampal pyramidal cells by up to 20%.

In the rat, the last stage of brain development, the so-called growth spurt, occurs in the first weeks after birth (Dobbing and Sands, 1971; 1979). In this vulnerable period there is a maturation of myelin, growth of axons and dendrites, multiplication of glial structures, and the formation and maturation of synaptic connections. In comparison, in human infants the growth spurt takes place in the last months of fetal life and lasts up to the second postnatal year (Dobbing, 1970). Because of the postnatal growth spurt of the rat central nervous system some authors administered ethanol to rat pups postnatally. With an inhalation method Bauer-Moffett and Altman (1975, 1977) found an impaired cerebellar maturation with a significant loss of Purkinje cells and a loss of granular cells which was most pronounced after exposure of the animals throughout the lactating period. Subsequently the method of neonatal alcohol exposure was improved (Diaz and Samson, 1980; Samson and Diaz, 1982; Samson et al., 1982). Young rats fed postnatally from day 4 to day 7 with alcohol via an intragastric cannula showed no changes in body weight but a reduction in total brain weight by up to 19% in comparison to control animals. Samson et al. (1982) reported that the microcephaly which severely affected the cerebellum was caused neither by alcohol withdrawal nor zinc deficiency (Samson and Diaz, 1982) but probably by the toxicity of ethanol.

Chemical investigations

Intrauterine and postnatal growth deficiency, the main symptom of FAS, may be caused not only by a direct toxic effect of alcohol on the fetus but also by alterations of maternal and fetal metabolism. Rawat (1975) reported a decrease of cerebral ribosomal protein biosynthesis by up to 30% in the offspring of alcohol-drinking dams. Furthermore, he reported a decrease of total RNA and DNA in neonates whose mothers received alcohol during the lactating period. An inhibitional effect of alcohol on fetal and neonatal protein biosynthesis was observed in liver (Rawat, 1976) and heart (Rawat, 1979). Alterations of protein metabolism in the brain were also observed in adult animals (Noble and Tewari, 1973, 1975; Tewari and Noble, 1976; Tewari et al., 1978). In addition, alcohol administration to pregnant and lactating dams causes a significant decrease of acetylcholine levels in the brain (Rawat, 1976a) and a reduced activity of catecholamine-metabolizing enzymes (Detering et al., 1979). Kornguth et al. (1979) reported reduced serum thyroxine (T_4) levels, together with a retarded cerebellar development in rat FAS. This alteration in endocrinological function may explain the impaired neuronal maturation because hypothyroidism in the postnatal period causes cerebral and cerebellar hypotrophy (Balázs et al., 1968; Nicolson and Altman, 1972).

Malone et al. (1978) observed in rat FAS a decrease in the proteolipid concentration in fractions of mitochondria and nerve endings. Important results were described by Lancaster et al. (1982). After alcohol administration during pregnancy the offspring showed a lower birth weight, delayed eye opening and a reduction of myelin synthesis by about 30%. Interestingly, myelin synthesis recovered in the postnatal period.

Neurohistological investigations

In my own experiments, in which alcohol was administered in the daily drinking water (Volk, 1977), the offspring of alcohol-drinking dams displayed a retarded postnatal weight gain and impaired histogenesis of the central nervous system. Some of the experimental animals showed a hydrocephalus internus ex vacuo (Fig. 8.1). However, these malformations occurred rarely. Because the application of alcohol in the daily drinking water might be nutritionally unbalanced (Lieber and DeCarli, 1972, 1974), we switched over to liquid diet models. In these experiments (Volk et al., 1980a, b, 1981) we focussed on the development of the cerebellum (Altman, 1982, 1972a–c; Larsell, 1970) using histological and electron microscopic techniques. Some of the data from these experiments concerning rat FAS are described here. Firstly alcohol was given to dams before and during pregnancy, secondly alcohol was administered to dams prior to and during pregnancy and in the postnatal period (lactating period). I shall deal with each in turn.

Material and methods
Female nulliparous Wistar rats with initial body weights between 180 and 200 g were housed in plastic cages. Four weeks before mating, they received the liquid diet 'Stardit' in special drinking tubes which allow a very exact feeding of the animals (Fig. 8.2).The diet was supplemented by vitamins 'Multivitamin-Kombinationspulver' and minerals. 20% of the daily calories were supplied by alcohol. Measurements of blood

168

alcohol levels of experimental animals (Bernt and Gutmann, 1970) revealed that values in day and night profiles were mostly lower than 0.1 mg/ml.

After 4 weeks the animals were mated; a positive vaginal smear was used to determine the first day of pregnancy. Controls were housed in the same way as the experimental group. Instead of alcohol these animals received the liquid diet together with isocaloric amounts of sucrose and equal amounts of vitamins. Both groups were pair-fed. After birth the offspring of experimental and control groups did not show significant differences in birth weight and postnatal weight gain. At 3, 4, 7, 12, 17 and 21 days, eight controls and experimental animals were prepared for histological and electron microscopic investigations. The two groups showed no differences in the postnatal development of the central nervous system. Next we nearly doubled the alcohol content of the liquid diet 'Stardit' which was again vitamin-supplemented. 20 female nulliparous Wistar rats (200 g) received a liquid diet in which about 38% of the daily calories were supplied by alcohol 4 weeks before mating and during pregnancy. Blood alcohol levels of the animals were up to 1.6 mg/ml. Controls received isocaloric amounts of sucrose. The animals of both groups were pair-fed and after birth the litter size of the two groups was standardized to eight animals.

Again at 3, 4, 7, 12, 17 and 21 days, eight experimental animals and controls were fixed by vascular perfusion via the left heart (Volk et al., 1981). After dissection of the brain and the spinal cord, midsagittal sections of the entire vermis (Larsell, 1970)

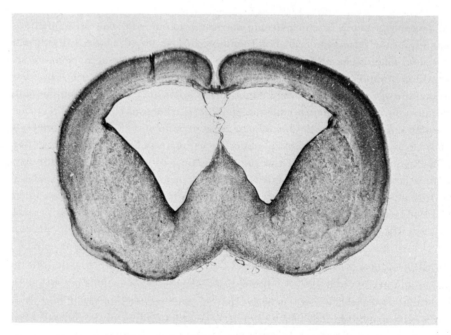

Fig. 8.1. 4 day old experimental animal. Frontal section showing a hydrocephalus internus ex vacuo and a cavum septi pellucidi: Nissl stain, × 12.

169

were embedded in Araldite. 1-μm sections were stained with methylene blue (Richardson et al., 1960). We used a semiautomatic image analysing system MOP AM03 (Kontron Messgeräte GmbH, D-8057 Eching, FRG) for counting the Purkinje cell nuclei of folia 5 and 8 of the vermis (Altman, 1972a–c). Parts of the cerebellum (lob. 5, 8), parietal cortex (Area 3), hypothalamus, thalamus and spinal cord were prepared for histological and electron microscopic investigations. We used uranyl acetate and lead citrate for staining the thin sections. From 7 day old experimental animals and controls small tissue blocks of the ventral part of lobe 8 were stained with ethanolic phosphotungstic acid (EPTA) and embedded in Epon 812 (Aghajanian and Bloom, 1967; Bloom and Aghajanian, 1968). Because the EPTA solution penetrates tissue

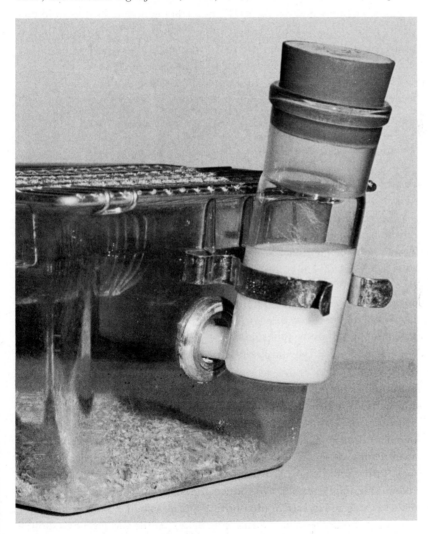

Fig. 8.2. Special drinking bottle filled with liquid diet.

very slowly we kept the tissue samples with EPTA in a slight vacuum at room temperature and obtained homogenous staining results at EM level. Furthermore, cerebellar tissue of 7 day old animals of both groups was prepared in order to visualize membrane-bound Concanavalin A (Con A) binding glycoproteins. For fluorescence studies 50-μm thick sections of the cerebellum were incubated with FITC Con A according to Zanetta et al. (1978). At the EM level, we used Con A peroxidase (HRP-Con A) and followed the methods of Bernhard and Avrameas (1971) and Graham and Karnovsky (1966). Samples stained by the HRP-Con A method were postfixed in 1% OSO_4 and embedded in Araldite. For electron microscopy we used a Zeiss EM 9A.

In view of the postnatal growth spurt of the rat central nervous system (Davison and Dobbing, 1968; Dobbing and Sands, 1971), in further experiments the liquid diet (38% of the daily calories supplied by alcohol) was administered 4 weeks prior to, and during pregnancy and in the postnatal period. Experimental animals and controls were pair-fed, vitamin supplemented and housed individually (Volk et al., 1981). The highest blood alcohol levels were up to 2.0 mg/ml. Postnatally at day 3, 4, 7, 12, 17 and 21, eight experimental animals and controls were fixed by perfusion. Entire sections of the cerebellar vermis, small samples of the cerebellar and parietal cortex, thalamus and spinal cord were embedded for histological morphometric and electron microscopic investigations.

Results of alcohol prior to and during pregnancy
In our alcohol-exposed groups (38% of the daily calories supplied by alcohol), we often observed a reduced litter size of alcohol-drinking dams, an increased neonatal mortality and a more or less retarded weight gain in the postnatal period. However, the weight differences between controls and experimental animals were of transient character (Volk, 1977; Volk et al., 1981). After 4 weeks we could not find significant weight differences between the offspring of alcohol-exposed animals and controls. The only malformations observed were hydrocephali interni ex vacuo. They were extremely rare and comparable to those (Fig. 8.1) we found in previous experiments. After birth some of the offspring looked dystrophic and displayed a dry and squamous skin. Similar features were described by Tze and Lee (1975).

Cerebellar development   In morphometric studies of some cerebellar lobuli (5 and 8) we could not find differences in the number of Purkinje cells between controls and experimental animals. In 7 day old experimental animals, the nuclear diameter of Purkinje cells was significantly smaller; 5 days later this difference had disappeared.

In our histological investigations in 4 day old controls, we found the Purkinje cells (PCs) lying in a single line (Fig. 8.3A) with well-developed apical cytoplasm. In 4 day old experimental animals (Fig. 8.3B), PCs were smaller with a less developed apical cone. Furthermore, in experimental animals the external granular cell layer and the molecular layer were thinner than in controls (Fig. 8.3A). At the EM level PCs showed fewer cytoplasmic organelles than the controls. In some experimental animals (7 and

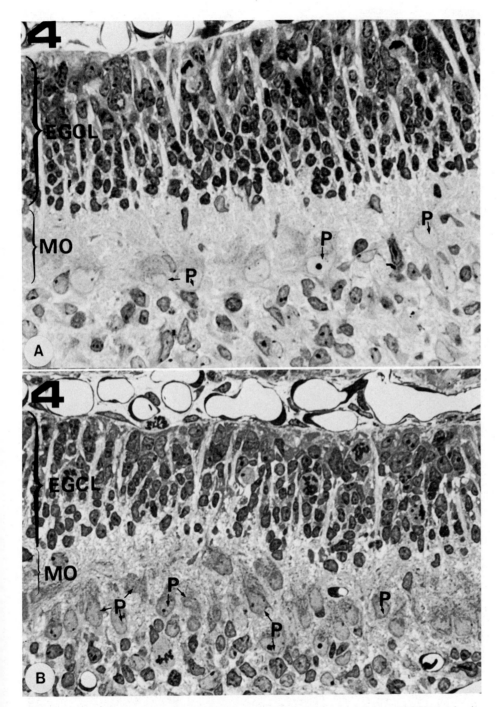

Fig. 8.3. (A) 4 day old control animal. Vermis (lob. 8). External granular cell layer (EGCL), molecular layer (MO) and Purkinje cells (P). The number in the left upper corner shows the age of the animal. (B) 4 day old experimental animal (Vermis, lob. 8). EGCL, MO and P are less developed than in controls. Semithin sections. methylene blue, × 600.

172

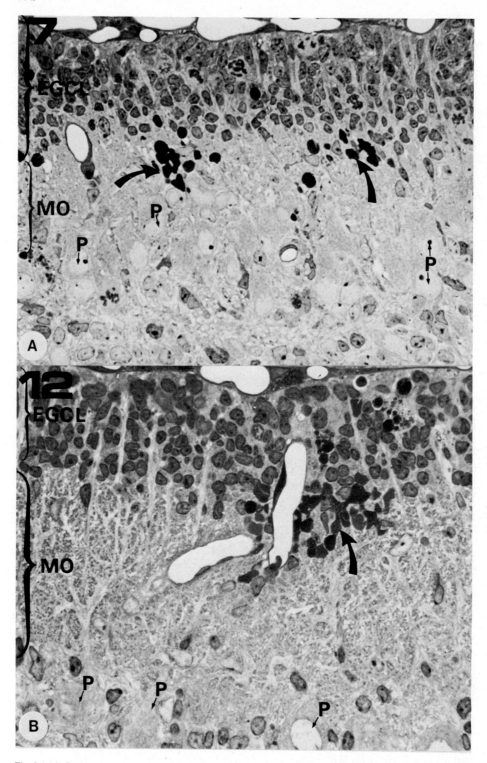

Fig. 8.4.(A, B) 7 and 12 day old experimental animals. Vermis (lob. 8). Beneath the external granular cell layer (EGCL) and in the molecular layer (MO)perivascular hemorrhages (thick curved arrows). In A, Purkinje cells (P) are lying in a scattered line. Semithin section, methylene blue, × 600.

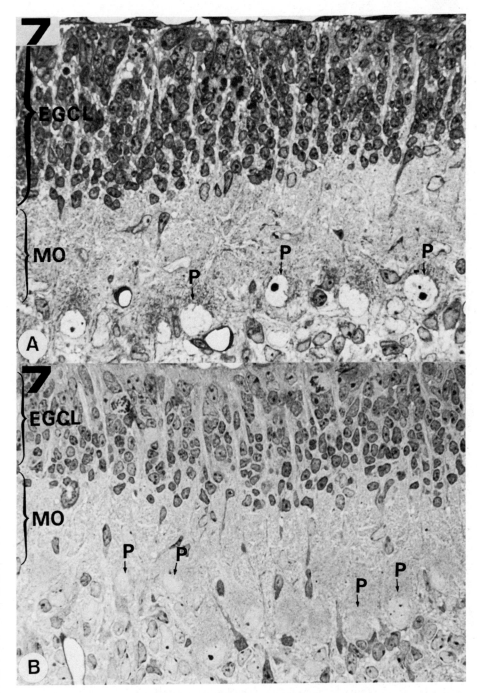

Fig. 8.5. (A) 7 day old control. Vermis (lob. 8). The external granular cell layer (EGCL) shows some mitoses. Molecular layer (MO) and Purkinje cells (P) are well developed. (B) 7 day old experimental animal. Vermis (lob. 8). EGCL and MO are thinner than in A. Purkinje cells show an immature cytoplasm. Semithin sections, methylene blue, × 600.

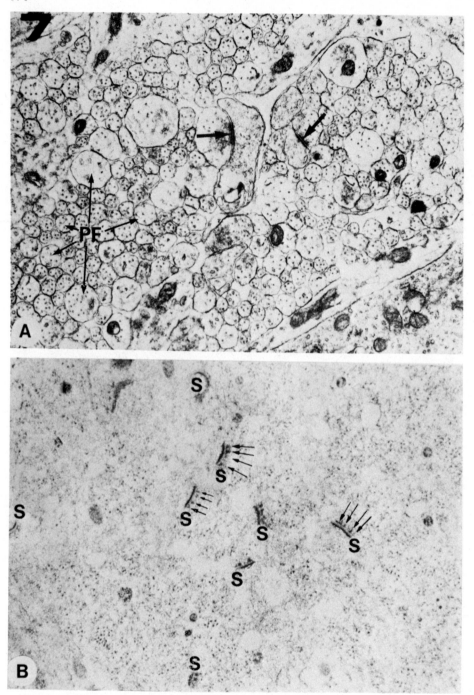

Fig. 8.6. (A) 7 day old control. Vermis (lob. 8). In sagittal section parallel fibres (PF) show synaptic contact with dendritic spines of Purkinje cells (arrows). Electron micrograph, × 12 000. (B) 7 day old control. Vermis (lob. 8). Molecular layer after staining with ethanolic phosphotungstic acid (EPTA). Only synaptic contacts are visualized (S) with dense projections (arrows) and postsynaptic band. Electron micrograph, × 12 000.

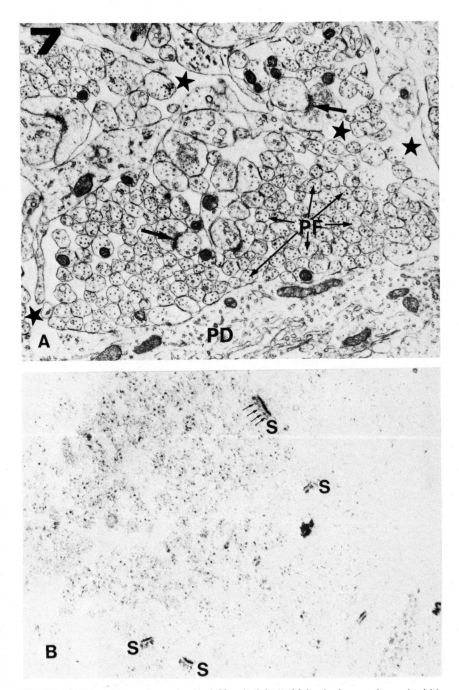

Fig. 8.7. (A) 7 day old experimental animal. Vermis (lob. 8). Molecular layer with axo-dendritic synapses (thick arrows) between Purkinje cells and parallel fibres (PF). Extracellular space is marked with an asterisk. In the lower part of the picture a Purkinje cell dendrite (PD). Electron micrograph, × 12 000. (B) 7 day old experimental animal. Molecular layer stained with phosphotungstic acid (EPTA). Synaptic contacts (S) show dense projections (arrows) and postsynaptic bands. Electron micrograph, × 12 000.

12 day old), we observed perivascular hemorrhages in the cerebellar cortex (Fig. 8.4). We never saw such alterations in the control animals. According to cell pyknoses in the external granular cell layer, offspring of alcohol-drinking dams at days 7 and 12 displayed more degenerating embryonal granular cells than controls. At 7 days of age, Purkinje cells in the controls showed well-developed primary dendrites and a round nucleus (Fig. 8.5A). Many mitoses were seen in the broad external granular cell layer (Fig. 8.5A). In the 7 day old experimental animals, the primary dendrites of PCs were less developed. Furthermore the diameters of nuclei and nucleoli of PCs were smaller (Fig. 8.5A). In comparison to the controls, the external granular cell layer and molecular layer were less developed (Fig. 8.5B). In 7 day old controls the molecular layer in EM investigations revealed well-stained synapses between parallel fibers and Purkinje cell spines (Fig. 8.6A). In EPTA staining, active zones displayed dense projections, cleft material and postsynaptic bands (Fig. 8.6B). Often we observed synaptic junctions with three and four dense projections. In the middle of the line between the inner surface of the external granular cell layer and the Purkinje cell layer, we counted EPTA-stained active synaptic zones as the mean number/50 μm^2 and found a mean of 3.3 synapses. Similar values were reported by Bloom (1972) and Woodward et al. (1971)

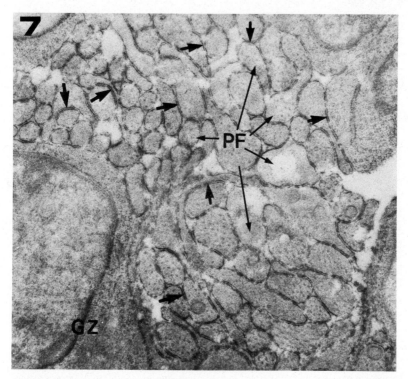

Fig. 8.8. 7 day old control. Vermis (lob. 8). Molecular layer with a migrating external granular cell (GZ) and parallel fibers (PF). Unstained section after HRP-Con A treatment. Plasma membranes of parallel fibers show intensively HRP Con A-reaction products (thick arrows). Electron micrograph, × 13 000.

in the cerebellum. In contrast, the 7 day old experimental animals revealed a marked extracellular space (Fig. 8.7A) in the molecular layer. In the EPTA stain (Fig. 8.7B) we counted 2.8 active zones as the mean number/50 μm^2. Furthermore, the dense projections of experimental animals were irregularly formed and active zones with four dense projections were fewer in number compared to the controls. However, the differences between the two groups were not statistically significant. Because of this we moved on to measuring 17 and 21 day old animals which are more suitable for quantitative investigations.

Our ultrastructural observations of a disturbed cerebellar synaptic differentiation in the FAS of the rat correspond with previous investigations which showed a vulnerability of the cerebellum to prenatal and postnatal alcohol administration (Volk, 1977, 1981; Kornguth et al., 1979; Samson and Diaz, 1982). These alterations may probably explain some of the neurological deficits in FAS which have been reported (Abel, 1982; Riley et al., 1980). In further investigations, I think one should focus on synaptic development in the FAS, and quantitative studies in different areas of the cerebellum and cerebrum should measure not only the number of synapses but also the differentiation of presynaptic areas and the formation of the synaptic curvature (Dyson and Jones, 1976; Devon and Jones, 1979; Jones and Dyson, 1981).

In some of our 7 day old experimental animals and controls we tried to visualize Con A-binding glycoproteins in the molecular layer of the cerebellum. First investigations showed an intensive labelling by fluorescent Con A (FITC, Con A) and Con A-peroxidase (HRP-Con A) in the molecular layer of controls (Fig. 8.8). Experimental animals, however, were less labelled in the molecular layer. These preliminary results indicate a decrease of lectin-binding capacity in the cerebellum in the FAS. During the postnatal development of the rat, the binding of Con A in the molecular layer of the cerebellum, which indicates the presence of glycoproteins, is transient and has its highest values in the first three postnatal weeks (Zanetta et al., 1978). Con A is bound to the white matter, the plasma membrane of parallel fibers, the external granular cell layer (Zanetta et al., 1978) and the synaptic cleft (Bittiger and Schnebli, 1974). Thus, a decrease of membrane-bound glycoproteins which are involved in neuronal recognition and differentiation may alter the interaction of growing processes and disturb the formation and differentiation of synapses (Volk, 1980). Further investigations are required to confirm this hypothesis.

Besides the impaired development of Purkinje cells and the delayed maturation of synapses in the molecular layer the internal granular cell layer is also involved. In 12 and 17 day old control animals, the mossy fiber rosettes were well differentiated (Fig. 8.9), whereas mossy fibers of experimental animals displayed degenerative changes such as glycogen inclusions (Fig. 8.10) and showed less organelles like mitochondria and synaptic vesicles. Furthermore, the diameter of mossy fibers in 12 day old experimental animals was smaller in comparison with the controls. In lobuli 5 and 8 of 12 and 17 day old experimental animals we observed a delayed thinning of the external granular cell layer (EGCL), which was significantly broader in experimental animals.

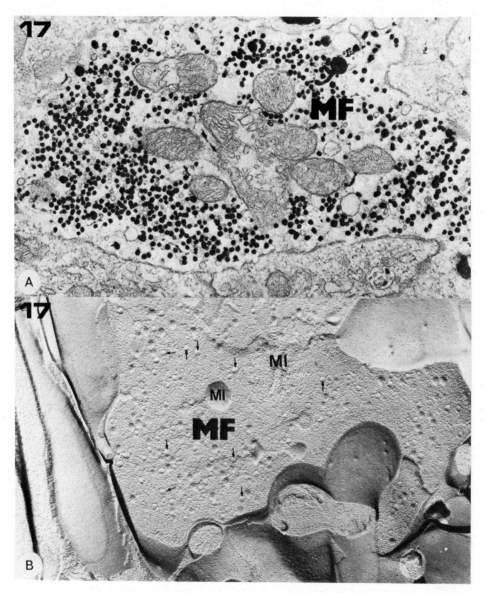

Fig. 8.9. *(A)* 17 day old control. Vermis (lob. 8). Mossy fibre terminal (MF) in the internal granular cell layer with abundant black stained synaptic vesicles and central cluster of organelles. Osmium-zinc iodide stain according to Vrensen and DeGroot (1974). Electron micrograph, × 30 000. (B) 17 day old control. Vermis (lob. 8). Freeze-fractured mossy fibre (MF) with broken and unbroken mitochondria (MI) and synaptic vesicles (arrows). For the method of fracturing see Volk (1983). Electron micrograph, original magnification × 35 000; publisher's reduction factor 82%.

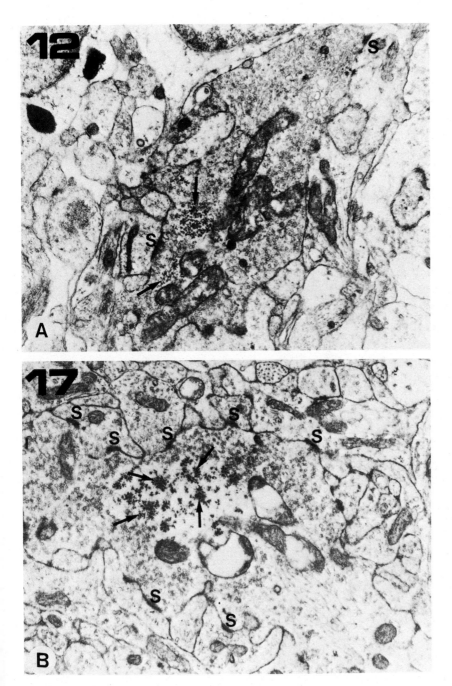

Fig. 8.10. (A) 12 day old experimental animal. Vermis (lob. 8). Internal granular cell layer with cerebellar glomerulus. The mossy rosette shows accumulation of glycogen (arrows). In the periphery synaptic contacts (S). Electron micrograph, × 12 400. (B) 17 day old experimental animal. Vermis (lob. 8). Mossy fibre rosette with glycogen inclusions (arrows) and synaptic contacts (S). Electron micrograph, 12 400.

180

Kornguth et al. (1979) described a similar retardation in the FAS of the rat. At the age of 21 days, offspring of alcohol-drinking dams displayed a persistent EGCL which disappeared a few days later. In a previous report (Volk et al., 1981), we investigated at EM level the development of Purkinje cells in the FAS and found no differences between control and experimental animals at 17 and 21 days.

It appears unlikely that a direct malnutrition has developed in our dams after pair-feeding a vitamin-supplemented diet. However, we cannot exclude completely an altered maternal behavior towards the offspring postnatally. Preliminary results of

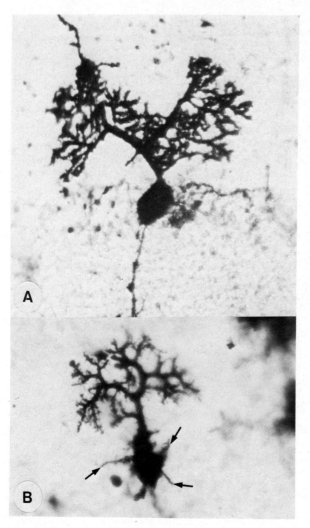

Fig. 8.11. (A) 12 day old control. Vermis. Golgi stained Purkinje cell with dendritic branching. (B) 12 day old experimental animal. Vermis. Purkinje cell with reduced dendritic branching and extrasomal dendrites (arrows). The micrographs were generously provided by Dr. Stoltenburg-Didinger et al. (1982).

further experiments show that the cerebellar cortex also displays a delayed development after surrogate fostering of offspring after birth. Similar features were reported
by Stoltenburg-Didinger et al. (1982), who observed an impaired dendritic branching
of Purkinje cells (Fig. 8.11) in the FAS of the rat.

Parietal Cortex   As to the maturation of the cortex, first results show that in 7 and
12 day old experimental animals nuclei of neurons in layers III and V of the parietal
cortex (Area 3) are smaller than those of controls. Moreover, in 7 day old experimental
animals perivascular hemorrhages and an increasing amount of pyknoses occurred.

Results of alcohol prior to and during pregnancy, and in the lactation period
Similar to previous experiments we observed a decrease of stillbirths and a diminished

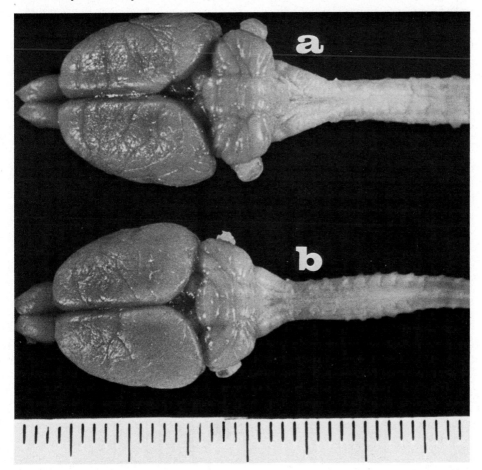

Fig. 8.12. (A) 10 week old control. Preparation of the central nervous system with spinal cord. (b) 10 week
old experimental animal (alcohol prior to, during pregnancy and in the lactating period). Cerebrum and
cerebellum are underdeveloped in comparison to (a).

birth weight. However, the postnatal weight gain of experimental animals was extremely retarded, and at 25 days of age the weight differences between controls and experimental animals were about 40%. After weaning, we kept some of the animals of both groups up to 10 weeks. During that time experimental animals could not catch up on their developmental deficit (Fig. 8.12). Similar to previous reports (Volk et al., 1981), we counted Purkinje cells in lobuli 5 and 8 of 7 day old experimental animals and observed a reduction of PCs of about 10% (Fig. 8.13). Furthermore, cerebella of experimental animals revealed perivascular hemorrhages in the molecular layer and in the internal granular cell layer. The Purkinje cell development was retarded. PCs of 12 day old experimental animals were immature with huge amounts of free ribosomes (Fig. 8.14) and an undeveloped rough endoplasmic reticulum. In some areas we found PCs with apical cytoplasmic cones which resembled PCs of 7 day old controls. Despite the dramatic weight differences between the animals of both groups, PCs displayed only slight differences electron microscopically in the proliferation of the rough endoplasmic reticulum (Figs. 8.15 and 8.16). In this experiment we also noticed a disturbed synaptogenesis (Volk et al., 1980a). These features are described and discussed in detail elsewhere (Volk, 1984).

First investigations of the cerebral cortex showed much more severe alterations than in the previous group in which alcohol was given prior to and during pregnancy. Again we found perivascular hemorrhages (Fig. 8.17), abundant pyknoses and a significant decrease of nuclear diameter in neurons of the parietal and frontal lobe. Our results also show an irreversible developmental delay with loss of Purkinje cells, impaired neurohistological differentiation and disturbed cytoarchitecture of the cerebrum. Similar features were reported in the cerebellum after alcohol vapor inhalation by suckling rats (Bauer-Moffett and Altman, 1975, 1977). Furthermore, Yanai and

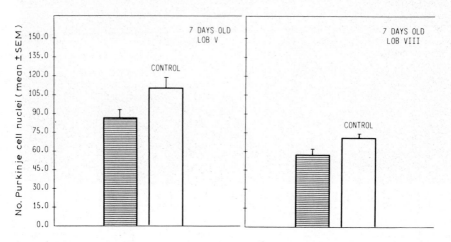

Fig. 8.13. This figure shows mean ± SEM of the number of Purkinje cell nuclei in the lob. V and VIII of 7 day old controls and experimental animals. There is a significant difference ($p < 0.01$) between the two groups (Student's t-test).

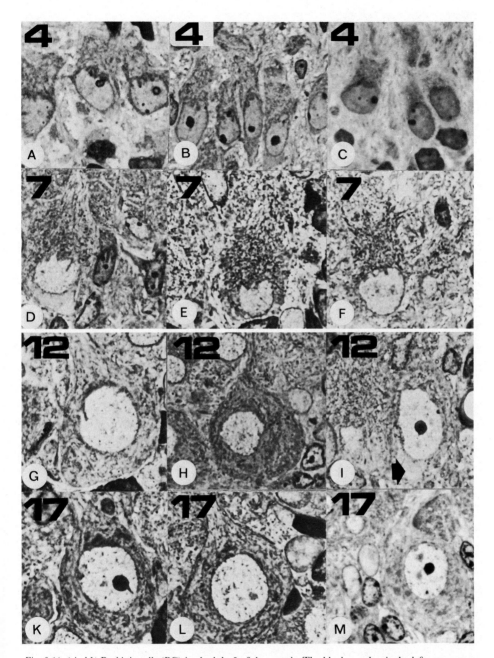

Fig. 8.14. (A–M) Purkinje cells (PC) in the lob. 5 of the vermis. The black number is the left upper corner means the age of the animals. (A, D, G, K) controls; (B, E, H, L) experimental animals (alcohol prior to and during pregnancy. (C, F, I, M)experimental animals (alcohol prior to, during pregnancy and in the lactating period). A is more developed than B and C. E and F show an immature cytoplasm. In I there are accumulations of free ribosomes. Between G and H, and between K, L and M there are no differences. Semithin sections, methylene blue, phase-contrast, original magnification × 1400; publisher's reduction factor 83%.

184

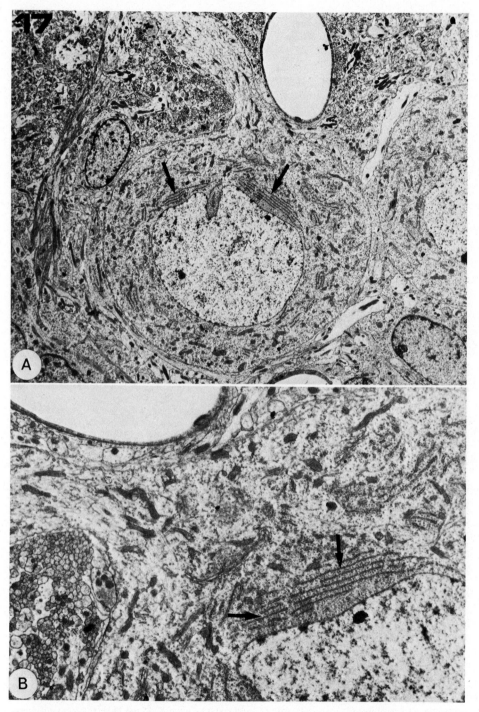

Fig. 8.15. (A) 17 day old control. Vermis (lob. 8). Purkinje cell (PC) with well differentiated rough endoplasmic reticulum (arrows). Electron micrograph, × 3400. (B) Higher power view of A. × 6800.

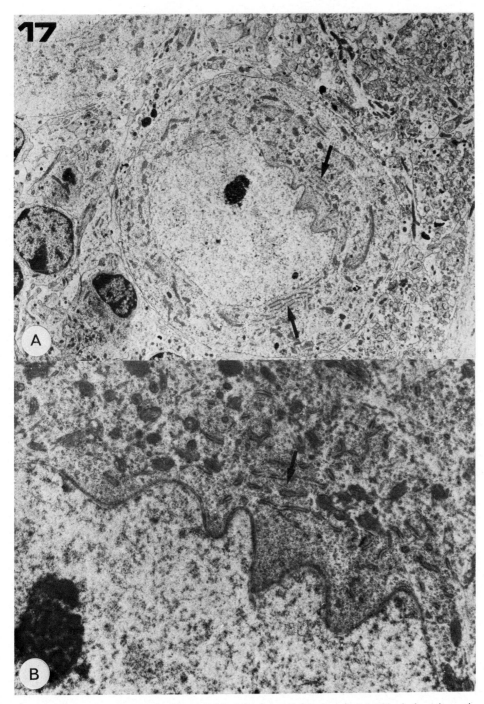

Fig. 8.16. (A) 17 day old experimental animal (alcohol prior to, during pregnancy and in the lactating period; vermis lob. 8). Purkinje cell with fragments of the rough endoplasmic reticulum (arrows). Electron micrograph, × 3400. (B) Higher power view of A with membranes of the endoplasmic reticulum. Electron micrograph, × 12 400.

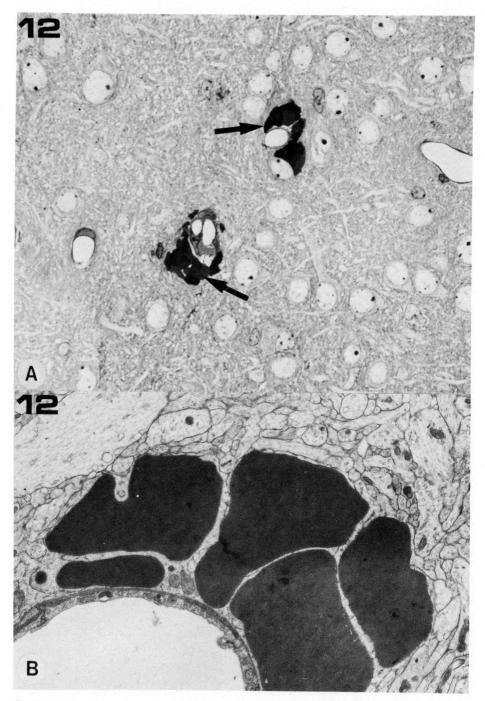

Fig. 8.17. 12 day old experimental animal (alcohol prior to, during pregnancy and in the lactating period). Parietal cortex (area 3) with perivascular hemorrhages (arrows). Semithin section, Methylene blue, × 300. (B) Electron micrograph of A. A small vessel with erythrocytes in the sourrounding tissue, × 6000.

Bergman (1981) and Yanai et al. (1979) observed neuronal deficits in the cerebellum and hippocampus after prenatal and neonatal exposure to phenobarbital. However, these cerebellar and cerebral alterations are not caused by alcohol alone which might have been ingested by the offspring via their mother's milk. It must be considered that alcohol decreases maternal milk production (Fuchs, 1969) and this might disturb post-natal development and the recovery of the offspring. Thus it is well known nutritional deficits during the growth spurt of mice and rats lead to dramatic reduction in brain development with permanent neuronal loss (Barnes and Altman, 1973; Winick, 1976). For neonatal alcohol administration the method of Samson and Diaz (1982) avoids these problems by using intragastric administration with a cannula.

Conclusions

Chronic alcohol exposure of rats before and during pregnancy leads to slight differences in birth weight between experimental animals and controls and retarded weight gain in the offspring of alcohol-drinking mothers. Morphometric analyses of different parts of the cerebellar cortex reveal no reduction of Purkinje cells but a decrease of synapses and an impaired synaptic maturation. The cerebral cortex also shows a delayed differentiation of neurons.

In the human FAS, postnatal growth deficiency and mental retardation are the main clinical features (Majewski, 1980). Because inadequate nutrition with protein and vitamin deficiency is usually associated with chronic alcoholism (Thomson, 1982), symptoms of the FAS such as developmental delay and growth deficiency may be enhanced by nutritional deficits. Therefore, in experimental models of the FAS, alcohol should not only be administered during pregnancy and postnatally but also prior to pregnancy. A delayed neurohistological differentiation and impaired synaptic maturation in the cerebral and cerebellar cortex are the most striking features we observed in our experiments. This might be the morphological substrate of microcephaly and mental retardation of the human fetal alcohol syndrome.

However, it is not possible to explain our results only by the specific neurotoxicity of alcohol. In our chronic model the developmental delay observed might be of multifactorial origin. Alcohol-induced alteration of myelination, changes in protein metabolism, deficits in specific transmitters and hormones, the energy cost of maternal alcohol oxidation (Pirola and Lieber, 1972) and other maternal nutritional factors could contribute to intrauterine hypotrophy and delayed postnatal development.

Acknowledgments

Dedicated to Georg Volk, M.D. on the occasion of his 85th birthday.

This work was supported by grants of the Deutsche Forschungsgemeinschaft

(DFG) VO 272/4-3. Presented in part at the International Congress of Neurotoxicology, Varese, Italy, 27–30 September, 1979, and at the 13th C.J.N.P. Congress Jerusalem, Israel, 20–25 June, 1982.

References

Abel, E.L. (1978) Effects of ethanol on pregnant rats and their offspring. Psychopharmacology 57, 5–11.

Abel, E.L. (1980) Fetal alcohol syndrome: bahavioral teratology. Psychol. Bull. 87, 29–50.

Abel, E.L. (1982) In utero alcohol exposure and developmental delay of response inhibition. Alcoholism 6, 369–376.

Aghajanian, G.K. and Bloom, F.E. (1967) The formation of synaptic junctions in developing rat brain: a quantitative electron microscopic study. Brain Res. 6, 716–727.

Åkesson, C. (1974) Autoradiographic studies on the distribution of ^{14}C-2-Ethanol and its non-volatile metabolites in the pregnant mouse. Arch. Int. Pharmacodyn. 209, 296–304.

Altman, J. (1972a) Postnatal development of the cerebellar cortex in the rat. I. The external germinal layer and the transitional molecular layer. J. Comp. Neurol. 145, 353–398.

Altman, J. (1972b) Postnatal development of the cerebellar cortex in the rat. II. Phases in the maturation of purkinje cells and of the molecular layer. J. Comp. Neurol. 145, 399–464.

Altman, J. (1972c) Postnatal development of the cerebellar cortex in the rat. III. Maturation of the components of the granular layer. J. Comp. Neurol. 145, 465–514.

Altman, J. (1982) Morphological development of the rat cerebellum. In: The Cerebellum – New Vistas (Palay, S.L. and Chan-Palay, V., eds.) Springer-Verlag, Heidelberg.

Balázs, R., Kovács, S., Teichgräber, P., Cocks, W.A. and Eayrs, J.T. (1968) Biochemical effects of thyroid deficiency on the developing brain. J. Neurochem. 15, 1335–1349.

Barnes, D. and Altman, J. (1973) Effects of two levels of gestational-lactational undernutrition on the post-weaning growth of the rat cerebellum. Exp. Neurol. 38, 420–428.

Barnes, D.E. and Walker, D.W. (1981) Prenatal ethanol exposure permanently reduces the number of pyramidal neurons in rat hippocampus. Dev. Brain Res. 1, 333–340.

Bauer-Moffett, C. and Altman, J. (1975) Ethanol-induced reduction in cerebellar growth of infant rats. Exp. Neurol. 48, 378–382.

Bauer-Moffett, C. and Altman, J. (1977) The effect of ethanol chronically administered to preweanling rats on cerebellar development: a morphological study. Brain Res. 119, 249–268.

Berlinkoff, S. and Hall Jr., O.W. (1950) Intravenous alcohol during labor. Am. J. Obstet. Gynecol. 59, 429–432.

Bernhard, W. and Avrameas, S. (1971) Ultrastructural visualization of cellular carbohydrate components by means of concanavalin A. Exp. Cell Res. 64, 232–236.

Bernt, E. and Gutmann, J. (1970) Äthanol: Bestimmung mit Alkohol-Dehydrogenase and NAD. In: Methoden der enzymatischen Analyse (Bergmeyer, H.U., ed.) Verlag Chemie, Weinheim.

Bierich, J.R., Majewski, F., Michaelis, R. and Tillner, J. (1976) Über das embryo-fetale Alkoholsyndrom. J. Pediat. 121, 155–177.

Bittiger, H. and Schnebli, H.P. (1974) Binding of concanavalin A and ricin to synaptic junctions of rat brain. Nature 249, 370–371.

Bloom, F.E. (1972) The formation of synaptic junctions in developing rat brain. In: Structure and Function of Synapses (Pappas, G.D. and Purpura, D.P., eds.) Raven Press, New York.

Bloom, F.E. and Aghajanian, K. (1968) Fine structural and cytochemical analysis of the staining of synaptic junctions with phosphotungstic acid. J. Ultrast. Res. 23, 316–375.

Chernoff, G.F. (1977) The fetal alcohol syndrome in mice: A animal model. Teratology 15, 223–230.

Chernoff, G.F. (1980) Introduction: A teratologist's view of the fetal alcohol syndrome. In: Alcoholism, Vol. VII. (Galanter, M., ed.) Grune and Stratton, New York, pp. 5–13.

Clarren, S.K. and Smith, D.W. (1978) The fetal alcohol syndrome. N. Engl. J. Med. 298, 1063–1067.

Cohen, G. (1977) A mechanism for altered adrenergic activity in alcoholism. In: Alcohol and Opiates (Blum, K., ed.) Academic Press, New York, pp. 141–155.

Collins, M.A. (1977) Identification of isoquinoline alkaloids during alcohol intoxication. In: Alcohol and Opiates (Blum, K., ed.) Academic Press, New York, pp. 155–167.

Collins, M.A. and Bigdeli, M.G. (1975) Tetrahydroisoquinolines in vivo. I. Rat brain-formation of Salsolinol, a condensation product of dopamine and acetaldehyde under certain conditions during ethanol intoxication. Life Sci. 16, 585–602.

Davison, A.N. and Dobbing, J. (1968) The developing brain. In: Applied Neurochemistry (Davison, A.N. and Dobbing, J., eds.) Davis, Philadelphia, PA.

Deitrich, R.A. and Erwin, V.G. (1975) Involvement of biogenic amine metabolism in ethanol addiction. Fed. Proc. 34, 1962–1969.

Diaz, J. and Samson, H.H. (1980) Impaired brain growth in neonatal rats exposed to ethanol. Science 208, 751–753.

Detering, N.K., Ozand, P.T. and Karahasan, A. (1979) The effects of ethanol on development in the rat. In: (Neuhoff, V., ed.) Proceedings of the European Society for Neurochemistry, Verlag Chemie, Weinheim, p. 444.

Devon, R.M. and Jones, D.G. (1979) Synaptic terminal parameters in unanaesthetized rat cerebellar cortex. Cell Tissue Res. 203, 189–200.

Dobbing, J. (1970) Undernutrition and the developing brain: the relevance of animal models to the human problem. Am. J. Dis. Child. 120, 411–415.

Dobbing, J. and Sands, J. (1971) Vulnerability of developing brain. IX. The effect of nutritional growth retardation on the timing of the brain growth-spurt. Biol. Neonate 19, 363–378.

Dobbing, J. and Sands, J. (1979) Comparative aspects of the brain growth spurt. Early Hum. Dev. 3, 79–83.

Dyson, S.E. and Jones, D.G. (1976) Some effects of undernutrition on synaptic development – A quantitative ultrastructural study. Brain Res. 114, 365–378.

Dyson, S.E. and Jones, D.G. (1976a) The morphological categorization of developing of synaptic junctions. Cell. Tiss. Res. 167, 363–371.

Ellis, F.W. and Pick, J.R. (1976) Beagle model of the fetal alcohol syndrome. Pharmacologist 18, 190.

Fetchko, A.M., Weber, J.E., Carrol, J.H., Thomas, G.J. and Pittsburgh, P.A. (1951) Intravenous alcohol used for preinduction analgesia in obstetrics. Am. J. Obstet. Gynecol. 62, 662–664.

Fuchs, A.R. (1969) Ethanol and the inhibition of oxytocin release in the lactating rats. Acta Endocrinol. 62, 546–554.

Gärtner, U. and Rydén, G. (1972) The elimination of alcohol in the premature infant. Acta Paediat. Scand. 61, 720.

Graham, R.C. and Carnovsky, M.J. (1966) The early stages of absorption of injected horseradish peroxidase in the proximal tubules of mouse kidney: ultrastructural cytochemistry by a new technique. J. Histochem. Cytochem. 14, 291–302.

Haddad, R. and Dumas, R.M. (1982) Teratogenicity of binge drinking: comparative susceptibility of C57BL/6J and CBA/J mice to teratogenic effects of a single oral dose of ethanol. Alcoholism Clin. Exp. Res. 6, 298.

Henderson, G.I. and Schenker, S. (1979) The effect of maternal alcohol consumption on the viability and visceral development in the newborn rat. Res. Commun. Chem. Pathol. Pharmacol. 16, 15–32.

Henderson, G.I., Hoyumpa, A.M., McClain, C. and Schenker, S. (1979) The effects of chronic and acute alcohol administration on fetal development in the rat. Alcoholism Clin. Exp. Res. 3, 99–106.

Ho, B.T., Fritchie, G.E., Idänpään-Heikkilä, J.E. and McIsaac, W.M. (1972) Placental transfer and tissue distribution of ethanol-1-^{14}C. A radioautographic study in monkeys and hamsters. Q. J. Stud. Alcohol 33, 485–493.

190

Hollstedt, C. and Rydberg, U. (1970) Ethanol metabolism in the growing rat. Arch. Int. Pharmakodyn. Ther. 188, 341–348.

Idanpään-Heikklä, J., Jouppila, P., Akerblom, H.K., Isoaho, R., Kauppila, E. and Koivisto, M. (1972) Elimination and metabolic effects of ethanol in mother, fetus and newborn infant. Am. J. Obstet. Gynecol. 112, 1.

Isselbacher, K.J. and Carter, E.A. (1973) Ethanol metabolism: Oxidative and peroxidative mechanismus. Drug Metab. Dispos. 1, 449–454.

Jones, D.G. and Dyson, S.E. (1981) The influence of protein restriction, rehabilitation and changing nutritional status on synaptic development: a quantitative study in rat brain. Brain Res. 208, 97–111.

Jones, K.L. and Smith, D.W. (1973) Recognition of the fetal alcohol syndrome in early infancy. Lancet ii, 999.

Jones, K.L., Smith, D.W., Ulleland, C.N. and Streissguth, A.P. (1973) Pattern of malformation in offspring of chronic alcoholic mothers. Lancet i, 1267–1271.

Jones, K.L. and Smith, D.W. (1975) The fetal alcohol syndrome. Teratology 12, 1–10.

Kesäniemi, Y.A. and Sippel, H.W. (1975) Placental and foetal metabolism of acetaldehyde in rat. I. Contents of ethanol and acetaldehyde in placenta and foetus of the pregnant rat during ethanol oxidation. Acta Pharmacol. Toxicol. 37, 43–48.

Kornguth, S.E., Rutledge, J.J. Sunderland, E. Siegel, F., Carlson, I., Smollens, J., Juhl, U. and Young, B. (1979) Impeded cerebellar development and reduced serum thyroxine levels associated with fetal alcohol intoxication. Brain Res. 177, 347–360.

Kronick, J.B. (1976) Teratogenic effects of ethyl alcohol administered to pregnant mice. J. Obstet. Gynecol. 124, 676–680.

Lancaster, F.E., Mayur, B.K., Patsalos, P.N., Samorajski, T. and Wiggins, R.C. (1982) The synthesis of myelin and brain subcellular membrane proteins in the offspring of rats fed ethanol during pregnancy. Brain Res. 235, 105–113.

Larsell, O. (1970) The Comparative Anatomy and Histology of the Cerebellum from Monotremes through Apes (Jansen, J.,ed.) University of Minnesota Press, MN.

Leiber, B. (1977) Das bedeutendste teratogene Agens der Gegenwart: Alkohol. Medizin 5, 345.

Lemoine, P. Harousseau, H., Bortyru, J. and Menuet, J.C. (1968) Les enfants des parents alcooliques: anomalies observées apropos de 127 cas. Arch. Fr. Pediatr. 25, 831.

Lieber, C.S. (1975) Interference of ethanol in hepatic cellular metabolism. Ann. NY. Acad. Sci. 252, 24–50.

Lieber, C.S. and DeCarli, L.M. (1972) The role of the hepatic microsomal ethanol oxidizing system (MEOS) for ethanol metabolism in vivo. J. Pharmacol. Exp. Ther. 181, 279–287.

Lieber, C.S. and DeCarli, L.M. (1974) An experimental model of alcohol feeding and liver injury in the baboon. J. Med. Primatol. 3, 153–163.

Lieber, C.S., Jones, D.P. and DeCarli, L.M. (1965) Effects of prolonged ethanol intake: Production of fatty liver despite adequate diets. J. Clin. Invest. 44, 1009–1021.

Majewski, F. (1980) Untersuchungen zur Alkoholembryopathie. Thieme, Copythek, Stuttgart.

Majewski, F., Bierich, J.R. Löser, H., Michaelis, R., Leiber, B. and Bettecken, F. (1976) Zur Klinik und Pathogenese der Alkohol-Embryopathie. Münch. Med. Wschr. 118, 1635–1642.

Malone, M.J., Szoke, M.C. and Rosman, N.P. (1978) Pathogenesis of fetal alcohol syndrome: reduction of brain lipid-soluble protein. Neurology 28, 348.

Mann, L.J., Bhakthavathsalan, A., Liu, M. and Makowski, Ph. (1975) Placental transport of alcohol and its effect on maternal and fetal acid-base balance. Am. J. Obstet. Gynecol. 122, 837–844.

Martin, J.C., Martin, D.C., Lund, L.A. and Streissguth, A.P. (1977) Maternal alcohol ingestion and cigarette smoking and their effects on newborn conditioning. Alcoholism 1, 243–247.

Moser, K., Papenberg, J. and von Wartburg, J.P. (1969) Heterogenität und Organverteilung der Alkoholdehydrogenase bei verschiedenen Spezies. Enzymol. Biol. Clin. 9, 447–558.

Nicolson, J.L.and Altman, J. (1972) The effects of early hypo- and hyperthyroidism on the development of rat cerebellar cortex. I. Cell proliferation and differentiation. Brain Res. 44, 13–23.

Noble, E.P. and Tewari, S. (1973) Protein and ribonucleic acid metabolism in brains of mice following chronic alcohol consumption. New York Acad. Sci. 215, 333–345.

Noble, E.P. and Tewari, S. (1975) Ethanol and brain ribosomes. Fed. Proc. 34, 1942–1947.

Papara-Nicholson, D. and Telford, J.R. (1957) Effects of alcohol on reproduction and fetal development in guinea pigs. Anat. Rec. 127, 438.

Peiffer, J., Majewski, F., Fischbach, H., Bierich, J.R. and Volk, B. (1979) Alcohol embryo- and fetopathy; neuropathology of 3 children and 3 fetuses. J. Neurol. Sci. 41, 125–137.

Priola, R.C. and Lieber, C.S. (1972) The energy cost of the metabolism of drugs, including ethanol. Pharmacology 7, 185–196.

Pikkarainen, P.H. and Räiha, N.C.R. (1967) Development of alcohol dehydrogenase activity in the human liver. Pediatr. Res. 1, 165.

Räiha, N.C.R., Koskinen, M. and Pikkarainen, P. (1967) Developmental changes in alcohol dehydrogenase activity in rat and guinea-pig liver. Biochem. J. 103, 623–626.

Randall, C.L. and Taylor, W.J. (1979) Prenatal ethanol exposure in mice: teratogenic effects. Teratology 19, 305–312.

Randall, C.L., Taylor, W.J. and Walker, D.W. (1977) Ethanol-induced malformations in mice. Alcohol. Clin. Exp. Res. 1, 219–224.

Raskin, N.H. and Sokoloff, L. (1968) Brain alcohol dehydrogenase. Science 162, 131–132.

Rawat, A.K. (1975) Ribosomal protein synthesis in the fetal and neonatal rat brain as influenced by maternal ethanol consumption. Res. Commun. Chem. Pathol. Pharmacol. 12, 723–732.

Rawat, A.K. (1976a) Effect of maternal ethanol consumption on fetal and neonatal rat hepatic protein synthesis. Biochem. J. 160, 653–651.

Rawat, A.K. (1976) Neurochemical consequences of ethanol on the nervous system. Int. Rev. Neurobiol. 19, 123–172.

Rawat, A.K. (1979) Derangement in cardiac protein metabolism in fetal alcohol syndrome. Res. Commun. Chem. Pathol. Pharmacol. 25, 365–375.

Rawat, A.K. and Kuriyama, K. (1972) Ethanol oxidation: Effect on the redox state of brain in the mouse. Science 176, 1133–1135.

Richardson, K.C., Jarett, L. and Finke, E.H. (1960) Embedding in epoxy resins for ultrathin sectioning in electron microscopy. Stain Technol. 35, 313–323.

Riley, E.P., Lochry, E.A. and Shapiro, N.R. (1980) Alcohol-induced behavioral teratogenesis: an animal model. In: Animal Models in Alcohol Research (Eriksson. K., Sinclair, J.D. and Kiianmaa, K., eds.) Academic Press, New York, pp. 393–399.

Ryan, M. (1837) The Philosophy of Marriage in its Social, Moral and Physical Relations. Churchill, London.

Samson, H.H. and Diaz, J. (1982) Effects of neonatal ethanol exposure on brain development in rodents. In: Fetal Alcohol Syndrome, (Abel, E.I., ed.) CRC Press Florida, Vol. III, Animal Studies. pp. 131–150.

Samson, H.H., Grant, K.A., Coggan, S. and Sachs, V.M. (1982) Ethanol induced microcephaly in the neonatal rat: occurrence without withdrawal. Neurobehav. Toxicol. Teratol. 4, 115–116.

Sandor, St. (1968) The influence of aethyl-alcohol on the development of the chick embryo. II. Rev. Roum. Embryol. Cytol. Sér. Embryol. 5, 167–171.

Sandor, St. and Elias, St. (1968) The influence of aethylalcohol on the development of the chick embryo. Rev. Roum. Embryol. Cytol. Sér. Embryol. 5, 151–167.

Semaille-Vilette, Ch. and Semaille, P.P. (1977) Le syndrome d'alcoholism foetal. A propos de 47 observations. Thèse de médicine, Lille, 1976. Zit. Nouv. Press. Méd. 6. 1763.

Shoemaker, W.J. and Bloom, F.E. (1977) Effect of undernutrition on brain morphology. In: Nutrition and the Brain, Vol. 2, (Wurtman, R.J. and Wurtman, J.J., eds.) Raven Press, New York, pp. 147–192.

Sippel, H.W. and Kesäniemi, Y.A. (1975) Placental and foetal metabolism of acetaldehyde in rat. II. Studies on metabolism of acetaldehyde in the isolated placenta and foetus. Acta Pharmacol. Toxicol. 37, 49–55.

Stockard, Ch.R. (1910) The influence of alcohol and other anaesthetics on embryonic development. Am. J. Anat. 10, 369–392.

Stoltenburg-Didinger, G., Spohr, H.L. and Chahoud, I. (1982) Animal studies of postnatal brain development in fetal alcohol syndrome. IXth International Congress of Neuropathology, Vienna, Sept. 5–10, Abstract B 3–20.

Streissguth, A.P., Landesman-Dwyer, S., Martin, J.C. and Smith, D.W. (1980) Teratogenetic effects of alcohol in humans and laboratory animals. Science 209, 353–361.

Sulik, K.K., Johnston, M.C. and Webb, M.A. (1981) Fetal alcohol syndrome: embryogenesis in a mouse model. Science 214, 936–938.

Sullivan, W.C. (1899) A note on the influence of maternal inebriety on the offspring. J. Ment. Sci. 45, 489–503.

Swanberg, K.M. and Crumpacker, D.W. (1977) Genetic differences in reproductive fitness and offspring viability in mice exposed to alcohol during gestation. Behav. Biol. 20, 122–127.

Tenbrinck, M.S. and Buchin, Y.S. (1975) Fetal alcohol syndrome. Report of a case. J. Am. Med. Assoc. 232, 1144–1147.

Teschke, R. and Lieber, C.S. (1978) Biochemie und Pathophysiologie des Alkoholstoffwechsels. Leber Magen Darm 8, 237–345.

Teschke, R., Hasumura, Y. and Lieber, C.S. (1974) NADPH-dependent oxidation of methanol, ethanol, propanol and butanol by hepatic microsomes. Biochem. Biophys. Res. Commun. 60, 851.

Tewari, S. and Noble, E.P. (1976) Chronic ethanol ingestion by rodents: Effects on brain RNA. In: Alcohol and Abnormal Protein Biosynthesis; Biochemical and Clinical. (Rothschild, M.A., Oratz, M. and Schreiber, S.S., eds.) Pergamon Press, New York, pp. 421–448.

Tewari, S., Murray, S. and Noble, E.P. (1978) Studies on the effects of chronic ethanol injection on the properties of rat brain ribosomes. J. Neurosci. Res. 3, 375–389.

Thomson, A.D. (1982) Alcohol related structural brain changes. Brit. Med. Bull. 38, 87–94.

Tze, W.J. and Lee, M. (1975) Adverse Effects of maternal alcohol consumption on pregnancy and foetal growth in rats. Nature 257, 479–480.

Ulleland, C., Wennberg, R.P., Igo, R.P. and Smith, N.J. (1970) The offspring of alcoholic mothers. Pediatr. Res. 4, 474.

Volk, B. (1977) Delayed cerebellar histogenesis in 'embryo-fetal alcohol syndrome'. Light microscopic study of the rat cerebellum. Acta Neuropathol. 39, 157–163.

Volk, B. (1980) Tierexperimentelle Studien zur Alkoholembryofetopathie. Histologische und elektronenmikroskopische Untersuchungen am Kleinhirn der Ratte. Habilitationsschrift, Universität Heidelberg.

Volk, B., Berlet, H.H. and Maletz, J. (1980a) The influence of alcohol on cerebellar histo- and synaptogenesis. Light and electron microscopic histochemical and neurochemical investigations of the rat cerebellar cortex. Drug Alcohol Depend. 6, 67.

Volk, B. Maletz, J. Tiedemann, M., Ilzenhöfer, H., Berlet, H.H. (1980b) Impaired development of synaptic junctions of rat brain in fetal alcohol syndrome. Morphological and biochemical studies. In: Proceedings of the Third Meeting of the European Society of Neurochemistry, Ljubljana (Brzin, M., Sket, D. and Bachelard, H., eds.) Pergamon Press, Oxford, p. 407.

Volk, B., Maletz, M., Tiedemann, M., Mall, G., Klein, C. and Berlet, H.H. (1981) Impaired maturation of Purkinje cells in the fetal alcohol syndrome of the rat. Light and electron microscopic investigations. Acta Neuropathol. 54, 19–29.

Volk, B. (1983) A freeze fracture study on membranous cytoplasmic bodies (MCBs) in GM$_2$ gangliosidosis. In: Lysosomal Diseases of the Nervous System (Cervos-Navarro, J., ed.) Raven Press, New York, in press.

Volk, B. (1984) Cerebellar histogenesis and synaptic maturation following pre- and postnatal alcohol administration. An electron microscopic investigation of the rat cerebellar cortex. Acta Neuropathol. in press.

Vrensen, G. and DeGroot, D. (1974) Osmium-zinc iodide staining and the quantitative study of central synapses. Brain Res. 74, 131–142.

Wagner, L., Wagner, G. and Guerrero, J. (1970) Effect of alcohol on premature newborn infants. Am. J. Obstet. Gynecol. 108, 308–315.

Waltman, R. and Iniquez, E.S. (1972) Placental transfer of ethanol and its elimination at term. Obstet. Gynecol. 40, 180–185.

Winick, M. (1976) Malnutrition and Brain Development. Oxford University Press, Oxford.

Woodward, D.J., Hoffer, B.J., Siggins, G.R. and Bloom, F.E. (1971) The ontogenetic development of synaptic junctions, synaptic activation and responsiveness to neurotransmitter substances in the rat cerebella Purkinje cells. Brain Res. 34, 73–97.

Yanai, J. and Bergman, A. (1981) Neuronal deficits after neonatal exposure to phenobarbital. Exp. Neurol. 73, 199–208.

Yanai, J. and Ginsburg, B.E. (1977) A developmental study of ethanol effect on behavior and physical development in mice. Alcoholism 1, 325–333.

Yanai, J., Roselli-Austin, L. and Tabakoff, B. (1979) Neuronal deficits in mice following prenatal exposure to phenobarbital. Exp. Neurol. 64, 237–244.

Zanetta, J.P., Roussel, G., Ghandour, M.S., Vincendon, G. and Gombos, G. (1978) Postnatal development of rat cerebellum. Massive and transient accumulation of concanavalin A binding glycoprotein in parallel fiber axolemma. Brain Res. 142, 301–319.

Section III

DRUGS OF USE AND ABUSE
B. OPIOIDS AND MARIHUANA

Neurobehavioral Teratology
edited by Joseph Yanai
© Elsevier Science Publishers BV 1984

9

An Overview of the Neurobehavioral Sequelae of Perinatal Opioid Exposure

Ian S. Zagon and Patricia J. McLaughlin

Department of Anatomy, The Milton S. Hershey Medical Center, The Pennsylvania State University, Hershey, PA 17033, USA

THE use of opium dates back to antiquity, and natural and synthetic forms of opium have been employed in religious, medicinal, social, and personal contexts (Blum, 1970; Macht, 1915; Musto, 1973; Terry and Pellens, 1928). An important correlate to opioid consumption by pregnant women is the passive dependence of the fetus. [The term *opioid* is used in the generic sense (Jaffe and Martin, 1980; Wikler, 1980) and refers to a group of exogenous and endogenous substances, natural or synthetic in origin, that possess opium- or morphine-like properties. The term *dependence* is used to indicate a state of psychological and/or physiological dependence on a drug and follows the recommendation of the World Health Organization's Expert Committee on Addiction-Producing Drugs (1973).]

It is unclear how long ago this corollary was recognized. Hippocrates (see Martin, 1893) mentions opium in connection with 'uterine suffocation', perhaps alluding to opium's toxicity on the embryo or fetus. Certainly by the late 1800s (Zagon et al., 1982), clinical reports were in evidence describing the unusual behavior of the fetus and the neonate as a consequence of opium consumption. Férè (1883) and Fürst (1889) first noted clinical findings in the fetus, as manifested by violent kicking of the fetus when the mother was denied opioids. Infants involved with 'congenital morphinism', 'congenital narcotic addiction', or 'chronic opium intoxication' were reported to exhibit excessive nervousness, rapid breathing and convulsive movements shortly after birth, with death occurring within the first week of life (Menninger-Lerchenthal, 1934; Terry and Pellens, 1928). A tragic example of chronic maternal opium use, and one illustrating the perplexity and confusion of physicians at that time, was recorded by Petty (1913). A woman with 2 normal children was prescribed an 'elixir of opium' to prevent a miscarriage during her third pregnancy. The woman developed the 'opium habit' and although the newborn child appeared normal, the infant died of convulsions within 48 h of birth. Subsequently, all of the infants resulting from this woman's next 14 pregnancies also died within 3 days of birth. The same physician attended her in all these confinements, and both the mother and physician looked upon the death of the children as a 'natural consequence of the mother's condition and inevitable'. The child resulting from her 18th pregnancy lived. In this case, she was attended by another physician who 'understood the necessity of protecting it [the infant] from the shock incident to the abrupt withdrawal of the opiate' and prescribed treatment with paregoric.

A review of the early literature not only provides historical perspective to the field of perinatal opioid dependence, but also shows the extraordinary inquisitiveness and insightfulness on the part of some investigators. Collectively, these early reports represent an impressive amount of information that merits recognition and appreciation. In 1895, for example, Bureau found that morphine could pass through the human placenta. Sainsbury (1909) reported that 'the morphinist father tends to beget children whose vitality is, from the beginning, not only seriously impaired, but specifically biased'. The passage of opium into breast milk was clearly understood. Moreover, these early workers recognized that enough opium was contained in breast milk to alleviate withdrawal (Laase, 1919; Langstein, 1930; Petty, 1912, 1913; Van Kleek, 1920) or to even invoke drug dependency in a normal infant breast-fed by a woman that becomes dependent on heroin after parturition (Lichtenstein, 1915). The importance of therapeutic support by administration of morphine, heroin or paregoric to prevent withdrawal was also published repeatedly (Menninger-Lerchenthal, 1934; Terry and Pellens, 1928). Even the long-term implications of perinatal opioid exposure did not go unnoticed by these early investigators. Wilson and Eshner, writing in the American Textbook of Applied Therapeutics (1896), stated that 'The ultimate prognosis as to the child's [maternally exposed to opium] growing up is, however, 'bad' and this may be considered fortunate, as the moral and mental strength of these children is so far below par as to make them liable to much subsequent suffering'. And, in a discussion following the presentation of a paper by Earle (1888) concerning the adverse effects of fetal opioid exposure, a number of participants reported the association of neurobiological abnormalities in offspring (including adults) maternally exposed to opium.

The incidence of perinatal opioid dependency in earlier periods, and even up to recent times, has been difficult to gauge. In a number of instances in the early literature the authors refer to the 'rare' occurrence of such situations (Perlstein, 1947; Petty, 1913). However, opioid dependency of the newborn infant may have been more common than the literature would suggest. The use of opium to 'quiet' children has been the practice in a number of cultures. According to Marfori (cited in Menninger-Ler-chenthal, 1934), most children in India formerly received opium to the age of 5 years. From 1875 to 1959, Cobrinik and colleagues (1959) have estimated the publication of 204 case reports and an additional 100 cases that have unrecorded histories. Graham-Mulhall (1926) reported that in 1921 the Department of Narcotic Control of the State of New York received 55 requests for advice on the handling of newborn 'addicts'. Graham-Mulhall (1926) also states that in a 1-year period over 800 pregnant women consuming opioids were registered in New York. Finally, the response to a questionaire sent to physicians by the Committee on Drug Addiction in 1921 revealed that 9% of 570 physicians reported observing 'congenital narcotic addiction' (Terry and Pellens, 1928).

Despite the fact that heroin was widely available shortly after the turn of the century, morphine appears to be used almost exclusively in the cases reported up to the 1950s. The publication of the paper of Goodfriend et al. (1956), documenting nine cases of heroin-dependent babies, signaled a change in drug usage. Moreover, the 1950s marked an upturn in clinical interest in perinatal opioid dependency. Between 1951 and 1960, almost twice as many reports concerning this subject were issued than in any other previous 10 year period (Zagon et al., 1982). Yet another trend in the type of drug utilized began to occur after Dole and Nyswander's (1965) advocation of the methadone maintenance treatment program as an alternative to heroin dependency. Numerous reports (Blatman and Lipsitz, 1972; Blinick, 1968; Blinick et al., 1976; Pierson et al., 1972; Wallach et al., 1969; Zelson et al., 1973) followed that documented methadone's interaction in the fetus and neonate, and this area of investigation has continued to be one of intense interest (see Zagon et al., 1982).

Paralleling the change from consumption of morphine to the utilization of heroin and methadone that took place since the 1950s, a dramatic increase in the number of births of opioid-dependent women has been recorded. In a single municipal hospital in New York City, for example, only 22 infants were delivered by heroin-dependent mothers from 1955 to 1959, but 26 infants were delivered during 1960 alone (Zelson, 1975) and in this same hospital, a six-fold increase in drug-dependent babies was recorded between 1960 (1 in 164 births) and 1972 (1 in 27 births). A similar rise in the number of opioid dependent babies was found in a Philadelphia hospital (Finnegan, 1975). In 1969, one infant in 184 was born to a drug-dependent mother. However, by 1972, the incidence was 1 in 16 and, by 1973, one infant in 14. The exact magnitude of the number of infants exposed to opioids is difficult to determine. One estimate (Carr, 1975) places the birth rate of heroin and methadone dependent mothers at 3000 per year in New York City, with approximately 100 000 children in New York City already exposed to these drugs in early life. If one estimates that New York City has one-third to one-half of the total number of chronic heroin and methadone users in the United States (Carr, 1975; Salerno, 1977), then one could extrapolate 6000–9000 births/year to opioid-consuming women, and a total population of 200 000–300 000 children in the US that were born of females chronically using heroin or methadone. Placed within the context of the average number of births in the US every year (roughly 3.5 million), our calculations suggest that at least 1 in 1000 births is by a mother using heroin or methadone. This would be comparable to estimates of the incidence of the fetal alcohol syndrome (Clarren and Smith, 1978). Taking our estimates one step further, a population of 230 000 children exposed perinatally to opioids would represent 1 in 1000 people in the US (assuming a total population of 230 million). These numbers would indicate that a very large group of individuals may be at risk. Of course, given the unreported use of opioids by pregnant women and the possible influence exerted by paternal opiate consumption, the incidence might even be far greater. If exposure to opioids in early life does compromise physical or mental well-being, then the children raised by opioid-dependent mothers may pose serious social and public health problems.

In view of the incidence of perinatal opioid dependency and the obvious trauma inflicted upon the fetus and neonate by withdrawal, assessment of the risks involved with opioid exposure during early life on the developing infant and child, as well as the long-term consequences in adults perinatally subjected to these compounds, has become of great concern to health-care professionals and laymen alike. The purpose of this chapter is to review the clinical and laboratory information in this area, with special reference to the neurobehavioral sequelae involved with opioid dependency of the fetus and neonate. Findings from these studies will be interpreted in light of other neurobiological investigations in order to address the issue of etiology.

Clinical observations

Even before birth the offspring of opioid-dependent women are subjected to a host of potential problems. Many of the influences encountered not only hold danger for the fetus, but for the infant, child and adult as well. In regard to medical complications (Table 9.1), infectious diseases, nutritional deficits, and high incidence of veneral disease have been identified with chronic opioid consumption during pregnancy. Obstetrical complications (Table 9.2) include toxemia of pregnancy and intrauterine growth retardation. Additionally, spontaneous miscarriage, abortion and stillbirths are suspected of being higher than normal and bear closer investigation (Salerno, 1977). Although little attention has been paid to weight gain in pregnant women consuming

Table 9.1. Medical complications encountered in women dependent on opioids

Anemia	Pulmonary embolism	Gonorrhea
Bacteremia	Urinary tract infection	Herpes
Endocarditis	Tetanus	Hepatitis
Cellulitis	Pneumonia	Thrombophlebitis
Edema	Tuberculosis	Malnutrition
Septicemia	Syphilis	

Table 9.2. Obstetrical complications associated with opioid dependency

Abortion	Intrauterine growth retardation	Postpartum hemorrhage
Abruptio placentae	Placental insufficiency	Toxemia
Breech presentation	Premature rupture of membranes	
Intrauterine death	Premature labor	

opioids, Stryker (1977) has recorded perceptibly lower maternal weights at delivery in women enrolled in a methadone program. Many of these coassociated medical and obstetrical complications are secondary to the life style and habits of the pregnant addict (Perlmutter, 1974). And, of course, prenatal care, which constitutes the basis of programs to reduce maternal and fetal hazards, often goes neglected as a result of the intense dependency on drugs. The use of methadone as a substitute for heroin is more acceptable in this regard, since the pregnant women is placed in touch with health professionals that encourage prenatal care.

A decrease in birthweight in infants born to heroin-dependent mothers has been reported (Finnegan et al., 1972; Wilson et al., 1979; Zelson et al., 1971), with many of these low birthweight infants being small for gestational age. Although low birthweights were long suspected to be related to poor maternal nutrition and health, the growth delays associated with prenatal heroin exposure do not appear to be related to maternal nutrition or prenatal care (Connaughton et al., 1975; Naeye et al., 1973; Ramer et al., 1973). On the other hand, infants born to mothers maintained on methadone are reported to have higher birthweights and greater gestational ages than those exposed to heroin, although mean weight is still less than among non drug-dependent controls (Kandall et al., 1974; Zelson et al., 1973).

No studies have conclusively documented an association of maternal opioid dependency with congenital malformations, although some incidences (e.g. congenital heart defects, inguinal hernias) have been reported (Ostrea and Chavez, 1979; Reddy et al., 1971; Stone et al., 1971; Terry and Pellens, 1928). Chromosomal aberrations have been reported to be increased in infants exposed to heroin (Abrams, 1975; Amarose and Norusis, 1976), but not necessarily in those subjected to methadone (Abrams, 1975). An increased incidence of the sudden infant death syndrome (SIDS) has been found to be associated with opioid exposure (Chavez et al., 1979; Finnegan, 1979; Finnegan and Reeser, 1978), but it has not been determined whether it is a direct or indirect effect (Finnegan, 1979). Some hypotheses that have been suggested for the association of SIDS in opioid-exposed neonates include: disturbances of the autonomic nervous system of the neonate during the abstinence syndrome and its subsequent treatment, chronic fetal hypoxia, and infection (Finnegan, 1979)

Two prominent physiological effects of intrauterine opioid exposure on the neonate are worthy of mention. First, a lower incidence and severity of neonatal jaundice have been reported among heroin-exposed infants (Zelson et al., 1973; Nathenson et al., 1972). However, it is not clear whether this is a direct effect of in utero exposure to narcotics (which are not effective enzyme inducers) or an influence from other maternally abused substances (e.g. barbiturates) on the enzymes involved in bilirubin metabolism (Finnegan, 1979). Secondly, premature infants of heroin-dependent mothers often have a lower than expected incidence of respiratory distress syndrome (Glass et al., 1971). Since opioid-exposed infants also may exhibit a 'shift to the right' in the oxyhemaglobin dissociation curve (Glass et al., 1972), some investigators (Glass and Evans, 1977) have suggested that the enhanced ability of red blood cells to deliver more oxygen to tissues in these infants may contribute to the decreased incidence of respiratory distress syndrome.

The incidence of stillbirths and neonatality in the opioid-exposed population generally appears to be increased in comparison to control data (Finnegan, 1976; Fricker and Segal, 1978; Ostrea and Chavez, 1979; Perlmutter, 1967; Rementeria and Lotongkhum, 1977; Rementeria and Nuang, 1973). This higher mortality rate is not necessarily related to the neonatal withdrawal syndrome (Fricker and Segal, 1978; Ostrea and Chavez, 1979) with intrauterine asphyxia, prematurity, aspiration pneumonia (especially meconium aspiration), and hyaline membrane disease being the most important problems cited (Ostrea and Chavez, 1979).

Unfortunately very few studies have pursued details of postmortem examination of drug-dependent infants. Nesbitt (1957) has suggested that heroin can cause histological changes within the brain during fetal life. In the most complete study to date, Rorke and colleagues (1977) performed neuropathological studies on 10 infants exposed to heroin or methadone. Of eight categories of lesions recorded, three were thought to bear some relationship to maternal drug dependence and were not seen in severely ill infants of similar gestational ages. These included: gliosis (5/10), foci of old infarction (4/10), and brain developmental retardation (3/10). Other lesions identified included those common to high risk neonates: germinal plate hemorrhage (7/10), acute necrosis with and without hemorrhages (5/10), germinal plate cysts (4/10), and subarachnoid hemorrhage (3/10). This evidence would suggest that in addition to a host of non-specific secondary gestational complications, primary and specific effects of addictive drugs on the developing nervous system do occur.

It has been estimated that 60–90% of infants born to mothers chronically consuming opioids manifest some degree of withdrawal (Desmond and Wilson, 1975; Perlmutter, 1974; Zelson et al., 1971; Ramer and Lodge, 1975; Rosen and Pippenger, 1975). The common signs and symptoms characterizing the neonatal abstinence syndrome are summarized in Table 9.3. At birth, most passively dependent infants, whether born to heroin or methadone using mothers, appear physically and behaviorally normal. The withdrawal syndrome usually develops from 24 to 72 h after delivery (Desmond and Wilson, 1975; Ramer et al., 1973; Zelson, 1975), but cases with delayed onset of symptomology occurring from 2 to 4 weeks after birth have been reported (Kandall and Gartner, 1974). Fetal accumulation and delayed excretion of the drugs may account for the late presentation of symptoms (Kandall and Gartner, 1974). The type of drug or drugs utilized by the mother, drug dosage, timing of the dose before delivery, the character of labor, the type and amount of anesthesia and analgesia given dur-

Table 9.3. Signs and symptoms of neonatal abstinence in order of frequency
Adapted from Finnegan (1979). Data reflect observations of 138 infants made at Philadelphia General
Hospital between 1974 and 1976.

	Frequency (%)		Frequency (%)
Tremors	96	Hyperactive, more reflexive	62
High-pitched cry	95	Diarrhea	51
Sneezing	83	Sweating	49
Increased muscle tone	82	Excoriation	43
Frantic sucking of fists	79	Mottling	33
Reguritation	74	Nasal congestion	33
Sleeps less than 2 h after feeding	66	Frequent yawning	30
Respiratory rate greater than 60/min	66	Fever	29
Poor feeding	65		

ing labor, the maturity, nutrition, and presence or absence of intrinsic disease in the infant may all play a role in determining the time of onset in the individual infant (Desmond and Wilson, 1975). Efforts to correlate maternal opioid dose and the severity of neonatal withdrawal has proved inconclusive (Harper et al., 1977; Ostrea et al., 1976; Rosen and Pippenger, 1975; Zelson et al., 1971, 1973). However, the average length of hospitalization at the time of birth for opioid-dependent groups is often significantly increased from controls (e.g., Wilson et al., 1979), reflecting the more severe morbidity of these groups.

Although follow-up investigations on the opioid-exposed infant are few, there are indications of persistent effects of the drugs beyond the perinatal period. Early symptoms such as diarrhea, irregular sleep patterns and irritability may continue in attenuated form for up to 6 months after birth (Desmond and Wilson, 1975; Ramer and Lodge, 1975; Wilson, 1975; Wilson et al., 1973).

Depending on the severity of the withdrawal syndrome, treatment may be required. Paregoric, phenobarbital, diazepam and chlorpromazine are among the most commonly used agents (Kahn et al., 1969; Nathenson et al., 1972). The period of drug treatment may last from a few days to several months (Zelson et al., 1970). The advisability of breast feeding by women on narcotics remains a question. Opioids are known to be contained in the breast milk (Blinick et al., 1974, 1975; Kreek, 1975) and reports abound describing 'addictive' effects in infants consuming opioid-containing milk (Menninger-Lerchenthal, 1934; Terry and Pellens, 1928). In view of the peculiarities of the blood-brain barrier during perinatal development, and the fact that only nanogram and picogram amounts of drug are needed to occupy the opiate receptors, even small quantities of opioids in the milk may be capable of influencing the infant.

Utilizing 'classical' neurological tests, Davis and Shanks (1975) have drawn one of the more comprehensive pictures of the opioid-dependent infant. These babies exhibit central nervous system hyperexcitability, with irritability, tremors and hypertonicity, impaired nutritive sucking, vomiting, severe sleep deficit, hyperthermia and tachypnea. Autonomic dysfunction varies from vasomotor lability and diaphoresis to the less frequent diarrhea. In the early weeks after birth, these authors noted "almost univer-sally" lability of "states", with frequent shifts through the various stages of sleep and wakefulness that are often precipitated by environment or possibly internal stimuli. Sleep was disturbed in quality and quantity at the expense of decreased quiet, or non-REM sleep. An increased oral drive, with non-nutritive sucking in a tireless, sometimes frantic manner was also commonly observed.

Hyperactivity, a sign of irritability, was a persistent finding, and was found to en-dure through the early school age. These symptoms appeared to be an exaggerated relationship of motor behavior changes with changes of body posture. When the infant was supine and unrestrained, Davis and Shanks (1975) observed movements that assumed a jerky, purposeless, 'en masse' character, apparently perpetuated by unchecked proprioceptive stimuli. Early infantile automations and postural reflexes (e.g. crawling) were intact, but usually exaggerated. Some reflexes (e.g. tonic neck re-flex) were found to be accelerated in their maturational sequencing. Increasingly com-plex milestones such as crawling, weight bearing and standing were frequently acceler-ated, but the rate of this advance appeared to slacken with the increasing complexity of the milestone.

Some investigators (Chasnoff et al., 1980, 1982; Davis and Shanks, 1975; Kron et al., 1977; Lodge, 1976, Lodge et al., 1975; Marcus et al., 1982; Ramer and Lodge, 1975; Soule et al., 1974; Strauss et al., 1975, 1979a; Zarin-Ackerman, 1976), working with opioid-exposed infants, have utilized the Brazelton Neonatal Behavioral Assess-ment Scale (BNBAS) in an effort to quantify infant response to external stimuli, motor organization and ability to regulate state of consciousness. This instrument is particu-larly valuable since it assesses behaviors directly pertinent to the neonatal withdrawal syndrome (e.g. irritability, consolability), and taps generally significant adaptive capa-cities such as habituations to stimuli during sleep and attentiveness during alert peri-ods.

The picture that emerges from these studies dramatizes the impaired ability of opioid-dependent babies to adequately organize their response to environment, with a lessened capacity to attend and react to noxious stimuli and to habituate to disturb-ing events (Davis and Shanks, 1975). Newborns exposed perinatally to opioids appear to be significantly more tremulous, irritable, adept at placing their hands into or near their mouths, and behaviorally labile. These neonates were also less cuddly and tended to manifest less smooth or mature motor movements, probably as a consequence of their greater irritability (Strauss et al., 1975). Although these infants cried more often in response to stimulation than did non-dependent infants, they were as capable of self-quieting and responding to soothing intervention as normal neonates.

Infant performance on the response decrement scales of the BNBAS assesses the rapidity and degree of habituation to stimuli. Response decrement has been suggested as an index of cognitive maturity and central nervous system integrity (Bowes et al., 1970). Infants born of opioid-using mothers exhibited a depressed response decrement to light, a stimulus known to be aversive to adults during opioid withdrawal. In regard to orientation of early cognitive behavior and the development of mother-infant inter-action pattern, opioid-dependent infants were less often and less extensively in alert stages than non-dependent infants. Visual and auditory orientation were most often cited as problem areas (e.g. Chasnoff et al., 1982; Soule et al., 1974). Thus these opioid-exposed infants were less available for interaction with the nonsocial stimuli used in examination. The inability to attend to new stimuli and process information in opioid-dependent infants has been suggested to be a preliminary indication of possi-ble future cognitive dysfunction.

A number of workers (Chasnoff et al., 1980, 1982; Marcus et al., 1982) have tried more closely to examine performance on the Brazelton test as a means of deciphering the specific effects of narcotics on the neonate. Chasnoff and colleagues (1982) found that methadone-dependent infants demonstrated even poorer state organization than polydrug-exposed infants. Moreover, only methadone infants exhibited difficulties in orientation response and motor maturity. Marcus et al. (1982) have examined the re-lationship between motor and state functioning in perinatal narcotic dependence and found that motor function was a clearer discrimination between methadone- and non-methadone-dependent children than state functioning. These authors suggest the be-havioral problems in methadone infants may not be due to generalized central nervous system irritability, but may be more differential, being seen in neuromuscular func-tioning in particular.

The BNBAS not only allows elucidation of specific aspects of the infants developing behavioral organization but, by implication, the behavior elicited from care-givers as well (Bell, 1974). Strauss and colleagues (1975) make note of this important point. They state that the major differences between dependent and non-dependent neonates are found for variables which define two primary behavioral dimensions on the Brazel-ton scale: orientation responsiveness and excitability. Both have substantial impact on care-giver's perceptions of infants and, depending on their extent and duration of man-ifestation, may have long-term consequences for the development of infant caregiver interaction patterns.

The question of when normalization occurs on the BNBAS for opioid-exposed neo-nates has been addressed by a number of investigators. Kaplan et al. (1978) found alertness to be within normal limits at 28 days of age, but tremulousness was noted to remain significantly elevated at that time. Strauss et al. (1976) have also reported normalization of all behaviors on the BNBAS by the first month of life except for tre-mulousness. Strauss and colleagues (1979a) have also found that infants requiring pharmacotherapy remain tremulous at one month, as opposed to normal behavior of non-drug-dependent infants and opioid-dependent babies who did not require phar-macotherapy. Of course, it must be recognized that the BNBAS was designed to be sensitive through the period of the first few days of life, rather than through the period of the first month of life (Sameroff, 1979). Thus, only gross behavioral dysfunction is most likely to be detected in one month olds, and finer-grained tests are needed to de-tect more subtle neurobehavioral changes.

A number of investigators have chosen to transcend the BNBAS and examine specific neurobehavioral aspects of neonates passively dependent on opioids. One area of interest has been the characteristic pattern of lability of states in which sleep is disturbed. Schulman (1969) and Dinges et al. (1980) have found a significant decrease in quiet sleep and increased rapid eye movement (REM) sleep in opioid exposed neonates, a profile shared among newborns at high risk for central nervous system impairment. Sisson et al. (1974) also found a decrease in quiet sleep, but also reported a decrease in REM sleep. REM sleep could be increased if withdrawal was treated by chlorpromazine therapy. Sisson concluded that since REM sleep is an important time of neuronal protein synthesis, treatment of withdrawal is essential not only to relieve symptoms but to promote normal and necessary sleep patterns required for brain development.

Another way of obtaining a more comprehensive profile of behavior in the neonate perinatally exposed to opioids has been the pursuit of the pattern of disorganized feeding behavior. Kron and colleagues (1976) have reported an uncoordinated and ineffectual sucking reflex as a major manifestation of neonatal opioid abstinence. Interestingly, the sucking behavior of infants born to mothers attending methadone clinics was significantly more depressed than that of infants born to street addicts. The behavioral difference between babies of methadone and street addicts may be due to the differential pharmacology of the narcotic agents used (e.g. relative potency and time course of action). Another interesting finding in Kron's study was that pretreatment of the abstinence syndrome with paregoric, but not phenobarbital or diazepam, normalized sucking behavior. Strauss et al. (1979a), in discussing Kron's work, points out that the sucking response can be used to study attention, perceptual development, and learning through much of infancy. Strauss stresses that this is a period in which cognitive development is occurring but one in which the objective behavioral repertoire of humans is limited.

A third line of investigation concerning the behavior of the neonate maternally exposed to opioids has been the delineation of the electrophysiological properties of heroin, methadone, and methadone-heroin dependent groups. Lodge et al. (1975) found that the neonatal withdrawal period was characterized by heightened auditory responsiveness and orientation, lowered overall alertness, and poor attentiveness to and following presentation of visual stimuli. Electroencephalographic recordings revealed high frequency dysynchronous activity that suggested central nervous system irritability. Analysis of evoked response data provided evidence for a low arousal value of visual stimulation in vertex frequency characteristics and poorly defined occipital responses that correspond to the diminished visual attention noted behaviorally. Lodge and colleagues (1975) feel that it is the arousal feature of visual input, rather than sensory processing, which distinguishes opioid-exposed and normal infants.

In terms of neurological status, some investigators have reported few differences between narcotic-dependent and control groups (Johnson and Rosen, 1982; Kaltenbach et al., 1979; Green and Zarin-Ackerman, 1977; Ting et al., 1974, 1978). However, Rosen and Johnson (1982a), in an examination of children up to 18 months of age delivered by methadone-maintained mothers reported a number of neurologic abnormalities. The most common were tone discrepancies, developmental delays, and eye problems. Between 6 and 12 months of age, delays in sitting and in the development of transfer ability and fine motor coordination were seen. At 18 months, no real language development was detected. Moreover, the children continued to have strabismus and nystagmus, a finding reported by others (Chavez et al., 1979)

Neurodevelopment of infants beyond the withdrawal period has also been examined by Wilson and colleagues (1973, 1981). In one of the earliest reports (Wilson et al., 1973) concerned with following the neurobehavioral ontogeny of children subjected perinatally to opioids, Wilson made a detailed study of 30 heroin-exposed infants ranging in age from 3 to 34 months. Adaptive behavior, language, performance and personal-social development in these children were fairly comparable to controls. Motor development was noted to be normal, but gross motor coordination was often found to be more advanced than fine motor coordination. Six children of 1 year, all placed in stable foster homes, demonstrated disturbances of activity level or attention span or both, with associated sleep disturbances, temper tantrums, and low tolerance to frustration. At 12 to 18 months, Wilson and colleagues encountered the onset of hyperactivity. Activity levels and attention spans were abnormal and adaptive performance was erratic and performance age was difficult to assess. These children completed occasional age-specific tasks with swift precision, suggesting normal potential, but they lacked the persistence necessary to complete the majority of tasks. Wilson relates one case in which a "hyperkinetic patient completed all required tasks and responded promptly to directions despite constant motor activity, which included climbing on and creeping under the examination table and chair". Abnormal or equivocal neurological findings were noted in five patients at their last visit (6–34 months old), including: hypo- and hypertonicity, asymmetrical handedness, and fine motor delay and disability. In a subsequent article (Wilson, 1981) on the neurobehavioral development of heroin or methadone-exposed infants during the first year, muscle tone (particularly of the extensor muscles) was increased in the heroin group, and differed significantly from the methadone group. Wilson noted that fine motor coordination of both methadone and heroin-exposed offspring was significantly poorer than that of drug-free controls.

A number of investigators have used the Bayley Scales of Infant Behavior for measurements of mental and motor development to determine whether differences occur between opioid-dependent and non-dependent children. The Bayley items are organized according to standardized age norms and consist of social responses (e.g. social smile), cognitive response (e.g. orienting to an object and grasping it), and gross motor responses (e.g. sitting with slight support). The results from this examination do not show a consistent pattern. Some workers (Johnson and Rosen, 1982; Blatman and Lipsitz, 1972; Chasnoff et al., 1980; Green and Zarin-Ackerman, 1977; Zarin-Ackerman, 1976) have found that results with children subjected perinatally to opioids are within the normal range. Wilson et al. (1981) found that scores on the mental development index (MDI) and motor development index (PDI) were within normal range for heroin- and methadone-exposed infants during the first year of life. However, the scores on the PDI for the methadone-subjected children were lower than those of the heroin-exposed group and significantly lower than those of drug-free groups. Wilson called attention to the less attentive nature of both the methadone and heroin infants. Kaltenbach et al. (1979) examined methadone-exposed children of 1 and 2 years of age on the MDI. Although scores were within the normal range of mental development, the 2 year olds showed a significantly higher failure rate on three specific items: naming of two objects, pointing to five pictures, and naming of three objects. Kaltenbach suggests that subtle differences in cognitive behavior are occurring that may be occluded by summary scores. Rosen and Johnson (1982a), examined methadone-exposed infants up to 18 months of age and found normal, but lower scores on the MDI and PDI at 6 months. By 12 months of age, and again at 18 months, the methadone children were significantly below the control population in both indices, particularly the PDI. Moreover, the comparison subjects also passed the Bayley language milestone earlier than methadone subjects did. Strauss and colleagues (1976) also have found that opioid-dependent infants exhibited delays in the PDI. In contrast, some researchers have reported higher PDI scores (Lodge, 1976; Ramer and Lodge, 1975). Davis and Shanks (1975) have examined opioid-subjected infants between 2 and 25 months of age and recorded normal scores in the first 8 to 12 months but, after 15 months, a borderline to definite lag in mental development was noted. This delay in MDI was thought to be related primarily to poor verbal ability in these children. In fact, Davis and Shanks (1975) estimated that these children were 2–4 months below the norm in language development. Ramer and Lodge (1975) and Lodge (1976) have also recorded a lower MDI for methadone children, and suggest that this may be due to poor attentiveness to visual stimuli and lack of sustained visual following.

In regard to other parameters of behavioral development, opioid-subjected infants tested on the Gesell scales (Finnegan et al., 1977; Ting et al., 1974; Wilson et al. 1973), Merrill-Palmer test and Peabody Picture Vocabulary Test (Blatman and Lipsitz, 1972), as well as on the Object Permanence Scales (Johnson and Rosen, 1982a), appeared to be normal. A number of workers have reported disorders in speech and/or language development (Blatman and Lipsitz, 1972; Nichtern, 1973; Sardemann et al., 1976) in children subjected to opioids, although Lodge (1976) reported relative strength in the realm of language for children exposed to methadone.

There are only a handful of investigations on children maternally subjected to opioids that extend beyond the first few years of childhood. Nichtern (1973), examining a population of children born to heroin-dependent mothers, recorded observations on some children that were up to 15 years of age. Many of the children appeared to manifest some problems with their capacity for human relationships, demonstrating excessive adult-peer interactions, poor socialization, and the use of withdrawal in attempting to deal with these problems. Nichtern also found a general reduction of responsiveness in these children so that they functioned below their potential. And finally, some of these children demonstrated a variety of learning problems, with discrepancies between their mental ages and their performance and achievement levels.

In regard to children perinatally exposed to methadone, Lodge (1976) has examined 3–5 year olds born of mothers maintained on methadone and found scores on the Stanford Binet Intelligence Scale to be within normal range. Rosen and Johnson (1982b), in a 3 year follow up study of children exposed in utero to methadone, found overall performance on the Merrill-Palmer Scale of Mental Tests not to differ from the control group, but they did find significantly more low scores for the methadone children. Moreover, these authors found other signs of impaired development, including smaller head circumferences, strabismus and/or nystagmus, and abnormalities in muscle tone, coordination and language. Examination of 5 year old children of methadone-treated women using the McCarthy Scale of Children's Abilities also revealed no differences in cognitive or perceptual performance (Strauss et al., 1979), although these children (and a matched non-drug dependent group) performed below normative expectations. These children also did not differ in observed characteristics of home environment or patterns of child or caregiving behavior in a playroom observation, but children who had been transplacentally exposed to narcotics behaved less maturely and were more inappropriately active during psychological testing. Strauss found a cluster of behavioral differences related to greater task-irrelevant activity of methadone children while in a testing situation. He suggests that in structured and demanding situations, the qualities of attentiveness and motor inhibition may be a domain in which opioid-exposed children might reveal particular vulnerabilities.

The only study investigating the long-term neurobehavioral implications of exposure to heroin during early life has been the report of Wilson et al. (1979). In this study, 3–6 year old children of heroin-dependent mothers were compared to three other groups (drug environment, high-risk, socioeconomic) matched for age, race, sex, birthweight and socioeconomic status. On a battery of psychometric tests, the heroin-exposed group scored within normal ranges, but this group often did significantly poorer than those of comparison groups. On the Illinois Test of Psycholinguistic Abilities, mean values for the heroin-exposed and drug environment groups were below combined group means on the subtest for auditory memory, while heroin-exposed and high-risk groups were below group means on visual closure. On the psycholinguistic quotient, the socioeconomic group had a significantly higher score than the mean of all three other groups. The mean IQ as determined by the Columbia Mental Maturity Scale did not differ between groups, nor did the parents' perceptions of the function of their child as measured by the Minnesota Child Development Inventory. On the McCarthy Scales of Children's Abilities, heroin-exposed children performed poorer than comparison groups on the General Cognitive Index and on three of five subtests: perceptual performance, quantitative, and memory.

Wilson did not find any problems with speech and language function, but on a battery of perceptual measures, visual, tactile and auditory perception were poorer in the heroin-exposed group than in the 'combined control groups'. Finally, in regard to be-havior, the heroin-exposed group was rated by parents as having greater difficulty in areas of self adjustment, social adjustment, and physical adjustment. Items of particu-lar note included: uncontrollable temper, impulsiveness, poor self-confidence, aggress-iveness, and difficulty making and keeping friends. A subjective evaluation of the child's activity level during physical examination ranked the heroin-exposed group as significantly more active than any other group. However, on ratings of attention, co-operation and alertness, and activity level as rated by review of videotaped sessions, by ultrasonic equipment, or by the rocking chair counter, no differences between any of the groups were encountered. Based on these results, Wilson suggests that consistent patterns of low functioning by the heroin-exposed target group occurs in all modalities of the perceptual battery, indicating a problem common to the general process of per-ception rather than specific sensory deficit. She feels that the behavioral problems recorded may be manifestations of "impaired attention and organizational abilities".

Although the primary focus of this chapter is on the behavioral sequelae found in children born of narcotic-dependent women, it would be remiss not to give consider-ation to the somatic growth of these children. Some studies (Blatman and Lipsitz, 1972) have found growth parameters to be comparable to that of control populations, while others (Strauss et al., 1976; Wilson et al., 1981; Finnegan et al., 1977) have recorded lower (but not statistically reliable) values for offspring exposed to opioids. There are a substantial number of reports (Wilson et al., 1973, 1979; Wilson, 1975; Ting et al., 1974, 1978; Rosen and Johnson, 1982a, b; Chasnoff et al., 1982) document-ing delayed growth properties associated with perinatal opioid exposure. Wilson and colleagues (1973, 1975, 1979) have recorded marked growth impairment in children up to 6 years of age that were transplacentally subjected to heroin. This delay in soma-tic development took the form of noticeably lower body weights, body lengths (height) and head circumferences. Wilson (1975) feels that nutrition may not necessarily be related to this retardation, since these infants and children often had an abnormally high caloric intake. A similar pattern of growth deficits has been reported for children born to mothers receiving methadone. Wilson (1975) found normal intrauterine growth for these individuals, but body lengths and head circumferences of 25% of the 13 patients measured had fallen below the tenth percentile after 9 months of life. Ting et al. (1974, 1978) have found head circumference measurements of methadone chil-dren to remain within 2 standard deviations, but 26% of 25 children (ages 6–41 months) were below the 3rd percentile in stature as compared to none in the control group. Chasnoff et al. (1980) have reported that mean birthweight and length to be at the 10th percentile for methadone infants, and head circumference to be at the 5th percentile, with deficits remaining until 4–6 months. At this time, withdrawal appears to subside and an accelerated growth pattern can be noted. Finally, Rosen and John-son (1982a, b) found decreases in head circumference that were prominent in metha-done-exposed children of up to 3 years of age, but relatively few differences in body weight or height were observed.

Data collection and interpretation in most areas of human research are usually fraught with difficulties. In the study of perinatal opioid exposure and human development, the potential for problems is compounded. A number of fundamental issues can be delineated. First, the licit and illicit use of opioids so alters psychological, behavioral and physiological processes that it raises the drug to a paramount position in the life of any user. No better testimony to the distorted perspective of these individuals need be given than to consider that the mother disregards the health of her child by consuming these substances during pregnancy. Given the adaption of each individual to such a situation, it is understandable why the complexity of evaluating a single person, much less a group of individuals, reaches extraordinary heights. Secondly, investigations on the effects of opioid exposure on the developing human actually involves the study of two individuals: the mother and her offspring. In some cases, other individuals (e.g. caregivers) may be involved as well. The interaction of these forces only serves to make the isolation of any one influence a very difficult task. In recent years the role of confounding variables in the field of perinatal opioid exposure and development has not been overlooked. Recognition and discussion about problems in experimental design and interpretation have become increasingly apparent (e.g. Householder et al., 1982; Strauss et al., 1979a, b; Wilson et al., 1979, 1981; Aylward, 1982). Although it is beyond the scope of this chapter to appraise critically each of the studies mentioned in this review of the clinical literature, it is imperative that the limitations in these investigations be appreciated. In Table 9.4, a catalogue of some of these factors (many of which overlap with one another) are presented.

The list of confounding variables may appear to be overwhelming. However, one cannot simply dismiss the published reports cited in this review, nor say that such studies are of little utility. Rather, one should be aware that although the goal of clinical research may indeed be to determine the existence of a linear relationship between cause and effect, this type of distinction may be unattainable. Perhaps experimental designs of this sort often may be better framed as correlational, thereby inferring an association between variables rather than a delineation of cause and effect (see Aylward, 1982; Kaltenbach et al., 1979; Householder et al., 1982). Thus in the case of opioid exposure and human development, we may eventually have to be satisfied with the knowledge that we are dealing with a cumulative effect from an overall potentially detrimental milieu in which opioids are a prime, but not necessarily the sole factor in the etiology and pathogenesis of any damaging sequelae encountered.

In view of the clinical literature, and despite the confounding variables that can be enumerated, it is important to realize that opioid consumption by the pregnant woman places the fetus, neonate, infant, and child at considerable risk for injury. An underlying litany of somatic and neurobiological disturbances can be detected in the literature. Given this risk in early life, a period crucial to developmental processes, it would not be unreasonable to suspect long-term repercussions that could compromise the mental and/or physical well-being of the adult.

Laboratory observations

General observations on pregnancy and progeny

The effects of perinatal opioid exposure on neurobehavioral development of laboratory animals have been an active area of investigation in recent years (see Zagon et al., 1982). A variety of protocols has been employed in these investigations, each utilizing different routes of administration, drug dosages, and schedules of treatment (Tables 9.5–9.7). Maternal exposure to opioids appears to have little effect on estrous cycle, fertility, length of gestation and parturition (e.g. Zagon and McLaughlin, 1977a, b), although some investigators working with methadone have mentioned difficulties with conception (Buchenauer et al., 1974), a protraction of the gestational period (Buchenauer et al., 1974; Chandler et al., 1975), and positional malformations of the fetus (Chandler et al., 1975). Maternal body weight often tends to be reduced in pregnant animals chronically treated with opioids (McGinty and Ford, 1980; Ford and Rhines, 1979; Hutchings et al., 1976; Markham et al., 1971; Middaugh and Simpson, 1980; Seidler et al., 1982; White et al., 1978; Zagon and MacLaughlin, 1977a, b), however these weight deficits do not appear to be caused by insufficient nutritional status (Ford and Rhines, 1979; White et al., 1978). The effect of opioids on maternal viability is related to the type of opioid studied, the dosage employed, and the experimental de-

Table 9.4. Confounding influences often present in clinical studies on opioid-dependent women and their offspring

Polydrug and substance abuse prior to, during, and after pregnancy: opioids, alcohol, caffeine, nicotine, stimulants, tranquilizers, hallucinogens	Length of hospitalization at parturition
	Neonatal withdrawal; occurrence(s), severity, duration, treatment
Evaluation and procedures for monitoring polydrug and substance abuse; e.g. reliability of self-reporting, compliance, frequency of urine analysis	Rehospitalization of the child
	Exposure to opioids postnatally; breast milk, treatment for withdrawal
Drug dosage	Breast feeding; transmission of drugs, maternal-infant bonding
Rehabilitation: drug withdrawal, methadone maintenance	'Parenting'
Episodic withdrawal during pregnancy	Adoption or fostering
General 'lifestyle', e.g. prostitution	Mother-infant/child interaction
Health	Paternal influence
Age	'Environmental' factors
Parity	Age of child investigated
Dietary habits and nutritional status	Sample selection; randomization, availability and number of subjects
Obstetrical and postpartum medications and complications	Statistical analysis
Socioeconomic status	Inconsistency in criteria evaluated
Race	Subjectivity of reporting (e.g. neonatal withdrawal syndrome)
Demographics	Type of tests used for investigation
Genetic background	Use of summary scores vs analysis of individual test items
Prenatal care	Structuring of appropriate comparison groups
Postnatal care	'Drop-out' rate of patients in study

Table 9.5. Protocols of laboratory studies concerning perinatal opioid exposure and neurobehavioral development: morphine and heroin
In studies where dosages are escalated, only the final dosage is given. *indicates direct treatment of offspring.

Authors	Species	Dosage	Route	Treatment schedule	Experimental group(s)
Caza and Spear (1980)	rat	0.1, 0.5, 1, 5 mg/kg morphine	sc	*acute injection on postnatal days 10, 17, or 24	postnatal
Davis and Lin (1972)	rat	45 mg/kg morphine	sc	days 5–18 of gestation	prenatal
Friedler (1977)	mouse	240 mg/kg morphine	sc	5 day exposure occurring at least 6 days prior to mating	pregestational
Glick, et al. (1977)	rat	0.5 g/l morphine	po	day 1 of gestation → day 15 of lactation	prenatal-postnatal
Kirby (1979)	rat	1.25, 5, 10, 20, 40 mg/kg morphine	sc	days 7–18 of gestation (20 mg/kg, twice daily) or acute injection on day 18 of gestation (other dosages)	prenatal
Kirby (1981)	rat	10 mg/kg morphine	sc	acute injection on days 15–21	
Kirby and Holtzman (1982)	rat	20 mg/kg morphine	sc	days 12–21 of gestation (5 mg/kg every 6 h or 10 mg/kg every 12 h)	prenatal
		3.2 mg/kg dextrorphanol or levorphanol	sc	days 12–21 of gestation (0.8 mg/kg every 6 h)	
LaPointe and Nosal (1982)	rat	56 mg/kg morphine	ip	5 days prior to mating → day 16 of gestation (through weaning)	prenatal, postnatal, and prenatal-postnatal
Lasky et al. (1977)	rat	5 mg/kg heroin	ip	5 days prior to mating → weaning (5 mg/kg once daily or 2.5 mg/kg twice daily)	prenatal-postnatal
McGinty and Ford (1976)	rat	0.3 mg/ml morphine	po	days 15 of gestation → weaning	prenatal-postnatal
Newby-Schmidt and Norton (1981a)	chick	20 mg/kg egg morphine	air sac	days 12–19 or 16–19 of incubation	in ovo
Newby-Schmidt and Norton (1981b)	chick	20 mg/kg egg morphine	air sac	days 12–19 of incubation	in ovo
		1 mg/kg chick	ip	*acute injection on days 1–2 or 4–5	postnatal
Peters (1978)	rat	7.5 mg/kg morphine	ip	7 days prior to mating → weaning	prenatal-postnatal
Sobrian (1977)	rat	40 mg/kg morphine	sc	5 days prior to mating → day 15 of lactation	prenatal-postnatal
Sonderegger and Zimmermann (1976)	rat	4, 8, 16 mg/kg morphine	sc	*days 0–7, 8–14 or 15–22 of lactation (twice daily)	postnatal
Sonderegger et al. (1979)	rat	75 mg morphine	sc implant	*implantation on day 5 or 11	postnatal

214

Table 9.6. Drug protocols in laboratory studies concerning perinatal opioid exposure and neurobehavioral development: methadone and NLAAM
In studies where dosages are escalated, only the final dosage is given. *indicates direct treatment of offspring.

Authors	Species	Dosage	Route	Treatment schedule	Experimental group(s)
Freeman (1980)	rat	4 or 16 mg/kg methadone	sc	days 8–22 of gestation	prenatal
Friedler (1977)	mouse	20 mg/kg methadone	sc	5 days exposure occurring at least 6 days prior to mating (twice daily)	pregestational
Grove et al. (1979)	rat	0.125 mg/ml methadone	po	day 1 of gestation → weaning cross-fostered at birth	prenatal, postnatal, and prenatal-postnatal
Hutchings et al. (1979a)	rat	10 or 15 mg/kg methadone	po	days 8–22 of gestation	prenatal
Hutchings et al. (1980)	rat	5, 7.5 or 10 mg/kg methadone	po	days 8–22 of gestation	prenatal
Hutchings et al. (1979b)	rat	10 mg/kg methadone	po	days 8–22 of gestation	prenatal
McGinty and Ford (1976)	rat	0.35 mg/kg methadone	po	day 15 of gestation → weaning	prenatal-postnatal
Middaugh and Simpson (1980)	mouse	2.5, 5 or 10 mg/kg methadone	sc	days 15–22 of gestation	prenatal (but nursed on biological mothers)
Peters (1977, 1978)	rat	5 mg/kg methadone	ip	7 days prior to mating → weaning	prenatal-postnatal
Rech et al. (1980)	rat	10 mg/kg methadone	sc	day 5 or gestation → weaning cross-fostered at birth	prenatal, postnatal, and prenatal-postnatal
Soyka et al. (1978)	rat	10 mg/kg methadone	sc	12 days prior to mating	pregestational
Thompson and Zagon (1982)	rat	5 mg/kg methadone	ip	5 days prior to mating → weaning (cross-fostered at birth)	prenatal, postnatal, and prenatal-postnatal
Van Wagoner et al. (1981)	rat	5 mg/kg methadone	ip	5 days prior to mating → weaning (cross-fostered at birth)	prenatal, postnatal, and prenatal-postnatal
Walz (1981)	rat	15 mg/kg methadone	po	60 days prior to mating → weaning (both sexes exposed prior to mating)	prenatal-postnatal
Zagon and McLaughlin (1978)	rat	5 mg/kg methadone	ip	5 days prior to mating → weaning (cross-fostered at birth)	prenatal, postnatal, and prenatal-postnatal
Zagon et al. (1979a)	rat	5 mg/kg methadone	ip	5 days prior to mating → weaning (cross-fostered at birth)	prenatal, postnatal, and prenatal-postnatal
Zagon et al. (1979b)	rat	5 mg/kg methadone	ip	5 days prior to mating → weaning (cross-fostered at birth)	prenatal, postnatal, and prenatal-postnatal (females only)
Zagon and McLaughlin (1981a)	rat	5 mg/kg methadone	ip	5 days prior to mating → weaning (cross-fostered at birth)	prenatal, postnatal, and prenatal-postnatal
Kuwahara and Sparber (1981)	chick	2.5 or 3.4 mg/kg egg 1-α-noracetylmethadol	intra-chorion	acute injection on day 3 of incubation	in ovo
Kuwahara and Sparber (1982)	chick	2.5, 5, 10 mg/kg egg	intra-chorion	acute injection on day 3 of incubation	in ovo
		0.15, 0.3, 0.5 mg chick 1-α-noracetylmethadol	ip	*days 1–2	postnatal

Table 9.7. Protocols of laboratory studies concerning perinatal opioid exposure and neurobehavioral development: endorphins and opiate antagonists
In studies where dosages are escalated, only the final dosage is given. *indicates direct treatment of offspring.

Authors	Species	Dosage	Route	Treatment schedule	Experimental group(s)
Kastin et al. (1980)	rat	80 μg/kg Met-enkephalin	sc	*days 1–7 of lactation	postnatal
Harry and Rosecrans (1979)	rat	1 mg/ml naltrexone	po	days 0–21 of gestation	prenatal
				day 0 of gestation → weaning	prenatal-postnatal
Paul et al. (1978)	rat	20 to 60 mg/kg naltrexone	sc	*days 3–20 of lactation	postnatal
Vorhees (1981)	rat	40 mg/kg naloxone	ip	days 7–20 of gestation (20 mg/kg, twice daily)	prenatal (but nursed on biological mothers)

sign utilized (e.g. Buchenauer et al., 1974; Hutchings et al., 1976; Zagon and McLaughlin, 1977a, b). In general, maternal exposure to morphine (Davis and Lin, 1972; LaPointe and Nosal, 1982; Sobrian, 1977), methadone (Freeman, 1980; Hutchings et al., 1979a, b; Soyka et al., 1978; Zagon and McLaughlin, 1977b, c), and naloxone (Voorhess, 1981) does not have a detrimental effect on litter size, although Hutchings et al. (1979b) and Middaugh and Simpson (1980) have reported decreases in litter size with higer doses of methadone. Transplacental exposure to morphine (Harpel and Gautieri, 1968; Arcuri and Gautieri, 1973; Geber and Schramm, 1975), methadone (Jurand, 1973; Geber and Schramm, 1975), and heroin (Geber and Schramm, 1975) have been recorded to be teratogenic, with a variety of central nervous system lesions often occurring. However, teratogenicity seems to be associated with high drug dosages that are administered acutely or over a short period of time, rather than with lower dosages of opioids administered chronically (Zagon and McLaughlin, 1977a, b; Hutchings et al., 1976). In papers providing information on the number of stillborns delivered by opioid-treated mothers, some studies report a marked increase in stillborns that is often associated with high drug dosages (Freeman, 1980; Grove et al., 1979; Hutchings et al., 1980; Sobrian, 1977), while many reveal no problems (Davis and Lin, 1972; Hutchings et al., 1979a, b; Middaugh and Simpson, 1980; Newby-Schmidt and Norton, 1981; Zagon and McLaughlin, 1977a, b, c).

The effect of transplacental exposure to opioids on infant viability is generally determined by whether or not the neonates continue to receive opioids postnatally (e.g. breast milk). Pups that do not continue to receive opioids often appeared to be hypersensitive to stimuli and experience tremors at birth, with a marked infant mortality often found in the first few days of life for those pups exposed to either morphine (Davis and Lin, 1972; Sobrian, 1977), heroin (Zagon and McLaughlin, 1982c), methadone (Freeman, 1980; Hutchings et al., 1979a, b, 1980; Rech et al., 1980; Soyka et al., 1978; Zagon and McLaughlin, 1977c), and NLAAM (Lichtblau and Sparber, 1981). Beyond the first few days, the incidence or mortality is usually not elevated from controls.

Fetal behavior
A consistent finding in perinatal opioid research is a reduction in spontaneous activity of the 'fetus' as recorded in rats and chicks (Table 9.8). This effect is sensitive to naloxone, since the administration of opioid antagonists results in an increase in spontaneous activity (Kirby, 1981; Kirby and Holtzman, 1982; Newby-Schmidt and Norton, 1981; Kuwahara and Sparber, 1981).

Preweaning behavior
During the first week of life, the behavior of animals prenatally exposed to opioids is characterized by abnormal increases in tremors and head-shakes (Zagon and McLaughlin, 1977c) and in activity levels (Hutchings et al., 1980) (Table 9.9). Since the timetable of behavioral maturation in rodents is well-known, evaluation of the

Table 9.8. Effects of opioids on behavior monitored in ovo or in utero

Arrows indicate the direction of significant change from controls for all opioid-treated groups studied or those specified within parentheses; NS = not significant.

Author	Age examined		Behavior
Morphine			
Kirby (1979)	18 days in utero	↓	spontaneous activity
Kirby (1981)	15–21 days in utero	↓	spontaneous activity
Kirby and Holtzman (1982)	18–20 days in utero	↓	spontaneous activity (twice daily injection group)
NLAAM			
Newby-Schmidt and Norton (1981)	16 days in ovo	NS	spontaneous activity
Kuwahara and Sparber (1981)	19 days in ovo	↓	spontaneous activity

ontogenetic pattern in the preweaning period offers a valuable means for studying opioid-related actions on the developing nervous system. The results of these investigations show delays in the expression of gross motor development, the appearance of certain physical characteristics, and/or the maturation of both simple and complex sensory and motor behaviors (see Table 9.10). These delays may take the form of retardation in the age of initial appearance of a particular behavior, the age at which 50% and 100% of the animals express a specific behavioral parameter, and the time difference between the age at which a behavioral characteristic was first observed and the age at which a maximal number of animals displayed a specific activity (i.e. maturational range). Disturbances related to vision, audition, locomotion, exploration and emotionality are among the most notable.

A distinct difference between opioid agonists and antagonists can be observed in

Table 9.9. Effects of opioids on behavior in the preweaning period (days 0–21)

Arrows represent direction of significant change from controls for either all opioid-treated groups studied or those specified within parentheses. NS = not significant.

Author	Age examined		Behavior
Morphine			
Caza and Spear (1980)	10 days	↓	open field–locomotion (0.5, 1, 5 mg/kg groups)
		↑	catalepsy (5 mg/kg group)
		NS	gnawing
		NS	grooming, sniffing, rearing
	17 days	↑	open field–locomotion (0.5 mg/kg group)
		↓	open field–locomotion (5 mg/kg group)
		↑	catalepsy (5 mg/kg group)
		NS	gnawing, grooming, sniffing, rearing
	24 days	NS	open field–locomotion
		↑	gnawing (5 mg/kg group)
		NS	grooming, sniffing, rearing

Table 9.9 Contd.

Author	Age examined	Behavior	
Friedler (1977)	0–21 days	↓	(delayed) ear and eye opening
LaPointe and Nosal (1982)	0–21 days	NS	battery of sensorimotor reflexes except:
		↓	(delayed) eye opening (prenatal)
		↓	frequency of pivoting (prenatal-postnatal)
		↓	respiratory rate (0–3 days)
		↑	frequency of crying (0–3 days)
		↑	restlessness (0–3 days)
McGinty and Ford (1976)	0–21 days	↓	open field–ambulation
		↓	(delayed) reflex and motor skill development
		↓	(delayed) ear, eye, vaginal opening, hair covering
Newby-Schmidt and Norton (1981a)	1, 2 days	↑	neuromuscular weakness (16–19 day group)
	7 days	↑	disruption of stride (16–19 day group)
Newby-Schmidt and Norton (1981b)	1, 2 days	NS	distress vocalization
	4, 5 days	↑	distress vocalization
Sobrian (1977)	1, 5, 10 days	NS	activity monitor
	15, 20, 25, 30 days	↑	activity monitor

Methadone

Author	Age examined	Behavior	
Friedler (1977)	0–21 days	↓	(delayed) ear and eye opening
Hutchings et al. (1979a)	17, 22 days	↑	activity monitor, 3 littermates/group (10 mg/kg group)
		↑	number of rest-activity fluctuations, 3 littermates/group (10 mg/kg group)
Hutchings et al. (1980)	2 days	↓	activity monitor, 8–10 littermates/group (10 mg/kg group)
	5 days	↑	activity monitor, 8–10 littermates/group (5 mg/kg group)
	14–32 days	NS	activity monitor, 8–10 littermates/group
Hutchings et al. (1979b)	0–21 days	NS	time of eye opening and hair covering
McGinty and Ford (1976)	11 days	↓	open field–ambulation
	0–21 days	↓	(delayed) reflex and motor skill development
		↓	(delayed) ear, eye, and vaginal opening, hair covering
Walz (1981)	0–21 days	↓	(delayed) reflex ontogeny
	0–14 days	↓	open field–exploration
	14–21 days	↑	open field–exploration
	10–21 days	↓	open field–defecation
Zagon and McLaughlin (1978)	2–19 days	↓	(delayed) reflex and spontaneous motor development, physical characteristics (see Table 9.10)

NLAAM

Author	Age examined	Behavior	
Kuwahara and Sparber (1982)	3, 4 days	↓	open field–escape jumps, ambulation (prenatal, postnatal groups)
		↓	(retarded) acquisition of detour performance (5 mg/kg prenatal group)
		↑	frequency of distress vocalizations (5 mg/kg prenatal group)

Naltrexone

Author	Age examined	Behavior	
Paul (1978)	3–21 days	NS	reflexive behavioral ontogeny

Naloxone

Author	Age examined	Behavior	
Vorhees (1981)	3–21 days	NS	appearance of eye and vaginal opening, lower incisor eruption, and testicular descent
		↑	(accelerated) appearance of upper incisor eruption
		↑	(accelerated) capability of surface righting, swimming
		NS	open field (rearing, defecation, grooming)
		↑	(facilitated) startle response
		↑	(facilitated) olfactory orientation

Table 9.10. Summary of sensorimotor and physical parameters in preweaning rats maternally subjected to methadone

Age is the day when 50% of all animals (pups from both control and experimental groups) displayed a particular behavior. Arrows indicate the direction of significant change from controls; NS = not significant. Modified from data presented in Zagon and McLaughlin (1978a).

Parameter	Age (days)	Treatment group		
		Prenatal	Postnatal	Prenatal-postnatal
A. *Spontaneous motor*				
Unilaterial head turn with no return	2	NS	↓	↓
Unilateral head turn to left and return	5	↓	NS	NS
Head raise	8	↓	NS	NS
Pivoting 360°	8	↓	↓	NS
Foreleg and hindleg movement	11	↓	NS	NS
Head, foreleg, hindleg movement	12	NS	↓	NS
Walking	13	↓	↓	NS
B. *Reflex tests*				
Startle	3	↓	↓	↓
Righting reflex	3	NS	↓	NS
Pain – paw withdrawal	5	↓	NS	NS
Bar grasping	11	↓	NS	NS
Tail hanging	12	↓	↓	↓
Edge aversion	12	NS	↓	NS
Visual orientation	15	↓	↓	↓
Auditory reflex	16	NS	NS	↓
C. *Physical development*				
Incisor eruption	9	↓	↓	NS
Hair covering	11	↓	↓	NS
Ear opening	13	↓	↓	↓
Eye opening	14	↓	NS	NS

measurements of preweaning activity. Whereas the opioid agonists generally delay development, opioid antagonists accelerate the appearance of some characteristics (Paul et al., 1978; Vorhees, 1981).

Behavior in the weanling

A number of studies (Table 9.11) have explored sensory and motor capabilities during the period shortly after weaning (days 21–44). With the exception of Davis and Lin's (1972) findings of increased ambulatory activity and emotionality in morphine-treated animals, pups exposed perinatally to morphine, heroin and methadone generally exhibit less activity and decreased emotionality relative to control offspring. In regard to methadone treatments, Zagon and McLaughlin (1981a) found an abnormally high incidence of wet-dog shakes and head-shake behaviors during this period that resembled drug withdrawal. Rodents exposed to opioid antagonists (naltrexone, naloxone) appear to be comparable to controls in behavioral parameters monitored thus far.

Table 9.11. Effects of opioids on behavior in the weanling period (days 22–44)

Arrows represent direction of significant change from controls for either all opioid-treated groups studied or those specified within parentheses. NS = not significant.

Author	Behavior	
Morphine		
Davis and Lin (1972)	↑	open field–ambulation rearing
	↓	open field–defecation
	NS	open field–face washing
	NS	activity cage
Friedler (1977)	↓	activity monitor–running, rearing (males)
	↓	open field–exploration
Sonderegger et al. (1979)	NS	open field–ambulation, defecation
Heroin		
Lasky et al. (1977)	NS	open field–ambulation
	NS	activity cage
	NS	activity wheel
	↓	latency to step down from an elevated platform
Methadone		
Freeman (1980)	↓	activity cage–ambulation (16 mg/kg groups)
	NS	activity cage–defecation
Friedler (1977)	↓	activity monitor–running, rearing (males)
	↓	open field–exploration (males)
Grove et al. (1979)	↓	activity cage
	↓	open field–ambulation, rearing (prenatal and prenatal-postnatal groups)
	NS	open field–defecation
Middaugh and Simpson (1980)	↓	open field–ambulation
	↓	reactivity to stimulus presentation (5 mg/kg females)
Peters (1977)	↑	shock avoidance, latency
Zagon et al. (1979a)	↓	open field–ambulation
	↓	activity cage
	NS	activity wheel
	↑	latency to step down from an elevated platform (prenatal group)
Zagon and McLaughlin (1981a)	↑	withdrawal, head shakes (prenatal, postnatal groups)
Naltrexone		
Harry and Rosecrans (1979)	NS	activity cage
Paul et al. (1978)	NS	open field–ambulation
Naloxone		
Vorhees (1981)	NS	activity wheel
	NS	M-maze (discrimination water maze)
	NS	open field–ambulation

Behavior in the young adult

In contrast to the hypoactivity in opioid-treated pups at weaning, young adults (days 45–89) generally were hyperactive and more emotional (Table 9.12). During this period, Zagon and McLaughlin (1981a) have found that methadone-exposed offspring often exhibit head-shake and wet-dog shake behaviors, suggesting a protracted phase

Table 9.12. Effects of opioids on behavior in young adult animals (days 45–89)

Arrows represent direction of significant change from controls for either all opioid-treated groups studied or those specified within parentheses. NS = not significant.

Author	Behavior
Morphine	
Davis and Lin (1972)	↑ open field activity–ambulation, rearing
	NS open field–defecation, face washing
	↑ activity cage
	NS audiogenic seizures
Peters (1978)	NS food maze
	↑ treadmill (females)
	↑ shock avoidance–latency
Sonderegger et al. (1979)	↑ errors in Lashley III maze
Methadone	
Grove et al. (1979)	↑ open field–ambulation (prenatal group, prenatal-postnatal group)
	NS open field–rearing, defecation
	↑ activity cage
Hutchings et al. (1979b)	NS acquisition level pressing
	NS variable interval reinforcement
	NS auditory-visual discrimination
	NS response inhibition in a punishment paradigm
Peters (1978)	NS food maze
	NS treadmill (males)
	↑ shock avoidance, latency
	↑ treadmill (females)
Soyka et al. (1978)	↑ open field–ambulation
	↓ open field–defecation
Zagon et al. (1979a)	↑ open field–ambulation (prenatal, postnatal groups)
	↑ activity cage (postnatal, prenatal-postnatal groups)
	↑ activity wheel (postnatal group)
	↓ latency to step down from an elevated platform (prenatal, prenatal-postnatal)
Zagon and McLaughlin (1981a)	↑ withdrawal, head shakes
	↑ withdrawal, wet-dog shakes (postnatal, prenatal-postnatal groups)
Naloxone	
Vorhees (1981)	↑ Biel maze, number of errors
	NS active avoidance
	NS passive avoidance
	NS T-maze (spontaneous alternation)
	NS food grasping
	NS activity wheel

of withdrawal in these animals. Preliminary evidence also indicates that methadone- and morphine-exposed rats may demonstrate learning disabilities (Peters, 1978).

Behavior in the mature adult

The effects of exposure to opioids in early life on adult behavior are presented in Table 9.13. Adult rats appear to have a lasting impairment in the ability to acquire fear

Table 9.13. Effects of opioids on behavior in mature adult animals (days 90 and over)

Arrows represent direction of significant change from controls for either all opioid-treated groups studied or those specified within parentheses. NS = not significant.

Author		Behavior
Morphine		
Glick et al. (1977)	↑	(facilitation) self-administration behavior
Sonderegger and Zimmermann (1976)	↓	conditioned suppression
Methadone		
Middaugh and Simpson (1980)	NS	acquisition of lever response (5 mg/kg group)
	↑	fixed ratio reinforcement
Rech et al. (1980)	↑	active avoidance 'massed' trials
Soyka et al. (1978)	NS	open field–emotionality
	NS	conditioned avoidance
Thompson and Zagon (1982)	↓	social dominance (water-deprivation test)
Van Wagoner et al. (1980)	↓	discrimination learning (prenatal, postnatal groups)
	NS	discrimination learning (prenatal-postnatal group)
Zagon and McLaughlin (1981a)	↑	withdrawal, head shakes
Zagon et al. (1979b)	↓	active avoidance 'spaced' trials (prenatal, prenatal-postnatal groups)
	NS	passive avoidance
	↓	food-reward light-dark discrimination maze (prenatal, postnatal groups)
Enkephalin		
Kastin et al. (1980)	↑	(facilitation) maze performance
Naltrexone		
Harry and Rosecrans (1979)	↑	rate of extinction, modified conditioned emotional response

(Sonderegger and Zimmerman, 1976), a reduction in social dominance (Thompson and Zagon, 1982), problems in learning (Middaugh and Simpson, 1980; Van Wagoner et al., 1980; Zagon et al., 1979b), and a facilitation towards self-administrative behavior (Rech et al., 1977). However, unlike perinatal exposure to morphine or methadone, rats subjected to enkephalins in the preweaning period exhibited a facilitation in learning ability (Kastin et al., 1980).

Physiological correlations

In addition to the neurobehavioral effects enumerated, some mention should be made of other aspects of biological function perturbed by perinatal exposure to opioids. Some of the most prominent alterations associated with opioid exposure in early life have been somatic growth retardation (e.g. McLaughlin and Zagon, 1980; McLaughlin et al., 1978; Slotkin et al., 1976, 1980; Zagon and McLaughlin, 1977c), smaller brain dimensions (Zagon and McLaughlin, 1977c, 1978), and deficits in organ weight(McLaughlin and Zagon, 1980; McLaughlin et al., 1978). Physiological dysfunction concerning disturbances in thermoregulation (Thompson and Zagon, 1981;

Thompson et al., 1979), nociceptive thresholds (Zagon and McLaughlin, 1980b, 1981b, 1982a), and aberrant response to drug (Zagon and McLaughlin, 1981a) have also been cited.

Methodological considerations of laboratory models

Just as with clinical studies, laboratory experiments may be fraught with difficulties in design and interpretation. Data collected in laboratory investigations can only be as meaningful to the subject at hand as the strategy utilized in addressing a question and to the quality of research performed. Although it is not within the purview of this chapter critically to assess each of the laboratory studies mentioned, I think it is important to draw the reader's attention to some of those factors which are crucial in obtaining the most relevant information to the clinical problem.

A prominent characteristic of maternal opioid consumption in humans is the regular use of opioids prior to and during pregnancy. To be consistent with this pattern of human consumption, it would be most advantageous in laboratory models to initiate drug exposure as early as possible, preferably beginning before mating and continuing throughout gestation. In humans, tolerance and physical dependence usually accompany the regular use of opioids. In the laboratory situation, some degree of tolerance to the adverse physiological effects following initial exposure to opioids (e.g. depressed ventilation) would therefore be an essential component in experimental design. The presence of tolerance also would be desirable in order to minimize the contribution of other factors (e.g. hypoxia) that could form the basis of neurobehavioral abnormalities and obfuscate the deciphering of influences related to long-term drug consumption. Of equal importance to evidence showing tolerance would be documentation of physical dependence in the mother, and especially in the neonate. Such information could be derived from experiments which determined the presence of the abstinence syndrome following removal of the drug or upon administration of an opioid antagonist such as naloxone.

An important aspect of clinical practice (particularly in the methadone maintenance program) that must be kept in mind in laboratory experiments is the prevention of episodic withdrawal. This situation could occur when the dosage of drug is inadequate to maintain a dependent state. Rementeria and Lotongkhum (1977), for example, suggest that an increase in methadone dosage during later stages of pregnancy should be considered in order to compensate for the methadone utilized by the growing fetus. As noted by Zuspan and colleagues (1975), failure to adjust the dosage near term may lead to drug craving in the pregnant woman and to fetal distress. Thus, in the realm of laboratory experimentation, documentation of the absence of episodic withdrawal is required, perhaps by inspection of maternal behavior at intervals throughout a 24-h period. Such observations would eliminate the confounding variable of in utero withdrawal when examining the effects of long-term opioid consumption on offspring. A related point in this regard is the necessity of adjusting drug dosage for body weight. This procedure is predicated on the basis of dosage/volume distribution, and is mandatory to control the pharmacological regimen in order to provide meaningful data for within- or between-group comparisons.

Two other factors that are unrelated to the clinical situation, but which would shed light on the etiology of opioid action, should be mentioned. First, the experiments in which the stereospecific relationship of opioids is explored would be quite valuable in determining the specificity of opioid response. Second, the capability of blocking the effects of opioid agonists by concomitant administration of an antagonist would indicate whether the effect of a particular opioid resides at the level of the opiate receptor.

Finally, and perhaps most importantly, is the resemblance of the clinical findings to those obtained in laboratory experiments. An affirmative answer in this regard would provide considerable strength to the laboratory model at hand.

Conclusions

In the preceding sections of this review, the effects of opioids on the developing organism have been examined. A number of striking parallels between clinical and laboratory findings emerge from this information. In brief, these include: passive dependency of the fetus on opioids, occurrence of the neonatal abstinence syndrome, high rate of morbidity and mortality if the neonate is not given supportive therapy for withdrawal, protracted and/or subacute withdrawal, sleep disturbances in the neonate, delays in sensorimotor development, retardation in somatic growth, smaller head circumferences in humans/smaller brain sizes in laboratory animals, delays in walking, problems in visual and/or auditory systems, abnormalities in neuropathological studies indicating aberrations in neuro-ontogeny, less alert, poor attention spans in early phases of development, hyperactivity in later phases of development, learning disabilities, and social problems.

It is evident from the laboratory and clinical studies reviewed that exposure to opioids during early life is associated with adverse neurobehavioral sequelae. However, the mechanisms through which the effects are produced remain unclear. Laboratory studies do indicate that opioid-exposed offspring have deficits in brain cell number, as well as alterations in brain RNA and protein concentrations and content (Zagon and McLaughlin, 1977d, 1978b). Furthermore, changes in polyamine metabolism (Slotkin et al., 1976, 1979) and in the ontogeny of catecholaminergic systems, as well as a retardation in the synaptic development of 5-hydroxytryptamine, dopamine, and epinephrine neurons in the nervous system have been recorded (McGinty and Ford, 1980; Rech et al., 1980; Slotkin, 1982). Morphological studies indicate that the timetable of neurogenesis is dependent on the schedule of drug exposure (gestation and/or lactation) (Zagon and McLaughlin, 1982d), and that prenatal exposure to opioids is associated with reductions in cortical thickness and number of cells in the neocortex during the first 2 weeks of rat development, as well as neuronal density changes/unit area in the hippocampus up to postnatal day 28 in the rat (Ford and Rhines, 1979).

It does appear from a review of the laboratory and clinical literature (Ford and Rhines, 1979; Zagon and McLaughlin, 1982b; McLaughlin and Zagon, 1980; Naeye et al., 1973; Seidler et al., 1982; White et al., 1978; Raye et al., 1977; Smith et al., 1977) that neither maternal undernutrition nor inadequate nutrition of the offspring form the etiological basis for opioid related problems. Moreover, hypoxia due to opioid consumption does not appear to be responsible for the sequelae observed (White and Zagon, 1979).

Two of the most important observations to date that may lead to a better understanding of the etiology of neurobehavioral dysfunction are concerned with the pharmacological nature of opioid action on the developing organism. First, opioids have been reported to exert a stereospecific effect on growth in animals (Smith et al., 1977; Crofford and Smith, 1973), suggesting that opioid action is extremely specific. Secondly, the effects of opioids on development have been shown to be blocked by concomitant administration of opioid antagonists (e.g. naloxone) (Crofford and Smith, 1973; Hui et al., 1978; Smith et al., 1977), indicating that opioid agonist action resides at the level of the opiate receptor. It is known that opiate receptors evolve during the perinatal period (Bardo et al., 1982; Clendeninn et al., 1976; Garcin and Coyle, 1978) and opioids selectively accumulate in the brains of fetal rats (Peters et al., 1972) and preweaning rats (Shah and Donald, 1979), presumably because developing animals have an increased permeability of the blood-brain barrier. Based on these observations, it may be conjectured that opioids alter developmental processes in the brain by interacting with the opiate receptor. The opiate receptor in turn may be linked to fundamental processes (e.g. cyclic nucleotides) (Sharma et al., 1977; Lampert et al., 1976; Brandt et al., 1976) essential to cell proliferation, migration and differentiation that could lead to cell deficits, aberrant morphological patterns and neurochemical disturbances. Moreover, cellular events may be adversely affected not only by the presence of the drug, but also by the absence of drug (i.e. in utero and/or neonatal withdrawal). Any one or a combination of these factors may result in neurodysgenesis that ultimately could be responsible for the behavioral and physiological irregularities observed.

Acknowledgements

The preparation of this chapter, as well as the authors' work summarized in this article, were supported by the National Institute on Drug Abuse (Grant DA-01618). We are grateful to Ms. Dixi Weaver for technical assistance.

References

Abrams, C.A.L. (1975) Cytogenetic risks to the offspring of pregnant addicts. Addict. Dis. 2, 63–77.

Amarose, A.P. and Norusis, M.J. (1976) Cytogenetics of methadone-managed and heroin addicted pregnant women and their newborn infants. Am. J. Obstet. Gynecol. 124, 635–639.

Arcuri, P.A. and Gautieri, R.F. (1973) Morphine-induced fetal malformations. III. Possible mechanisms of action. J. Pharm. Sci. 62, 1626–1634.

Aylward, G.P. (1982) Methadone outcome studies: is it more than the methadone? J. Pediat. 101, 214–215.

Bardo, M.T., Bhatnagar, R.K., Gebhart, G.F. and Hughes, R.A. (1982) Opiate receptor development in midbrain and forebrain of posthatch chicks. Dev. Brain Res. 3, 668–673.

Beil, R.Q. (1974) Contributions of human infants to caregiving and social interaction. In: (Lewis, M. and Rosenblum, L.A., eds.) The Effect of the Infant on its Caregiver. Wiley, New York.

Blatman, S. and P.J. Lipsitz (1972) Children of women maintained on methadone: accidental methadone poisoning of children. In: Proceedings of the Fourth National Conference on Methadone Treatment, NAPAN, New York, pp. 175–176.

Blinick, G. (1968) Menstrual function and pregnancy in narcotic addicts treated with methadone. Nature 219, 180.

Blinick, G., Inturrisi, C.E., Jerez, E. and Wallach, R.C. (1974) Amniotic fluid methadone in women maintained on methadone. Mt. Sinai J. Med. 41, 254–259.

Blinick, G., Inturrisi, C.E., Jerez, E. and Wallach, R.C. (1975) Methadone assays in pregnant women and progeny. Am. J. Obstet. Gynecol. 121, 617–621.

Blinick, G., Wallach, R.C. Jerez, E. and Ackerman, B.D. (1976) Drug addiction in pregnancy and the neonate. Am. J. Obstet. Gynecol. 125, 135–142.

Blum, R.H. (1970) A history of opium. In: Society and Drugs. I. Social and Cultural Observations, Jossey-Bass Inc., San Fransisco, pp. 45–58.

Bowes, W.A., Brackbill, Y., Conway, E. and Steinschneider, A. (1970) The effects of obstetrical medication on fetus and infant. Monog. Soc. Res. Child. Dev. 35, Serial No. 137.

Brandt, M., Gullis, R.J., Fischer, K., Buchen, C., Hamprecht, B., Moröder, L. and Wünsch, E. (1976) Enkephalin regulates the levels of cyclic nucleotides in neuroblastoma X glioma hybrid cells. Nature 262, 311–313.

Buchenauer, D., Turnbow, M. and Peters, M.A. (1974) Effect of chronic methadone administation on pregnant rats and their offspring. J. Pharmacol. Exp. Ther. 189, 66–71.

Bureau, A. (1895) Accouchement d'une morphinomane: prevue chimique du passage de la morphine à travers le placenta: reflexions. Bull Mem. Soc. Obstet. Gynecol. 356–362.

Carr, J.N. (1975) Drug patterns among drug-addicted mothers: incidence, variance in use, and effects on children. Pediat. Ann. 4, 408–417.

Caza, P.A. and Spear, L.P. (1980) Ontogenesis of morphine-induced behavior in the rat. Pharmacol. Biochem. Behav. 13, 45–50.

Chandler, J.M., Robie, P., Schoolar, J. and Desmond, M.M. (1975) The effects of methadone on maternal-fetal interactions in the rat. J. Pharmacol. Exp. Ther. 192, 549–554.

Chasnoff, I.J., Hatcher, R. and Burns, W.J. (1980) Early growth patterns of methadone-addicted infants. Am. J. Dis. Child. 134, 1049–1051.

Chasnoff, I.J., Hatcher, R. and Burns, W.J. (1982) Polydrug- and methadone-addicted newborns: a continuum of impairment? Pediatrics 70, 210–213.

Chavez, C.J., Ostrea, E.M., Stryker, J.C. and Smialek, Z. (1979) Sudden infant death syndrome among infants of drug-dependent mothers. J. Pediat. 95, 407–409.

Clarren, S. and Smith D. (1978) The fetal alcohol syndrome. M. Engl. J. Med. 298, 1063.

Clendeninn, N.J., Petraitis, M. and Simon, E.J. (1976) Ontological development of opiate receptors in rodent brain. Brain Res. 118, 157–160.

Cobrinik, R.W., Hood, T. and Chusid, E. (1959) The effect of maternal narcotic addiction on the newborn infant. Pediatrics 24, 288–304.

Connaughton, J.F., Finnegan, L.P., Schut, J. and Emich, J.P. (1975) Current concepts in the management of the pregnant opiate addict. Addict. Dis. 2, 21–35.

Crofford, M. and Smith, A.A. (1973) Growth retardation in young mice treated with dl-methadone. Science 181, 947–949.

Davis, M.M. and Shanks, B. (1975) Neurological aspects of perinatal narcotic addiction and methadone treatment. Addict. Dis. 2, 213–226.

Davis, W.M. and Lin, C.H. (1972) Prenatal morphine effects on survival and behavior of rat offspring. Res. Commun. Chem. Pathol. Pharmacol. 3, 205–214.

Desmond, M.M. and Wilson, G.S. (1975) Neonatal abstinence syndrome: recognition and diagnosis. Addict. Dis. 2, 112–121.

Dinges, D.F., Davis, M.M. and Glass, P. (1980) Fetal exposure to narcotics: neonatal sleep as a measure of nervous system disturbance. Science 209, 619–621.

Dole, V.P. and Nyswander, M. (1965) A medical treatment for diacetylmorphine (heroin) addiction. J. Am. Med. Assoc. 193: 646–650.

Earle, F.B. (1888) Maternal opium habit and infant mortality. M. Standard (Chicago) 3, 2.

Férè, Ch. (1883) De la morphinomanie au point de vue de la grossesse et de la né du foetus. Comm. Soc. Biol. Sem. Méd. 294.

Finnegan, L.P. (1975) Narcotics dependence in pregnancy. J. Psychedel. Drugs 7, 299–311.

Finnegan, L.P. (1976) Clinical effects of pharmacologic agents on pregnancy, the fetus, and the neonate. Ann. N.Y. Acad. Sci. 281, 74–89.

Finnegan, L.P. (1979) In utero opiate dependence and sudden infant death syndrome. Clin. Perinatol. 6, 163–180.

Finnegan, L.P. and Reeser, D.S. (1978) Opiate use in pregnancy: a possible causative factor in the sudden infant death syndrome. Committee on Problems of Drug Dependence (40th Annual Scientific Meeting), Baltimore, MD, pp. 340–350.

Finnegan, L.P., Connaughton, J.F. Emich, J.P. and Wieland, W. (1972) Comprehensive care of the pregnant addict and its effect on maternal and infant outcome. In: Committee on Problems of Drug Dependence (34th Annual Scientific Meeting), Ann Arbor, MI, pp. 372–390.

Finnegan, L.P., Reeser, D.S., Ting, R.Y., Rozenzwerg, M. and Keller, A. (1977) Growth and development of children born to women maintained on methadone during pregnancy. Pediat. Res. 11, 377.

Ford, D. and Rhines, R. (1979) Prenatal exposure to methadone HCl in relationship to body and brain growth in the rat. Acta Neurol. Scand. 59, 248–262.

Freeman, P.R. (1980) Methadone exposure in utero: effects on open-field activity in weanling rats. Int. J. Neurosci. 11, 295–300.

Fricker, H.S. and Segal, S. (1978) Narcotic addiction, pregnancy, and the newborn. Am. J. Dis. Child. 132, 360–366.

Friedler, G. (1977) Effect of pregestational morphine and methadone administration to mice on the development of their offspring. Fed. Proc. 36, 1001.

Fürst, C. (1889) Wien. Klin. Wschr. 191–220.

Garcin, F. and Coyle, J.T. (1978) The ontogenetic development of the opiate receptor and enkephalin in rat brain. Neuropsychopharmacology 2, 1379–1385.

Geber, W.F. and Schramm, L.C. (1975) Congenital malformations of the central nervous system produced by narcotic analgesics in the hamster. Am. J. Obstet. Gynecol. 123, 705–713.

Glass, L. and Evans, H.E. (1977) Physiological effects of intrauterine exposure to narcotics. In: Drug Abuse in Pregnancy and Neonatal Effects. (Rementería, J.L., ed.) C.V. Mosby Co., St. Louis, MO, pp. 108–115.

Glass, L., Rajegowda, B.K. and Evans, H.E. (1971) Absence of respiratory distress syndrome in premature infants of heroin-addicted mothers. Lancet ii, 685–686.

Glass, L., Rajegowda, B.K., Kahn, E.J. and Floyd, M.V. (1972) Effect of heroin withdrawal on respiratory rate and acid-base status in the newborn. N. Engl. J. Med. 286, 746–748.

228

Glick, S.D. Strumpf, A.J. and Zimmerberg, B. (1977)Effect of in utero administration of morphine on the subsequent development of self-administration behavior. Brain Res. 132, 194–196.

Goodfriend, M.J., Shey, I.A. and Klein, M.D. (1956) The effects of maternal narcotic addiction on the newborn. Am. J. Obstet. Gynecol. 71, 29–36.

Graham-Mulhall, S. (1926) Opium the Demon Flower. Harold Vinal, New York, (reprinted in 1981 by Arno Press Inc.).

Green, M. and Zarin-Ackerman, J. (1977) Effect of prenatal exposure to narcotics on CNS function of the child. In: Drug Abuse in Pregnancy and Neonatal Effects, (Rementería, J.L., ed.) C.V. Mosby Co., St. Louis, MO, pp. 145–156.

Grove, L.V., Etkin, M.K. and Rosecrans, J.A. (1979) Behavioral effects of fetal and neonatal exposure to methadone in the rat. Neurobehav. Toxicol. 1, 87–95.

Harpel, H.S. and Gautieri, R.F. (1968) Morphine induced fetal malformations. I. Exencephaly and axial skeletal fusions. J. Pharm. Sci. 57, 1590–1597.

Harper, R.G. Solish, G., Feingold, F., Gersten-Woolf, N. and Sokal, M.M. (1977) Predictors of the severity of neonatal methadone withdrawal. Pediat. Res. 11, 417.

Harry, G.J. and Rosecrans, J.A. (1979) Behavioral effects of perinatal naltrexone exposure: a preliminary investigation. Pharmacol. Biochem. Behav. 11 (Suppl.), 19–22.

Householder, J., Hatcher, R., Burns, W. and Chasnoff, I. (1982) Infants born to narcotic-addicted mothers. Psychol. Bull. 92, 453–468.

Hui, F.W. Krikum, E. and Smith, A.A. (1978) Inhibition of d,1-methadone of RNA and protein synthesis in neonatal mice: antagonism by naloxone or naltrexone. Eur. J. Pharmacol. 49, 87–93.

Hutchings, D.E., Hunt, H.F., Towey, J.P., Rosen, T.S. and Gorinson, H.S. (1976) Methadone during pregnancy in the rat: dose level effects on maternal and perinatal mortality and growth in the offspring. J. Pharmacol. Exp. Ther. 197, 171–179.

Hutchings, D.E., Feraru, E., Gorinson, H.S. and Golden, R.R. (1979a) Effects of prenatal methadone on the rest-activity cycle of the pre-weanling rat. Neurobehav. Toxicol. 1, 33–40.

Hutchings, D.E., Towey, J.P., Gorinson, H.S. and Hunt, H.F. (1979b) Methadone during pregnancy: assessment of behavioral effects in the rat offspring. J. Pharmacol. Exp. Ther. 208, 106–112.

Hutchings, D.E., Towey, J.P. and Bodnarenko, S.R. (1980) Effects of prenatal methadone on the activity level in the pre-weanling rat. Neurobehav. Toxicol. 2, 331–335.

Jaffe, J.H. and Martin, W.R. (1980) Opioid analgesics and antagonists. In: The Pharmacological Basis of Therapeutics (Gilman, A.G., Goodman, L.S., and Gilman, A., eds.) 6th ed., MacMillan, New York, pp. 494–534.

Johnson, H.L. and Rosen, T.S. (1982) Prenatal methadone exposure: effects on behavior in early infancy. Pediat. Pharmacol. 2, 113–120.

Jurand, A. (1973) Teratogenic activity of methadone hydrochloride in mouse and chick embryos. J. Embryol. Exp. Morphol. 30, 449–458.

Kahn, E.F., Neumann, L.L. and Polk, G.A. (1969) The course of the heroin withdrawal syndrome in newborn infants treated with phenobarbital or chlorpromazine. J. Pediat. 75, 495–500.

Kaltenbach, K., Graziani, L.T. and Finnegan, L.P. (1979) Methadone exposure in utero: developmental cstate at one and two years of age. Pharmacol. Biochem. Behav. 11 (Suppl.), 15–17.

Kandall, S.R. (1977) Late complications in passively addicted infants. In: Drug Abuse in Pregnancy and Neonatal Effects (Rementeria, J.L., ed.) C.V. Mosby Co., St. Louis, MO, pp. 116–128.

Kandall, S.R. and Gartner, L.M. (1974) Late presentation of drug withdrawal symptoms in newborns. Am. J. Dis. Child. 127, 58–61.

Kandall, S.R., Gartner, L.M. and Berle, B.B. (1974) Birthweights and maternal narcotic use. Pediat. Res. 8, 364.

Kaplan, S.L., Kron, R.E., Phoenix, M.D. and Finnegan, L.P. (1978) Brazelton neonatal assessment at three and twenty-eight days of age: a study of passively addicted infants, high risk infants, and normal infants. In: Critical Concerns in the Field of Drug Abuse (Schecter, A., Alksne, H. and Kaufman, E., eds.) Marcel Dekker, New York, pp. 726–730.

Kastin, A.J., Kostrzewa, R.M., Schally, A.V. and Coy, D.H. (1980) Neonatal administration of met-enke-phalin facilitates maze performance of adult rats. Pharmacol. Biochem. Behav. 13, 883–886.

Kirby, M.L. (1979) Effects of morphine on spontaneous activity of 18-day rat fetus. Dev. Neurosci. 2, 238–244.

Kirby, M.L. (1981) Effects of morphine and naloxone on spontaneous activity of fetal rats. Exp. Neurol. 73, 430–439.

Kirby, M.L. and Holtzman, S.G. (1982) Effects of chronic opiate administration on spontaneous activity of fetal rats. Pharmacol. Biochem. Behav. 16, 263–269.

Kreek, M.J. (1975) Pharmacologic modalities of therapy: methadone maintenance and the rise of narcotic antagonists. In: Heroin Dependency. (Stimmel, B., ed.) Stratton Int. Medical Book Co., New York, pp. 232–290.

Kron, R.E., Litt, M., Phoenix, M.D. and Finnegan, L.P. (1976) Neonatal narcotic abstinence: effects of pharmacotherapeutic agents and maternal drug usage on nutritive sucking behavior. J. Pediat. 88, 637–641.

Kron, R.E., Kaplan, S.L., Phoenix, M.D. and Finnegan, L.P. (1977) Behavior of infants born to narcotic addicted mothers: effects of prenatal and postnatal drugs. In: Drug Abuse in Pregnancy and Neona-tal Effects (Rementería, J.L., ed.) C.V. Mosby Co., St. Louis, MO, pp. 129–144.

Kuwahara, M.D. and Sparber, S.B. (1981) Prenatal withdrawal from opiates interferes with hatching of otherwise viable chick fetuses. Science 212, 945–947.

Kuwahara, M.D. and Sparber, S.B. (1982) Behavioral consequences of embryonic or early postnatal expo-sure to 1-α-noracetyl methadol (NLAAM) in the domestic chicken. Neurobehav. Toxicol. Teratol. 4, 323–329.

Laase, C.F.J. (1919) Narcotic drug addiction in the newborn, report of a case. Am. Med. 25, 283–286.

Lampert, A., Nirenberg, M., and Klee, W.A. (1976) Tolerance and dependence evoked by an endogenous opiate peptide. Proc. Natl. Acad. Sci. USA 73, 3165–3167.

Langstein, L. (1930) Über das schicksal von morphiumsuchtigen frauen geborener saüglinge. Med. Klin. 26, 500–501.

LaPointe, G. and Nosal, G. (1982) Morphine treatment during rat pregnancy: neonatal and preweaning consequences. Biol. Neonate 42, 22–30.

Lasky, D.I., Zagon, I.S. and McLaughlin, P.J. (1977) Effect of maternally administered heroin on the motor activity of rat offspring. Pharmacol. Biochem. Behav. 7, 281–284.

Lichtenstein, P.M. (1915) Infant drug addiction. N.Y. Med. J. 15, 905.

Lodge, A. (1977) Developmental findings with infants born to mothers on methadone maintenance: a preli-minary report. In: NIDA Symposium on Comprehensive Health Care for Addicted Families and Their Children. (Beschner, G. and Brotman, R., ed.) U.S. Government Printing Office, Wash-ington, DC. pp. 79–85.

Lodge, A., Marcus, M.M. and Ramer, C.M. (1975) Neonatal addiction: a two-year study. II. Behavioral and electrophysiological characteristics of the addicted neonate. Addict. Dis. 2, 235–255.

Macht, D.I. (1915) The history of opium and some of its preparations and alkaloids. J. Am. Med. Assoc. 64, 477–481.

Marcus, J., Hans, S.L. and Jeremy, R.J. (1982) Differential motor and state functioning in newborns of women on methadone. Neurobehav. Toxicol. Teratol. 4, 459–462.

Marfori, P. (1930) Gli stupefacenti (Veleni del cervello) nei loro effetti individuali e sociali. Profilassi e cura delle tossico-manie. V. Idelson, Naples (cited in Menninger-Lerchenthal, 1934).

Markham, J.K., Emmerson, J. and Owen, N.W. (1971) Teratogenicity studies of methadone HCl in rats and rabbits. Nature 233, 342–343.

Martin, E. (1893) L'opium, ses abus, mangeurs et fumerus d'opium morphinomanes. Paris.

McGinty, J.F. and Ford, D.H. (1976) The effects of maternal morphine or methadone intake on the growth reflex development and maze behavior of rat offspring. In: Tissue Responses to Addictive Drugs. (Ford, D.H. and Clouet, D.H., eds.) Spectrum Publications, New York, pp. 611–629.

McGinty, J.F. and Ford, D.H. (1980) Effects of prenatal methadone in rat brain catecholamines. Dev. Neurosci. 3, 224–234.

McLaughlin, P.J. and Zagon, I.S. (1980) Body and organ development of young rats maternally exposed to methadone. Biol. Neonate 38, 185–196.

McLaughlin, P.J., Zagon, I.S. and White, W.J. (1978) Perinatal methadone exposure in rats: effects on body and organ development. Biol. Neonate 34, 48–54.

Menninger-Lerchenthal, E. (1934) Die morphinkrankheit der neugeboren morphinstischer mutter. Monatsschr. Kinderheilkd. 60, 182–193.

Middaugh, L.D. and Simpson, L.W. (1980) Prenatal maternal methadone effects on pregnant C57BL/6 mice and their offspring. Neurobehav. Toxicol. 2, 307–313.

Musto, D.F. (1973) The American Disease. Yale University Press, New Haven, CT.

Naeye, R.L., Blanc, W., LeBlanc, W. and Khatamee, M.A. (1973) Fetal complications of maternal heroin addiction: abnormal growth, infections, and episodes of stress. J. Pediat. 83, 1055–1061.

Natherson, G., Cohen, M.I., Litt, I.F. and McNamara, H. (1972) The effect of maternal heroin addiction on neonatal jaundice. J. Pediat. 81, 899–903.

Newby-Schmidt, M.B. and Norton, S. (1981a) Alterations of chick locomotion produced by morphine treatment in ovo. Neurotoxicology 2, 743–748.

Newby-Schmidt, M.B. and Norton, S. (1981b) Development of opiate tolerance in the chick embryo. Pharmacol. Biochem. Behav. 15, 773–778.

Nichtern, S. (1973) The children of drug users. J. Am. Acad. Child. Psychiat. 12, 24–31.

Ostrea, E.M. and Chavez, C.J. (1979) Perinatal problems (excluding neonatal withdrawal) in maternal drug addiction. A study of 830 cases. J. Pediat. 94, 292–295.

Ostrea, E.M., Chavez, C.J. and Strauss, M.E. (1976) A study of factors that influence the severity of neonatal narcotic withdrawal. J. Pediat. 88, 642–645.

Paul, L., Diaz, J. and Bailey, B. (1978) Behavioral effects of chronic narcotic antagonist administration to infant rats. Neuropharmacology 17, 655–657.

Perlmutter, J.F. (1967) Drug addiction in pregnant women. Am. J. Obstet. Gynecol. 99, 569–572.

Perlmutter, J.F. (1974) Heroin addiction and pregnancy. Obstet. Gynec. Surv. 29, 439–446.

Perlstein, M.A. (1947) Congenital morphinism. A rare cause of convulsions in the newborn. JAMA 135, 633.

Peters, M.A. (1977) The effect of maternally administered methadone on brain development in the offspring. J. Pharmacol. Exp. Ther. 203, 340–346.

Peters, M.A. (1978) A comparative study on the behavioral response of offspring of female rats chronically treated with methadone and morphine. Proc. West. Pharmacol. Soc. 21, 411–418.

Peters, M.A., Turnbow, M. and Buchenauer, D. (1972) The distribution of methadone in the nonpregnant, pregnant and fetal rat after acute methadone treatment. J. Pharmac. Exp. Ther. 181, 273–278.

Petty, G.E. (1912) Congenital morphinism with report of cases: general treatment of morphinism. Memphis M. Monthly 32, 37–63.

Petty, G.E. (1913) Narcotic Drug Diseases and Allied Ailments, J.A. Davis Co., Tennessee.

Pierson, P.S., Howard, P. and Kleber, H.D. (1972) Sudden death in infants born to methadone-maintained addicts. JAMA 220, 1733–1734.

Ramer, B.S., Webb, G.A. Ramer, C.M. and Mondanaro, J. (1973) Treatment experiences with the pregnant addict. In: Proc. 5th Natl. Conf. Meth. Treat., NAPAN, New York, pp. 1138–1145.

Ramer, C.M. and Lodge, A. (1975) Neonatal Addiction: a two-year study. Part I. Clinical and developmental characteristics of infants of mothers on methadone maintenance. Addict. Dis. 2, 227–234.

Raye, J.R., Dubin, J.W. and Blechner, J.N. (1977) Fetal growth retardation following maternal morphine administration: nutritional or drug effect? Biol. Neonate 32, 222–228.

Rech, R.H., Lomuscio, G. and Algeri, S. (1980) Methadone exposure in utero: effects on brain biogenic amines and behavior. Neurobehav. Toxicol. 2, 75–78.

Reddy, A.M. Harper, R.G. and Stern, G. (1971) Observations in heroin and methadone withdrawal in the newborn. Pediatrics 48, 353–358.

Rementería, J.L. and Lotongkhum, L. (1977) The fetus of the drug-addicted woman: conception, fetal wastage, and complications. In: Drug Abuse in Pregnancy and Neonatal Effects (Rementería, J.L., ed.) C.V. Mosby Co., St. Louis, MO, pp. 3–18.

Rementería, J.L. and Nuang, N.N. (1973) Narcotic withdrawal in pregnancy: stillbirth incidence with a case report. Am. J. Obstet. Gynecol. 116, 1152–1156.

Rorke, L.B., Reeser, D.S. and Finnegan, L.P. (1977) Pathological findings in the nervous system of infants born to substance abusing women. In: Committee on Problems of Drug Dependence (39th Annual Scientific Meeting), Cambridge, MA, pp. 551–571.

Rosen, T.S. and Johnson, H.L. (1982a) Children of methadone-maintained mothers: follow-up to 18 months of age. J. Pediat. 101, 192–196.

Rosen, T.S. and Johnson, H.L. (1982b) In utero methadone exposure – three year follow-up. Pediat. Res. 16, 130A.

Rosen, T.S. and Pippenger, C.E. (1975) Disposition of methadone and its relationship to severity of withdrawal in the newborn. Addict. Dis. 2, 169–178.

Sainsbury, H. (1909) Drugs and the Drug Habit. Methuen Co., London.

Salerno, L.J. (1977) Prenatal care. In: Drug Abuse in Pregnancy and Neonatal Effects (Rementería, J.L., ed.) C.V. Mosby Co., St. Louis, MO, pp. 19–29.

Sameroff, A.J. (1979) Organization and Stability of Newborn Behavior: A Commentary on the Brazelton Neonatal Behavior Scale. Univ. Chicago Press, Chicago.

Sardemann, H., Madsen, K.S. and Friis-Hansen, B. (1976) Follow-up of children of drug-addicted mothers. Arch. Dis. Child. 51, 131–134.

Schulman, C.A. (1969) Alterations of the sleep cycle in heroin-addicted and 'suspect' newborns. Neuropadiatrie 1, 89–100.

Seidler, F.J., Whitmore, W.L. and Slotkin, T.A. (1982) Delays in growth and biochemical development of rat brain caused by maternal methadone administration: are the alterations in synaptogenesis and cellular maturation independent of reduced maternal food intake? Dev. Neurosci. 5, 13–18.

Shah, N.S. and Donald, A.G. (1979) Pharmacological effects and metabolic fate of levo-methadone during post-natal development in rat. J. Pharmacol. Exp. Ther. 208, 491–497.

Sharma, S.K., Klee, W.A. and Nirenberg, M. (1977) Opiate-dependent modulation of adenylate cyclase. Proc. Natl. Acad. Sci. USA 74, 3365–3369.

Sisson, T.R.C., Wickler, M., Tsai, P. and Rao, I.P. (1974) Effect of narcotic withdrawal on neonatal sleep patterns. Pediat. Res. 8, 451.

Slotkin, T.A., Lau, C. and Bartolome, M. (1976) Effects of neonatal or maternal methadone administration on ornithine decarboxylase activity in brain and heart of developing rats. J. Pharmacol. Exp. Ther. 199, 141–148.

Slotkin, T.A., Whitmore, W.L., Salvaggio, M. and Seidler, F.J. (1979) Perinatal methadone addiction affects brain synaptic development of biogenic amine systems in the rat. Life Sci. 24, 1223–1230.

Slotkin, T.A., Seidler, F.J. and Whitmore, W.L. (1980) Effects of maternal methadone administration on ornithine decarboxylase in brain and heart of the offspring: relationships of enzyme activity to dose and to growth impairment in the rat. Life Sci. 26, 861–867.

Slotkin, T.A., Weigel, S.J., Whitmore, W.L. and Seidler, F.J. (1982) Maternal methadone administration: deficit in development of α-noradrenergic responses in developing rat brain as assessed by norepinephrine stimulation of ^{33}Pi incorporation into phospholipids in vivo. Biochem. Pharmacol. 31, 1899–1902.

Smith, A.A., Hui, F.W. and Crofford, M.J. (1977) Inhibition of growth in young mice treated with d,l-methadone. Eur. J. Pharmacol. 43, 307–314.

Sobrian, S.K. (1977) Prenatal morphine administration alters behavioral development in the rat. Pharmacol. Biochem. Behav. 7, 285–288.

Sonderegger, T. and Zimmermann, E. (1976) Persistent effects of neonatal narcotic addiction in the rat.

In: Tissue responses to Addictive Drugs (Ford, D.H. and Clouet, D.H., eds.) Spectrum Publications, New York, pp. 589–609.

Sonderegger, T., O'Shea, S. and Zimmermann, E. (1979) Consequences in adult female rats of neonatal morphine pellet implantation. Neurobehav. Toxicol. 1, 161–167.

Soule, A.B., Standley, K., Copans, S.A. and Davis, M. (1974) Clinical uses of the Brazelton neonatal scale. Pediatrics 54, 583–586.

Soyka, L.F., Peterson, J.M. and Joffe, J.M. (1978) Lethal and sublethal effects on the progeny of male rats treated with methadone. Toxicol. Appl. Pharmacol. 45, 797–807.

Stone, M.L., Salerno, L.J., Green, M. and Zelson, C. (1971) Narcotic addiction in pregnancies. Am. J. Obstet. Gynecol. 109, 716–723.

Strauss, M.E., Lessen-Firestone, J.K., Starr, R.H. and Ostrea, E.M. (1975) Behavior of narcotic-addicted newborns. Child. Dev. 46, 887–893.

Strauss, M.E., Andresko, M., Stryker, J.C. and Wardell J.N. (1976) Relationship of neonatal withdrawal to maternal methadone dose. Am. J. Drug Alcohol Abuse 3, 339–345.

Strauss, M.E., Lessen-Firestone, J.K., Chavez, C.J. and Stryker, J.C. (1979a) Psychological characteristics and development of narcotic addicted infants. NIDA Conf. Genetic, Perinatal, and Developmental Effects of Abused Substances, Airlie, VA.

Strauss, M.E., Lessen-Firestone, J.K., Chavez, C.J. and Stryker, J.C. (1979b) Children of methadone-treated women at five years of age. Pharmacol. Biochem. Behav. 11 (suppl.), 3–6.

Stryker, J.C. (1977) A unique situation – two people must be considered: an overview of the Hutzel Hospital Program. In: NIDA Symposium on Comprehensive Health Care for Addicted Families and Their Children (Beschner, G. and Brotman, R., eds.) U.S. Government Printing Office, Washington, DC, pp. 24–37.

Terry, C.E. and Pellens, M. (1970). The Opium Problem. Patterson Smith., New Jersey, pp. 312–348. (Orginally published in 1928 by the Bureau of Social Hygiene, Inc.)

Thompson, C.I. and Zagon, I.S. (1981) Long-term thermoregulatory changes following perinatal methadone exposure in rats. Pharmacol. Biochem. Behav. 14, 653–659.

Thompson, C.I. and Zagon, I.S. (1982) Decreased dominance in adult rats perinatally exposed to methadone. Eastern Psychological Association, Baltimore, MD.

Thompson, C.I., Zagon, I.S. and McLaughlin, P.J. (1979) Impaired thermal regulation in juvenile rats following perinatal methadone exposure. Pharmacol. Biochem. Behav. 10, 551–556.

Ting, R., Keller, A., Berman, P. and Finnegan, L.P. (1974) Follow-up studies of infants born to methadone-dependent mothers. Pediat. Res. 8, 346.

Ting, R.Y., Keller, A. and Finnegan, L.P. (1978) Physical neurological and developmental assessment of infants born to methadone dependent mothers. In: Drug Abuse: Modern Trends, Issues, and Perspectives (Schecter, A., Alksne, H., Kaufman, E., Shorty, V., Henderson, A. and Lowinson, J.H., eds.) Marcel Dekker, New York, pp. 632–641. (presented at the 2nd Natl. Drug Abuse Conf., New Orleans, LA, 1975).

Van Kleek, L.A. (1920) Symptoms of morphine withdrawal in an infant. Am. Med. 15, 51–52.

Van Wagoner, S., Risser, J., Moyer, M. and Lasky, D. (1980) Effect of maternally administered methadone on discrimination learning of rat offspring. Percept. Motor Skill 50, 1119–1124.

Vesbitt, R. (1957) Perinatal Loss in Modern Obstetrics, F.A. Davis Co., Philadelphia, PA, p. 159.

Vorhees, C.V. (1981) Effects of prenatal naloxone exposure on postnatal behavioral development of rats. Neurobehav. Toxicol. Teratol. 3, 295–301.

Wallach, R.C., Jerez, E. and Blinick, G. (1969) Pregnancy and menstrual function in narcotics addicts treated with methadone. Am. J. Obstet. Gynecol. 105, 1226–1229.

Walz, M.A. (1981) Behavioral and metabolic alterations in progeny of methadone-treated rats. Doctoral Dissertation, University of Mississippi, MS.

White, W.J. and Zagon, I.S. (1979) Acute and chronic methadone exposure in adult rats: studies on arterial blood gas concentrations and pH. J. Pharmacol. Exp. Ther. 209, 451–455.

White, W.J., Zagon, I.S. and McLaughlin, P.J. (1978) Effects of chronic methadone treatment on maternal body weight and food and water consumption in rats. Pharmacology 17, 227–232.

Wikler, A. (Ed.) (1980) Opioid Dependence. Mechanisms and Treatment. Plenum Press, New York, p. 255.

Wilson, G.S. (1975) Somatic growth effects of perinatal addiction. Addict. Dis. 2, 333–345.

Wilson, G.S., Desmond, M.M. and Verniaud, W.M. (1973) Early development of infants of heroin-addicted mothers. Am. J. Dis. Child. 126, 457–462.

Wilson, G.S., McGreary, R., Kean, J. and Baxter, J.C. (1979) The development of preschool children of heroin-addicted mothers: a controlled study. Pediatrics 63, 135–141.

Wilson, G.S., Desmond, M.M. and Wait, R.B. (1981) Follow-up of methadone-treated and untreated narcotic-dependent women and their infants: health, developmental, and social implications. J. Pediatr. 98, 716–722.

Wilson, J.C. and Eshner, A.A. (1896) American Textbook of Applied Therapeutics. W.B. Saunders, New York.

World Health Organization Expert Committee on Drug Dependence (1973) 20th Annual Report, WHO Tech. Report Series 516, Geneva.

Zagon, I.S. and McLaughlin, P.J. (1977a) Effects of chronic morphine administration on pregnant rats and their offspring. Pharmacology 15, 302–310.

Zagon, I.S. and McLaughlin, P.J. (1977b) Effect on chronic maternal methadone exposure on perinatal development. Biol. Neonate 31, 271–282.

Zagon, I.S. and McLaughlin, P.J. (1977c) The effects of different schedules of methadone treatment on rat brain development. Exp. Neurol. 56, 538–552.

Zagon, I.S. and McLaughlin, P.J. (1977d) Methadone and brain development. Experientia 33, 1486–1487.

Zagon, I.S. and McLaughlin, P.J. (1978a) Perinatal methadone exposure and its influence on the behavioral ontogeny of rats. Pharmacol. Biochem. Behav. 9, 665–672.

Zagon, I.S. and McLaughlin, P.J. (1978b) Perinatal methadone exposure and brain development: a biochemical study. J. Neurochem. 31, 49–54.

Zagon, I.S. and McLaughlin, P.J. (1980a) Motor activity and learning ability in rats perinatally exposed to methadone. NIDA Res. Monogr. 27, 121–127.

Zagon, I.S. and McLaughlin, P.J. (1980b) Protracted analgesia in young and adult rats maternally exposed to methadone. Experientia 36, 329–330.

Zagon, I.S. and McLaughlin, P.J. (1981a) Withdrawal-like symptoms in young and adult rats maternally exposed to methadone. Pharmacol. Biochem. Behav. 15, 887–894.

Zagon, I.S. and McLaughlin, P.J. (1981b) Enhanced sensitivity to methadone in adult rats perinatally exposed to methadone. Life Sci. 29, 1137–1142.

Zagon, I.S. and McLaughlin, P.J. (1982a) Analgesia in young and adult rats perinatally exposed to methadone. Neurobehav. Toxicol. Teratol. 4, 455–457.

Zagon, I.S. and McLaughlin, P.J. (1982b) Comparative effects of postnatal undernutrition and methadone exposure on protein and nucleic acid contents of the brain and cerebellum in rats. Dev. Neurosci. 5, 385–393.

Zagon, I.S. and McLaughlin, P.J. (1982c) The effects of chronic heroin exposure in pregnant rats and their offspring. NIDA Res. Monogr. 41, 488–494.

Zagon, I.S. and McLaughlin, P.J. (1982d) Neuronal cell deficits following maternal exposure to methadone in rats. Experientia 38, 1214–1216.

Zagon, I.S., McLaughlin, P.J. and Thompson, C.I. (1979a) Development of motor activity in young rats following perinatal methadone exposure. Pharmacol. Biochem. Behav. 10, 743–749.

Zagon, I.S., McLaughlin, P.J. and Thompson, C.I. (1979b) Learning ability in adult female rats perinatally exposed to methadone. Pharmacol. Biochem. Behav. 10, 889–894.

Zagon, I.S., McLaughlin, P.J., Weaver, D.J. and Zagon, E. (1982) Opiates, endorphins and the developing organism: a comprehensive bibliography. Neurosci. Biobehav. Rev. 6, 439–479.

Zarin-Ackerman, J. (1976) Developmental assessment of all infants born to the family care program,

234

1975–1976. In: NIDA Symposium on Comprehensive Health Care for Addicted Families and their Children (Beschner, G. and Brotman, R. eds.) U.S. Government Printing Office, Washington, DC, 99–106.

Zelson, C. (1975) Acute management of neonatal addiction. Addict. Dis. 2, 159–168.

Zelson, C., Kahn, E.J., Neumann, L. and Polk, G. (1970) Heroin withdrawal syndrome. J. Pediat. 76, 483.

Zelson, C., Rubio, E. and Wasserman, E. (1971) Neonatal narcotic addiction – 10-year observation. Pediatrics 18, 178–189.

Zelson, C., Lee, S.T. and Casalino, M. (1973) Neonatal narcotic addiction. N. Engl. J. Med. 289, 1216–1220.

Zuspan, F.P., Gumpel, J.A., Mejia-Zelaya, A., Madden, J., Davis, R., Filer, M. and Tiamson, A. (1975) Fetal stress from methadone withdrawal. Am. J. Obstet. Gynecol. 122, 43–46.

Neurobehavioral Teratology
edited by Joseph Yanai
© Elsevier Science Publishers BV 1984

10

ALTERATIONS IN FETAL AND ADULT RESPONSIVENESS TO OPIATES FOLLOWING VARIOUS SCHEDULES OF PRENATAL MORPHINE EXPOSURE

Margaret L. Kirby

Department of Anatomy, Medical College of Georgia, Augusta, GA 30909, USA

MATERNAL drug dependence presents an extremely high risk to a suprisingly large number of children. In 1975, Carr estimated that the number of children affected by maternal drug dependence might be as high as 10% of the total population (Carr, 1975). However, the risk may not be confined to children of habitual drug abusers. Any pharmacological intervention which affects the developing nervous system carries certain risks. It has been suggested that there may be subtle, permanent effects on learning and motor activity of the offspring after a single injection of an opiate to suppress pain during normal labor. (Morrison et al, 1976; Stechler, 1964; Aleksandrowicz and Aleksandrowicz, 1974; Satran and Rosen, 1966; Conway and Brackbill, 1970). This presents an alarming problem to medicine and to potential parents because of the frequent clinical use of narcotics during labor and delivery.

The effects of opiate exposure during development range from gross abnormalities and fetal and neonatal death to reduced somatic and brain weights and subtle behavioral abnormalities of the offspring depending on the particular opiate and the dose (Jurand, 1973; Strauss et al., 1976; Iliucci and Gautieri, 1970; Harpel and Gautieri, 1968; Geber and Schramm, 1974, 1975; Geber, 1967; Ford and Rhines, 1979; Davis and Lin, 1972; Buchenauer et al., 1974). In a long-term study of offspring of women who were maintained on methadone during pregnancy, Wilson has described the

236

somatic and psychological profile of these children from birth through the preschool years. Most of the persistent changes she has reported reflect subtle psychological problems such as hyperactivity, problems with social adjustment, difficulty concentrating, abnormal agressiveness and sleep disturbances (Wilson et al., 1973; Wilson and McCreary 1976; Wilson, 1974; Wilson et al., 1979). In recent years, interest has focused on these subtle abnormalities because of their potential for clinical treatment. It seems logical to assume that at least some of the problems associated with subtle long-term changes in a child's psychological profile might be due to disruption of the neural systems which mediate responsiveness to these drugs in the adult. Thus, one of the most productive ways to discover subtle behavioral abnormalities induced by drug exposure during development is by examination of the offspring's response to acute administration of the same drug long after the initial period of exposure. Because of ethical constraints it has not been possible to test human offspring for residual abnormal responsiveness to the opiates to which they were exposed prior to birth. Therefore, studies have been performed in animal models.

Responsiveness to morphine in rats

Normal adult rats

Acute administration of morphine in normal adult animals causes measurable changes in animal behavior. In order to appreciate changes in responsiveness to opiates caused by perinatal opiate exposure, it seems appropriate to review the changes in behavior of normal adult animals following acute administration of morphine. The two parameters of behavior which are usually measured following acute morphine administration are spontaneous motility and response latency to pain. Thus, I will confine myself to a discussion of morphine's effects on nociceptive relfexes and motor activity in the rat.

Morphine has complex effects on spontaneous activity of adult rats. These effects include mixed depressant and stimulant components that are time- and dose-related. Low to moderate doses of morphine (1–5 mg/kg) produce hyperactivity lasting 1–2 h followed by a return to normal activity. Higher doses (10–40 mg/kg) have biphasic effects: an initial depression of activity followed by a period of hyperactivity. The duration of the depressant effect increases as a function of the dose of morphine (Oka and Hosoya, 1976; Gellert and Holtzman, 1978; Bubaum et al., 1973; Babbini and Davis, 1972; Ayhan and Randrup, 1973).

Morphine causes a depression of the simple somatic polysynaptic reflexes as well as the monosynaptic reflexes. The polysynaptic reflexes are depressed by smaller doses of morphine than the monosynaptic reflexes (Wikler 1945; 1950). Depression of reflexes causes an increase in the time between the stimulus and the response (response latency). Thus by depressing the polysynaptic reflexes, morphine causes an increase in the response latency to a painful stimulus.

Changes following perinatal exposure to opiates

Several laboratories have demonstrated that opiate exposure at various times during development will alter adult motor activity and responsiveness to opiates. Friedler (1974a, 1974b) treated female mice, as well as male or female rats for 5 consecutive days with high doses of morphine. The animals were bred to a non-drug exposed animal 5 days after the last morphine injection, and the adult offspring were found to be tolerant to the analgetic effect of morphine. Morphine administration to rats during early (O'Callaghan and Holtzman, 1976, 1977) or late gestation (Steele and Jöhannesson, 1975; Jöhannesson et al., 1972; Jöhannesson and Becker, 1972, 1973) produced tolerance to the analgetic effect of opiates in the offspring that can persist for as long as 11 weeks postnatally. Zimmerman et al. (1974) treated neonatal rats with morphine during the prepuberal period and found that these animals were tolerant to the analgetic effect of morphine at 30 days of age. Bardo and Hughes (1981) demonstrated single dose tolerance to morphine-induced analgesia by injecting 1 day old rats with morphine and testing them on the hot plate at 26 days. They found shorter response latencies in hot plate tests indicating that the animals were tolerant to morphine even though they had been injected only one time (3 weeks) previously.

In contrast, Zagon and McLaughlin (1980, 1981) have shown that adult rats (120 days of age) which had been exposed to methadone perinatally had increased baseline (prior to any drug administration) hot-plate latencies and increased analgetic responses to acute methadone administration. This indicates increased sensitivity to opiates which is opposite to tolerance.

Motor activity is affected in the offspring as well. Sobrian (1977) found that morphine administration prenatally caused the offspring to be significantly more active between 10 and 30 days postnatally. Zagon et al. (1979) found a similar increase in activity at somewhat later ages after perinatal exposure to methadone. Bardo and Hughes (1981) found that rats at 26 days were hypoactive following a single morphine injection on day 1 postnatally.

Normal fetal rats

Although much data has accumulated showing normal adult responsiveness to acute opiate administration and the long-lasting changes produced by opiate-exposure during development, we have only recently become aware of fetal responsiveness to opiates.

Zuspan et al. (1975) cite an FDA document which stated that methadone-treated patients should be withdrawn from the drug 21 days after pregnancy is verified. During the withdrawal program intrauterine fetal death frequently occurred. This was attributed to fetal withdrawal since violent intrauterine movements preceded stillbirth (Zuspan et al., 1975). The FDA later modified the recommendation to withdrawal only during the first trimester or not at all (Zuspan et al., 1975). This glaring example illustrates our basic ignorance of the effects of opiates during development. It should be obvious that a study of fetal responsiveness to opiates in an animal model could help prevent future incidents of this type. Just such an animal model is available and has been used in my laboratory to test the effects of opiates on fetal spontaneous activity and reflexes.

By the 17th day of gestation, the rat fetus exhibits both polysynaptic reflexes and spontaneous activity (Narayanan et al., 1971). Although morphine does not cross the placenta in appreciable quantities during the first two-thirds of gestation it readily passes the placenta during late gestation when reflexes and spontaneous activity occur (Table 10.1) (Kirby, 1979a; Sanner and Woods, 1965; Blane and Dobbs, 1967; Davis and Fenimore, 1978).

Table 10.1. Morphine concentration in fetal and maternal tissues at various times after subcutaneous injections of morphine to the mother
Variation is expressed as SEM. Values are ng/g wet wt. Data reprinted from Kirby, M.L. (1979) Proc. Soc. Exp. Biol. Med. 162, 287–290.

Day of gestation	Hours after injection				
	1/2	1	2	6	12
Fetal tissue					
11	9.9 ± 1.9	63.5 ± 8.5	54.1 ± 9.8	43.4 ± 8.5	2.2 ± 1.5
13	192.5 ± 29.1	179.8 ± 21.3	168.7 ± 19.6	15.0 ± 5.0	11.0 ± 4.5
15	243.9 ± 17.1	405.9 ± 10.3	396.0 ± 13.0	85.4 ± 5.6	64.7 ± 3.6
17	176.2 ± 9.1	714.2 ± 31.8	461.2 ± 15.4	76.7 ± 3.7	54.3 ± 8.1
19	356.4 ± 2.0	519.6 ± 17.9	367.5 ± 21.4	183.7 ± 9.8	76.5 ± 6.4
Placenta	746.4 ± 41.4	1092.2 ± 100.9	721.7 ± 73.3	182.4 ± 17.5	100.5 ± 6.4

In rats, acute morphine administration to the mother causes a depression of fetal spontaneous activity and polysynaptic reflexes (Kirby, 1979b). The depression in fetal spontaneous activity is dose-dependent between 1.25 mg/kg and 20 mg/kg, where the maximum depression of activity occurs. Fetal activity is about 70% below normal following 20 mg/kg of morphine administered to the mother. Presumably this depression of spontaneous activity and reflexes is mediated by spinal opiate receptors which appear at about 16 days of gestation (Fig. 10.1) Kirby, 1981a, 1981b).

Although the adult response to morphine is complex, the fetal response to morphine appears to be limited to dose-dependent depression of activity. Presumably, this is due to the fact that the fetal nervous system is still relatively simple and that polysynaptic reflexes and spontaneous activity are controlled mostly within the spinal cord (Kirby, 1981b) with very little supraspinal input. As other neural systems grow into the spinal cord and begin to function the complex adult response appears. With this view of neural layering underlying the increasingly complex response to morphine, it is possible to envision various types of insult depending on the state of functional development of the nervous system. The existence of critical periods for the effects of drugs on development has been postulated previously (Gauron and Rowley, 1972).

Since the spinal cord undergoes most of its development during the last third of gestation and is known to contain opiate receptors and to mediate fetal responses to morphine, my coworkers and I have been interested in determining whether specific spinal systems can be altered by chronic opiate administration during this decisive period in spinal cord development.

Changes in responsiveness to opiates caused by morphine treatment prenatally

Experimental design

Several factors must be taken into consideration in designing an appropriate experimental paradigm. The first involves the timing of the drug exposure. For the experiments which will be described, morphine was administered on days 12–21 of gestation to coincide with major events in spinal cord development. The next important consid-

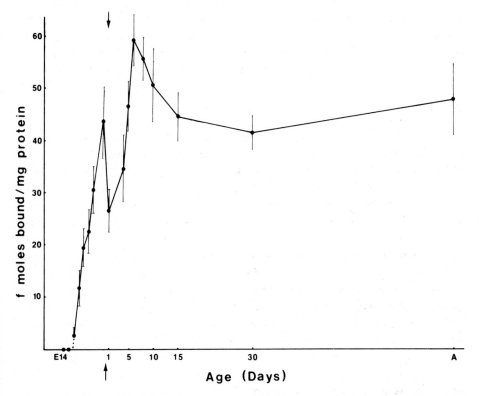

Fig. 10.1. Diprenorphine binding to opiate receptors in the developing rat spinal cord. Each point represents the mean (± SEM) of a minimum of 20 whole spinal cords from animals in 5 different litters, assayed on a minimum of 3 different days. Arrows indicate parturition. Homogenate was incubated with 5 nM [³H]-diprenorphine with either 1 μM levorphanol or dextrophan according to Hiller et al. (1978). Binding cannot be measured prior to 16 days gestation but increases rapidly thereafter. The adult complement of receptors is present by 15 days postnatally. (Reprinted from Kirby, M.L. (1981) Brain Res. 205, 400–404.)

eration is the frequency of injections. Since the half-life of morphine in fetal tissues is about 3 h (this changes somewhat with chronic injections, Yeh and Woods, 1970; Kirby, 1979a), a 12–24 h delay between injections would introduce an extra variable into the experiment because of maternal withdrawal. However, injections every 6 h, although preventing withdrawal, would certainly be stressful, which could cause changes in behavioral measures (Hutchings and Gibbon, 1970; Ader and Conklin, 1963). Both injection schedules have been used in the following experiments: All animals were injected every 6 h, although one morphine treatment group received its daily dose of morphine in two injections (10 mg/kg per injection), with saline injected in the alternate injections (this group is designated M10 × 2), while the other morphine treatment group received 5 mg/kg per injection every 6 h (M5 × 4). Thus, each group received 20 mg/kg per day injected subcutaneously. This dose was chosen because it is not a teratogenic dose but is considered analgetic in these injection increments in the rat (Cicero et al., 1974).

Two control groups have been used. The first was a saline-injected group and the second a pair-fed group. The saline group was injected with 1 ml of saline every 6 h while the pair-fed animals were not injected but were restricted to an amount of lab chow comparable to that eaten ad lib by the morphine-injected animals (pair-fed controls). Generally, the morphine-injected dams ate 20–30% less than the saline-injected dams.

Changes in fetal responsiveness

Spontaneous fetal activity was measured following morphine and naloxone challenge on the 18th–20th days of gestation. In both control and pair-fed animals, activity was depressed equally following maternal morphine injection (Fig. 10.2). Fetuses exposed to 10 mg/kg of morphine two times daily showed the same depression of activity as control and pair-fed fetuses, while fetuses exposed to 5 mg/kg of morphine four times daily showed much less sensitivity to morphine and thus were considered to be tolerant.

All fetuses exposed to biologically active opiates had extended periods of vigorous hyperactivity when the mothers were injected with naloxone (Fig. 10.3). Fetuses exposed to saline or dextrorphan, or pairfed, did not exhibit this hyperactivity on exposure to naloxone. Thus, the hyperactivity seen in this situation is a withdrawal sign in fetuses. Hyperactivity has been reported along with increased heart rate as withdrawal signs in human fetuses when withdrawal is attempted during the third trimester (Stryker, 1979).

Changes in neonatal and adult responsiveness

As mentioned above, fetuses exposed every 6 h to 5 mg/kg of morphine from day 12 of gestation developed tolerance to morphine by days 18–20 of gestation. If identically treated dams are allowed to withdraw and to deliver their pups, it is possible to determine whether tolerance persists into adulthood. Hot-plate testing of the offspring at

30 days postnatally showed no change in the baseline latencies, and morphine produced similar dose-related increases in response latency in all groups of offspring. However, the hot-plate test for analgesia involves supraspinal participation in the reflex response. It was pointed out above that the period of drug exposure coincided with the period of intense development of the spinal cord. Thus a better test would be one which involved the spinal cord only. The tail-flick test for analgesia elicits a polysynaptic reflex thought to be mediated wholly within the spinal cord. This test would give an assessment of morphine-induced changes in a specified area of the nervous system caused by morphine exposure during development.

Using tail-flick testing for analgesia at 60 days postnatally, the baseline latencies remained the same, but the animals treated with 5 mg/kg four times daily showed increased sensitivity to morphine's analgetic effect (Kirby et al., 1982). This is in contrast to animals exposed to 10 mg/kg of morphine twice daily. These animals were not tolerant to morphine prenatally and did not show altered responsiveness to morphine postnatally (Fig. 10.4).

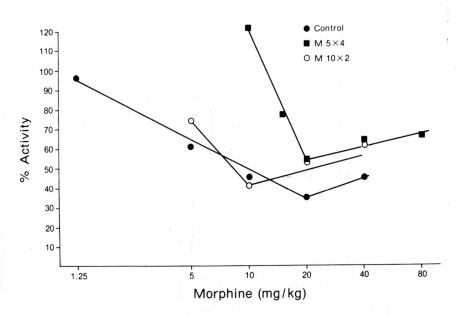

Fig. 10.2. Spontaneous activity of 18–20 day rat fetuses following acute injection of morphine. Activity after morphine injection is expressed as % of control activity (e.g. activity prior to morphine injection). The dams had been pretreated from days 12 to 18–20 of gestation on the following drug injection schedules: 1 cc of saline every 6 h (control); 5 mg/kg of morphine every 6 h (M5 × 4); or 10 mg/kg of morphine every 12 h with saline being injected at alternate 12-h intervals (M10 × 2). Spontaneous activity decreases in a dose dependent fashion up to 20 mg/kg of morphine. Pretreatment with 5 mg/kg of morphine every 6 h causes development to tolerance to morphine's effect on spontaneous activity while pretreatment with 10 mg/kg every 12 h does not result in tolerance. (Reprinted from Kirby, M.L. and Holtzman, S.C. (1982) Pharmacol. Biochem. Behav. 16, 263–269.)

Changes in spinal cord receptors and morphology

Interestingly, both of these groups of morphine-treated animals had abnormal spinal opiate receptor numbers (Table 10.2). During the prenatal period both groups had fewer receptors, while as adults the opiate receptor concentration was above normal (Kirby, 1982b). Thus, there was no apparent relationship between the concentration of opiate receptors in the spinal cord and behavioral responsiveness to morphine.

Since the period of drug exposure coincides with very rapid growth of the spinal cord, I have attempted to discover morphological correlates of these behavioral and biochemical changes. Preliminary measurements have been completed (Table 10.3). The spinal volume in morphine-treated 18-day fetuses was found to be reduced by 20% from control while spinal volume in pair-fed fetuses was also reduced, but only by 10% (Kirby, 1980). By the 6th day postnatally the spinal volume was reduced in

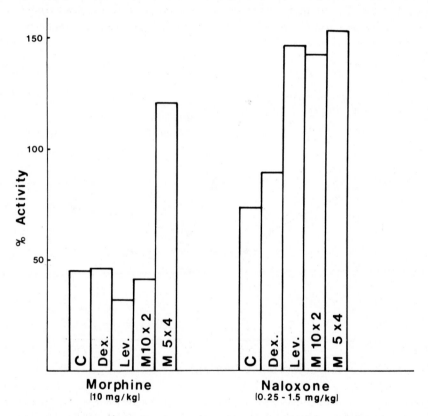

Fig. 10.3. Spontaneous activity of 18–20 day rat fetuses following morphine (10 mg/kg) or naloxone (0.25–1.5 mg/kg) injection during the observation period. Activity after the injection is expressed as % of control (activity prior to the injection). The dams were pretreated from day 12 of gestation with saline every 6 h (C); 5 mg/kg of morphine every 6 h (M5 × 4); 10 mg/kg of morphine every 12 h (M10 × 2); 0.8 mg/kg of dextrorphan every 6 h (Dex; an inactive opiate); or 0.8 mg/kg of levorphanol every 6 h (Lev; the active form of Dex). (Reprinted from Kirby, M.L. and Holtzman, S.G. (1982) Pharmacol. Biochem. Behav. 16, 263–269.)

morphine-treated and pair-fed animals by 16–17%. This difference can be attributed to a 16–17% decrease in the gray volume in these groups. The gray matter suffers the largest reduction in the dorsal horn (Kirby, 1982a).

On the 15th day postnatally the spinal volume was not different from controls, but the gray to white ratio was increased in morphine-treated offspring. The altered gray/white ratio is primarily due to a decrease in white volume in the morphine-treated offspring (Kirby, 1982a). Since volumes in pair-fed animals were reduced at 18 days gestation and 6 days postnatally, it must be concluded that the reduction in spinal volume in morphine-treated animals is at least partly due to maternal undernutrition during the last half of gestation.

However, the retardation in spinal cord development caused by undernutrition is compounded by treatment with morphine. The pattern of recovery in the morphine-treated animals seems to indicate that morphine's retardant effect is not selective for gray or white matter but that the fastest-growing area is most affected. This would support the idea that morphine retards growth by affecting cellular processes generally (Clouet and Ratner, 1967) rather than affecting cells via opiate receptors which are concentrated in fairly discrete areas of the spinal cord, e.g. the dorsal horn (Lamotte et al., 1976; Hiller et al., 1978). Whether more subtle morphological changes can be recognized in the dorsal horn of morphine-treated animals alone remains to be seen.

On the other hand, results from pre- and postnatal behavioral testing seem to indi-

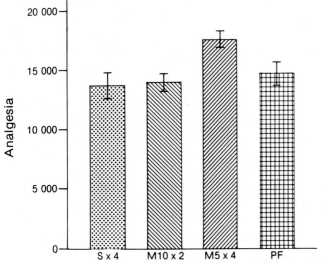

Fig. 10.4. The analgesic effect of 10 mg/kg of morphine on 60 day postnatal offspring of dams treated with morphine from days 12 to 21 of gestation on the following drug injection schedule: 1 ml of saline every 6 h (S × 4); 10 mg/kg of morphine every 12 h (M10 × 2); 5 mg/kg of morphine every 6 h (M5 × 4); pair-fed with the morphine-injected animals (PF). Analgesia was assessed every 20 min following the morphine injection and a time-effect curve was constructed for each group. The area under each curve was calculated. Each bar represents the mean area bounded by the analgesia curve ± SEM. M5 × 4 is significantly different from the other groups ($p > 0.05$). (Reprinted from Kirby, M.L. et al. (1982) Pharmacol. Biochem Behav. 17, 1161–1164.)

Table 10.2. Changes in K_D and B_{max} in [^{3}H]naloxone binding in the spinal cord following prenatal morphine exposure

Reprinted from Kirby, M. L. Neuropharmacology 22, 303–307 (1983).

	K_D (nM)	% Change	B_{max} (fmol)	% Change
E21				
S × 4	7.07 ± 1.81		166.1 ± 15.2	
PF	7.11 ± 0.63		170.9 ± 5.7	
M10 × 2	7.85 ± 2.75	↑ 11%	145.4 ± 10.2	↓ 12%
M5 × 4	7.29 ± 1.20	↑ 4%	130.2 ± 7.7	↓ 22%
P60				
S × 4	3.16 ± 0.32		76.4 ± 4.14	
PF	3.13 ± 0.25		81.4 ± 1.73	
M10 × 2	4.51 ± 0.74	↑ 43%	107.5 ± 7.93	↑ 41%
M5 × 4	4.86 ± 0.66	↑ 50%	107.6 ± 6.50	↑ 41%

cate that morphine does affect the development of specific opiate-sensitive pathways. It is enigmatic that opiate receptor development is altered in both groups of morphine-exposed animals, while responsiveness to morphine changes with only one of the injection schedules. The obvious conclusion is that total receptor population is not important in influencing the behavioral effects of morphine. The key word here is *total*. We cannot exclude the possibility that the behavioral responses measured are mediated by a small population of active receptors or by a subtype or even a ratio of receptor subtypes. Several subtypes of opiate receptors have been identified pharmacologically and biochemically, including the mu, delta and kappa receptors which are thought to mediate analgesia in the spinal cord (Chang and Cuatrecasas, 1979; Smith and Simon, 1980; Martin et al., 1976).

In conclusion it appears that the effects of opiates on developing animals differ widely depending on small variations in experimental design. In particular, the experiments presented above demonstrate that the injection schedule may be as important as the total daily dose of morphine in producing behavioral teratogenesis. In general, things such as animal strain, critical periods, drug choice, drug injection schedule, choice of test and postnatal duration of test administration are of critical importance in designing and interpreting experiments of this type.

Table 10.3. Hemisegment volumes

Data from Kirby, M. L. Brain Res. 202, 143–150 (1980) and Dev. Brain Res. 6, 211–217 (1983).

	18 day gestation (mm^2)	P6 (mm^2)	P15 (mm^2)
Saline-injected	0.2839 ± 0.0015	0.7677 ± 0.0359	1.4473 ± 0.0782
Pairfed	0.2563 ± 0.0090	0.6376 ± 0.0265	1.5260 ± 0.0673
M5 × 4	0.2238 ± 0.0086	0.6558 ± 0.0198	1.4529 ± 0.0632
M10 × 2		0.6593 ± 0.0179	1.4597 ± 0.0862

It is apparent from this discussion that it is important to continue our inquiry into the effects of opiates on development since the widespread use of these drugs potentially affects us all.

Acknowledgments

This work was supported by PHS grant DA 02060. I would like to take this opportunity to thank several collaborators: Drs. Stephen Holtzman, Robert Aronstam, Sarah DeRossett and Dale E. Bockman for their continued help on these projects, Janet Whittle and George Forbes for technical assistance, Martin Kirby for critical comments and Rosemary Widener and Pat O'Meara for typing this manuscript.

References

Ader, R. and Conklin, P.M. (1963) Handling of pregnant rats. Effects on emotionality of their offspring. Science 142, 411–412.

Aleksandowicz, M.K. and Aleksandrowicz, D.R. (1974) Obstetrical pain-relieving drugs as predictors of infant behavior variability. Child Dev. 45, 935–945.

Ayhan, I.H. and Randrup, A. (1973) Behavioural and pharmacological studies on morphine-induced excitation of rats. Psychopharmacologia 29, 317–328.

Babbini, M. and Davis, W.M. (1972) Time-dose relationships for locomotor activity effects of morphine after acute or repeated treatment. Brit. J. Pharmacol. 46, 213–224.

Bardo, M.T. and Hughes, R.A. (1981) Single-dose tolerance to morphine-induced analgesic and hypoactive effects in infant rats. Dev. Psychobiol. 14, 415–423.

Blane, G.F. and Dobbs, H.E. (1967) Distribution of tritium-labelled etorphine (M99) and dihydromorphine in pregnant rats at term. Brit. J. Pharmacol. Chemother. 30, 166–172.

Bubaum, D.M., Yarbrough, G.G. and Carter, M.E. (1973) Biogenic amines and narcotic effects. I. Modification of morphine-induced analgesia and motor activity after alteration of cerebral amine levels. J. Pharmacol. Exp. Ther. 185, 317–327.

Buchenauer, D., Turnbow, M. and Peters, M.A. (1974) Effect of chronic methadone administration on pregnant rats and their offspring. J. Pharmacol. Exp. Ther. 189, 66–71.

Carr, J.N. (1975) Drug patterns among drug-addicted mothers. Incidence, variance in use, and effects on children. Pediatr. Ann. 4, 408–417.

Chang, K.-J. and Cuatrecasas, P. (1979) Multiple opiate receptors, enkephalins and morphine bind to receptors of different specificity. J. Biol. Chem. 254, 2610–2618.

Cicero, T.J., Meyer, E.R. and Smithloff, B.R. (1974) Alpha adrenergic blocking agents: antinociceptive activity and enhancement of morphine-induced analgesia. J. Pharmacol. Exp. Ther. 189, 72–82.

Clouet, D.H. and Ratner, M. (1967) The effect of the administration of morphine on the incorporation of (C^{14}) leucine into protein of rat brain. Brain Res. 4, 33–43.

Conway, E. and Brackbill, Y. (1970) Delivery medication and infant outcome: an empirical study. Soc. Res. Child. Dev. Monogr. 35, Serial 137, 24–34.

Davis, C.M. and Fenimore, D.C. (1978) The placental transfer and maternofetal disposition of methadone in monkeys. J. Pharmacol. Exp. Ther. 205, 577–586.

Davis, W.M. and Lin, C.H. (1972) Prenatal morphine effects on survival and behavior of rat offspring. Res. Comm. Chem. Pathol. Pharmacol. 3, 205–214.

Ford, D.H. and Rhines, R.K. (1979) Prenatal exposure to methadone HCl in relationship to body and brain growth in the rat. Acta. Neurol. Scand. 59, 248–262.

Friedler, G. (1974a) Long-term effects of opiates. In: Perinatal Pharmacology: Problems and Priorities (Hwang, J.C., ed.) Raven Press, New York, pp. 207–219.

Friedler, G. (1974b) Effect of pregestational morphine administration to mice on behavior of their offspring. Pharmacologist 16, 203.

Gauron, E.F. and Rowley, V.N. (1972) Critical periods for drug administration effects in infancy. Psychopharmacologia 26, 73–78.

Geber, W.F. (1967) Congenital malformations induced by mescaline, lysergic acid diethylamide and bromolysergic acid in the hamster. Science. 158, 265.

Geber, W.F. and Schramm, L.C. (1974) Postpartum weight alteration in hamster offspring from females injected during pregnancy with either heroin, methadone, or composite drug mixture, or mescaline. Am. J. Obstet. Gynecol. 120, 1105–1111.

Geber, W.F. and Schramm, L.C. (1975) Congenital malformations of the central nervous system produced by narcotic analgesics in the hamster. Am. J. Obstet. Gynecol. 123, 705–713.

Gellert, V.F. and Holtzman, S.G. (1978) Development and maintenance of morphine tolerance and dependence in the rat by scheduled access to morphine drinking solutions. J. Pharmacol. Exp. Ther. 205, 536–546.

Harpel, H.S. and Gautieri, R.F. (1968) Morphine-induced fetal malformations. I. Exencephaly and axial skeletal fusions. J. Pharm. Sci. 57, 1590–1597.

Hiller, J.M., Simon, E.J., Crain, S.M. and Peterson, E.R. (1978) Opiate receptors in cultures of fetal mouse dorsal root ganglia (DRG) and spinal cord: predominance in DRG neurites. Brain Res. 145, 396–400.

Hutchings, D.E. and Gibbon, J. (1970) Preliminary study of behavioral and teratogenic effects of two 'stress' procedures administered during different periods of gestation in the rat. Psychol. Rep. 26, 239–246.

Iuliucci, J.D. and Gautieri, R.F. (1970) Morphine-induced fetal malformations. II. Influence of histamine and diphenhydramine. J. Pharm. Sci. 60, 420–425.

Jöhannesson, T. and Becker, B.A. (1972) The effects of maternally administered morphine on rat foetal development and resultant tolerance to the analgesic effect of morphine. Acta. Pharmacol. Toxicol. 31, 305–313.

Jöhannesson, T. and Becker, B.A. (1973) Morphine analgesia in rats at various ages. Acta. Pharmacol. Toxicol. 33, 429–441.

Jöhannesson, T., Steele, W.G. and Becker, B.A. (1972) Infusion of morphine in maternal rats at near-term: Maternal and foetal distribution and effects on analgesia, brain DNA, RNA and protein. Acta. Pharmacol. Toxicol. 31, 353–363.

Jurand, A. (1973) Teratogenic activity of methadone HCl in mouse and chick embryos. J. Embryol. Exp. Morphol. 30, 449–458.

Kirby, M.L. (1979a) Morphine in fetuses after maternal injection: Increasing concentration with advancing gestational age. Proc. Soc. Biol. Med. 162, 287–290.

Kirby, M.L. (1979b) Effects of morphine on spontaneous activity of 18-day rat fetus. Dev. Neurosci. 2, 238–244.

Kirby, M.L. (1980) Reduction of fetal rat spinal cord volumes following maternal morphine injection. Brain Res. 202, 143–150.

Kirby, M.L. (1981a) Development of opiate receptor binding in rat spinal cord. Brain Res. 205, 400–404.

Kirby, M.L. (1981b) Effects of morphine and naloxone on fetal rat spontaneous activity. Exp. Neurol. 73, 430–439.

Kirby, M.L. (1983a) Recovery of spinal cord volume following prenatal exposure to morphine. Dev. Brain Res. 6, 211–217.

Kirby, M.L. (1983b) Changes in (^{3}H)-naloxone binding in spinal cord of rats treated prenatally with morphine. Neuropharmacology 22, 303–307.

Kirby, M.L. and Holtzman, S.G. (1982) Effects of chronic opiate administration on spontaneous activity of fetal rats. Pharmacol. Biochem. Behav. 16, 263–269.

Kirby, M.L., DeRossett, S.E. and Holtzman, S.G. (1983) Enhanced analgesic response to morphine in adult rats exposed to morphine prenatally. Pharmacol. Biochem. Behav. 17, 1161–1164.

Lamotte, C., Pert, C.B. and Snyder, S.H. (1976) Opiate receptor binding in primate spinal cord. Distribution and changes after dorsal root section. Brain Res. 112, 407–412.

Martin, W.R., Eades, C.G., Thompson, J.A., Huppler, R.E. and Gilbert, P.E. (1976) The effects of morphine and nalorphine-like drugs in the nondependent and morphine-dependent chronic spinal dog. J. Pharmacol. Exp. Ther. 197, 517–532.

Morrison, J.C., Whybrew, W.D., Rosser, S.I., Bucovay, E.T., Wiser, W.L. and Fish, S.A. (1976) Metabolites of meperidine in the fetal and maternal serum. Am. J. Obstet. Gynecol. 126, 997–1002.

Narayanan, C.H., Fox, M.W. and Hamburger, V. (1971) Prenatal development of spontaneous and evoked activity in the rat (Rattus norwegicus albinos). Behaviour 40, 100–134.

O'Callaghan, J.P. and Holtzman, S.G. (1976) Prenatal administration of morphine to the rat: Tolerance to the analgesic effect of morphine in the offspring. J. Pharmacol. Exp. Ther. 197, 533–544.

O'Callaghan, J.P. and Holtzman, S.G. (1977) Prenatal administration of levorphanol or dextrophan to the rat: Analgesic effect of morphine in the offspring. J. Pharmacol. Exp. Ther. 200, 255–262.

Oka, T. and Hosoya, E. (1976) Effects of humoral modulators and naloxone on morphine-induced changes in the spontaneous locomotor activity of the rat. Psychopharmacology 47, 243–248.

Sanner, J.H. and Woods, L.A. (1965) Comparative distribution of tritium-labelled dihydromorphine between maternal and fetal rats. J. Pharmacol. Exp. Ther. 148, 176–184.

Satran, R. and Rosen, M.G. (1966) Effect of meperidine administered during labor on the neonatal EEG. Electroenceph. Clin. Neurophysiol. 21, 404–405.

Smith, J.R. and Simon, E.J. (1980) Selective protection of sterospecific enkephalin and opiate binding against inactivation by N-ethylmalimide: Evidence for two classes of opiate receptors. Proc. Natl. Acad. Sci. USA 77, 281–824.

Sobrian, S.K. (1977) Prenatal morphine administration alters behavioral development in the rat. Pharmacol. Biochem. Behav. 7, 285–288.

Stechler, G. (1964) Newborn attention as affected by medication during labor. Science 144, 315–316.

Steele, W.J. and Jöhannesson, T. (1975) Effects of prenatally-administered morphine on brain development and resultant tolerance to the analgesic effect of morphine in offspring of morphine treated rats. Acta Pharmacol. Toxicol. 36, 243–256.

Strauss, M.E., Starr, R.H., Ostrea, E.M., Chavez, C.J. and Stryker, J.C. (1976) Behavioral concomitants of prenatal addiction to narcotics. J. Pediatr. 89, 842–846.

Stryker, J.C. (1979) Novel methodology to assess abstinence syndrome in utero. A preliminary report. Conference on Genetic, Perinatal and Developmental Effects of Abused Substances, NIDA, Airlie, Virginia.

Wikler, A. (1945) Effects of morphine, nembutal, ether, and eserine on two-neuron and multineuron reflexes in the cat. Proc. Soc. Exp. Biol. Med. 58, 193–196.

Wikler, A. (1950) Sites and mechanisms of action of morphine and related drugs in the central nervous system. J. Pharmacol. Exp. Ther. 2, 435–506.

Wilson, G.S. (1975) Somatic growth effects of perinatal addiction. Addict. Disease 2, 333.

Wilson, G.S. and McCreary, R. (1976) A controlled study of preschool children of heroin addicts – their growth, development and behavior. Pediat. Res. 10, 309.

Wilson, G.S., Desmond, M.M. and Verniaud, W.M. (1973) Early development of infants of heroin-addicted mothers. Am. J. Dis. Child.. 126, 457–462.

Wilson, G.S., McCreary, R., Kean, J. and Baxter, J.C. (1979) The development of preschool children of heroin-addicted mothers: A controlled study. Pediatrics 63, 135–141.

Yeh, S.Y. and Woods, L.A. (1970) Maternal and fetal distribution of H^3-dihydromorphine in the tolerant and non-tolerant rat. J. Pharmacol. Exp. Ther. 174, 9–13.

248

Zagon, I.S. and McLaughlin, P.J. (1980) Protracted analgesia in young and adult rats maternally exposed to methadone. Experientia 36, 329–330.

Zagon, I.S. and McLaughlin, P.J. (1981) Enhanced sensitivity to methadone in adult rats perinatally exposed to methadone. Life. Sci. 29, 1137–1142.

Zagon, I.S., McLaughlin, P.J. and Thompson, C.I. (1979) Development of motor activity in young rats following perinatal methadone exposure. Pharmacol. Biochem. Behav. 10, 743–749.

Zimmerman, E., Branch, B., Taylor, A.N., Young, J. and Pang, C.N. (1974) Long-lasting effects of prepuberal administration of morphine in adult rats. In: Narcotics and the Hypothalamus (Zimmerman, E. and George, R., eds.) Raven Press, New York, pp. 183–194.

Zuspan, F.P., Gumpel, J.A., Mejia-Zelaya, A., Madden, J., Davis, R., Filer, M. and Tiamson, A. (1975) Fetal stress from methadone withdrawal. Am. J. Ostet. Gynecol. 122, 43–46.

Neurobehavioral Teratology
edited by Joseph Yanai
© Elsevier Science Publishers BV 1984

11

NEUROBEHAVIORAL DEVELOPMENT OF CHILDREN EXPOSED IN UTERO TO OPIOID DRUGS

Sydney L. Hans[1], Joseph Marcus[1], Rita J. Jeremy[1] and Judith G. Auerbach[2]

[1] Department of Psychiatry and Unit for Research in Child Psychiatry and Development, The University of Chicago, 950 East 59th Street, Box 411, Chicago, IL 60637, USA and [2] Department of Psychology, The Hebrew University of Jerusalem, Israel

ALTHOUGH it was widely believed that the placental barrier protected unborn children from harmful effects of substances in the maternal blood stream, such tragedies as thalidomide infants born without limbs and children left malformed and mentally retarded by their mothers' alcoholism forced a re-evaluation of this assumption. Many chemicals ingested by pregnant women can and do cause birth defects of both body and mind. In the past decade there has been growing public concern about the effects of various toxins on the human fetus. It is now standard obstetrical practice to recommend that pregnant women avoid all drugs (including alcohol, caffeine and nicotine), many chemicals in the workplace, and foods containing certain additives and pollutants. Although research on the teratological effects of different substances lags behind the need for information, a substantial body of data is now accumulating on certain chemicals.

Opioid drugs are one type of substance whose teratological effects are being researched. As early as a century ago, medical journals carried isolated case reports of infants of morphine-using women who were born addicted (cf. Ghodse et al., 1977). Today heroin use is an enormous and steadily increasing social problem in many countries of the world. There are hundreds of thousands of heroin addicts in the United States alone, and of the women involved, almost all are of childbearing age (Carr, 1975). Heroin addicts in the US obtain their drugs illegally and at great expense. A large proportion are from lower socio-economic strata, and their drug abuse further depletes their limited physical, medical and social-emotional resources. Heroin users must structure their lifestyle around drug procurement, and that usually involves criminal activity. In women, this most commonly takes the form of prostitution.

In the United States, chronic heroin addicts who seek treatment are often admitted to government-funded methadone maintenance programs where they receive free daily oral doses of methadone, a synthetic opioid. The drug is dispensed in a clinic setting that may also provide a variety of social services and medical supervision to its clients. In general, people maintained on methadone lead more stable lives than they did as heroin addicts and are assured of better pharmacological control of their habit (cf. Marcus et al., 1983).

Because opioids can pass through the placental barrier (Blinick et al., 1975), the potential effects of maternal drug use on the developing fetus are many. The literature reports that pregnancies of opioid-dependent women are often complicated by problems such as toxemia, maternal syphilis and hepatitis, placental problems, abnormal presentation, and fetal distress; infants are of small size at birth and show increased risk for neonatal morbidity and mortality (Finnegan, 1975; Rementeria and Lotongkhum, 1977; Perlmutter, 1974). Most strikingly, however, children of opioid-addicted women are themselves born addicted and go through a period of withdrawal from the drug. Evidence suggests that some of the medical risks to the children are lessened by maternal methadone maintenance, presumably because of the better medical care and more careful monitoring of the drug use rather than any pharmacological properties of the drug itself (Connaughton et al., 1975; Strauss et al., 1974; Zelson, 1973).

The offspring of opioid-dependent women are not only at risk for medical problems. This chapter describes the behavior of children born to women who used opioid drugs, primarily heroin and methadone, during their pregnancies. We shall discuss both behavioral signs during the neonatal withdrawal period as well as longer term behavioral development.

Clinical assessments of the early neonatal period

Within 1–3 days of birth, most infants born to opioid-addicted women show clinical signs of withdrawal (Desmond and Wilson, 1975; Pierog, 1977; Zelson et al., 1971). These signs include a large number of behavioral and physiological symptoms that are indicators of both nonspecific central and autonomic nervous system dysfunctioning. Among the more frequently observed signs of neonatal abstinence are: high-pitched crying, poor sleeping, hyperactive reflexes, tremors, hypertonus, convulsions, frantic sucking of fists, poor feeding, regurgitation, diarrhea, dehydration, yawning, sneezing, nasal stuffiness, sweating, skin mottling, fever, rapid respiration, and excoriation of skin.

Data systematically comparing the behavior of opioid exposed and non-exposed neonates have been published from only six different samples*: (1) Soule et al., 1974 [DC]; (2) Strauss et al., 1975, 1976 [MI]; (3) Kron et al., 1975, 1977 [PA]; (4) Lodge et al., 1975 [CA]; (5) Chasnoff et al., 1980, 1982 [IL-NW]; and (6) our own study, Marcus et al., 1982a; Jeremy and Hans, 1982 [IL-UC].

In each of these studies, infant behavior during the first week of life was evaluated using the Neonatal Behavioral Assessment Scale (NBAS) (Brazelton, 1973). The NBAS is a widely used instrument in clinical research that was designed to assess a cross-section of neonatal behaviors, particularly those behaviors that are likely to have consequences for caregiving exchanges and for the establishment of an affectionate bond between the infant and his or her caregivers. The behaviors assessed are ones that can typically be observed in newborns without using special equipment or professional skills.

The core of the NBAS consists of 26 items measured on 9-point scales. Five other items (known as the Kansas supplements) are also sometimes administered (Horowitz et al., 1978). Analyses of the structure of the examination from a variety of samples (Sameroff, 1978) plus our own analyses in a sample including methadone-exposed neonates (Jeremy and Hans, 1982) have indicated that there are eight types of items. *Arousal* items measure the infant's highest observed state of arousal, how quickly into the examination the infant becomes upset, the number of situations in which the infant becomes upset, the amount of spontaneous activity, and the number of swings in arousal state shown by the infant during the examination. *Quieting* items measure the success with which the infant self quiets and the ease with which s/he can be consoled by the examiner. The *hand-to-mouth* item measures the success with which the infant can bring his/her hand to the mouth. In most samples, but not those composed of methadone-exposed infants, this ability is highly associated with self-quieting skill. *Motor control* items measure the jerkiness and tremulousness of the infant's movements. *Tone* items measure the tone (rigidity) of the infant's whole body, strength of neck and shoulders, and resistance to molding while being held. *Defensive movement* items measure the infant's success at removing a cloth placed over the face. *Alertness* items measure the degree to which the infant will turn his/her head to various auditory and visual stimuli and assesses length and quality of sustained periods of alertness. *Response decrement* items assess the speed with which the sleeping infant habituates to repetitions of light, sound and tactile stimuli; it is assumed that rapid habituation to repetition is adaptive.

In the samples assessed neonatally on the NBAS (as well as those of the other major

*There are eight major research groups that have reported data comparing the behavioral development of children born to opioid-using women with that of children whose mothers used no drugs. Throughout this chapter, these research groups will be identified by the following abbreviations: (1) District of Columbia; National Institute of Child Health and Human Development [DC], (2) Detroit, Michigan; Hutzel Hospital and Wayne State University School of Medicine [MI], (3) Philadelphia, Pennsylvania; University of Pennsylvania School of Medicine [PA]. (4) San Fransisco, California; Children's Hospital of San Francisco [CA], (5) Chicago, Illinois; Northwestern University Medical School, [IL-NW], (6) Chicago, Illinois; The University of Chicago Pritzker School of Medicine [IL-UC], (7) Houston, Texas; Baylor College of Medicine [TX], and (8) New York, New York; Columbia University College of Physicians and Surgeons [NY].

research groups), opioid-group infants were generally the offspring of methadone-maintained women; but at least two samples included some children whose mothers were non-treated heroin addicts [CA, PA], and others contained a subgroup of metha-done-maintained women who continued to use heroin and other narcotic or nonnarcotic street drugs [CA, NY, TX, IL-UC]. Given the frequency of illicit drug use by people maintained on methadone (cf. McGlothin and Anglin, 1981), it is also likely that some methadone-maintained women from the other samples also used street drugs. Dosages of methadone varied from sample to sample, reflecting the different practices of methadone-treatment facilities from state to state and year to year. Some women were enrolled in low-dose programs where daily doses were typically less than 20 mg and never more than 40 mg [IL-NW, IL-UC, MI]. The philosophy of such programs is to maintain women at the minimum medication level needed to prevent withdrawal symptoms. Other women were enrolled in high-dose programs (PA, NY, TX) where the philosophy is to maintain women at a level high enough that, due to blocking from methadone, effects of other opioids such as heroin would be minimally felt. Consequently, the temptation to return to the use of street drugs is minimized (Dole, 1980).

Studies also varied in the type of treatment administered to opioid-withdrawing infants. The first line of treatment for neonatal narcotic abstinence is usually soothing, use of pacifiers, and swaddling. Severe withdrawal is treated pharmacologically, although rates of pharmacologic intervention vary widely from hospital to hospital. Medications of choice include diazepam, phenobarbital, paregoric and chlorpromazine. In the samples of NBAS-examined infants, the proportion of infants being treated pharmacologically at the time of behavioral examination varied from zero [DC, IL-UC, MI] to over 50% [PA, CA].

Infants in the comparison groups also varied considerably from study to study. In one sample [DC], they were an existing group of different race, socioeconomic status, and, presumably, measured by a different examiner from the opioid group. In another sample [PA], they were high-risk infants whose mothers did not use drugs. In three samples [MI, IL-NW, IL-UC], they were matched to the opioid group infants by a variety of criteria, including in some combination in each study: race, socioeconomic status, parity, mother's age, gestational age, birthweight, Apgar scores, obstetric medication, maternal education, maternal alcohol use and cigarette smoking. From reports, it appears that in only one of the studies [IL-UC] were the examiners blind to information about whether the infants' mothers were opioid addicted. The top part of Table 11.1 summarizes the characteristics of the neonates assessed in each of the six published samples. Opioid and control groups varied considerably across studies on a variety of factors and varied in the degree to which they were matched within studies. Studies also differed in the ways in which they analyzed data and the degree to which data were fully reported.

Following is a summary of results from the studies reporting NBAS assessments of opioid-exposed neonates. The results will be presented in terms of the eight categories of neurobehavioral functioning assessed by the NBAS that were described previously.

Table 11.1. Summary of reported differences between opioid-exposed and comparison infants on the Neonatal Behavior Assessment Scale

Sample	DC	MI	PA	CA	IL-NW	IL-UC
Total no. opioid infants	19	46	23	29	39	27
No. treated opioid infants	0	0	13	15	12	0
Methadone dose in mg/day						
Mean	?	16	45	28	15	19
Range	?	?–40	10–100	5–60	5–40	5–40
Total no. comparison infants	41	46	10	10	27	44
Day of testing	3	1,2	3–7	1–25	2	2[a]
Areas of functioning with reported differences in group means						
Arousal	×	×	×	×	×	×
Quieting		×			×	
Hand-to-mouth		×		×		×
Motor control	×	×	×		×	×
Tone	×			×		×
Defensive movements						
Alertness/orientation	×[b]	×[bc]		×[b]	×	[c]
Response decrement	×[d]	×[d]				

[a] A small number of the opioid-group infants were tested at older ages, up to the 5th day.
[b] Opioid-group infants were less alert, particularly for visual orientation.
[c] More missing data were reported for opioid-group infants.
[d] Opioid-group infants were slower to habituate only on the light stimulus.

The bottom part of Table 11.1 provides a very brief summary of these results, indicating those areas of functioning in which group differences were reported in each of the six studies.

(1) All six studies reported that opioid-exposed infants were more aroused at the time of testing than comparison-group infants. Opioid-withdrawing infants were more quickly aroused to higher degrees of upset by less obnoxious stimuli. Such behavior may be interpreted by parents or other caregivers as negative and directed purposefully by the infant toward them. Caregivers need to be educated about expectations of typical behavior that may be exhibited by opioid-exposed infants soon after birth, and advised about ways of handling such infants that could attenuate the severity of the overt symptoms of neonatal narcotics withdrawal.

(2) Two of the six studies [PA, IL-NW] reported that opioid-group infants required higher levels of intervention to console than did comparison-group infants; two groups of investigators [DC, IL-UC] commented on the good consolability of most opioid infants and the quickness of their responsiveness to soothing by handling, use of a pacifier or swaddling. These contradictory findings cannot be completely reconciled here, but progress toward their interpretation can only be made with additional knowledge about the NBAS scales. The consolability item on the NBAS is rated only if the infant reaches and stays in the highest state of upset. When an infant is in the highest state of arousal, the tester tries a series of manoeuvers, in a prescribed order from minimal

to maximal handling, aimed at reducing the infant's upset. A score of 9 indicates a baby who is consolable at the sight of the examiner's face (a minimal intervention); a 7, by the touch of the examiner; 5, by picking up; 4, by rocking; 2, by use of a pacifier in addition to previous measures (maximal handling that succeeds); and 1, by no means. The order of administration follows from presentation of face alone to swaddling and insertion of pacifier, as needed. Note that a lower score indicates that more intrusive intervention is required for consolation, not necessarily that consolation takes longer or is more difficult for the caregiver.

Analyses of consolability assessed by the NBAS have typically been based on scores with large proportions of missing data. Some infants never reach high states of upset; others are able to quiet themselves; and others, although very upset early in the examination, are so tired by the time the consolability item is administered that they become drowsy or fall asleep. Thus the finding of differences in consolability between opioid-exposed and comparison groups is difficult to interpret. Those infants who can be scored may not be representative of their groups, and reasons for missing data may vary between groups.

Reported mean scores from the NBAS consolability item were 5.9 [IL-UC], 5.4 [CA], 6.7 [MI], and 4.5 [IL-NW] for the opioid-group neonates. Thus of those opioid group infants who needed consolation, most could be consoled simply by being held.

These scores suggest that perhaps the upset of most infants withdrawing from opioid drugs could be managed by non-pharmacological means of intervention if hospital staffing patterns would permit individual attention to infants. The NBAS requires the examiner systematically to attempt a variety of means of consolation with an infant. Nurses should also be encouraged to do so, and the mothers should be given instruction on various techniques of consolation. We feel the data suggest that once a caregiver learns the infant's preferences, the highly aroused infant may in fact be responsive to her ministrations and reinforcing for her efforts.

(3) Half of the studies [MI, CA, IL-UC] reported more bringing of hands to mouth in opioid-exposed infants. This is consistent with anecdotal reports of frantic fist sucking in infants going through narcotics abstinence. This behavior appears in the opioid infants not to be an organized sophisticated attempt at self regulation, but rather a frenzied, automatic response.

(4) Five out of the six studies reported that opioid-exposed infants have poorer motor control: their limb movements tend to be jerky and tremulous.

(5) Half of the studies [DC, CA, IL-UC] reported differences between opioid-exposed and comparison infants in muscle tone. The general body tone of opioid-exposed infants tends toward hypertonicity.

(6) None of the studies reported any differences between opioid and comparison infants in ability to defend themselves against obstruction of the face. This finding is interesting because it suggests that the high incidence of Sudden Infant Death Syndrome in methadone-exposed infants (Finnegan, 1979; Pierson et al., 1972; Rajegowda et al., 1978; Chavez et al., 1979) is probably not related to these infants' inability to

protect themselves from objects in the environment covering the face (Anderson and Rosenblith, 1971).

(7) On the NBAS, most of the information from which judgments of alertness are made comes from a series of tasks, called orientation tasks, in which the infant is expected to turn his/her head in the direction of auditory or visual stimuli. Four of the studies [DC, MI, CA, IL-NW] reported poorer mean levels of performance by opioid-exposed infants on these items. We [IL-UC] found no mean differences between opioid and comparison infants in their overall levels of alertness and responsivity to stimuli. However, our data show much higher rates of missing data on the orientation items for the opioid-group infants, indicating that they were less likely to be in awake, non-crying states than comparison infants. The only other study to report sample sizes for items (Strauss et al., 1975) also reported more missing data on the orientation items in the opioid group (almost 50%).

The NBAS is a molar instrument which was not designed to yield fine-grained results about specific cognitive processes. Failure to perform well on these items could have two different causes: (1) failure to be in the proper non-crying, non-sleeping, receptive state of arousal and (2) failure to perceive and respond correctly to information even when alert. We suspect that opioid-group infants perform poorly because of problems in arousal rather than perception or motor responsiveness. This hypothesis is given support by studies with monkeys that show the greatest density of cortical opiate receptors near those areas associated with the limbic system and in the frontal lobe (Wise and Herkenham, 1982; Lewis et al., 1981). These are areas involved in modulation of arousal and allocation of attention rather than primary sensory processing. One should also note that differences in alertness between the samples could be due to the inclusion of medicated infants in the opioid groups. A less responsive baby could be the result of diazepam or phenobarbital administered post-natally rather than an opioid pre-natally.

An interesting pattern of results on the orientation items was reported by three research groups [DC, MI, and CA]. Opioid-group infants were less responsive primarily to items requiring orientation to visual stimuli. They showed normal response patterns to items that used only auditory stimulation. This pattern is analogous to reports by opioid-withdrawing adults of acute aversion to light. We [IL-UC] did not find differences between opioid-exposed and comparison newborns; both groups were somewhat better on auditory than visual orientation items.

(8) Two studies [DC, MI] report that opioid-exposed infants were slower than comparison infants to show a response decrement to light. On this item the examiner records the sleeping infant's magnitude of response as a flashlight beam is passed across the eyes. This slowness of the opioid infants to habituate to the light stimulus could again be related to a sensitivity to light associated with withdrawal.

Summary. The pattern of results from the six samples suggests that opioid-exposed infants tend to be much more easily aroused and aroused to higher levels than other newborns. This behavior is similar to the increased irritability reported by adults with-

256

drawing from opioid drugs. In addition, opioid-exposed newborns show poorer motor control (tremulousness and jerkiness) and higher muscle tonus – both signs of increased CNS irritability and similar to motoric symptoms reported in adults experiencing narcotics abstinence. Results are somewhat ambiguous with respect to consolability, partially due to the structure of the NBAS examination. Consolability results do indicate that, while opioid-group infants differ from comparison infants, opioid-group infants are highly responsive to soothing by a variety of techniques. There is also ambiguity in interpretation of alertness data. Opioid babies are less likely to be in alert states during testing, possibly due to higher states of arousal when non-medicated or drowsiness when medicated, but it is not clear that when they are alert, the quality of their perception or responsiveness is any poorer. The only suggestion of a deficit in a specific aspect of information processing is that opioid-exposed neonates attend less well to visual than auditory stimuli and habituate less quickly to presentation of light than auditory stimuli. This result may be analogous to hypersensitivity to light often experienced by adults withdrawing from opioids.

Laboratory assessments of the early neonatal period

A number of neonatal differences in behavior between opioid-exposed and comparison infants have been investigated using laboratory, usually electrophysiological, assessment procedures.

Blinick and his colleagues (Blinick et al., 1971) performed sound spectrographs of cries made in the delivery room by 31 infants born to drug-addicted mothers and a large comparison group. Over half of the infants born to drug-addicted mothers had abnormal cry spectrograms compared to only 11% of the comparison infants. Drug-exposed infants, even most of those whose cries were considered normal, tended to have high-pitched cries. These results are consistent with clinical reports of high-pitched cries in withdrawing neonates. The authors suggest that group differences in pitch are most likely due to differences in the tonus of the laryngeal musculature.

Kron and his colleagues (Kron et al., 1977, 1976, 1975; Kaplan et al., 1975) [PA] have measured sucking behavior in opioid-exposed infants using a special nursing instrument that monitors sucking rate, sucking pressure, amount of nutrient consumed, and percentage of time during the experiment that the infant is actively sucking. Forty-three infants born to opioid-dependent women were monitored twice daily just prior to scheduled feedings for three days beginning at 24–36 h of age. The infants born to opioid-dependent women showed depressed sucking rates (22 sucks per minute) in contrast to a comparison group of 10 infants (40 sucks per minute). The opioid-group infants also sucked with less pressure and consumed less nutrient during the trials than comparison infants. Although most of the infants were tested while being pharmacologically treated, those infants tested in the absence of drug treatment showed comparably depressed rates of sucking. There were also sucking differences as a function of the treatment drug administered. Infants treated with barbiturate drugs showed sucking rates near zero; those treated with opioid drugs (paregoric) showed sucking rates near normal. When the barbiturates were discontinued, sucking rates improved within several days.

Marcus and Hans (1982) [IL-UC] investigated the muscle tone of opioid-exposed infants using a quantified electromyography procedure. EMG was recorded from the limbs of 18 opioid-exposed neonates during periods of rest and of passive movement of the limbs. Compared to 26 comparison infants, the opioid-exposed infants showed higher electrical output from both arms and legs, both while at rest and during limb manipulation. This is congruent with clinical and NBAS reports of hypertonicity in withdrawing infants.

Infant sleep patterns typically show cycles of active sleep (characterized by rapid eye movements [REM], body movement, variable heart rate, low voltage fast wave EEG, variable respiration) followed by periods of quiet sleep (characterized by high voltage slow wave EEG activity, regular heart rate and respiration, infrequent body movement, and absence of REM). Schulman (1969) monitored sleep states for 45 minutes in 8 neonates born to heroin-addicted women in 8 normal comparison infants. During active sleep heroin-group infants showed greater REM and body movement activity than comparison infants. Unlike comparison infants, heroin-group infants rarely entered a quiet sleep phase during the testing session. Dinges et al. (1980) monitored sleep in 28 neonates born to women maintained on methadone (some with concomitant heroin use) and 30 comparison neonates. Drug-exposed newborns averaged less quiet sleep and more active sleep than did the comparison infants.

Lodge et al. (1975) [CA] examined their sample of 29 opioid-exposed and 10 comparison infants in an evoked potential paradigm. Occipital and temporal lobe EEG activity was monitored during exposure to repeated visual (light and checkerboard) and auditory (click) stimuli and averaged across 50 trials for each type of stimulus. The auditory data were measured mostly during sleep states; most (sic) of the visual data were collected with infants in awake states. Both auditory and visual evoked potentials from the opioid-exposed group were 'more irregular and more unreliable' than those of the comparison group. Desynchronized high frequency activity was often present in the addicted infants' EEG's even during seemingly quiet sleep. Both visual and auditory evoked potentials were characterized by early, sharp, high amplitude components in the opioid group. The authors felt that these characteristics most likely reflected greater CNS irritability in the opioid-exposed neonates. Differences in response frequencies were found only in the vertex region responses and only to visual stimuli; opioid infants showed lowered vertex but normal occipital arousal responses to light stimulation. The authors concluded that the opioid-exposed infants showed adequate auditory processing, but abnormal visual processing that, given the regional response pattern, was most likely a reflection of poor modulation of arousal rather than deficits in sensory abilities.

Summary. In general, laboratory assessments of opioid-exposed neonates confirm results found by clinical observations. During the first few days of life these infants suck poorly, are hypertonic, have high-pitched cries possibly due to abnormal tone of the laryngeal muscles, and show abnormal sleep patterns, generally with an abnormally great percentage of time spent in the more highly aroused sleep state. Also paralleling clinical observation in the same sample, evoked potential studies found response peculiarities to visual but not to auditory stimuli. These differences were localized in brain regions whose functions are primarily modulation of arousal patterns rather than sensory processing. This supports our earlier suggestion that group differences in NBAS orientation/alertness items were due primarily to the inappropriate states of arousal rather than to deficits in sensation or perception.

Effects of maternal drug dosage and type on neonatal abstinence

Issues of major concern to those who manage the methadone use of pregnant women are how maternal drug dosage affects the behavior of the newborn infant and how methadone-treated pregnancies compare to those of untreated addicts. A number of studies examining the relation between maternal methadone dosage and neonatal behavior have reported small to moderate degrees of association between drug dosage and severity of infant withdrawal symptoms (cf. Ostrea Jr. et al., 1976; Madden et al., 1977), emphasizing that infants whose mothers receive less than 20 mg of methadone a day are much less likely to need treatment for the symptoms of withdrawal. Many studies, however, have reported no correlation between dosage and behavior (cf. Newman et al., 1975; Finnegan et al., 1975). Such negative results do not necessarily mean that dosage has no effect on severity of withdrawal. The narrow range of doses administered at any one methadone clinic studied and the high incidence of abuse of other opioid drugs by women maintained on methadone would diminish the likelihood of finding an empirical association between methadone dosage and severity of withdrawal.

The differential effects of methadone and heroin use on neonatal behavior have been considered in a number of reports. Kron et al., (1977) [PA] found that methadone infants had poorer sucking rates than heroin infants; there were no differences between the groups on the NBAS. Lodge et al. (1975) reported that for most NBAS items and their electrophysiological measures, heroin infants were more like controls than were methadone infants; infants whose mothers used both heroin and methadone showed the worst behavior. Chasnoff et al. (1982) [IL-NW] found that methadone neonates had poorer state control and responsivity to stimuli than the polydrug infants, many of whose mothers used heroin. Ostrea Jr. et al. (1976) found that methadone-group infants had worse withdrawal symptoms than heroin infants, but only if their mothers were receiving more than 20 mg of methadone per day. At first glance, it appears that methadone causes more severe withdrawal symptoms in infants than does heroin. It is likely, however, that these results are due to dosage effects rather than to the pharmacological properties of the drugs. Because methadone-maintained women regularly receive pure methadone, they receive higher and more consistent levels of opioids than do street addicts who take diluted, impure drugs on irregular schedules as they can be afforded. Many methadone-maintained women are using street drugs in addition to methadone. Consequently, it is impossible to compare directly the relative severity of withdrawal from the two drugs without better scientific control of drug dosage and mixing.

No one has yet presented convincing evidence that heroin and methadone withdrawal have different types of behavioral symptoms in the neonate, although there is some evidence that methadone withdrawal may have a somewhat delayed onset and a longer duration of action than heroin (Kandall and Gartner, 1974; Lipsitz and Blatman, 1974). Such a pattern is consistent with observations of opioid withdrawal in adults – that withdrawal of methadone produces a syndrome qualitatively similar to that of heroin, but it develops more slowly and is more prolonged, probably due to the high tissue-binding capabilities of methadone (cf. Jaffe, 1980; Jaffe and Martin, 1980).

Changes during the neonatal period

There is little systematic research on the diminution of withdrawal symptoms during the course of the first month of life. While at the time of release from hospital (usually around 1 week post-partum) opioid-exposed infants are typically no longer showing the acute withdrawal symptoms, not all symptoms have disappeared. There are reports in the research literature of late onset of acute withdrawal in children who showed only mild symptoms during their hospital stay (Kandall and Gartner, 1974). Only two of the NBAS studies described previously repeated the examination at the end of the neonatal period. Strauss et al. (1976) [MI] reassessed a third of their sample at one month of age using the NBAS. They reported that the opioid-exposed infants differed from a comparison group in only one area; motor control. Opioid-group infants remained more tremulous at one month. Jeremy and Hans (1982) [IL-UC] found no strong group differences between opioid and comparison infants at 1 month. In all areas of the NBAS the two groups converged by one month of age (Fig. 11.1 plots mean scores for the two groups), with opioid-group infants becoming more alert, less stiff, and smoother in their movements. They also became *more* irritable, as did the comparison infants. Thus while the average behavior of opioid-exposed infants has become near normal by one month, their high level of arousal – the aspect of their behavior most likely to have an aversive effect on their interaction with their caregivers – has actually increased. We also note that, while in these data there were no differences in group means at one month, several individual infants had patterns of behavior that were still characteristic of the acute phase of opioid withdrawal (Marcus et al., 1982b).

Follow up into infancy past the neonatal period

While information about the behavioral effects of in utero exposure to opioid drugs on the neonate is important for the medical management of the child during the immediate post-partum period, it is usually assumed that the dramatic behavioral abnormalities of this period are primarily transitory symptoms of withdrawal rather than signs of permanent neurological dysfunctioning. Teratological effects for which long term intervention might be required can only be assessed at later ages, after withdrawal symptoms have presumably subsided.

The most frequently used instrument for assessing the mental and motor skills of infants past the neonatal period is the Bayley Scales of Infant Development (Bayley, 1969). Its three parts are the Mental Record, the Psychomotor Record, and the Infant

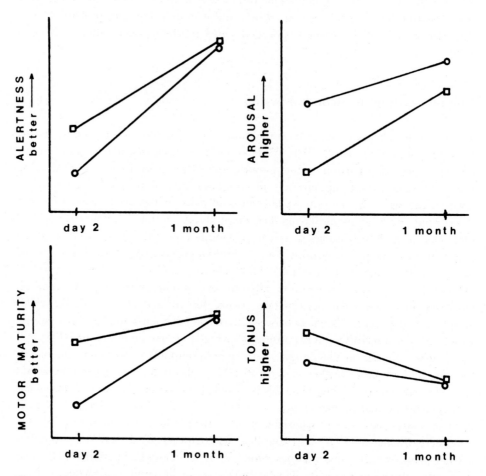

Fig. 11.1. Neurobehavioral changes during the neonatal period as assessed by The Neonatal Behavioral Assessment Scale. Methadone exposed = ○; comparison = □.

Behavior Record (IBR). The first two consist of specific skill items arranged in order of difficulty and scored as pass or fail, with summative scores that can be converted to normalized scores (analogous to IQ): the Mental Development Index (MDI) and the Psychomotor Development Index (PDI). In contrast, the IBR makes global, qualitative judgments of various aspects of the infant's functioning rather than assessing particular skills.

A number of samples of opioid-exposed infants have been assessed on the Bayley Scales, but only five have reported comparisons to a sample of drug-free infants matched for socioeconomic status: (1) Strauss et al. (1976) [MI], (2) Kaltenbach et al. (1979) [PA], (3) Wilson et al. (1981) [TX], (4) Rosen and Johnson (1982) [NY], and (5) our own data [IL-UC]. We feel comparison groups are essential because the Bayley Scales were standardized 20 years ago on a relatively small sample of children (less than 100) at each age and one cannot assume that scores of 100 actually represent the average functioning of infants today. In addition, the Bayley standardization sample infants reflect a wide national, racial and socioeconomic distribution, while studies of opioid-exposed infants generally have an overrepresentation of black infants from poor homes. Both race and socioeconomic status have been shown to affect Bayley scores, with black children showing higher levels of motor skill during the first year of life (Bayley, 1965) and poor children showing steadily declining scores after the first year of life (Ginsburg, 1973).

Table 11.2 lists mean MDI and PDI scores for infants assessed in the five samples

Table 11.2. Summary of differences between opioid-exposed and comparison infants on the Bayley Mental and Psychomotor Scales

Sample:	MI		PA		TX		NY		IL-UC	
	Opioid	Comparison	Opioid	Comparison	Opioid	Comparison	Opioid	Comparison	Opioid	Comparison
Number of infants:	25	26	27	16	64	55	45	25	19	23
Mean MDI										
3 months	112	115								
4 months									110	115
6 months	116	114					45	101		
8 months									113	124
9 months					98	106				
12 months	113	115	103	108			98	107	108	107
18 months							96	106	89	98
Mean PDI										
3 months	119	117								
4 months									117	118
6 months	109	112			101	105				
8 months									112	115
9 months					91	99				
12 months	103	110					95	103	104	108
18 months							93	105	105	103

on the Bayley Scales. In the three samples with longitudinal data, both opioid and comparison infants show a trend for decreasing scores, especially PDI scores during the first year. Across the studies, there is a general tendency for opioid-exposed infants to perform more poorly than comparison-group infants. For the 12 MDI comparisons reported, in 10 cases the opioid infants had lower mean scores. For the 11 PDI comparisons reported, in 9 cases the opioid infants had lower mean scores. If one were to use a nonparametric statistic on these proportions, they would indicate a greater than chance probability of poorer functioning in the opioid-group infants.

The MDI and PDI scales of the Bayley Scales are measures of skill acquisition, they measure *whether* certain skills are performed. The Bayley IBR, on the other hand, measures more clinical aspects of behavior, *how* the skills are performed. Only two of the above studies have reported Bayley IBR data on opioid-exposed and comparison infants.

Wilson et al. (1981) [TX] found that their 9 month old opioid-exposed infants showed poorer fine-motor coordination and shorter span of attention than comparison infants.

Our own work is the only other source of data on the IBR and the only one with longitudinal assessments reported (Marcus et al., 1982b; Jeremy et al., 1982) [IL-UC]. Fig. 11.2 plots the mean scores for opioid and comparison infants from 4 to 18 months on sums of IBR items in the areas of activity, motor coordination and attention. The activity level of all infants increased greatly from 4 to 18 months. A difference that was found between methadone and comparison infants at 4 months, with methadone infants being more active, disappeared at the later ages. While motor coordination improved with age for all infants, at all ages the mean motor coordination scores were poorer for methadone-group infants, although substantially so only at 4 months. All infants showed dramatic increases in attention between 4 and 8 months. At all ages, methadone-group infants had lower mean levels of attention; this is significantly so only at 12 months.

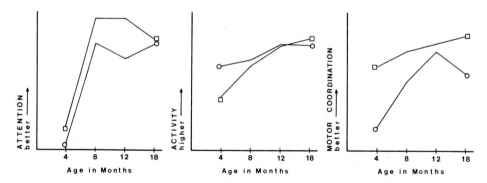

Fig. 11.2. Neurobehavioral changes from 4 to 18 months of age as assessed by the Bayley Infant Behavior Record. Methadone-exposed = ○; comparison = □.

Summary. As a group, infants born to opioid-using women show a small lag in the acquisition of developmental skills as measured by standardized tests. Greater differences are observed in more qualitative measures of infant behavior such as those assessed on the Infant Behavior Record. Behaviors that are emerging as characteristics of infants exposed in utero to opioids are poor motor coordination, high activity level, and poor attention. Studies have also found high activity level in rats exposed prenatally to methadone (Hutchings et al., 1979; Zagon et al., 1979). The differences in motor coordination and activity observed with the IBR seem to be especially pronounced early in the first year of life and may be subtle signs of continuing withdrawal from opioid drugs. Differences in attentional functioning seem to emerge later and may be the early signs of a new, more permanent neurobehavioral syndrome, in some of the children, of, perhaps, a type of attentional deficit disorder (DMS-III, 1982).

Follow up into early childhood

Past the period of infancy, follow up data on children who were exposed to opioids in utero become scarce. Kaltenbach et al. (1978) compared the performance of a small sample of 4 year old children who were exposed to methadone in utero ($n = 9$) and comparison children ($n = 12$) on the Wechsler Preschool and Primary Scale of Intelligence (WPPSI) and tests of perception, language skills, and neurological functioning. The authors concluded that there were no statistically significant differences between the groups, although the mean performance of the methadone-group infants on the WPPSI (84.3) was seven points lower than that of the comparison group (91.5).

Wilson et al. (1979) [TX] reported on the behavior of twenty-two 3–6 year old children whose mothers were addicted to heroin during their pregnancies. Contrasted with comparison-group children, the opioid-exposed children showed poorer performance on the auditory memory portion of the Illinois Test of Perceptual Abilities, three of the subscales of the McCarthy Scales of Children's Abilities (Perceptual-Performance, Quantitative, and Memory) (McCarthy, 1972), and on several perceptual tasks. Parent ratings indicated that the heroin-exposed children had greater adjustment difficulties, including uncontrollable temper tantrums and impulsivity.

Strauss et al. (1979) [MI] examined 33 children of drug-dependent women and a comparison group on the McCarthy Scales at five years of age. They concluded that there were no differences between the groups on any of the subscales. However, examiners' clinical ratings of the children showed that the children of the drug-dependent women were more active and energetic during testing, showed more task-irrelevant activity, and tended to show poorer fine-motor coordination.

Summary. While data are few, the pattern of behavior emerging in older children is provocative. As was seen in the infant data, the older offspring of drug-using women also have a number of the characteristics of attentional deficit disorder: high activity, impulsivity, poor self-control, poor motor coordination, and poor performance on cognitive tests requiring focused attention.

Longitudinal Analysis

Longitudinal design is the most powerful research tool available in the field of child development. It is the only method that provides information about individual identity and the temporal patterning of developmental changes. One of the primary goals of at-risk research is to learn how to identify at an early age those children who will have behavioral problems later. This goal can be reached only through longitudinal data collection and analysis. Although most of the major studies of the offspring of drug-abusing mothers described in this chapter used longitudinal or partially longitudinal sampling, only our group at The University of Chicago has reported longitudinal analyses of data that examine patterns of continuity across age (Marcus et al., 1982b). Below is one such analysis examining behavioral continuity between 4 and 12 months of age.

Method   Infants studied were the first cohort of participants in a longitudinal study of effects of in utero methadone exposure on child development. The sample was a group of black infants whose mothers were being treated in methadone maintenance programs on the south side of Chicago, IL $(n = 16)$ and a comparison group $(n = 23)$ whose mothers were of similar age and socioeconomic background but had no history of drug use or alcohol abuse. Data from early infancy in this cohort have been reported in a number of sources (Marcus et al., 1982a,b, 1983; Bernstein et al., 1983a,b; Jeremy and Bernstein 1984). At 4 and 12 months of age, infants were administered the Bayley Scales of Infant Development by examiners who did not know whether infants were part of the methadone or comparison group, and who did not have information about infants' behavior at the earlier ages.

Analysis   The Bayley IBR consists of 30 items rated on 2-, 5- and 9-point scales by the examiner at completion of the testing session. Items on the IBR measure at least three areas of neurobehavioral functioning: attention, activity level, and motor coordination. Three psychologists were asked to select items from the IBR that they thought were exemplars of these types of functioning. From this item pool, items representing the three areas were selected according to the following criteria: that all items within a category were monotonically related to one another both within the methadone and comparison groups and at both 4 and 12 months. On this basis the following items were selected to represent each category: *Attention*, responsiveness to objects (No. 8); goal directedness (No. 11); attention span (No. 12) and reactivity (No. 15): *Activity level*, activity (No. 14) and energy (No. 25): and *Motor coordination*, gross motor coordination (No. 26) and fine motor coordination (No. 27). (Sums of these items were reported earlier in this chapter in Fig. 11.2.)

In order to look at the structural relationships of these variables, Partial Order Scalogram Analysis by Coordinates (POSAC) (Shye, 1980) was performed in two dimensions using an input profile for each child of these eight IBR variables as assessed at

4 months of age. In this analysis, the energy items showed no clear regionality and the POSAC was recomputed using an input profile of only the four attention and two motor coordination items. The resulting two dimensional space is displayed in Fig. 11.3. POSAC arranges subjects in space along a joint direction with the most poorly functioning infants at the lower left and the best-functioning infants at the upper right. The resulting POSAC space yielded two factors: motor coordination items along the horizontal axis and attention items along the vertical axis. In this figure, methadone-group infants are indicated by circles and comparison-group infants by squares. The POSAC space revealed strong discrimination between a subgroup of methadone infants and the remaining infants, with those showing poorest motor coordination being almost exclusively methadone infants. A broken line on the figure highlights the discrimination of this subgroup of poorly functioning methadone infants. Seven methadone-group infants and no comparison-group infants are in that region of the POSAC space.

A similar POSAC was computed on the attention and motor coordination profiles at 12 months of age. Again, the resulting space yielded two factors: motor coordination items on the horizontal axis and attention items on the vertical axis (see Fig. 11.4). The subject configuration showed sharp discrimination between methadone- and comparison-group infants. At this age, however, the attention direction is the better discriminator of the two groups. The infants functioning most poorly on the attention variables (at the bottom of the figure) were predominantly from the methadone group (9

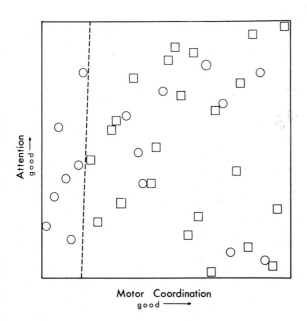

Fig. 11.3. POSAC of motor coordination and attention at 4 months as assessed by the Bayley Infant Behavior Record. Methadone-exposed = ○; comparison = □.

versus 3). The best functioning infants (at the right of the figure) were all from the comparison group (11 versus 0).

Since the goal of this exercise in longitudinal data analysis was not just to find discrimination between groups at one time point, but to find a rule for identifying at an early age (4 months) those children who will show poor functioning later (12 months), Pearson correlations were computed between the joint direction scores (along the good-to-poor diagonal) of the 4- and 12-month POSAC spaces. These joint direction scores were measures of overall functioning in attention and motor areas. For the comparison group the coefficient was $+0.26$; for the methadone group, $+0.10$. For neither group was this association strong enough to make clinically useful predictions from one age to another. Similarly, 4- to 12-month correlations of scores on the attention factor by itself (methadone, $r = +0.11$, control, $r = 0.13$) and the motor factor by itself (methadone, $r = +0.13$; control, $r = +0.21$) were also low.

In another attempt at cross-age prediction, we compared scores on the dimensions that were the best discriminators of the groups at the two ages. Here again, correlation coefficients between ages were not substantial and, in fact, were negative (methadone, $r = -0.28$; control, $r = -0.11$). However, there is an interesting pattern in the data for the methadone-group infants. (Fig. 11.5 plots motor coordination at 4 months by attention at 12 months for the methadone-group infants; broken lines correspond to those on Figs. 11.3 and 11.4.) All five of the methadone-group infants who showed good motor coordination at 4 months were showing poor attention by 12 months. This suggests the interesting possibility that good motoric functioning at 4 months in an

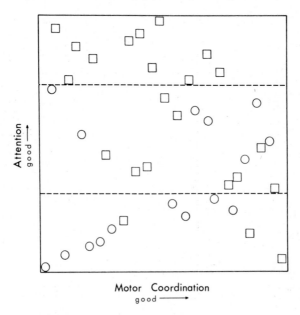

Fig. 11.4. POSAC of motor coordination and attention at 12 months as assessed by the Bayley Infant Behavior Record. Methadone-exposed = ○; comparison = □.

opioid-exposed infant is somehow unusual and does not necessarily mean that the child is displaying a generally good pattern of development. Perhaps the five children in question were born with constitutional characteristics that allowed them to very rapidly metabolize the methadone in their systems and hence show no signs of opioid withdrawal by 4 months. However these same underlying functional characteristics may have detrimental effects in other domains of the children's functioning, perhaps interfering with their ability to sustain careful attention to task and react appropriately to external stimuli at later ages. This finding is fragile because it is based on a very small number of children and the interpretation is highly speculative, but we present them to stimulate thought, to illustrate the potential that longitudinal analysis has for yielding interesting results, and to search for sources of replication.

Suggestions for future research

The behavior of neonates whose mothers used opioid drugs during pregnancy has been well described by several research groups. During the first week of life, these infants show a number of withdrawal signs, primarily related to arousal and motor control. Their abnormal arousal patterns are characterized by easy and frequent upset and inability to maintain an optimum state for processing environmental stimuli. Their signs of poor motor control include tremulousness, jerky limb movements, and hyper-

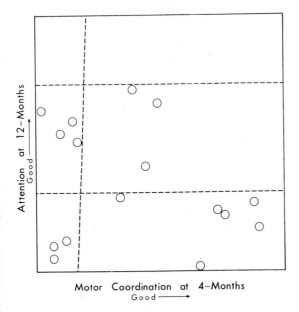

Fig. 11.5. Scatter plot of 4-month motor coordination with 12-month attention. Methadone-exposed = ○; comparison = □.

268

tonicity. By the end of the first month of life, these symptoms decrease dramatically in most infants.

Although the behavior of these children past the neonatal period has been less well studied, a few intriguing research results are emerging. Infants and children exposed in utero to opioid drugs have been described as having poor attention, high levels of activity, impulsive behavior, poor motor coordination, and specific perceptual-cognitive deficits. These behaviors are all among signs of attentional deficit disorders (ADD), perhaps the most common neurobehavioral disorders of childhood. ADD children show not only neurobehavioral deficits, but as they mature are likely to develop other behavior problems, including difficulties with emotional control, behavior problems in school, inappropriate responses to stress (such as depression or anxiety), and reckless or anti-social behavior, including alcohol and drug use as adults. However, such disorders are difficult to identify prior to entrance into school at which time children are placed in situations that require them to focus attention, inhibit activity, and comply to externally imposed norms. *A major research goal should be better data on the long-term behavioral sequelae of fetal exposure to opioids through follow up of the children in the existing longitudinal samples until at least middle childhood.*

A second major goal should be the analysis of data from the existing longitudinal samples so as to look at the patterns of individuals' behavior across time. The basic purpose of research on at-risk populations is to refine our abilities to identify at an early age children who will show problems later. It is only through longitudinal analysis that one can uncover such predictive relationships and identify the early behavior patterns characteristic of those individuals and subgroups who will show poor development. Relationships between early and later behavior are complex and must be studied in a manner that acknowledges their complexity. Such information is important because it will allow clinicians to know on which children to focus their interventions. Our own analysis presented in this chapter is only one small attempt to examine data longitudinally.

A third research goal should be the measurement of a wider number of behavioral outcomes in opioid-exposed children. Most existing studies have measured only a limited number and type of post-neonatal outcomes, usually standardized summative scores of rates of skill acquisition. These summative scores showed only weak discrimination of the opioid-exposed infants and children; in most cases, authors did not report which specific skills contributed to the discrimination. This review shows that, as discriminators of opioid-exposed infants, qualitative descriptors of behavior were generally better measures than rates of skill acquisition. We suggest that existing studies report more extensive analyses of qualitative data they have already collected (e.g. the Bayley IBR), and that future follow up studies include a rich variety of qualitative and clinical measures in addition to tests of developmental skills. A number of important types of measures are noticeably missing from existing follow-up studies of opioid-exposed children. Only one major study (Bernstein et al., 1983) reports on the social interactional skills of opioid infants and their mothers. No study reports biochemical or psychophysiological measures past the neonatal period. A wide variety of measures is needed to identify patterns of psychopathology or neurobehavioral dysfunctioning. Diagnoses cannot be made on the basis of a single developmental quotient score and effective intervention with children cannot be planned without knowledge of specific areas of deficit.

A fourth goal should be the better integration of behavioral and neurophysiological findings in children of opiate-using mothers. Most behavioral research on opioid-exposed infants has been conducted by pediatricians, child psychiatrists, and developmental psychologists. We encourage pharmacologists and neuro-scientists who read this review to add their insights to the intrepretation of the findings, to pursue research that will clarify results, and to join in collaborative efforts with behavioral scientists involved in the ongoing longitudinal studies of opioid-exposed children.

A final goal in the analysis of existing and future data must be consideration of the other factors that may be confounded with the direct toxicological action of opioid drugs on the child. Such factors are many and include maternal use of other drugs, paternal substance use, low parental intelligence, parental psychopathology, poor maternal nutrition, low family socio-economic status, poor family psychosocial supports, unstable relationship between the parents, low birthweight and perinatal complications (cf. Aylward, 1982). All of these factors are potentially associated with maternal opioid use and any could explain performance deficits or behavioral problems, or absence of expected problems, in opioid-exposed children. In research on human populations we have little control over all the factors that can act on the child. Despite this lack of control, we can still collect such information in order to be able to make predictions about human population and to study higher order cognitive and social behavior outcomes. Existing studies generally have reported little information about factors other than opioid use, even though these and other factors could be confounding interpretation of results. Such confounding is especially problematic when differences between opioid-exposed and comparison groups are not large to begin with, such as the differences in Bayley developmental scores between opioid-exposed and comparison infants.

There are at least four major possible causes for poor behavioral development in opioid-exposed children: (1) direct toxicological damage to the nervous system caused by opioid or other drug exposure, (2) damage caused by various perinatal problems or insults, (3) inheritance of familial temperament type, intellectual deficit, or psychopathology, and (4) the effects of an impoverished environment and, more particularly, poor mothering skills. Existing at-risk studies have attempted to match drug-exposed children to a group of comparison children on a variety of such background characteristics. However, no study can match on all characteristics that are likely to affect child development. It is important that future studies of opioid-exposed children assess as many of these characteristics as possible and consider them in their analyses. It is likely, and in fact some of our analyses are beginning to show (Marcus et al., 1983b), that maternal methadone use may cause neurobehavioral deficits in infants only when it is accompanied by very low family socioeconomic levels and poor maternal neurobehavioral functioning. Findings that are based on simultaneous consideration of parental drug use and other factors hold the most potential usefulness for enabling early identification of drug-exposed children at greatest risk for poor development.

In general, the direction of future research in the field of human behavioral teratology must be toward greater sophistication. We must acknowledge and embrace the variety of factors related to maternal drug abuse that can affect children and the variety of behaviors that can be affected. Research must move beyond the question of simply identifying the differences between groups of opioid-exposed and other children and must begin to address the more difficult problems of describing types or patterns of dysfunction typical of opioid-exposed children; of identifying subgroups of children most likely to show these patterns; of understanding the neurochemical and neurophysiological bases of these patterns and of isolating those variables that allow early prediction about children at highest risk. It is only by answering these last questions that we will generate information useful to clinicians who must identify individuals in need of prevention and intervention as well as select the best types of therapeutic approaches that would match specific needs to particular deficit patterns.

Acknowledgments

This work was supported by grants from NIDA (PHS 5 R18DA-01884) and Mr. Irving B. Harris to Joseph Marcus.

We thank our colleagues Victor J. Bernstein and Carrie B. Patterson for their contributions in the conception and execution of our study of infants born to methadone-maintained women. In addition, we acknowledge the help of Ora Aviezer, Paola Braucher, Barbara Byhouwer, Davina Clenna, Claire T. Dankoff, Karen Freel, Patricia Huetteman, Terrence Joyce, Susan D. Lutgendorf, Amy J. Morris, Wendy Rabinowitz-Munson, and Sandra Snook in the collection and analysis of data and preparation of this manuscript. Special thanks are extended to Professor Louis Guttman, The Hebrew University of Jerusalem, for his invaluable consultation on methodology and data analysis.

References

Anderson, R.B. and Rosenblith, J.F. (1971) Sudden unexpected death syndrome: Early indicators. Biol. Neonate 18, 395–406.
Aylward, G.P. (1982) Methadone outcome studies: Is it more than the methadone? J. Pediatr. 101, 214–215.
Bayley, N. (1965) Comparisons of mental and motor test scores for ages 1–15 months by sex, birth order, race, geographic location, and education of parents. Child Dev. 36, 379–411.
Bayley, N. (1969) Manual for the Bayley Scales of Infant Development. Psychological Corporation, New York.
Bernstein, V.J., Jeremy, R.J., Hans, S.L. and Marcus, J. (1983) A longitudinal study of offspring born to methadone-maintained women: II. Dyadic interaction and infant behavior at four months. Am. J. Alcohol Drug Abuse 10, in press.
Blinick, G., Inturrisi, C.E., Jerez, E. and Wallach, R.C. (1975) Methadone assays in pregnant women and progeny. Am. J. Obstet. Gynecol. 121, 617–621.

Blinick, G., Tavolga, W.N. and Antopol, W. (1971) Variations in birth cries of newborn infants from narcotic-addicted and normal mothers. Amer. J. Obstet. Gynecol. 110, 948–958.

Brazelton, T.B. (1973) Neonatal Behavioral Assessment Scale. Clinics in Developmental Medicine 50, Lippincott, Philadelphia, PA.

Carr, J.N. (1975) Drug patterns among drug-addicted mothers: Incidence, variance in use, and effects on children. Pediatr. Ann. 66–77.

Chasnoff, I.J., Hatcher, R. and Burns, W.J. (1980) Early growth patterns of methadone-addicted infants. Am. J. Dis. Child. 134, 1049–1051.

Chasnoff, I.J., Hatcher, R. and Burns, W.J. (1982) Polydrug- and methadone-addicted newborns: A continuum of impairment? Pediatrics 70, 210–213.

Chavez, C.J., Ostrea Jr., E.M., Stryker, J.C. and Smialek, Z. (1979) Sudden infant death syndrome among infants of drug-dependent mothers. J. Pediatr. 95, 407–409.

Connaughton, J.F., Finnegan, L.P., Schut, J. and Emich, J.P. (1975) Current concepts in the management of the pregnant opiate addict. Addict. Dis. 2, 21–35.

Desmond, M.M. and Wilson, G.S. (1975) Neonatal abstinence syndrome: Recognition and diagnosis. Addict. Dis. 2, 113–121.

Dinges, D.F., Davis, M.M. and Glass, P. (1980) Fetal exposure to narcotics: Neonatal sleep as a measure of nervous system disturbance. Science 209, 619–621.

Dole, V.P. (1980) Addictive behavior. Sci. Am. 243, 138–154.

DSM-III: Diagnostic and Statistical Manual of Mental Disorders (1980) American Psychiatric Association, Washington, D.C.

Finnegan, L.P. (1975) Narcotics dependence in pregnancy. J. Psychedelic Drugs 7, 299–311.

Finnegan, L.P. (1979) In utero opiate dependence and sudden infant death syndrome. Clin. Perinatol. 6, 163–180.

Finnegan, L.P., Connaughton, J.F. and Schut, J. (1975) Infants of drug-dependent women: Practical approaches for management. Proceedings of the 37th Annual Scientific Meeting of the Committee on Problems of Drug Dependence.

Finnegan, L.P., Kron, R.E., Connaughton, J.F. and Emich, J.P. (1975) Neonatal abstinence syndrome: Assessment and management. Addict. Dis. 2, 141–158.

Ginsburg, H. (1972) The Myth of the Deprived Child, Prentice-Hall, Englewood Cliffs, NJ.

Ghodse, A.H., Reed, J.L. and Mack, J.W. (1977) The effect of maternal narcotic addiction on the newborn infant. Psychol. Med. 7, 667–675.

Horowitz, F.D., Sullivan, J.W. and Linn, P. (1978) Stability and instability in the newborn infant: The quest for elusive threads. In: Organization and Stability of Newborn Behavior: A Commentary on the Brazelton Neonatal Behavioral Assessment Scale. (Sameroff, A.J., ed.) Monogr. Soc. Res. Child Dev. 43 (5–6), pp. 29–45.

Hutchings, D.E., Towey, J.P., Gorinson, H.S. and Hunt, H.F. (1979) Methadone during pregnancy: Assessment of behavioral effects in the rat offspring. J. Pharmacol. Exp. Ther. 208, 106–112.

Jaffe, J.H. (1980) Drug addiction and drug abuse. In: Goodman and Gilman's The Pharmacological Basis of Therapeutics, 6th edn. (Goodman, L.S. and Gilman, A.G., eds.) MacMillan, New York, pp. 535–584.

Jaffe, J.H. and Martin, W.R. (1980) Opioid analgesics and antagonists. In: Goodman and Gilman's The Pharmacological Basis of Therapeutics, 6th edn. (Gilman, A.G., Goodman, L.S. and Gilman, A., eds.) MacMillan, New York, pp. 494–534.

Jeremy, R.J. and Hans, S.L. (1982) Behavior of neonates exposed in utero to methadone as assessed on the Brazelton scale. Unpublished paper.

Jeremy, R.J. and Bernstein, V.J. (1984) Dyads at risk: Methadone-maintained women and their four-month-old infants. Child Dev. 55, in press.

Kaltenbach, K., Graziani, L.J. and Finnegan, L.P. (1978) Development of children born to women who received methadone during pregnancy. Pediatr. Res. 12, 372.

Kaltenbach, K., Graziani, L.J. and Finnegan, L.P. (1979) Methadone exposure in utero: Effects upon developmental status at 1 and 2 years of age. Pediatr. Res. 13, 332.

Kandall, S.R. and Gartner, L.M. (1974) Late presentation of drug withdrawal symptoms in newborns. Am. J. Dis. Child. 127, 58–61.

Kaplan, S.L., Kron, R.E., Litt, M., Finnegan, L.P. and Phoenix, M.D. (1975) Correlations between scores on the Brazelton Neonatal Behavioral Assessment Scale, measures of newborn sucking behavior, and birthweight in infants born to narcotic addicted mothers. In: Aberrant Development in Infancy: Human and Animal Studies (Ellis, N.R., ed.) Erlbaum, Hillsdale, NJ, pp. 139–148.

Kron, R.E., Kaplan, S.L., Finnegan, L.P., Litt, M. and Phoenix, M.D. (1975) The assessment of behavioral change in infants undergoing narcotic withdrawal: Comparative data from clinical and objective methods. Addict. Dis. 2, 257–275.

Kron, R.E., Kaplan, S.L., Phoenix, M.D. and Finnegan, L.P. (1977) Behavior of infants born to drug-dependent mothers: Effects of prenatal and postnatal drugs. In: (Rementeria, J.L., ed.) Drug Abuse in Pregnancy and Neonatal Effects, Moseley, Saint Louis, MO, pp. 129–144.

Kron, R.E., Litt, M., Phoenix, M.D. and Finnegan, L.P. (1976) Neonatal narcotic abstinence: Effects of pharmacotherapeutic agents and maternal drug usage on nutritive sucking behavior. J. Pediatr. 88, 637–641.

Lewis, M.E., Mishkin, M., Bragin, E., Brown, R.M., Pert, C.B. and Pert, A. (1981) Opiate receptor gradients in monkey cerebral cortex: Correspondence with sensory processing hierarchies. Science 211, 1166–1169.

Lipsitz, P.J. and Blatman, S. (1974) Newborn infants of mothers on methadone maintenance. N.Y. State Med. J. 74, 994–999.

Lodge, A., Marcus, M.M. and Ramer, C.M. (1975) Behavioral and electrophysiological characteristics of the addicted neonate. Addict. Dis. 2, 235–255.

Madden, J.D., Chappel, J.N. Zuspan, F., Gumpel, J., Mejia, A. and Davis, R. (1977) Observation and treatment of neonatal narcotic withdrawal. Am. J. Obstet. Gynecol. 127, 199–201.

Marcus, J. and Hans, S.L. (1982) Electromyographic assessment of neonatal muscle tone. Psychiat. Res. 6, 31–40.

Marcus, J., Hans, S.L. and Jeremy, R.J. (1982a) Differential motor and state functioning in newborns of women on methadone. Neurobehav. Toxicol. Teratol. 4, 459–462.

Marcus, J., Hans, S.L. and Jeremy, R.J. (1982b) Patterns of 1-day and 4-month motor functioning in infants of women on methadone. Neurobehav. Toxicol. Teratol. 4, 473–476.

Marcus, J., Hans, S.L., Patterson, C.B. and Morris, A.J. (1983a) A longitudinal study of offspring born to methadone-maintained women: I. Design, methodology and description of women's resources for functioning. Am. J. Alcohol Drug Abuse 10, in press.

Marcus, J., Hans, S.L. and Jeremy, R.J. (1983b) A longitudinal study of offspring born to methadone-maintained women: III. Effects of multiple risk factors on development at four, eight, and twelve months. Am. J. Alcohol Drug Abuse 10, in press.

McCarthy, D. (1972) Manual for the McCarthy Scales of Children's Abilities. Psychological Corporation, New York.

McGlothlin, W.H. and Anglin, M.D. (1981) Long-term follow-up of clients of high- and low-dose methadone programs. Arch. Gen. Psychiat. 38, 1055–1063.

Newman, R.G., Bashkow, S. and Calko, D. (1975) Results of 313 consecutive live births of infants delivered to patients in the New York City Methadone Maintenance Treatment Program. Am. J. Obstet. Gynecol. 121, 233–237.

Ostrea, Jr., E.M., Chavez, C.J. and Strauss, M.E. (1976) A study of factors that influence the severity of neonatal narcotic withdrawal. J. Pediatr. 88, 642–645.

Perlmutter, J.F. (1974) Heroin addiction and pregnancy. Obstet. Gynecol. Survey 29, 439–446.

Pierog, S. (1977) The infant in narcotic withdrawal: Clinical picture. In: (Rementeria, J.L., ed.) Drug Abuse in Pregnancy and Neonatal Effects, Moseley, Saint Louis, MO, pp. 95–102.

Pierson, P.S., Howard, P. and Kleber, H.D. (1972) Sudden deaths in infants born to methadone-maintained addicts. J. Am. Med. Assoc. 220, 1733–1734.

Rajegowda, B.K., Kandall, S.R. and Falciglia, H. (1978) Sudden unexpected death in infants of narcotic-dependent mothers. Early Human Dev. 2/3, 219–225.

Rementeria, J.L. and Lotongkhum, K. (1977) The fetus of the drug-addicted woman: Conception, fetal wastage and complications. In: (Rementeria, J.L., ed.) Drug Abuse in Pregnancy and Neonatal Effects, Moseley, Saint Louis, MO, pp. 1–18.

Rosen, T.V. and Johnson, H.L. (1982) Children of methadone-maintained mothers: Follow-up to 18 months of age. J. Pediatr. 101, 192–196.

Sameroff, A.J. (Ed.) (1978) Organization and stability of newborn behavior: A commentary on the Brazelton Neonatal Behavioral Assessment Scale. Monogr. Soc. Res. Child Dev. 43, (5–6).

Schulman, C.A. (1969) Alterations of the sleep cycle in heroin-addicted and 'suspect' newborns. Neuropaediatrie 1, 89–100.

Shye, S. (1980) Partial order scalogram analysis of the items by their scalogram generic roles: Description and computer programs for the two-dimensional case. The Israel Institute of Applied Social Research Publication No. 55/789/E.

Soule, A.B., III, Standley, K., Copans, S.A. and Davis, M. (1974) Clinical uses of the Brazelton Neonatal Scale. Pediatrics 54, 583–586.

Strauss, M.E., Andresko, M.A., Stryker, J.C., Wardell, J.N. and Dunkel, L.D. (1974) Methadone maintenance during pregnancy: Pregnancy, birth, and neonate characteristics. Am. J. Obstet. Gynecol. 120, 895–900.

Strauss, M.E., Lessen-Firestone, J.K., Chavez, C.J. and Stryker, J.C. (1979) Children of methadone-treated women at five years of age. Pharmacol. Biochem. Behav. 11, 3–6.

Strauss, M.E., Lessen-Firestone, J.K., Starr, R.H. and Ostrea Jr., E.M. (1975) Behavior of narcotics addicted newborns. Child Dev. 46, 887–893.

Strauss, M.E., Starr, R.H., Ostrea Jr., E.M., Chavez, C.J. and Stryker, J.C. (1976) Behavioral concomitants of prenatal addiction to narcotics. J. Pediatr. 89, 842–846.

Wilson, G.S., Desmond, M.M. and Wait, R.B. (1981) Follow-up of methadone-treated and untreated narcotic-dependent women and their infants: Health, developmental, and social implications. J. Pediatr. 98, 716–722.

Wilson, G.S., McCreary, R., Kean, J. and Baxter, J.C. (1979) The development of preschool children of heroin-addicted mothers: A controlled study. Pediatrics 63, 135–141.

Wise, S.P. and Herkenham, M. (1982) Opiate receptor distribution in the cerebral cortex of the rhesus monkey. Science 218, 387–389.

Zagon, I.S., McLaughlin, P.J. and Thompson, C.I. (1979) Development of motor activity in young rats following perinatal methadone exposure. Pharmacol. Biochem. Behav. 10, 743–749.

Zelson, C. (1973) Infant of the addicted mother. N. Engl. J. Med. 288, 1393–1395.

Zelson, C., Rubio, E. and Wasserman, E. (1971) Neonatal narcotic addiction: 10 year observation. Pediatrics 48, 178–189.

Neurobehavioral Teratology
edited by Joseph Yanai
© Elsevier Science Publishers BV 1984

12

Prenatal and Postnatal Consequences of Marihuana Use During Pregnancy

Peter A. Fried

Department of Psychology, Carleton University, Ottawa, K1S 5B6, Canada

Anecdotal reports of marihuana's effects on various aspects of reproduction go back several hundred years. As described by Abel (1980a) in his fascinating historical account of cannabis, eastern European folk medicine had, for several centuries, claimed that marihuana could be used to hasten delivery. Later, in a parallel vein in the 1840s, a physician returning to England after a nine-year career as surgeon and professor in an Indian medical college detailed the medicinal uses of the marihuana plant. One prominent attribute of the drug was its ability to increase the vigor of and decrease the time between contractions during labor. The earliest commissioned scientific report (Marijuana, Indian Hemp Drugs Commission, 1893–1894) discussed marihuana as both a sexual stimulant and, for ascetics , as a sexual inhibitor. The aphrodisiac properties of forms of cannabis are described in Arab literature of the 16th century and were also described in the mid-nineteenth century in the *U.S. Dispensatory*, the widely read pharmacopoeia of the time.

There have been some recent reports that link marihuana with increased sexual pleasure (see Abel, 1981) but it is not currently possible to separate the drug's effect from the drug users' overall lifestyles and values placed on sexual activity.

If one moves from the drug's possible role in the realm of anecdotal, psychological-related reproductive effects to marihuana's consequences on more objective reproductive measurements, one comes across a fairly large number of scientific reports. However, with only a few exceptions the information is restricted to studies carried out with animals and, until relatively recently, the dose levels used were typically much higher than those used by humans.

A number of laboratories using rodents have shown that Δ^9-tetrahydrocannabinol (THC), the principal psychoactive constituent of marihuana, or its metabolites crosses the placenta, although the amount found in the fetus (with the possible exception of hamsters) is relatively small (Idanpaan-Heikkila et al., 1969; Vardaris et al., 1976). More appears to cross the placenta early in gestation than late and, according to Kennedy and Waddell (1972), the highest levels are found in the central nervous system of the fetus. However, this finding of concentration of THC in the nervous system has not been found by other workers (e.g. Freudenthal et al., 1972).

Transfer of marihuana constituents from mother to infant is not only through the placenta. Findings from a number of animal studies consistently confirm that THC can be transferred via the milk of a lactating mother to her suckling offspring (Jakubovic et al., 1974; Raine et al., 1978; Dalterio and Bartke, 1979). This method of potential exposure of the neonate to cannabinoids takes on added importance in humans as the central nervous system (particularly glial and myelin growth) develops extensively post-natally (Morgane et al., 1978).

The term teratology has, in recent years, broadened from its traditional meaning. As originally used, teratology referred to the study of congenital malformations that were visible at birth and that were induced by exogenous agents during gestation. Today the definition casts a much wider net. It includes morphological, biochemical and behavioral anomalies that arise from drug exposure in utero and that are detected at birth or later.

The question of whether marihuana or its constituents has teratogenic properties cannot be answered by a simple yes or no. Not only is there the fairly obvious issue of dose level but there are also parameters such as species of animal used in the research, the route of administration and the source of plant material. The latter variable has been shown to be a factor in teratogenicity as climatic and growing conditions can greatly vary the proportion of some of the constituents of the marihuana plant and thereby affect the potency of the drug.

A number of studies have reported malformations in mice, rats, guinea pigs, hamsters and rabbits associated with in utero exposure to cannabis extracts during pregnancy, but in those studies in which THC content was specified the quantity of extract that produced effects was well beyond the range used by humans (reviews by Charlebois and Fried, 1979; Rosenkrantz, 1979; Abel, 1980b). When synthetic THC was used, congenital malformations were rarely seen, but at high doses (typically above 50 mg/kg) fetal and embryonic deaths did occur, particularly if the drug was administered early in gestation.

Interestingly, when THC was given to mice and rats via cannabis smoke in doses estimated to be considerably closer to human relevance (e.g. 3.8 mg/kg in Rosenkrantz, 1979), embryotoxicity (but not teratogenicity) was noted. Together, the results of the cannabis extract, the THC and the inhalation studies led to the conclusion that if there is an increased risk in terms of fetal mortality, constituents other than (or in addition to) THC are involved.

There have been two non-human primate studies that have examined marihuana and its potential effect upon the developing fetus. In one (Grilly et al., 1974) the reproductive histories were reported of eight chimpanzees with long-term exposure to marihuana who were mated either with each other or with drug-naive chimpanzees. In comparison to a non-drug colony, no differences in malformations or perinatal deaths were noted. On the other hand, in a more recent study, Sassenrath et al. (1979) reported data from 46 matings between 11 undrugged adult rhesus monkeys and eight breeders which had received daily oral doses of THC at 2.4 and 4.8 mg/kg for a 5-year period. There was an absence of frank teratology but, especially at the higher doses (roughly speaking equal to 16 joints of 2.5% THC per day, Rosenkrantz, 1979), there was a pregnancy loss four times higher in the treated animals than in the control animals that occurred at all stages of pregnancy and even during the neonatal period. In terms of malformations however both the viable and non-viable offspring were grossly normal in appearance.

In clinical single-case, retrospective reports there have been a variety of malformations noted in the offspring of pregnant women who were chronic users of marihuana (Carakushansky et al., 1969; Hecht et al., 1968). However, in all cases the women also had used LSD and other drugs and therefore the role of marihuana cannot be ascertained. Greenland in 1982 described the results of the effects of marihuana use in 35 pregnancies. The woman included in the investigation reported not using other illicit drugs and were recruited from two California pre-natal clinics. Compared to control subjects, significant differences in duration of labor (both protracted and prolonged) were observed as well as an increased incidence of meconium staining among the infants born to marihuana users. A subsequent study (Greenland, personal communication), which was designed to replicate the first, did not find that these adverse outcomes reached statistical significance. According to Greenland the principal difference in the two studies was the general higher levels of health and living conditions among the women who participated in the second study.

In one animal study (Charlebois and Fried, 1980) the potentiation of marihuana with other pregnancy risk factors has been demonstrated and is consistent with Greenland's observations. In Charlebois and Fried's study rats were exposed to either cannabis smoke, placebo smoke or no smoke while concurrently consuming one of three diets differing in protein concentration. Both the diet and drug treatments were administered 20 days prior to and throughout gestation. A number of dependent variables including stillbirths, litter destruction and post-natal deaths were potentiated by a combination of a low protein diet and cannabis smoke. Interestingly some physiological and developmental milestones that were delayed in the normal protein diet/cannabis smoke condition and were potentiated in the low protein/cannabis smoke condition were attenuated in the high protein diet/cannabis smoke condition.

Although low to moderate doses of cannabinoids administered prior to and/or throughout gestation or during critical periods of development, such as organogenesis, typically have not been found to produce any gross pre-natal effects, these same dose levels have resulted in more subtle developmental consequences. Rats born to mothers receiving 10 mg/kg of THC during days 10–12 of gestation were retarded in physical growth from day 4 post-natal to weaning (Borgen et al., 1973), and from birth to young adulthood when 16 mg/kg per day of cannabis was administered to the mothers throughout gestation via inhalation (Fried, 1976). Both Borgen et al. (1973) and Fried (1976) observed weight gain reduction in treated offspring fostered to untreated mothers and thus the effects were attributed to a direct pre-natal drug action on the developing fetus. However, Gianutsos and Abbatiello, who used dose levels of 250 mg/kg of cannabis extract administered on days 8–11 of gestation (1972), and Wright et al. who administered up to 5 mg/kg THC prior to and during gestation (1976), reported birth weight and growth rate up to young adulthood (65 days) to be unaffected by the drug. The ontogenetic appearance of several physiological features and reflexes has been shown to be delayed by pre-natal cannabinoid treatments. These include incisor eruption, eye opening and visual placing (Borgen et al., 1973; Fried, 1976).

A number of studies have focussed on the question of behavioral teratology and cannabis treatment, that is, whether behavioral deficits are induced by pre-natal cannabis exposure. The results are equivocal. Reflex development in rodents was delayed when high doses of THC were used (Borgen et al., 1973) but not when low doses were administered via inhalation (Fried, 1976; Charlebois and Fried, 1979). Open-field behavior in 1 week old rat pups was increased if exposure to THC occurred for two days mid-way during gestation (Borgen et al., 1973) but hypoactivity in an open field was found if the pups had been exposed to cannabis throughout gestation (Fried, 1976). In both of these open-field studies, when the pups were tested close to weaning, the drug effects had attenuated. Maze learning and passive avoidance performance have been found by some workers to be impaired by pre-natal exposure (Gianutsos and Abbatiello, 1972; Vardaris et al., 1976) and by other workers to be unaffected (Ulyeno, 1973; Charlebois and Fried, 1979; Abel, 1980). Differences in routes of administration, dosage, timing of fetal exposure, cross-fostering procedures and pair-feeding controls make it impossible to come to a definitive conclusion at this time.

Sassenrath and her co-workers (Golub et al., 1981), as a follow-up of the reproductive study with rhesus monkeys mentioned earlier (Sassenrath et al., 1979) examined the behavior of the offspring of monkeys who had received daily treatments of THC prior to and during pregnancy and throughout lactation. The types of behavior that were examined at one and two years of age included regulation of activity level, environmental responsiveness, problem solving and social interaction. The category of behavior that distinguished cannabis offspring from control offspring was visual attentiveness which was examined in a standardized test situation in which animals looked at projected slides. In comparison to the offspring of untreated mothers, the THC babies failed to habituate visually to novel visual stimuli. Because only five drug-treated animals were available for study, the researchers were not able to vary drug dose or timing of treatment parameters nor were they able to separate out whether the effect was a direct effect of pre-natal drug exposure on the developing fetal system or an indirect comparison mediated by altered maternal physiology and behavior.

In utero exposure to cannabinoids can result in long-term alterations in pituitary-gonadal function and sexual behavior. Dalterio and her co-workers (Dalterio and Bartke, 1979; Dalterio, 1980) have reported that oral doses of THC or cannabinol administered to mice late in pregnancy suppressed adult copulatory activity in their male offspring. Further, plasma concentration of luteinizing hormone was increased and testes weight was decreased in those males exposed prenatally to THC. Dalterio and her associates (Dalterio et al., 1980) have also found that in prenatally THC-exposed male mice the vas deferens at adulthood had a decreased sensitivity to norepinephrine or peptidyl opiates.

Gonadal alterations have also been noted in rats following in utero exposure to marihuana smoke by Fried and Charlebois (1979). Following pre-natal exposure, both male and female rats were significantly less fertile than cross-fostered controls. The males had smaller seminal vesicles and the females had smaller ovaries. Among those marihuana-exposed animals that did become pregnant there was an increased rate of resorptions and their offspring weighed less and were slower in some aspects of physiological development compared to control animals.

The advantages and indeed the necessity of animal studies in examining reproductive risk and alterations in post-natal development and behavior following fetal exposure to marihuana are self-evident. However, the final arbiter is certainly the human situation. As mentioned previously, objective published data based upon human pregnancy and marihuana use is extremely sparse and, at this time of writing is limited to the work of Greenland et al. (1982) relating to pregnancy complications and work from our own research facilities pertaining to the possible effects of in utero exposure upon neonatal neurological and behavioral status (e.g. Fried et al., 1980; Fried, 1980, 1982).

Since 1979 Fried and his associates have been collecting data from approximately 500 women in a prospective investigation carried out in the Ottawa, Canada region. Mothers-to-be were informed of the study by their obstetrician or notices in waiting rooms of pre-natal clinics in three of the largest hospitals in the city of Ottawa. Upon volunteering to participate, each subject was interviewed once during each of the trimesters remaining in her pregnancy. During each of the interviews, typically in the home of the mother-to-be, information that was collected included socio-demographic data, mother's health (both presently and prior to the pregnancy), father's health history, obstetrical history of previous pregnancies, a 24-h dietary recall, and past and present drug use with particular emphasis upon alcohol, cigarette and marihuana usage. For the drug histories, information was gathered about the year before pregnancy and each trimester of pregnancy.

The method of assessing such variables as nutrition and drug habits by interviewing raises the critical issue of both validity and reliability. Several factors are relevant. Despite the potential shortcomings of self-reporting questionnaires there is no practical alternative method of establishing the information needed for this type of investigation. However, a number of procedures are possible to enhance the probability of an accurate self-report. The same female interviewer 'followed' the mother-to-be during her entire pregnancy and a relaxed rapport was striven for. Strengthening the procedures was the fact that the questionnaire was repeated once during each trimester, permitting a test-retest reliability measure. Also there was a relatively short period of time for the women to have to recollect their drug use during pregnancy (i.e. 3 months).

It must be recognized that this self-report procedure, like any other, will likely result in an underestimation of actual drug usage (Smart, 1975) and therefore the information obtained must be viewed as probably representing conservative levels of use by pregnant women. As an additional attempt to increase validity, after the study had been underway approximately a year, the urine (collected at the time of the interviews) of those mothers reporting use of marihuana was subject to an enzyme immunoassay determination of cannabinoids and the presence of other drugs including amphetamines and opiates (Marks et al., 1980). Urine samples from randomly chosen women reporting no use of marihuana were analyzed at the same time so that the immunoassay procedures could be carried out in a blind fashion.

Because the range of marihuana use among the women in the sample was quite broad and was bimodal in distribution, the drug data were not treated as a continuous variable but were considered, instead, in terms of categories. As described elsewhere (Fried et al., 1980; Fried, 1980) four categories of marihuana use have been developed: the non-user; irregular user, one joint or less per week or exposure to the exhaled smoke of others; moderate user, two to five joints per week; and heavy user, more than five joints per week.

Among the total sample of 500 women, the average family income was just above $29 000, a figure that was very similar to that of the general population of the Ottawa area as reported by Statistics Canada. In addition to the sample being similar to the population from which it was drawn on an economic level, the women who volunteered were also similar in terms of age and parity with all women giving birth in the participating hospitals. The average age was 29 and the average parity was 0.7. In one respect the sample did differ from the general female population of Ottawa and that was along the dimension of formal education. Among the 500 women, 93% had at least a high school diploma and almost two-thirds had continued their education beyond high school. This degree of schooling was considerably higher than reported in the population from which the sample was drawn and likely reflects the selection bias of the recruitment procedures employed in the study.

In the volunteer sample 80% stated that they did not use any marihuana in the year before pregnancy, 13% used it irregularly, 3% smoked 2–5 joints per week and 4% smoked 6 or more joints per week. Once pregnant, usage declined but during each of the trimesters of pregnancy the percentages remained relatively consistent with,

90% reporting no use, 6% reporting irregular use, 1% smoking 2–5 joints and 3% reporting 6 or more joints per week.

Many but not all of the women who smoked marihuana to either a moderate or heavy extent during pregnancy differed from the remainder of the sample in a number of ways that might have an adverse effect on the course of pregnancy and on the development of the offspring. These potential confounding factors included a lower socio-economic level, less formal education and increased cigarette smoking. In addition, among the women in the 'heavy' marihuana category the average daily amount of alcohol consumed was significantly greater than that drunk by the remainder of the sample.

In terms of age the heavy marihuana users were a significant avarage of 3.2 years younger than the remainder of the sample. However, in terms of parity no differences were noted. Further, nutritional adequacy did not differ among the four categories of marihuana use.

Over the course of the study two general approaches have been utilized to examine the data: a multivariate analysis and a matched control procedure. In the latter case women who reported smoking either a moderate or heavy amount of marihuana were matched in terms of nicotine and alcohol habits. For the purposes of this matching both nicotine and alcohol use were categorized into three and four levels respectively as described elsewhere (Fried et al., 1980).

There were no differences between the marihuana users and their matched controls in terms of rate of miscarriages, type of presentation at birth, labor, Apgar status and the frequency of complications or major anomalies at birth. Whether there are increased minor anomalies associated with marihuana use is presently being investigated. No evidence of increased meconium staining among the newborn of the heavy marihuana users was noted. This is in contrast to the report by Greenland et al. (1982) but is consistent with Greenland's subsequent findings (personal communication) both of which were described earlier. It is noteworthy that the sample in the latter case was more similar in terms of ethnicity, education and general health to the Ottawa subjects than were the women in the published Greenland study.

Greenland observed an increased incidence of precipitate labor (less than 3 h) among the marihuana users in both of his studies (although statistical significance was not obtained in the second investigation). In the Ottawa study a similar trend was noted in that precipitate labor was observed in 23% of the heavy marihuana users as compared to 11% of the non-users. This association between marihuana use and shortened labor is consistent with historical anecdotes that have, over the past centuries, described how cannabis has been used as a method to increase the vigor of contractions and shorten labor (Abel, 1980a).

An additional pregnancy variable that was noted in the Ottawa study was an inverse dose response relationship between marihuana use and the length of gestation. An average use of marihuana six or more times per week during pregnancy was associated with a significant reduction of 1.1 weeks after statistically adjusting for nicotine, alcohol, parity, mother's pre-pregnancy weight and the sex of the child. With similar adjustments no reduction in birth weight was noted once gestational age was taken into account.

As described earlier animal work has indicated that cannabis constituents can alter a wide range of pituitary-ovarian and adrenal hormones (Dalterio and Bartke, 1979; Harclerode, 1980; Smith, 1980). There is also indirect evidence that THC can affect steroid production by the placenta (Harclerode, 1980). Although the underlying physiological nature of the shortened gestation length associated with heavy marihuana use can only be speculated upon at this stage of research, a likely candidate for the mechanism of action is marihuana's influence upon the reproductive hormonal system.

The Brazelton Neonatal Assessment Scale (Brazelton, 1973) was used to assess the newborn's capacity to interact and adjust to its environment. This examination was carried out at 60–80 h post-partum mid-way between feedings in a warm, quiet room free from sudden extraneous noises and located close to the nursery in the hospital. Behaviors that were observed included consolability, self-quieting, irritability, tremulousness, startle, activity, alertness, orientation to animate and inanimate visual and auditory stimuli, habituation to stimuli in various modalities, hand-to-mouth movements, pull-to-sit muscle tone, Moro reflex and lability of states. This variety of behavioral activities and states was assessed by two trained raters who were not aware of the mother's drug history.

A number of group differences emerged using the Brazelton procedures (Fried, 1980; 1982). A rather striking finding in view of the Golub et al. (1981) primate work described earlier was that smoking marihuana regularly during pregnancy was correlated with marked decrease in the likelihood of the offspring responding to a light repeatedly directed at their eyes. Among the 12 heaviest marihuana users, seven failed to respond to the light and two responded extremely weakly. The latter two babies did not habituate to the repeated light. Among the matched controls all but two responded vigorously and all responders habituated ($p < 0.001$). In the auditory modality there were no differences among the marihuana offspring and the matched controls. It is worth noting that, using the same Brazelton testing procedures, Finnigan (1981) observed that babies born to methadone-using mothers also responded poorly to visual stimuli but were not abnormal in their responsiveness to auditory stimulation.

Some other similarities to babies born to narcotic-using mothers were also observed among the babies born to the women who smoked marihuana regularly during pregnancy. These included significantly heightened tremors and startles. These behaviors were the most consistent and visible consequences of regular heavy marihuana consumption and, together with the altered habituation rate, may reflect neurological dysfunction.

However, unlike infants going through narcotic withdrawal, the marihuana babies were not more irritable than control infants and were readily consolable. Finally, at this age, no association between the degrees of activity or alertness and maternal marihuana use was observed.

At 9 and 30 days of age the Prechtl and Beintema (1969) neurological examination was given. This neurological inventory, using standardized techniques to elicit a comprehensive selection of reflexes and responses, is designed to measure subtle qualitative and quantitative differences in behavior. The altered responsiveness of the visual system persisted in those infants (particularly at 9 days of age) whose mothers smoked marihuana six or more times per week during their pregnancy. As part of the Prechtl test various extraocular movements were also examined and some abnormalities among the marihuana infants were noted. In order to pursue these 'soft' visual signs of the potential effect of intrauterine exposure to marihuana, a series of neurobehavioral and electrophysiological tests are presently being undertaken. Included in the neuro-ophthalmological battery are pupillary responses, gaze preponderance, tracking capability, opto-kinetic reflexes and visual evoked potentials to both patterned and non-patterned stimuli.

The Prechtl examination also revealed some motoric differences among the babies born to the heavy marihuana users that were most marked at the 9-day testing period. These included a continuation of the marked tremors that were observed when the infants were 3 or 4 days of age, an exaggerated Moro reflex, increased occurrence of athetoid movements and disinhibition in a number of motor tests. Like some of the observations made soon after birth, many of these behaviors are similar to those noted in infants undergoing narcotic withdrawal.

The Bayley Scale of Infant Development (1969) that includes mental, motor and behavioral temperament scales, has been administered to 6, 12 and 18 month old offspring of eight heavy users and four moderate users. The 'mental' portion of this scale assesses sensory perceptual abilities, early acquisition of object constancy memory, problem solving, vocalizations and the onset of words. The 'motor' portion is directed at assessing both gross and fine motor capabilities. Based on this very preliminary data and using both matched controls and normative scores, the performance of these relatively few babies did not suggest any negative effects associated with marihuana use during pregnancy. An evaluation of the babies' attitudes, interests and temperaments also failed to discriminate between those born to marihuana users and either those born to matched controls or normative scores based on a general population.

Overall, the data gathered from the Ottawa study is a preliminary step in attempting to determine the association between maternal marihuana use and its consequence upon the developing fetus. What has emerged to date is that in the neonate there are a number of neurobehavioral variables that are correlated with in utero marihuana exposure. Although it is not possible to control, either in terms of subject selection or by statistical manipulation, all the potential non-marihuana factors that may be contributing to the differences observed in the babies born to the heavy marihuana users, most of the more obvious ones have been taken into account. These include the non-marihuana drug habits, the history of previous pregnancies, socio-economic status and nutritional (including caffeine) intake.

The general observation that the measurable correlates in newborns of regular ma-

284

ternal marihuana use diminishes with age must must be interpreted cautiously. It is not at all clear whether this is the true state of affairs and arises because the neurological disturbances present at birth are transient and are either overcome or compensated for with maturity or whether the tests used at the later ages have a decreased discriminatory sensitivity to subtle differences that actually may exist. The hope and expectation is that by increasing the sample size, adding some further tests (some of which have been described earlier) and further follow-up of the infants will help clarify this important issue.

References

Abel, E.L. (1980a) Marihuana: The First Twelve Thousand Years. Plenum Press, New York.
Abel, E.L. (1980b) Prenatal exposure to cannabis: A critical review of effects on growth, development, and behavior. Behav. Neural Biol. 29, 137–156.
Abel, E.L. (1981) Marihuana and sex: A critical survey. Drug Alcohol Depend. 8, 1–22.
Bayley, N. (1969) Manual for the Bayley Scales of Infant Development. Psychological Corp., New York.
Borgen, L.A., Davis, W.M. and Pace, H.B. (1973) Effects of prenatal THC on the development of the rat offspring. Pharmacol. Biochem. Behav. 1, 203–206.
Brazelton, T.B. (1973) Neonatal Behavioral Assessment Scale. Heinemann, London.
Carakushansky, G., Neu, R.L. and Gardner, L.I. (1969) Lysergide and cannabis as possible teratogens in man. Lancet i, 150–151.
Charlebois, A.T. and Fried, P.A. (1980) The interactive effects of nutrition and cannabis upon rat perinatal development. Dev. Psychobiol. 13, 591–605.
Dalterio, S. (1980) Perinatal or adult exposure to cannabinoids alters male reproductive functions in mice. Pharmacol. Biochem. Behav. 12, 143–153.
Dalterio, S. and Bartke, A. (1979) Perinatal exposure to cannabinoids alters male reproductive function in mice. Science 205, 1420–1422.
Dalterio, S., Blum, K., Delallo, L., Sweeny, C., Briggs, A. and Bartke, A, (1980) Perinatal exposure to Δ^9-THC in mice: Altered enkephalin and norephinephrine sensitivity in vas deferens. Substance Alcohol Actions/Misuse 1, 467–478.
Finnigan, L.P. (1981) The effects of narcotics and alcohol on pregnancy and the newborn. Ann. N.Y. Acad. Sci. 362, 136–157.
Fried, P.A. (1976) Short and long-term effects of pre-natal cannabis inhalation upon rat offspring. Psychopharmacology 50, 185–291.
Fried, P.A. (1980) Marihuana use by pregnant women: Neurobehavioral effects in neonates. Drug Alcohol Depend. 6, 415–424.
Fried, P.A. (1982) Marihuana use by pregnant women and effects on offspring: An update. Neurobehav. Toxicol. Teratol. 4, 451–454.
Fried, P.A. and Charlebois, A.T. (1979) Cannabis administered during pregnancy: First- and second-generation effects in rats. Physiol. Psychol. 7, 307–310.
Fried, P.A., Watkinson, B., Grant, A. and Knights, R.M. (1980) Changing patterns of soft drug use prior to and during pregnancy: A prospective study. Drug Alcohol Depend. 6, 323–343.
Freudenthal, R.I., Martin, J. and Wall, M.E. (1972) Distribution of Δ^9-tetrahydrocannabinol in the mouse. Brit. J. Pharmacol. 44, 244–249.
Gianutsos, G. and Abbatiello, E.R. (1972) The effect of pre-natal Cannabis sativa on maze learning ability in the rat. Psychopharmacologie 27, 117–122.

Golub, M.S., Sassenrath, E.N. and Chapman, C.F. (1981) Regulation of visual attention in offspring of female monkeys treated chronically with $\varDelta^9$-tetrahydrocannabinol. Dev. Psychobiol. 14, 507–512.

Greenland, S., Staisch, K., Brown, N. and Gross, S. (1982) The effects of marihuana use during pregnancy. I. A preliminary epidemiologic study. Am. J. Obstet. Gynecol. 143, 408–413.

Grilly, D.M., Ferraro, D.P. and Brande, M.C. (1974) Observations on the reproductive activity of chimpanzees following long-term exposure to marihuana. Pharmacology 11, 304–307.

Harclerode, J. (1980) The effect of marijuana on reproduction and development. In Marihuana Research Findings, (Peterson, R.C., ed.) U.S. Govt. Printing Office, Washington, pp. 137–166.

Hecht, F., Beals, R., Lees, M., Jolly, H. and Roberts, P. (1968) Lysergic-acid-diethylamide and cannabis as possible teratogens in man. Lancet ii, 1087–1088.

Idanpaan-Heikkila, J., Fritchie, G.E., Englert, L.F., Ho, B.T. and McIsaac, W.M. (1969) Placental transfer of tritiated-1-$\varDelta^9$-tetrahydrocannabinol. New Engl. J. Med. 281, 330.

Jakubovic, A., Tait, R.M. and McGeer, P.L. (1974) Excretion of THC and its metabolites in ewe's milk. Toxicol. Appl. Pharmacol. 28, 38–43.

Joneja, M.G. (1976) A study of teratological effects of intravenous, subcutaneous, and intragastric administration of $\varDelta^9$-tetrahydrocannabinol in mice. Toxicol. Appl. Pharmacol. 36, 151–162.

Kennedy, J.S. and Waddell, W.J. (1972) Whole body autoradiography of the pregnant mouse after administration of ^{14}C-$\varDelta^9$-THC. Toxicol. Appl. Pharmacol. 22, 252–258.

Marijuana. Report of the Indian Hemp Drug Commission, 1893–1894. (1969) Reprinted by Thomas Jefferson, Silver Spring, MD.

Marks, V., Mould, G.P., O'Sullivan, M.J. and Teale, J.D. (1980) Monitoring of drug disposition by immunoassay. In: Progress in Drug Metabolism Vol. 5 (Bridges, J.W. and Chasseaud, L.F., eds.) Wiley, New York, pp. 255–310.

Morgane, P.J., Miller, M., Kemper, Stern, W., Forbes, W., Hall, R., Bronzio, J., Kissene, J., Hawrylewicz, E. and Resnick, O. (1978) The effects of protein malnutrition on the developing central nervous system in the rat. Neurosci. Biobehav. Rev. 2, 1–230.

Prechtl, H.F.R. and Beintema, D. (1969) Neurological examination of the full term infant. Clin. Dev. Med. 12, 1–101.

Raine, T.M., Wing, D.R. and Paton, W.D.M. (1978) The effects of $\varDelta^9$-tetrahydrocannabinol on mammary glands and growth, enzyme activity and plasma prolactin levels in the mouse. Eur. J. Pharmacol. 51, 11–17.

Rosenkrantz, H. (1979) Effects of cannabis on fetal development of rodents. In: Marihuana: Biological Effects (Nahas, G. and Paton, W.D., eds.) Pergamon Press, New York, pp. 479–499.

Sassenrath, E.N., Chapman, L.F. and Goo, G.P. (1979) Reproduction in rhesus monkeys chronically exposed to delta-9-tetrahydrocannabinol. In: Marihuana: Biological Effects (Nahas, G. and Paton, W.D., eds.) Permagon Press, New York, pp. 501–512.

Smart, R.G. (1975) Recent studies on the validity and reliability of self-reported drug use, 1970–1974. Can. J. Crim. Corr. 17, 326–333.

Smith, C.G. (1980) Effects of marihuana on neuroendocrine function. In: Marihuana Research Findings: 1980. Natl. Inst. Drug Abuse Monograph No. 31 (Peterson, E.C., ed.) U.S. Govt. Printing Office, Washington, pp. 120–136.

Uyeno, E.T. (1973) Delta-9-tetrahydrocannabinol administered during pregnancy of the rat. Proc. West. Pharmacol. Soc. 16, 64–67.

Vardaris, R.M., Weisz, D.J., Fazel, A. and Rawitch, A.B. (1976) Chronic administration of delta-9-tetrahydrocannabinol to pregnant rats: Studies of pup behavior and placental transfer. Pharmacol. Biochem. Behav. 4, 249–254.

Wright, P.L., Smith, S.H., Keplinger, M.L., Calandra, J.C. and Braude, M.C. (1976) Reproductive and teratologic studies with delta-9-tetrahydrocannabinol and crude marihuana extract. Toxicol. Appl. Pharmacol. 38, 223–237.

Section IV

SUBSTANCES ACTING ON NEUROTRANSMITTERS
AND THEIR RECEPTORS

Neurobehavioral Teratology
edited by Joseph Yanai
© Elsevier Science Publishers BV 1984

13

NEUROTRANSMITTERS IN DEVELOPMENT AS POSSIBLE SUBSTRATES FOR DRUGS OF USE AND ABUSE

Jean M. Lauder and Helmut Krebs

Department of Anatomy, School of Medicine, University of North Carolina at Chapel Hill,
111 Swing Building, 217H, Chapel Hill, NC 27514, USA

"... it is interesting to speculate on the possible metabolic origins and significance of the transmitters. Some of these substances, such as acetylcholine, occur in organisms under circumstances where they serve no apparent neural function. This suggests that the evolutionary appearance of the transmitters preceded that of the nervous system. Their hormonal function in modern organisms implies that they might have arisen as regulatory molecules-perhaps metabolic symbols, in the sense defined here. A possible clue to the biochemical origins of the neurotransmitters is provided by the fact that all the compounds currently accepted as transmitters are either amino acid metabolites-for example, the catecholamines, serotonin, γ-aminobutyric acid, acetylcholine-or are themselves amino acids (for example, glycine). Thus, perhaps the transmitters acted in primitive cells as intracellular symbols representing changes in environmental amino acid concentration. Eventually, these primordial nerve cells might have utilized the symbols in short-range intercellular (hormonal) roles, originally concerned with transducing information related to amino acid accumulation, and gradually with many other aspects of the environment." (Tomkins, 1975)

The hypothesis that particular neurotransmitters might have developmental functions prior to the evolutionary and developmental onset of neurotransmission derives from

Table 13.1. Non-transmission roles for neurotransmitters and neurohumors in development. Revised from Lauder et al., 1982a, by permission of Ankho Int. Inc.

Phase of development	Location	Organism	Neurotransmitter or neurohumor	Proposed function	References
Cleavage, gastrulation	Fertilized egg and early zygote	Sea urchin fish, amphibian, chick, rat, mouse	Acetylcholine, norepinephrine, epinephrine, dopamine, 5-hydroxytryptamine, (serotonin), 5-methoxytryptamine	Control of cell division and morphogenetic cell movements	Baker, 1965; Burden and Lawrence, 1973; Buznikov, 1980; Buznikov and Shmukler, 1981; Buznikov et al., 1964, 1968, 1970, 1972; Deeb, 1972; Emanuelsson, 1974; Gustafson and Toneby, 1970, 1971; Pienkowski, 1977; Toneby, 1977; Manukin et al., 1981.
Metamorphosis	Larvae	Abalone	GABA	Control of settling upon algal surface and metamorphosis	Morse et al., 1979
Morphogenesis, growth and regeneration	Head region, nerve and interstitial cells, cilia	Planaria, Hydra, Tetrahymena	Acetylcholine, serotonin, norepinephrine, dopamine, substance P	Promotion of morphogenetic and regenerative functions in protozoans and flatworms; inhibition of RNA synthesis (serotonin)	Blum, 1970; Franquinet, 1979, 1981; Müller et al., 1977; Taban and Cathieni, 1979; Rodriguez and Renaud, 1980.
Formation of neural tube and gut; torsion and flexure of the embryo; myogenesis	Notochord, neural plate, neural tube, gut, yolk sac, allantois	Frog, chick, rat, mouse	Acetylcholine, norepinephrine, dopamine, serotonin	Control of neural tube closure, cell division and cell differentiation, morphogenetic cell movements; myoblast differentiation	Allan and Newgreen, 1977; Boucek and Bourne, 1962; Burack and Badger, 1964; Caston, 1962; Cochard et al., 1978; Emanuelsson and Palén, 1975; Filogamo et al., 1978; Gérard et al., 1978; Gershon et al., 1979; Ignarro and Shideman, 1968a, b; Kirby and Gilmore, 1972; Lawrence Jr. and Burden, 1973; Palén et al., 1979; Schlumpf and Lichtensteiger, 1979; Schowing et al., 1977; Sims, 1977; Strudel et al., 1977a, b; Teitelman et al., 1978; Wallace, 1979, 1982; Curtis and Zalin, 1981.
Palate formation	Palatal shelves	Mouse	Acetylcholine, serotonin, GABA	Control of morphogenetic cell movements; cell migration	Kujawa and Zimmerman 1978; Clark et al., 1980; Venkatasubramanian et al., 1980; Wee et al., 1979, 1980; Zimmerman et al., 1980.
Brain organogenesis; retinal development	Neurons	Axolotl, frog, rat, mouse, rabbit, monkey, human	Acetylcholine, GABA, norepinephrine, dopamine, serotonin	Control of cell division, neuronal and glial differentiation, cell migration, synaptogenesis, other 'tropic functions'	Ahmad and Zamenhof, 1978; Bartels, 1971; Cadilhac and Pons, 1976; Chronwall and Wolff, 1980; Golden, 1972, 1973; Lauder and Bloom, 1974; Lauder and Krebs, 1976, 1978a, b; Lauder et al., 1980, 1982a; Levitt and Rakic, 1979; Lewis et al., 1977a; Maeda and Dresse, 1969; Olson et al., 1973; Olson and Seiger, 1972; Patel et al., 1979a; Schlumpf et al., 1977, 1980; Specht et al., 1978a, b, 1981; Taber Pierce, 1973; Vernadakis, 1973; Wolff et al., 1979; Yamamoto et al., 1980; Yew et al., 1974; Hogan and Coleman, 1981a, b; Tennyson et

the presence of these substances in primitive organisms and during key phases of embryogenesis and neurogenesis in higher organisms (Table 13.1). Proposed functions for these neurohumoral agents include: control of cell division and morphogenetic cell movements during early phases of embryogenesis, neural tube closure, palate formation, myoblast differentiation, regulation of cell differentiation during formation of the central nervous system (CNS), as well as involvement in such processes as metamorphosis, morphogenetic and regenerative processes in lower animals.

Monoamines and neurulation

The development of the CNS begins very early in gestation with the formation of the neural plate. Within hours of the induction of the neural ectoderm by the chordamesoderm, neural folds elevate at the lateral edges of the neural plate. As the neural folds near the midline, they fuse to form a continuous neural tube. Neurulation, the process of the formation of the neural tube, advances in both rostral and caudal directions from the initial point of contact of the neural folds and is complete with the closure of the rostral and caudal neuropores.

During this early period of neurogenesis, catecholamines and serotonin (5-HT) have been detected in chick embryos and implicated in the initial phases of nervous system development. In whole embryo extracts, the catecholamines norepinephrine and dopamine (NE, DA) have been biochemically measured as early as day one of incubation (Ignarro and Shideman, 1968a, b), whereas extracts of the notochord have revealed the presence of 5-HT as well as catecholamines (Strudel et al., 1977a, b). Various embryonic structures, discussed below, have been shown to accumulate these amines during the period of embryonic morphogenesis (Kirby and Gilmore, 1972; Lawrence and Burden, 1973; Wallace, 1979, 1982). This early presence of monoamines may influence the development of the chick embryo, as illustrated by the teratological effects of drugs which interfere with the metabolism of these transmitter substances. Alterations in catecholamine metabolism result in defects in neural tube closure and failure in the development of embryonic torsion and flexure (Lawrence and Burden,1973). Certain drugs which interfere with 5-HT synthesis, release and receptor interactions are also able to disturb the processes of blastoderm growth, primitive streak formation, neurulation, brain formation and somatogenesis (Jurand, 1980; Palén et al., 1979). The locations of these disturbances resulting from perturbations in monoamine metabolism may be related to the specific embryonic sites which concentrate the amines during morphogenesis .

Wallace (1979, 1982) has demonstrated sites of 5-HT and NE uptake and/or synthesis in the neural tube and notochord of chick embryos cultured with these compounds, using fluorescence histochemistry and anti-5-HT immunocytochemistry. In these studies, 5-HT uptake and synthesis was found in specific portions of the developing brain (within the floor plate of the mesencephalon and caudal myelencephalon) soon after neural tube closure. Similarly, sclerotome cells exhibited 5-HT soon after the somites began to exhibit morphological differentiation. In addition, caudal segments of the spinal cord and adjacent notochord developed the capacity to concentrate 5-HT in the region of the neural plate actively involved in closure. As progression of closure advanced caudally in the spinal cord, 5-HT accumulation observed in the floor

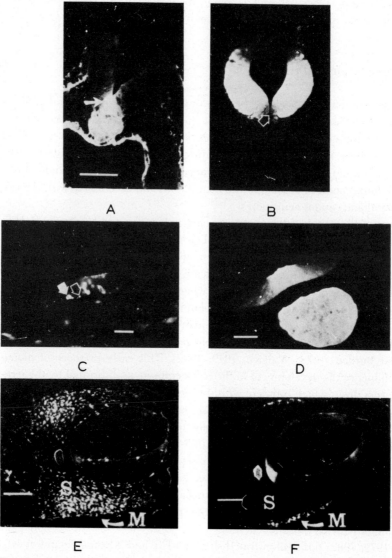

Fig. 13.1. Comparison between sites of serotonin (5-HT) and norepinephrine (NE) accumulation in the chick embryo following incubation in vitro with either of these compounds. A,C,E: Sites of 5-HT accumulation; B,D,F: Sites of NE accumulation. Note the different sites of accumulation and appearance of 5-HT and NE fluorescence at the same anatomical level of the neuraxis (A,B: caudal neuropore, stage 10 embryo; C,D: cervical level, stage 15 embryo; E,F: rostral somite level, stage 15 embryo). S: sclerotome; M: myotome. A,B,E,F: bars = 50 μm. C,D: bars = 20 μm. (From Wallace, 1979, by permission.)

plate of the neural tube and notochord also advanced caudally, remaining in the region of the closing caudal neuropore.

Over the same period, NE uptake initially appeared throughout the developing neural plate, with regions of increased accumulation found in progressively more caudal portions of the neural tube in apparent spatial and temporal coordination with the advance of neural tube closure. As the process of neurulation neared completion, the capacity of the neural tube to concentrate NE likewise ceased, again in a rostral to caudal sequence, with those areas initially completing closure losing this ability first. With a similar pattern, notochordal accumulation of NE was observed beneath regions of the developing brain and spread progressively into trunk portions of the chord over the period when the neural tube in the region of the spinal cord completed closure.

A comparison of embryonic sites concentrating either 5-HT or NE from the studies of Wallace (Fig. 13.1) demonstrated major differences in the location of these two neurotransmitters during the period of neurulation. Although an overlap in certain regions of the brain floor plate appeared temporarily, almost mutually exclusive patterns of accumulation were observed in the region of the caudal neuropore (Fig. 13.1A, B), as well as throughout the rostro-caudal extent of the notochord and within various components of the developing somites (Fig. 13.1E, F).

These findings raise the possibility that 5-HT and NE may play different roles in chick neurogenesis, possibly acting in concert to coordinate events leading to neural tube closure, brain organogenesis or somite differentiation, although such proposed actions are only speculative at present. The notochord may constitute a site of synthesis of monoamines in the early chick embryo (Kirby and Gilmore, 1972; Allan and Newgreen, 1977; Wallace, 1979, 1982), although yolk material has also been shown to contain catecholamines during early embryonic periods (Ignarro and Shideman, 1968a, b). Moreover, the malformations produced by drugs which interfere with 5-HT metabolism are associated with a delayed degradation of yolk granules which are thought to contain 5-HT and its precursor L-tryptophan (Emanuelsson, 1974). These granules, which are taken up into the neural plate and tube during neurulation (Santander and Cuadrado, 1976) could be a source of 5-HT for the developing nervous system in addition to the notochord. In the rat embryo, the yolk sac itself may be a source of monoamines for the early developing nervous system (Schlumpf and Lichtensteiger, 1979).

Serotonin as a differentiation signal during brain organogenesis

Introduction

The monoamines are early developing neurotransmitters which can be endogenously detected by the formaldehyde-induced fluorescence (FIF) method or immunocytochemistry shortly after or during formation of the neurons which will contain them, long before these cells themselves are innervated (Lauder and Bloom, 1974, 1975). In fact, monoamine neurons comprise some of the earliest forming neuronal populations in the entire brain, with the exception of a few brain stem nuclei. Further, most brain regions to which these neurons project are generated from one to several days later than the monoamine cells themselves (Lauder and Bloom, 1974).

These results, together with information from other studies indicating that the monoamines can promote differentiation of neuroblastoma and glioma cells in vitro, possibly via an effect on cyclic AMP (Gilman and Nirenberg, 1971; Oey, 1975; Pénit et al., 1977; Prasad and Gilmer, 1974; Sahu and Prasad, 1975; Schubert et al., 1976; Schwartz, 1976; Schwartz et al., 1973) raise the possibility that these neurotransmitter substances could act as humoral signals influencing initial phases of differentiation associated with the genesis of later developing neurons to which they will project. This might occur through cell-cell interactions between young monoamine neurons and proliferating germinal cells in the neural tube, or through an influence of circulating monoamines in the cerebrospinal fluid (CSF), vasculature or from the yolk sac.

Serotonin and neuronal genesis in the embryonic brain
In order to test the hypothesis that 5-HT neurons might exert an influence on the development of their target neurons during the time when the precursors of these neurons are ceasing cell proliferation and beginning to differentiate, we undertook a *pharmacological study* designed to inhibit 5-HT synthesis in the embryonic brain during that period when it might be used as such a signal (Lauder and Krebs, 1976, 1978a, b). Either *p*-chlorophenylalanine (pCPA) or physiological saline was injected ip into timed pregnant rats (Sprague-Dawley, Zivic Miller), beginning on day 8 of gestation (E8), and continued until the time of [³H]thymidine injection. Animals were born and lived to 30 days postnatal when they were prepared for autoradiography. The *time of neuronal genesis* (time of origin) of neurons in 44 different brain regions was determined by quantifying the proportion of heavily labelled cells in each neuronal population (those cells which ceased cell division on the day of [³H]thymidine injection).

The results of this pCPA study, in which we found delayed and/or prolonged neuronal genesis in many brain regions, were originally interpreted in terms of the effects of this treatment on '5-HT target cells', defined as neuronal populations which receive a 5-HT innervation in the adult, since no information was available concerning true embryonic target cells. These results seemed to indicate an effect of pCPA on time of neuronal genesis specifically in these so-called 5-HT target cell populations (Lauder and Krebs, 1976, 1978a, b). However, many of the neuronal populations defined as 'non-5-HT target cells' have now been found to contain limited numbers of 5-HT terminals in the adult brain (Steinbusch, 1981). Moreover, since the important issue is precisely which of these cells are targets of 5-HT neurons in the embryo, these data have now been reinterpreted in light of our recent immunocytochemical studies of the developing 5-HT system in the rat embryo and its relationship to proliferating neuroepithelial cells (Lauder et al., 1982a; Wallace and Lauder, 1983), in which we have been able to ascertain whether 5-HT axons grow into particular brain regions at the appropriate time to explain the results obtained in this pCPA study.

Figs. 13.2 and 13.3 illustrate the effects of maternal pCPA treatment on time of neuronal genesis in particular embryonic brain regions. Data from injected controls have been omitted from these graphs, since this treatment produced early neuronal genesis in all regions where pCPA effects were found, possibly due to chronic stress effects of daily ip injections of the pregnant rat. These effects are discussed in our earlier pCPA papers (Lauder and Krebs, 1976, 1978a, b) and need not be reiterated here, since they do not appear to serve as controls per se, but rather seem to comprise another experimental group.

Brain regions in the posterior diencephalon which are located directly in the path of (or close to) the major bundle of rostrally projecting 5-HT axons (Fig. 13.2), which appear to reach these parts of the presumptive neuroepithelium at or close to the beginning of neuronal genesis in each region, exhibit either suppression of the onset of neuronal genesis, suppression of neuronal genesis during the peak period, or prolongation of neuronal genesis .

Interestingly, certain hypothalamic regions (anterior ventral diencephalon) which are also in the direct path of rostrally projecting 5-HT axons showed no effect of the pCPA treatment. This may be related to the fact that 5-HT axons do not reach these

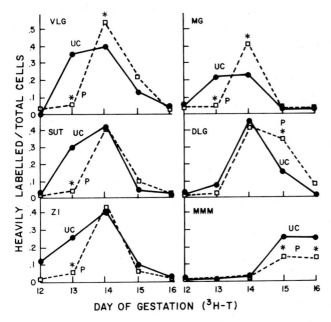

Fig. 13.2. Effects of maternal pCPA treatment on neuronal genesis (time of origin) in the posterior diencephalon. DLG, dorsal lateral geniculate; VLG, ventral lateral geniculate; SUT, subthalamic nucleus; ZI, zona incerta; MG, medial geniculate; MMM, medial mammillary nucleus; P= pCPA; UC= uninjected controls. In each brain region, 2–4 grid areas were sampled depending on the size of the cell·population. (1 grid area = 0.0144 mm²); n = 4 animals/treatment group per [³H]thymidine injection age. Differences between treatment groups were analyzed using Duncan's multiple F-test. Asterisks denote P significantly different from UC at $p < 0.01$. (From Lauder et al., 1982a, by permission of Ankho, Inc.)

regions until late in the time course of neuronal genesis(E15–E16), when most neurons have already been formed.

Biochemical studies designed to ascertain the specificity of the pCPA treatment have demonstrated that tryptophan hydroxylase activity (TPH) in embryonic rat brain is dramatically inhibited by this maternal drug treatment (Table 13.2) (Lauder et al., 1981). This inhibition indicates that the maternal pCPA treatment used in our neuronal genesis studies probably severely suppresses 5-HT synthesis in the embryonic brain. This finding is supported by further preliminary studies using high pressure liquid chromatography (Lauder, Towle, Mueller and Breese, unpublished results), which indicate that maternal pCPA treatment does significantly deplete 5-HT levels in the embryonic brain. Moreover, immunocytochemical studies presently in progress indicate decreased staining of 5-HT neurons in embryos from pCPA-treated mothers (Lauder and Towle, unpublished results).

Relationship between serotonergic neurons and proliferating cells in embryonic rat brain
The evidence provided by these pharmacological, biochemical and immunocytochemical studies led us to examine possible relationships of 5-HT neurons to proliferating neuroepithelial cells located in the ventricular zone adjacent to the developing 5-HT neuronal complex (B4–B9), as well as in regions through which rostrally projecting 5-HT axons pass on their way to the forebrain. In these studies, we used a combined anti-5-HT immunocytochemical/[³H]thymidine autoradiographic method to simulta-

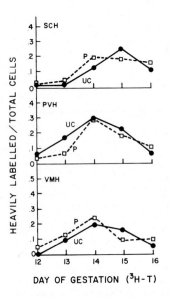

Fig. 13.3. Effects of maternal pCPA treatment on neuronal genesis in the anterior ventral diencephalon (hypothalamus). SCH: suprachiasmatic nucleus; PVH: paraventricular nucleus; VMH: ventromedial nucleus. Other abbreviations as described in legend to Fig. 2. (From Lauder et al., 1982a, by permission of Ankho, Inc.)

Table 13.2. Effects of various maternal treatments on embryonic rat tryptophan hydroxylase activity (whole head)

Values are means $\pm$ SEM. $*$ = A significant difference at $p < 0.01$ (t-test) for treatment mean compared to mean for normal controls. Numbers in parentheses indicate number of samples assayed. Each sample represents tissue pooled from 4 to 6 embryos. Treatments: DL-p-Chlorophenylalanine methyl-ester HCl (pCPA: 300 mg/kg in 2 ml saline ip on E8; 100 mg/kg in 1 ml ip, E9-killing); L-tryptophan (500 mg/kg in 2 ml 1 % carboxymethylcellulose, CMC, ip, E8-killing); hydrocortisone acetate (HCA: 20 mg/kg in 2 ml carboxymethylcellulose ip, E8-killing); corn (corn meal mixed with corn oil administered as sole dietary source ad libitum, E8-killing); stress (restraint in rat holder 15 min/day, E8-killing). Saline (1 ml ip, E8-killing). Day of insemination = E1.
(From Lauder et al., 1981, by permission of S. Karger.)

Treatment	Age of embryos (days) at killing	TPH activity (dpm $^{14}CO_2$/h per mg protein)	% of control
None (control	15	1.424 ± 72 (7)	100
Saline		1.365 ± 74 (8)	96
pCPA		128 ± 11 (6)	9*
L-Tryptophan		1.904 ± 105 (5)	134*
Corn		1.392 ± 42 (6)	98
HCA		1.407 ± 80 (4)	99
Restraint stress		1.382 ± 70 (6)	97
None (control)	17	1.618 ± 101 (6)	100
Saline		1.572 ± 92 (6)	97
pCPA		361 ± 20 (4)	22*
L-Tryptophan		2.122 ± 118 (6)	131*
Corn		1.780 ± 64 (6)	110
HCA		1.595 ± 68 (4)	99
Restraint stress		1.607 ± 72 (6)	99

neously localize 5-HT immunoreactive neurons and proliferating neuroepithelial cells in the same sections (Lauder et al., 1982b).

Since 5-HT neurons begin their own differentiation relatively early, both in terms of cessation of cell proliferation and neurotransmitter synthesis, it was to be expected that much proliferative activity would still be continuing in the adjacent ventricular zone, as these neurons begin to accumulate in the marginal zone on embryonic day 13 (E13; crown-rump length, CRL = 7 mm). Moreover, since 5-HT neurons send out processes as soon as they can be detected histochemically (Olson and Seiger, 1972) or immunocytochemically (Lauder et al., 1980), we constructed a model (Fig. 13.4A) to visualize how 5-HT neurons might engage in discrete cell-cell interactions with proliferating neuroepithelial cells in the ventricular zone. This model takes into account the fact that neuroepithelial cells undergo interkinetic nuclear migrations as they pass through the cell cycle (Sauer, 1936), such that their nuclei elevate to the outer boundaries of the ventricular zone during the G1 and S phases, then descend again towards the lumen during G2, finally rounding up for mitosis next to the lumenal surface. Architectonics such as those proposed in our model could allow for specific signalling between neuroepithelial cells and the more differentiated 5-HT neurons in their immediate vicinity.

298

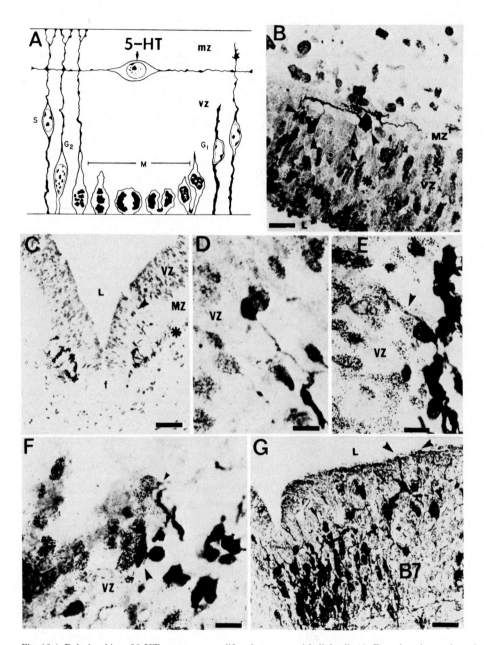

Fig. 13.4. Relationships of 5-HT neurons to proliferating neuroepithelial cells (A–F) and to the cerebrospinal fluid (G). (A): Hypothetical model of possible mode of interaction of 5-HT neurons located in the marginal zone (MZ) with proliferating neuroepithelial cells in the ventricular zone (VZ); S, G_2, M, G_1: phases of the cell cycle which neuroepithelial cells pass through as they undergo interkinetic nuclear migration. (B): embryonic day 13 (E13), crown-rump length (CRL) = 7 mm, sagittal plane, × 280. Bar = 36 μm. (C): E13–E14, CRL = 10 mm, transverse plane. Arrowhead designates cell shown in D. × 112. Bar = 90 μm. (D): E13–E14, CRL = 10 mm, transverse plane. 5-HT neuron apparently contacting proliferating

As shown in Fig. 13.4B, such an arrangement has been confirmed using our combined immunocytochemical/autoradiographic method in the E13 rat embryo (CRL 7 mm). At this age, a few 5-HT immunoreactive neurons can be seen dotting the marginal zone along an extent consisting approximately of the middle two-thirds of the B4–B9 complex. Interestingly, these small groups of neurons send out relatively long processes which fasciculate together as they course through the marginal zone adjacent to the perikarya of the proliferating neuroepithelial cells, which almost certainly send their apical processes through the path of these 5-HT fibers to reach the pial surface.

Within 12 h (E13–E14, CRL = 10 mm), many more 5-HT neurons have formed at the outer boundaries of the proliferating ventricular zone. As shown in Figs. 13.4C–F, some of these cells, in addition to sending rostrally projecting fibers through the marginal zone, also contact proliferating neuroepithelial cells directly, either by soma-somal interactions (Fig. 13.4C, D, F) or by varicose processes which extend into the ventricular zone (Fig. 13.4E).

Another possible way in which 5-HT neurons might influence the development of neuroepithelial cells could be through release of 5-HT into the CSF. This possibility is raised by the finding that some 5-HT neurons in the rostral aspect of the dorsal raphe nucleus send thick processes directly to the lumenal surface, as shown in Fig. 13.4G. It is conceivable that 5-HT, if released from these processes, could reach proliferating ventricular cells in brain regions not within the direct path of growing 5-HT axons.

Local cell-cell interactions between young 5-HT neurons and proliferating neuroepithelial cells might provide a mechanism whereby these neurons could exert an epigenetic influence upon less differentiated neuroepithelial cells in their vicinity. Alternatively, 5-HT might reach some parts of the neuroepithelium as a diffuse humoral signal carried in the CSF and influence the differentiation of more distantly located neuroepithelial cells not in direct physical contact with 5-HT neurons. Although the evidence is at best circumstantial, such relationships could be developmentally meaningful with respect to the differentiation of other 5-HT neurons, neurons of a different transmitter content located close to or even within the B4–B9 complex, or distant 5-HT target cells.

In a further attempt to gain insights into this dynamic developmental system through observations of necessarily static situations, we have traced the trajectories of rostrally projecting 5-HT axons of the B4–B9 complex through the diencephalon and

---

←

cell. × 640. Bar = 15 μm. (E): E13–E14, CRL = 10 mm, transverse plane. Arrowhead designates varicose process which appears to contact several proliferating cells in ventricular zone (VZ). × 700. Bar = 14 μm. (F): E13–E14, CRL = 10 mm, transverse plane. Large arrowhead designates 5-HT neuron in close contact with proliferating cell. Small arrowhead indicates thick process of 5-HT neuron looping close to proliferating cell. × 700. Bar = 14 μm. (B–F): [^{3}H]thymidine (40–60 Ci/mM, 10 μCi/g body weight) administered ip to pregnant rat on E14 (day 1 = day of insemination), 4 h prior to killing. (G): E15–E16, CRL = 14 mm, sagittal plane. Dorsal raphe nucleus (B7). Arrowheads designate thick processes of 5-HT neurons which may be in contact with the CSF since they extend through the ventricular zone to the lumen. × 170. Bar = 58 μm. f: floor plate of neural tube. Anti-5-HT immunocytochemistry (PAP method) and [^{3}H]thymidine autoradiography. (From Lauder et al., 1982a, by permission of Ankho, Inc.)

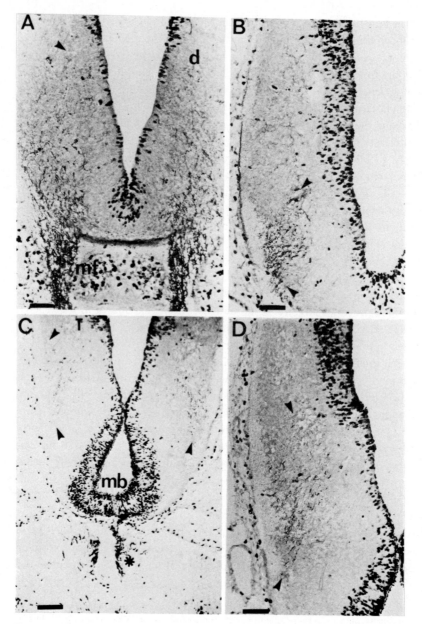

Fig. 13.5. Trajectory of rostrally projecting 5-HT axons relative to proliferative activity of the adjacent neuroepithelium. Note that location of fibers (designated by arrowheads) matches portion of neuroepithelium with least proliferative activity (E14–E15, CRL = 12 mm, sections horizontal to diencephalon, d). (A): Section through top of the mesencephalic flexure (mf). × 112. Bar = 90 μm. (B): Level ventral to A, cross-secting 5-HT axons as they pass ventrally into the posterior diencephalon. × 112. Bar = 90 μm. (C): Level ventral to B showing 5-HT axons in the vicinity of the developing mammillary body (mb). T: thalamus. × 70. Bar = 140 μm. Asterisk: 5-HT cell bodies cut in the transverse plane at the caudal end of the B4–B9 complex, near the pontine flexure. (D): Higher magnification of C. × 112. Bar = 90 μm. Anti-5-HT immunocytochemistry (PAP method) and [3H]thymidine autoradiography. [3H]Thymidine administered on E15 as described in Fig. 13.4. (From Lauder et al., 1982a, by permission of Ankho, Inc.)

have examined the proliferative activity of the neuroepithelium adjacent to these axons. As shown in Fig. 13.5, at E14–E15 (CRL = 12 mm), 5-HT axons seem to be located adjacent to a distinct segment of the neuroepithelium where proliferative activity is beginning to diminish, in contrast to the surrounding segments not adjacent to 5-HT axons where proliferation is more intense. This could indicate a cause-and-effect relationship between the presence of these fibers and such decreased proliferative activity. Alternatively, this could indicate that 5-HT axons grow into the most mature segment of the nearby diencephalon.

Possible roles for 5-HT during postnatal neurogenesis
Combined immunocytochemical-[^{3}H]thymidine autoradiographic studies as described above have been extended to the postnatal period in brain regions such as the cerebellum and hippocampus which are known to undergo much of their development after birth (Lauder et al., 1982b).

In the *cerebellum*, 5-HT axons have been observed growing into the white matter and regions of the deep cerebellar nuclei several days before birth. By postnatal day 2 (P2; Fig. 13.6A, B) a large number of these fibers can be seen in the white matter and especially in the presumptive internal granular layer (IGL). Serotonergic axons are also seen coursing into the molecular layer (ML) with occasional fibers running up to the proliferating external granular layer (EGL) which, however, they rarely penetrate. Other 5-HT fibers course parallel to the pia in the ML just beneath the EGL. Similar relationships are also observed in the P9 cerebellum (Fig. 13.6C, D) at a time when the bulk of granule cells are being generated from the EGL and migrating to the IGL.

Interactions between 5-HT axons and dividing cells in the IGL and ML (but not the EGL) are frequently seen in postnatal animals injected with [^{3}H]thymidine. Since the EGL is presumably the only source of proliferating neuronal precursor cells in the cerebellum, labeled cells in the IGL or ML in animals allowed to survive for only a few hours after injection of [^{3}H]thymidine must, by definition, be of glial rather than neuronal origin (Lewis et al., 1977b). Thus, 5-HT axons interact with glioblasts in the postnatally developing cerebellum, as demonstrated in Fig. 13.6. Although these relationships are more numerous at early postnatal ages (Fig. 13.6A, B), they are also found as late as the second week after birth (Fig. 13.6C, D). At this point, it is not clear whether 5-HT axons maintain these glial interactions into adulthood. However, it is possible that early relationships with 5-HT axons could affect the cellular activity of these glial cells (as suggested for norepinephrine in vitro; Nidess and Vernadakis, 1979), perhaps influencing the process of gliogenesis. Such developmental 5-HT neuronal-glial interactions might also be related to the expression of glial 5-HT receptors (Fillion et al., 1980) or uptake mechanisms which might be used in adult neuronal-glial interactions. Such issues must await clarification by future experimentation. It is already clear, however, that 5-HT axons are present during key phases of cerebellar development in locations which could allow them to exert their influence on such pro-

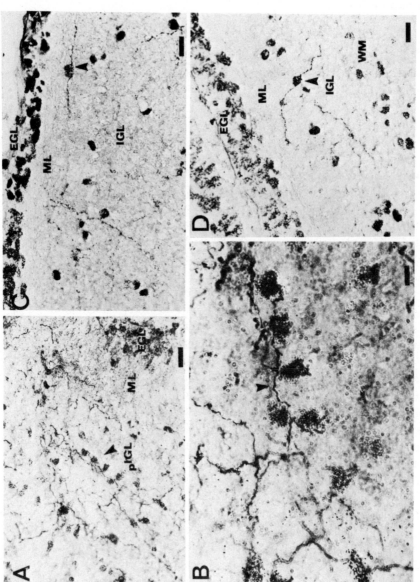

Fig. 13.6. Relationships of 5-HT axons to proliferating glioblasts in the developing cerebellum. (A): Postnatal day 2 (P2) coronal plane. Arrowhead denotes 5-HT axon running along 4 [³H]thymidine-labelled cells (×1120; bar = 4.5 μm) where small arrowhead designates this same fiber. pIGL: presumptive internal granular layer; ML: molecular layer; EGL: external granular layer. (C–D): P9, coronal plane, showing a sparser population of 5-HT axons which appear to contact (arrowheads) the occasional proliferating glioblasts which still remain in the IGL and ML. WM: white matter. ×280. Bar = 20 μm. [³H]Thymidine, 6.7 Ci/mM, 10 μCi/g body weight, injected subcutaneously on P2 or P9, survival 3–4 h. (From Lauder et al., 1982a, by permission of Anhas Inc.)

cesses as cell proliferation, migration of cells from the EGL or growth and differentiation of more mature cerebellar neurons such as the Purkinje cells.

It should be noted that axo-glial synapses during development have been reported in other systems (Grainger et al., 1968; Grainger and James, 1970; Henrikson and Vaughn, 1974; James and Tresman, 1969), but were interpreted as anomalities. More recently, however, axo-glial synapses have been found in cerebellar cultures and were interpreted as an indication of the plasticity of neuronal-glial interactions during development (Palacios-Prü et al., 1979).

In an experiment by Yamamoto et al. (1980), 5-HT neurons were transplanted into the fourth ventricle of the rat in the vicinity of the cerebellum at 4–14 days postnatally. These neurons survived and grew axons which somehow penetrated the cerebellum, causing a hyperinnervation of this region. Of particular interest in the present context is the fact that distinct disruptions of the Purkinje cell layer and clusters of ectopic granule cells were found in association with 5-HT axons, as if these fibers had altered the pattern of cell migration from the EGL and the lining up of Purkinje cells into a monolayer. Thus, this study also raises the possibility that 5-HT axons may be capable of influencing the differentiation of immature cells with which they come into contact during particular phases of cerebellar development.

In the developing *hippocampus*, serotonergic axons are first visible by E18 (Wallace and Lauder, 1983). Shortly after birth, fibers can be seen in the dentate gyrus (Fig. 13.7), where they contact labeled and unlabeled cells in [^{3}H]thymidine autoradiographs (Lauder et al., 1982a), particularly in the hilus region, which constitutes the main germinal zone for the granule cells (Bayer and Altman, 1974; Schlessinger et al., 1975). In addition, 5-HT fibers are frequently seen to traverse the granule cell layer during the first postnatal week. The serotonergic innervation of the dentate gyrus increases rapidly, such that a high density of fibers is seen in the hilus, granule cell layer and molecular layer by the end of the first postnatal week.

Thus, in the hippocampus as well as in the cerebellum, a 5-HT innervation is present in strategic locations during key phases of cell proliferation and differentiation. Such spatio-temporal relationships make these transmitter-containing axons good candidates for regulators of developmental functions in these brain regions.

In vitro studies of interactions between serotonergic neurons and proliferating cells
We began to explore these relationships in a dissociated cell culture system where serotonergic neurons from the embryonic rat brain are grown (together with other derivatives of the neuroepithelium) on a monolayer of non-neuronal cells (mainly astrocytes) or on polylysine alone. For these studies, E14 rat embryos (CRL = 10 mm) from timed pregnant Sprague-Dawley rats (Zivic Miller) are dissected to expose the brain, and a strip of tissue is removed between the mesenphalic and pontine flexures consisting of the ventral half of the metencephalon, including the floor plate, which contains the B4–B9 complex (Lauder et al., 1982a). This tissue is trypsinized and dissociated, then plated as a cell suspension either onto a layer of non-neuronal cells (mainly astro-

304

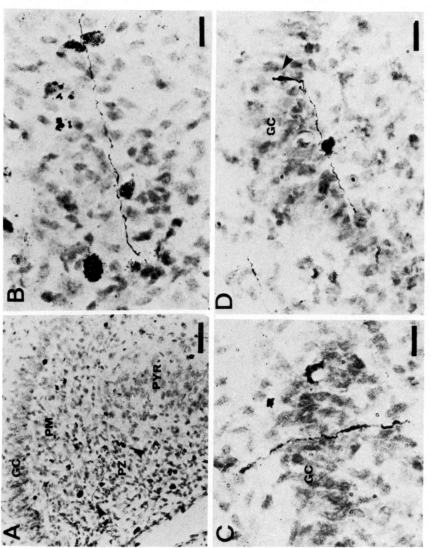

Fig. 13.7. 5-HT axons in the developing ventral hippocampus on postnatal day 2 (P2). (A): Arrowheads denote 5-HT axon in proliferative zone (PZ) of hilus of dentate gyrus (×44; bar = 220 μm). Same fiber is shown at higher magnification in B (×378; bar = 30 μm). PYR: pyramidal cell layer. [³H]Thymidine administered as in Fig. 13.4. PM: polymorph layer. (C,D): 5-HT axons in granule cell layer (GC). (D): Arrowhead points to apparent growth cone on 5-HT axon closely associated with proliferating cell at inner margin of the GC. (From Lauder et al., 1982a, by permission of Ankho, Inc.)

cytes) prepared according to McCarthy and DeVellis (1980) or directly onto polyly-sine-coated coverslips. These cultures are maintained in 12-well culture dishes containing Eagles basal medium, 10% fetal calf serum, 0.6% dextrose and penicillin/strepto-mycin. After several days, cultures are pulsed with [³H]thymidine, fixed, stained for immunocytochemistry and then prepared for autoradiography (Lauder et al., 1982b). It is also possible to stain these cultures with anti-5-HT and anti-GFAP simultaneously with or without [³H]thymidine autoradiography.

Using these methods, we have observed that 5-HT neurons seem to interact frequently with those cells identified as astrocytes (either derived from the embryonic brain or existing in the feeder layer of non-neuronal cells) due to their immunoreactivity with anti-glial fibrillary acidic protein (GFAP). If such cultures are also exposed to [³H]thymidine and prepared for autoradiography, it is clear that here as well as in the intact embryo 5-HT neurons interact closely with proliferating cells which, in this case, are either immature astrocytes or neuroepithelial cells (Fig. 13.8). In the future we hope to use this system to study the influence of 5-HT neurons on neuronal and glial precursor cell proliferation in vitro, as well as to explore the importance of neuronal-glial interactions for the differentiation of 5-HT neurons themselves.

Catecholamines and brain development

Other studies employing monoamine-depleting drugs such as 6-hydroxydopamine (6-OHDA) and reserpine have examined the possibility that catecholamines as well as serotonin might play roles in brain development. For example, Patel, Lewis and co-workers (Lewis et al., 1977a; Patel et al., 1977) found the administration of reserpine (which depletes both serotonin and catecholamines) from birth until 11 days postnatal produced changes in [³H]thymidine incorporation in forebrain and cerebellum, decreased glial cell proliferation in the subependymal layer of the lateral ventricle and caused a decreased mitotic index in the EGL of the cerebellum (location of neuronal precursor cells). Due to the presence of degenerating cells in such regions of cell proliferation, however, these workers interpreted their results as being due largely to toxic side effects of the drug. Nevertheless, in a more recent study using lower doses of reserpine (Patel et al., 1979), such side effects were in part ruled out, and yet a dose-dependent decrease in DNA synthesis was still observed (see Patel and Lewis, 1982 for a review of this and other related work). Therefore, although not unambiguous, these studies do lend support to the hypothesis that monoamines may play roles in the control of cell proliferation in the postnatally developing brain. Such a possibility is further strengthened by our own findings of interactions between the axons of 5-HT neurons and dividing glial or neuronal precursors in the postnatally developing cerebellum and hippocampus as discussed above (Figs. 13.6, 7).

In other studies employing 6-OHDA administration to neonates (which depletes catecholamines by destroying the nerve terminals containing them), defects in granule

306

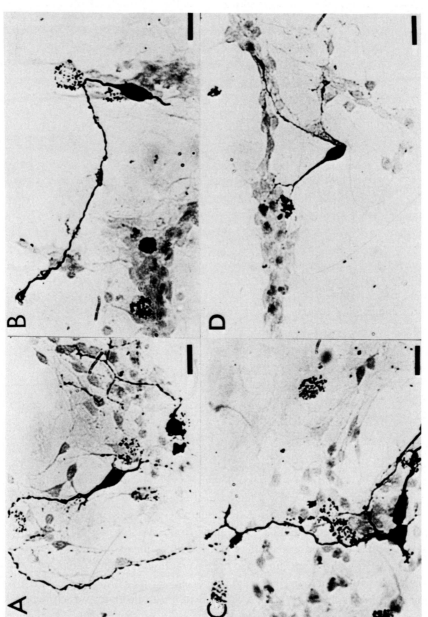

Fig. 13.8. Relationships of 5-HT neurons to proliferating neuroepithelial cells and non-neuronal cells in dissociated cultures derived from the metencephalon of the E14 rat embryo. A suspension of dissociated neural tube cells was plated onto a layer of non-neuronal cells (mainly astrocytes) growing on polylysine-coated coverslips (anti-5-HT immunocytochemistry, PAP method, and [³H]thymidine autoradiography). Bars =

cell migration, large deficits in granule cell numbers, abnormal foliation and fissuriza-
tion, and disorientation of Purkinje cell dendritic trees have been found in the developing cerebellum of drug-treated animals (Berry et al., 1980, 1981; Lovell, 1982; Sievers
et al., 1981). Again, it is not clear to what degree the effects of this treatment are the
results of cytotoxicity of the drug itself rather than resulting directly from the removal
of noradrenergic axons. However, in the study of Lovell (1982), much lower doses of
6-OHDA were used than in the other studies cited and no evidence of cytotoxicity
could be found. Although it is possible that some of the Purkinje cell dendritic tree
anomalies could be due to the absence of a large part of the granule cell population,
the effects on the granule cells themselves are interesting, especially if it can be demonstrated in future studies that NE fibers are in appropriate locations during cerebellar
development to explain such effects. Further evidence for an effect of catecholamine
neurons on cell migration in the cerebellum is found in the study of Rosenstein and
Brightman (1981), who transplanted fragments of superior cervical ganglia into the
postnatal rat cerebellum and found that EGL cells were either arrested at the brain
surface or migrated aberrantly to invade the graft. Basket cells and stellate cells were
also affected in addition to granule cells.

It should be noted here that in their study of the NE innervation of the chicken
cerebellum, Mugnaini and Dahl (1975) described a rich plexus of fibers in both the
IGL and ML. If NE fibers are present in these locations or in contact with the EGL
during granule cell genesis and migration, the above described effects of 6-OHDA
might be more easily interpretable. In fact, in a more recent study with an antiserum
to dopamine-β-hydroxylase (DBH), Verney et al. (1982) did show some thick, transient NE fibers in contact with the EGL, although these were not numerous.

In a prenatal study, Lidov and Molliver (1979) reported that injection of the rat
fetus with 6-OHDA on day 17 of gestation (E17) produced some abnormalities in cell
migration in cerebral cortex, such that distinct foci of ectopic neurons were found, but
since no other changes could be detected, this abnormality was also attributed to drug
toxicity. However, it should be noted that these 6-OHDA injections were done several
days after the arrival of NE fibers in the cortex, which may be too late to produce
clearcut effects on earlier cortical neurogenic events (Schlumpf et al., 1980). Moreover,
a more recent study, in which 6-OHDA administration caused extensive depletion of
NE in cerebral cortex, demonstrated dose-dependent changes in pyramidal cell dendritic arborizations, suggesting that NE axons may exert a neurotrophic role on cortical development during the period of most active dendritic growth, an effect which
may only be manifested upon complete removal of the NE innervation (Felten et al.,
1982).

With further reference to a possible trophic influence of NE fibers on dendritic
growth in the postnatally developing brain, several studies using either 6-OHDA or
locus coeruleus lesions should be mentioned (for review see Rakic and Goldman-
Rakic, 1982). In an early study, Maeda et al. (1974) reported that neonatal ablation
of the locus coeruleus resulted in an immature dendritic pattern for cerebral cortical

pyramidal cells of layer VI in animals sacrificed as young adults. In another study, Amaral et al. (1975) found that the dendrites of modified pyramidal cells in field CA4 of the hippocampus were abnormally long in adult rats treated with 6-OHDA as neonates. However, these results were not confirmed by Wendlandt et al. (1977). Based on these and other data, Berry et al. (1980) have speculated that monoamine fibers may help to induce dendritic outgrowth prenatally, although no clearcut evidence yet exists for such a function.

Kasamatsu and associates (Kasamatsu and Pettigrew, 1979; Kasamatsu et al., 1981; Kasamatsu et al., 1979) have recently reported that plasticity of the developing cat visual cortex seems to be influenced by NE, since 6-OHDA treatment of newborn kittens prevents the shift to ocular dominance normally seen after neonatal monocular deprivation. Microperfusion with NE, however, restores this plasticity and is restricted to the immediate vicinity of such perfusions. Moreover, it should be noted that microperfusions of NE can also restore this plasticity in monocularly deprived animals who presumably are past the 'critical period' for ocular dominance shifts. Of related interest is a study by Parnavelas and Blue (1982), who demonstrated a significant increase in synaptic density in cerebral cortex of rats in which the noradrenergic innervation has been eliminated postnatally by 6-OHDA, indicating that NE fibers could exert an inhibitory influence on cortical synaptogenesis. Two other studies using postnatal treatment with phenylalanine in combination with pCPA to simulate the condition of hyperphenylalaninemia (phenylketonuria; PKU) have reported changes in dendritic morphology of both cerebellar Purkinje cells and layer V pyramidal cells in cerebral cortex, which appear to be related to the distribution of monoaminergic nerve terminals, at least in the cerebellum (Hogan and Coleman, 1981a, b).

Summary

Thus, both positive and negative evidence now exists for roles of monoamines in pre- and postnatal brain development. However, evidence is now accumulating in favor of such developmental roles for these neurotransmitter substances. This is largely due to the realization that many of these effects may be subtle in nature and demonstrable only during appropriate 'critical periods'. The demonstration of such effects will necessitate rigorous experimental analyses to elucidate them, where present, and to distinguish them from artifacts which also will occur when neurotoxic agents must be employed, especially in high doses.

If neurotransmitters such as the monoamines do, in fact, play roles in key ontogenic processes such as neural tube formation, germinal cell proliferation, gliogenesis and neuronal differentiation, it is possible that drugs of use and abuse, which exert their actions in the adult brain via these neurotransmitter systems, could perturb these developmental events if present during those critical periods when such humoral influences are important for normal ontogeny.

References

Ahmad, G. and Zamenhof, S. (1978) Serotonin as a growth factor for chick embryo brain. Life Sci. 22, 963–970.

Allan, I.J. and Newgreen, D.F. (1977) Catecholamine accumulation in neural crest cells and the primary sympathetic chain. Am. J. Anat. 149, 413–421.

Amaral, D.G., Foss, J.A., Kellogg, C. and Woodward, D.J. (1975) Effects of subcutaneous administration of 6-hydroxydopamine (6-OHDA) in neonatal rats on dendritic morphology in the hippocampus. Neurosci. Abstr. 1, 789.

Baker, P.C. (1965) Changing serotonin levels in developing Xenopus laevis. Acta Embryol. Morphol. Exp. 8, 197–204.

Bartels, W. (1971) Die Ontogenese der aminhaltigen Neuronensysteme im Gehirn von Rana temporaria. Z. Zellforsch. 116, 94–118.

Bayer, S.A. and Altman, J. (1974) Hippocampal development in the rat: Cytogenesis and morphogenesis examined with autoradiography and low level X-irradiation. J. Comp. Neurol. 158, 55–80.

Berry, M., McConnell, P. and Sievers, J. (1980) Dendritic growth and the control of neuronal form. In: Current Topics in Developmental Biology (Hunt, R.K., Monroy, A. and Moscona, A.A., eds.) Academic, Press, New York, pp. 67–101.

Berry, M., Sievers, J. and Baumgarten, H.G. (1981) Adaption of the cerebellum to deafferentation. Prog. Brain Res. 53, 65–92.

Blum, J.J. (1970) Biogenic amines and metabolic control in tetrahymena. In: Biogenic Amines as Physiologic Regulators (Blum, J.J., ed.) Prentice-Hall, New Jersey, pp. 95–118.

Boucek, R.J. and Bourne, B.B. (1962) Catecholamines of the allantoic fluid in the developing chick embryo. Nature 193, 1181–1182.

Burack, W.R. and Badger, A. (1964) Sequential appearance of DOPA decarboxylase, dopamine-β-oxidase and norepinephrine N-methyltransferase activities in embryonic chick. Fed. Proc. 23, 561.

Burden, H.W. and Lawrence, I.E. (1973) Presence of biogenic amines in early rat development. Am. J. Anat. 136, 251–257.

Buznikov, G.A. (1980) Biogenic monoamines and acetylcholine in protozoa and metazoan embryos. In Neurotransmitters, Comparative Aspects (Salánki, J. and Turpaev, T.M., eds.) Akadémiai Kiadó, Budapest, pp. 7–29.

Buznikov, G.A. and Schmukler, Yu. B. (1981) Possible role of 'prenervous neurotransmitters' in cellular interactions of early embryogenesis: A hypothesis. Neurochem. Res. 6, 55–68.

Buznikov, G.A., Chudakova, I.V. and Znezdina, N.D. (1964) The role of neurohumors in early embryogenesis. I. Serotonin content of developing embryos of sea urchin and loach. J. Embryol. Exp. Mophol. 12, 563–573.

Buznikov, G.A., Chudakova, I.V., Berdysheva, L.V. and Vyazmina, N.M. (1968) The role of neurohumors in early embryogenesis. II. Acetylcholine and catecholamine content in developing embryos of sea urchin. J. Embryol. Exp. Morphol. 20, 119–128.

Buznikov, G.A., Kost, A.N., Kucherova, N.F., Mndzhoyan, A.L., Suvorov, N.N. and Berdysheva, L.V. (1970) The role of neurohumors in early embryogenesis. III. Pharmacological analysis of the role of neurohumors in cleavage divisions. J. Embryol. Morphol. 23, 549–569.

Buznikov, G.A., Sakharova, A.V., Manukhin, B.N. and Markova, L.V. (1972) The role of neurohumors in early embryogenesis. IV. Fluorometric and histochemical study in cleaving eggs and larvae of sea urchins. J. Embryol. Exp. Morphol. 27, 339–351.

Cadilhac, J. and Pons, F. (1976) Le développement prénatal des neurones a monoamines chez le rat. C. R. Soc. Biol. 170, 25–31.

Caston, J.D. (1962) Appearance of catecholamines during development of Rana pipiens. Dev. Biol. 5, 468–482.

Chronwall, B. and Wolff, J.R. (1980) Prenatal and postnatal development of GABA-accumulating cells in the occipital neocortex of rat. J.Comp. Neurol. 190, 187–208.

310

Clark, R.L., Venkatasubramanian, K., Wolf, J.M. and Zimmerman, E.F. (1980) Serotonin stimulation of protein caroboxymethylation and chemotaxis in palate. J. Cell Biol. 87, 55a.

Cochard, P., Goldstein, M. and Black, I. (1978) Ontogenetic appearance and disappearance of tyrosine hydroxylase and catecholamines in the rat embryo. Proc. Natl. Acad. Sci. USA 75(6), 2986–2990.

Curtis, D.H. and Zalin, R.J. (1981) Regulation of muscle differentiation: Stimulation of myoblast fusion in vitro by catecholamines. Science 214, 1355–1357.

Deeb, S.S. (1972) Inhibition of cleavage and hatching of sea urchin embryos by serotonin. J. Exp. Zool. 181, 79–86.

Emanuelsson, H. (1974) Localization of serotonin in cleavage embryos of *Ophryotrocha labronica* La Greca and Bacci. Wilhelm Roux' Arch. 175, 253–271.

Emanuelsson, H. and Palén, K. (1975) Effects of L-tryptophan on morphogenesis and growth in the early chick blastoderm. Wilhelm Roux' Arch. 177, 1–17.

Felten, D.L., Hallman, H. and Jonsson, G. (1982) Evidence for a neurotrophic role of noradrenaline in the postnatal development of rat cerebral cortex. J. Neurocytol. 11, 119–135.

Fillion, G., Beaudoin, D., Rousselle, J.C. and Jacob, J. (1980) [^{3}H]5-HT binding sites and adenylate cyclase in glial cell membrane fraction. Brain Res. 198, 361–374.

Filogamo, G., Peirone, S. and Sisto Daneo, L. (1978) How early do myoblast determination and fast and slow muscle fiber differentiation occur? In: Maturation of Neurotransmission (Vernadakis, A., Giacobini, E. and Filogamo, G., eds.) Karger, Basel, pp. 1–9.

Franquinet, P.R. (1979) Rôle de la sérotonine et des catécholamines dans la régénération de la planaire *Polycelis tenuis*. J. Embryol. Exp. Morphol. 51, 85–95.

Franquinet, R. and Martelly, I. (1981) Effects of serotonin and catecholamines on RNA synthesis in planarians; in vitro and in vivo studies. Cell Diff. 10, 201–209.

Gérard, A., Gérard, H. and Dollander, A. (1978) Capture et rétention de sérotonine tritiée par la chorde dorsale d'embryon de Poulet. C. R. Acad. Sci. Paris, Ser. D, 286, 891–894.

Gershon, D., Teitelman, G., Rothman, T.P., Joh, T.H. and Reis, D.J. (1979) Proliferation and lack of species and organ specificity in transient catecholaminergic cells of developing mammals. Soc. Neurosci. Abst. 5, 334.

Gilman, A.G. and Nirenberg, M. (1971) Effect of catecholamines on the adenosine 3':5'cyclic monophosphate concentrations of clonal satellite cells of neurons. Proc. Natl. Acad. Sci. USA 68, 2165–2168.

Golden, G.S. (1972) Embryologic demonstration of a nigro-striatal projection in the mouse. Brain Res. 44, 278–282.

Golden, G.S. (1973) Prenatal development of biogenic amine systems of the mouse brain. Dev. Biol. 33, 300–311.

Grainger, F. and James, D.W. (1970) Association of glial cells with terminal parts of neurite bundles extending from chick spinal cord in vitro. Z. Zellforsch. 108, 93–104.

Grainger, F., James, D.W. and Tresman, R.L. (1968) An electron-microscopic study of the early outgrowth from chick spinal cord in vitro. Z. Zellforsch. 90, 53–67.

Gustafson, T. and Toneby, M. (1970) On the role of serotonin and acetylcholine in sea urchin morphogenesis. Exp. Cell Res. 62, 102–117.

Gustafson, T. and Toneby, M. (1971) How genes control morphogenesis. Am. Sci. 59, 452–462.

Henrikson, C.K. and Vaughn, J.E. (1974) Fine structural relationship between neurites and radial glial processes in developing mouse spinal cord. J. Neurocytol. 3, 659–675.

Hogan, R.N. and Coleman, P.D. (1981a) Experimental hyperphenylalaninemia: dendritic alterations in motor cortex of rat. Exp. Neurol. 74, 218–233.

Hogan, R.N. and Coleman, P.D. (1981b) Experimental hyperphenylalaninemia: dendritic alterations in cerebellum of rat. Exp. Neurol. 74, 234–244.

Ignarro, L.J. and Shideman, F.E. (1968a) Appearance and concentrations of catecholamines and their biosynthesis in the embryonic and developing chick. J. Pharmacol. Exp. Ther. 159, 38–48.

Ignarro, L.J. and Shideman, F.E. (1968b) Norepinephrine and epinephrine in the embryo and embryonic heart of the chick: uptake and subcellular distribution. J. Pharmacol. Exp. Ther. 159, 49–58.

James, D.W. and Tresman, R.L. (1969) Synaptic profiles in the outgrowth from chick spinal cord in vitro. Z. Zellforsch. 10, 598–606.

Jurand, A. (1980) Malformations of the central nervous system induced by neurotropic drugs in mouse embryos. Dev. Growth Diff. 22, 61–70.

Kasamatsu, T. and Pettigrew, J.D. (1979) Preservation of binocularity after monocular deprivation in the striate cortex of kittens treated with 6-hydroxydopamine. J. Comp. Neurol. 185, 139–162.

Kasamatsu, T., Pettigrew, J.D. and Ary, M. (1979) Restoration of visual cortical plasticity by local microperfusion of norepinephrine. J. Comp. Neurol. 185, 163–182.

Kasamatsu, T., Pettigrew, J.D. and Ary, M. (1981) Cortical recovery from effects of monocular deprivation: Acceleration with norepinephrine and suppression with 6-hydroxydopamine. J. Neurophysiol. 45, 254–266.

Kirby, M.L. and Gilmore, S.A. (1972) A fluoresence study on the ability of the notochord of synthesize and store catecholamines in early chick embryos. Anat. Rec. 173, 469–478.

Kujawa, M.J. and Zimmerman, E.F. (1978) Palate cells in culture: 5-HT induced contraction and neural crest origin. Teratology 17, 29A.

Lauder, J.M. and Bloom, F.E. (1974) Ontogeny of monoamine neurons in the locus coeruleus, raphe nuclei and substantia nigra of the rat I. Cell differentiation. J. Comp. Neurol. 155, 469–481.

Lauder, J.M. and Bloom, F.E. (1975) Ontogeny of monoamine neurons in the locus coeruleus, raphe nuclei and substantia nigra of the rat II. Synaptogenesis. J. Comp. Neurol. 163, 251–264.

Lauder, J.M. and Krebs, H. (1976) Effects of p-chlorophenylalanine on time of neuronal origin during embryogenesis in the rat. Brain Res. 107, 638–644.

Lauder, J.M. and Krebs, H. (1978a) Serotonin as a differentiation signal in early neurogenesis. Dev. Neurosci. 1, 15–30.

Lauder, J.M. and Krebs, H. (1978b) Serotonin and early neurogenesis. In: Maturation of Neurotransmission (Vernadakis, A., Giacobini, E. and Filogamo, G., eds.) Karger, Basel, pp. 171–180.

Lauder, J.M., Sze, P.Y. and Krebs, H. (1981) Maternal influences on tryptophan hydroxylase activity in embryonic rat brain. Dev. Neurosci. 4, 291–295.

Lauder, J.M., Wallace, J.A. and Krebs, H. (1980) Serotonin as a timing mechanism in neuroembryogenesis. In: Progress in Psychoneuroendocrinology (Brambilla, F., Racagni, G. and de Wied, D., eds.) Elsevier, Amsterdam, pp. 539–556.

Lauder, J.M., Wallace, J.A., Krebs, H., Petrusz, P. and McCarthy, K. (1982a) In vivo and in vitro development of serotonergic neurons. Brain Res. Bull. 9, 605–625.

Lauder, J.M.., Petrusz, P., Wallace, J.A., DiNome, A., Wilkie, M.B. and McCarthy, K. (1982b) Combined sertonin immunocytochemistry and [³H]thymidine autoradiography: In vivo and in vitro methods. J. Histochem. Cytochem. 30, 788–793.

Lawrence Jr., I.E. and Burden, H.W. (1973) Catecholamines and morphogenesis of the chick neural tube and notochord. Am. J. Anat. 137, 199–208.

Levitt, P. and Rakic, P. (1979) Genesis of central monoamine (MA) neurons in the Rhesus monkey. Soc. Neurosci. Abst. 5, 341.

Lewis, P.D., Patel, A.J., Béndek, G. and Balázs, R. (1977a) Effect of reserpine on cell proliferation in the developing rat brain: a quantitative histological study. Brain Res. 129, 299–308.

Lewis, P.D., Fülöp, Z., Hajós, F., Balázs, R. and Woodhams, P.L. (1977b) Neuroglia in the internal granular layer of the developing rat cerebellar cortex. Neuropathol. Appl. Neurobiol. 3, 183–190,

Lidov, H.G.W. and Molliver, M.E. (1979) Neocortical development after prenatal lesions of noradrenergic projections. Neurosci. Abstr. 5, 341.

Lovell, K.L. (1982) Effects of 6-hydroxydopamine-induced norepinephrine depletion on cerebellar development. Dev. Neurosci. 5, 359–368.

Maeda, T. and Dresse, A. (1969) Recherches sur le développement du locus coeruleus. Etude des catécholamines au microscope de fluorescence. Acta Neurol. Belg. 69, 5–10.

Maeda, T., Tohyama, M. and Shimizu, N. (1974) Modification of postnatal development of neocortex in rat brain with experimental deprivation of locus coeruleus. Brain Res. 70, 515–520.

312

Manukhin, B.N., Volina, E.V., Markova, L.N., Rakić, L. and Buznikov, G.A. (1981) Biogenic monoamines in early embryos of sea urchins. Dev. Neurosci. 4, 322–328.

McCarthy, K.D. and DeVellis, J.D. (1980) Preparation of separate astroglial and oligodendroglial cell cultures from rat cerebral cortex. J. Cell Biol. 85, 890–902.

Morse, D.E., Hooker, N., Duncan, H. and Jensen, L. (1979) γ-Aminobutyric acid, a neurotransmitter, induces planktonic abalone larvae to settle and begin metamorphosis. Science 204, 407–410.

Mugnaini, E. and Dahl, A.-L. (1975) Mode of distribution of aminergic fibers in the cerebellar cortex of the chicken. J. Comp. Neurol. 162, 417–432.

Müller, W.A., Mitze, A., Wickhorst, J.-P. and Meier-Menge, H.M. (1977) Polar morphogenesis in early hydroid development: Action of caesium, of neurotransmitters and of an intrinsic head activator on pattern formation, Wilhelm Roux's Arch. 182, 311–328.

Nidess, R. and Vernadakis, A. (1979) Protein synthesis in neural cells in culture: Role of cell density and neurohumors. Mech. Aging Dev. 10, 39–52.

Oey, J. (1975) Noradrenaline induces morphological alterations in nucleated and enucleated rat C6 glioma cells. Nature 257, 317–319.

Olson, L. and Seiger, Å. (1972) Early prenatal ontogeny of central monoamine neurons in the rat: fluorescence histochemical observations. Z. Anat. Entwickl. Gesch. 137, 301–316.

Olson, L., Boreus, L.O. and Seiger, Å. (1973) Histochemical demonstration and mapping of 5-hydroxytryptamine and catecholamine-containing neuron systems in the human fetal brain. Z. Anat. Entwickl. Gesch. 139, 259–282.

Palacios-Prü, E., Palacios, L. and Mendoza, R.V. (1979) In vitro formation of neuroglial synapses. J. Neurosci. Res. 4, 115–122.

Palén, K., Thörneby, L. and Emanuelsson, H. (1979) Effects of serotonin anatagonists on chick embryogenesis. Wilhelm Roux's Arch. Dev. Biol. 187, 89–103.

Parnavelas, J.G. and Blue, M.E. (1982) The role of the noradrenergic system on the formation of synapses in the visual cortex of the rat. Dev. Brain Res. 3, 140–144.

Patel, A.J., Bailey, P. and Balázs, R. (1979) Effect of reserpine on cell proliferation and energy stores in the developing rat brain. Neuroscience 4, 139–143.

Patel, A.J., Béndek, G., Balázs, R. and Lewis, P.D. (1977) Effect of reserpine on cell proliferation in the developing rat brain: a biochemical study. Brain Res. 129, 283–297.

Patel, A.J. and Lewis, P.D. (1982) Effects on cell proliferation of pharmacological agents acting on the central nervous system. In: Mechanisms of Actions of Neurotoxic Substances (Prasad, K.N. and Vernadakis, A., eds.) Raven Press, New York, pp. 181–218.

Pénit, J., Cantau, B., Huot, J. and Jard, S. (1977) Adenylate cyclase from synchronized neuroblastoma cells: responsiveness to prostaglandin E_1, adenosine and dopamine during the cell cycle. Proc. Natl. Acad. Sci. USA 74, 1575–1579.

Pienkowski, M.M. (1977) Involvement of biogenic amines in control of early mouse embryos. Anat. Rec. 189(3), 550.

Prasad, K. and Gilmer, K.N. (1974) Demonstration of dopamine-sensitive adenylate cyclase in malignant neuroblastoma cells and change in sensitivity of adenylate cyclase to catecholamines in 'differentiated' cells. Proc. Natl. Acad. Sci. USA 71, 2525–2529.

Rakic, P. and Goldman-Rakic, P.S., eds. (1982) Development and modifiability of the cerebral cortex. Neurosci. Res. Prog. Bull. 20.

Rodriguez, N. and Renaud, F.L. (1980) On the possible role of serotonin in the regulation of regeneration of cilia. J. Cell Biol. 85, 242–247.

Rosenstein, J.M. and Brightman, M.W. (1981) Anomalous migration of central nervous tissue to transplanted autonomic ganglia. J. Neurocytol. 10, 387–409.

Sahu, S.K. and Prasad, K.N. (1975) Effects of neurotransmitters and prostaglandin E_1 on cyclic AMP levels in various clones of neuroblastoma cells in culture. J. Neurochem. 24, 1267–1269.

Santander, R.G. and Cuadrado, G.M. (1976) Ultrastructure of the neural canal closure in the chicken embryo. Acta Anat. 95, 368–383.

Sauer, F.C. (1936) The interkinetic migration of embryonic epithelial nuclei. J. Morphol. 60, 1–11.

Schlessinger, A.R., Cowan, W.M. and Gottlieb, D.I. (1975) An autoradiographic study of the time of origin and the pattern of granule cell migration in the dentate gyrus of the rat. J. Comp. Neurol. 159, 149–176.

Schlumpf, M. and Lichtensteiger, W. (1979) Catecholamines in the yolk sac epithelium of the rat. Anat. Embryol. 156, 177–187.

Schlumpf, M., Shoemaker, W.J., and Bloom, F.E. (1977) The development of catecholamine fibers in the prenatal cerebral cortex of the rat. Soc. Neurosci. Abstr. 3, 361.

Schlumpf, M., Shoemaker, W.J., and Bloom, F.E. (1980) Innervation of embryonic rat cerebral cortex by catecholamine-containing fibers. J. Comp. Neurol. 192, 361–376.

Schowing, J., Sprumont, P. and Van Toledo, B. (1977) Influence of L. 5-hydroxytryptophan on the development of the chick embryo. C. R. Acad. Sci. (Paris) 171(6), 1163–1166.

Schubert, D., Tarikas, H. and LaCorbiere, M. (1976) Neurotransmitter regulation of adenosine 3′,5′-monophosphate in clonal nerve, glia, and muscle cell lines. Science 30, 471–472.

Schwartz, J.P., Morris, N.R. and Breckenridge, B. McL. (1973) Adenosine 3′,5′-monophosphate in glial tumor cells. Alterations by 5-bromodeoxyuridine. J. Biol. Chem. 248, 2699–2704 (1973).

Sievers, J., Berry, M. and Baumgarten, H. (1981) The role of noradrenergic fibres in the control of postnatal cerebellar development. Brain Res. 207, 200–208.

Sims, T.J. (1977) The development of monoamine-containing neurons in the brain and spinal cord of the salamander, *Ambystoma mexicanum*. J. Comp. Neurol. 173, 319–336.

Specht, L.A., Pickel, V.M., Joh, T.H. and Reis, D.J. (1978a) Ultrastructure of the nigrostriatal system in early prenatal rat brain by immunochemical localization of tyrosine hydroxylase. Neurosci. Abstr. 4, 386.

Specht, L.A., Pickel, V.M., Joh, T.H. and Reis, D.J. (1978b) Immunocytochemical localization of tyrosine hydroxylase in processes within the ventricular zone of prenatal rat brain. Brain Res. 156, 315–321.

Specht, L.A., Pickel, V.M., Joh, T.H. and Reis, D.J. (1981) Light microscopic immunocytochemical localization of tyrosine hydroxylase in prenatal rat brain. I. Early ontogeny. J. Comp. Neurol. 199, 233–253.

Steinbusch, H.W.M. (1981) Distribution of serotonin-immunoreactivity in the central nervous system of the rat-cell bodies and terminals. Neuroscience 4, 557–618.

Strudel, G., Meiniel, P. and Gateau, G. (1977a) Recherches d'amines flurigenes dans les chordes d'embryons de Poulet traités par des cholinergiques. C. R. Acad. Sci. Paris 284, 1097–1100.

Strudel, G., Recasens, M. and Mandel, P. (1977b) Identification de cátecholamines et de sérotonine dans les chordes d'embryons de Poulet. C. R. Acad. Sci. Paris 284, 967–969.

Taban, C.H. and Cathieni, M. (1979) Localization of substance P-like immunoreactivity in *Hydra*. Experientia 35, 811–812.

Taber Pierce, E. (1973) Time of origin of neurons in the brainstem of the mouse. Prog. Brain Res. 40, 53–65.

Teitelman, G., Joh, T.H. and Reis, D.J. (1978) Transient expression of a noradrenergic phenotype in cells of the rat embryonic gut. Brain Res. 158, 229–234.

Tennyson, V.M., Barrett, R.E., Cohen, G., Cote, L., Heikkila, R. and Mytilineou, C. (1972) The developing neostriatum of the rabbit: Correlation of fluorescence histochemistry, electron microscopy, endogenous dopamine levels, and [H³]dopamine uptake. Brain Res. 46, 251–285.

Tennyson, V.M., Budininkas-Schoenebeck, M. and Gershon, P. (1982) Effects of chronic reserpine treatment on development of maturity of the putamen in fetal rabbits. Brain Res. Bull. 9, 651–662.

Tennyson, V.M., Mytilineou, C. and Barrett, R.E. (1973) Fluorescence and electron microscopic studies of the early development of the substantia nigra and area ventralis tegmenti in the fetal rabbit. J. Comp. Neurol. 149, 233–258.

Tennyson, V.M., Mytilineou, C., Heikkila, R., Barrett, R.E., Cole, L. and Cohen, G. (1975) Development of dopamine containing neuroblasts of the substantia nigra. In: The Golgi Centennial Symposium (Santini, M., ed.) Raven Press, New York, pp. 449–464.

314

Tomkins, G. (1975) The metabolic code. Science 189, 760-763.

Toneby, M. (1977) Functional Aspects of 5-Hydroxytryptamine and Dopamine in Early Embryogenesis of *Echinoidea* and *Asteroidea*. University of Stockholm, Stockholm.

Venkatasubramanian, K., Clark, R.L., Wolff, J.M. and Zimmerman, E.F. (1980) Translocation of palatal mesenchymal cells through a collagen gel matrix. J. Cell Biol. 87, 114a.

Vernadakis, A. (1973) Comparative studies of neurotransmitter substances in the maturing and aging central nervous system of the chicken. Prog. Brain Res. 40, 231-243.

Verney, C., Grzanna, R. and Farkas, E. (1982) Distribution of dopamine-beta-hydroxylase-like immunoreactive fibers in the rat cerebellar cortex during ontogeny. Dev. Neurosci. 5, 369-374.

Wallace, J.A. (1979) Biogenic amines in the development of the early chick embryo. Ph. D. Thesis, University of California, Davis, CA.

Wallace, J.A. (1982) Monoamines in the early chick embryo: Demonstration of serotonin synthesis and the regional distribution of serotonin-concentrating cells during morphogenesis. Am. J. Anat. 165, 261-276.

Wallace, J.A. and Lauder, J.M. (1983) Development of the serotonergic system in the rat embryo. Brain Res. Bull. 10, 459-479.

Wee, E.L., Babiarz, B.S., Zimmerman, S. and Zimmerman, E.F. (1979) Palate morphogenesis. IV. Effects of serotonin and its antagonists on rotation in embryo culture. J. Embryol. Exp. Morphol. 53, 75-90.

Wee, E.L., Phillips, N.J., Babiarz, B.S. and Zimmerman, E.F. (1980) Palate morphogenesis. V. Effects of cholinergic agonists and antagonists on rotation in embryo culture. J. Embryol. Exp. Morphol. 58, 177-193.

Wendlandt, T.J., Crow, T.J. and Stirling, R.V. (1977) The involvement of the noradrenergic system arising from the locus coeruleus in the postnatal development of the cortex in the rat brain. Brain Res. 125, 1-9.

Wolff, J.R., Rickmann, M. and Chronwall, B.M. (1979) Axo-glial synapses and GABA-accumulating glial cells in the embryonic neocortex of the rat. Cell Tissue Res. 201, 239-248.

Yamamoto, M., Chan-Palay, V., Steinbusch, H.W.M. and Palay, S.L. (1980) Hyperinnervation of arrested granule cells produced by the transplantation of monoamine-containing neurons into the fourth ventricle of rat. Anat. Embryol. 159, 1-15.

Yew, D.T., Ho, A.K.S. and Meyer, D.B. (1974) Effect of 6-hydroxydopamine on retinal development in the chick. Experientia 30, 1320-1322.

Zimmerman, E.F., Wee, E.L., Clark, R.L. and Venkatasubramanian, K. (1980) Neurotransmitter and teratogen involvement in cell mediated palatal elevation. In: International Symposium on Current Research Trends in Craniofacial Development (Christiansen, R.L. and Pratt, R.L., eds.) Elsevier/North-Holland, Amsterdam, pp. 187-202.

Neurobehavioral Teratology
edited by Joseph Yanai
© Elsevier Science Publishers BV 1984

14

AGE AT THE TIME OF TESTING RECONSIDERED IN NEUROBEHAVIORAL TERATOLOGICAL RESEARCH

Linda Patia Spear

Department of Psychology and Center for Neurobehavioral Sciences,
State University of New York at Binghamton, Binghamton, NY 13901, USA

T HE nervous system is particularly sus-
ceptible to chemical insults during its development. Such insults may produce no overt
signs of gross malformations and yet may have notable consequences on the fine structure of the nervous system that are manifest in altered behavior of the organism at
various times during the life span. When assessing the potential of a chemical agent
as a neurobehavioral teratogen, it is important to consider that the manifest effects
of a teratogen may vary substantially with testing age. For instance, three possible time
courses of the expression of a neurobehavioral teratogenic insult traditionally have
been emphasized (e.g. Adams and Buelke-Sam, 1981): (1) A potential neurobehavioral
teratogen may produce behavioral effects early in life due to an ontogenetic alteration
or delay in nervous system development that becomes less evident later in life as a result of compensatory ontogenetic growth. (2) A potential teratogen may produce an
alteration in behavior and the nervous system that becomes most evident in adulthood
at the time when the affected neuronal system normally would have matured into
playing an important role in brain function (i.e. the so-called 'growing into one's deficits', a term derived originally from studies of infant brain damage, e.g. Isaacson,
1975). (3) Another possibility is that a teratogen may produce subtle alterations that
are most evident later in life with the decline in neural function seen during the aging
process, leading in some cases to premature senescence or death (e.g. Spyker, 1975).

It is important to realize that these three are not the only possible age-specific manifestations of a neuroteratological insult. For example, it is possible that an insult-induced alteration in behavioral functioning may be discontinuous, appearing at a restricted time during development or, conversely, being less evident at a particular age than at younger or older ages. Such ontogenetic discontinuities in the behavioral manifestations of a neuroteratological insult may be a result of specific maturational events occurring at a particular time during ontogeny that may either mask or accentuate the expression of the underlying central nervous system alterations produced by the teratogen.

Consideration of testing age in neurobehavioral teratological research is important from several perspectives. For example, to determine the true teratogenic potential of a substance, it is critical to assess the long-term effects of the potential teratogen throughout the life span. Moreover, it is important to recognize that disparities reported among studies in the manifest effects of teratogens may be related partially to differences among studies in age at the time of testing. In addition to these rather pragmatic concerns, the ontogenetic pattern of manifest effects of teratogen also may be of import from a more theoretical perspective. The ontogenetic timing of appearance of behavioral manifestations induced by a teratogen may provide both suggestions as to the neural mechanisms by which these behavioral alterations are produced, as well as information potentially contributing to the further elucidation of general patterns of neural functioning and their development.

In spite of the importance of careful consideration of testing age as a variable in teratological research, relatively few studies have included a systematic manipulation of this significant factor. The largest proportion of studies in this area have assessed the animals in adulthood after chemical insults during development. This approach leaves unresolved the issues of which developmental processes lead to the structural and functional alterations evident at maturity. Of that research which has examined animals at different stages of their life span, most have used longitudinal designs where the performance on a different test is examined at each age. Though relatively cost-efficient, such longitudinal survey approaches are difficult to evaluate; significant differences found with one test at one age, and not with other tests at other ages, could be due to the sensitive nature of that particular test, or alternatively could be a result of testing at a particularly 'sensitive' age for expressing the effects of the insult, or possibly could be a function of both factors.

To illustrate the importance of testing age as a variable in neurobehavioral teratological studies, two general types of examples will be given in this chapter. Both examples will present discontinuities in the ontogenetic appearance of behavioral alterations induced by administration of neurobehavioral teratogens influencing the catecholaminergic systems. These two types of illustrative examples differ, however, in the nature of the ontogenetic discontinuities that are observed. The first example will present a teratogen-induced behavioral alteration appearing at a restricted time during development and not at younger or older ages. Conversely, in the second example, a temporary age-specific amelioration of the appearance of behavioral alterations induced by an ontogenetic insult will be discussed. These examples were chosen to demonstrate the importance and utility of systematic consideration of age at the time of testing as a variable in neurobehavioral teratological research.

Transient hyperactivity produced by neonatal 6-hydroxydopamine

6-Hydroxydopamine (6-OHDA) is a catecholaminergic neurotoxin that is particularly potent in permanently depleting forebrain catecholamines after administration during the neonatal period. Although 6-OHDA has neurotoxic effects on both dopaminergic and noradrenergic neuronal populations, the relative degree of depletion of each catecholamine can be selectively manipulated. For example, while central administration of moderate or substantial doses of 6-OHDA has a long-term neurotoxic effect on both the dopamine (DA) and norepinephrine (NE) neurotransmitter systems, central administration of low doses of 6-OHDA, or peripheral 6-OHDA administration, prior to the development of a blood-brain barrier to this substance, depletes NE while having little influence on DA levels (e.g. Smith et al., 1973; Schmidt and Bhatnagar, 1979). Pretreatment with a drug that inhibits NE uptake, demethylimipramine (DMI), prior to intracisternal or intraventricular 6-OHDA administration results in a fairly specific depletion of DA alone (Smith et al., 1973).

Several studies have reported that neonatal administration of 6-OHDA in DMI-pretreated rat pups induces a transient period of locomotor hyperactivity which first appears at approximately 15 days postnatally and dissipates shortly after weaning (Shaywitz et al., 1976a, b; Shaywitz et al., 1977; Pappas et al., 1980; Concannon and Schechter, 1982; Pappas et al., 1982). From the summary of these studies presented in Table 14.1, it is evident that this transient hyperactivity appearing after neonatal 6-OHDA and DMI treatment is an example of an ontogenetic discontinuity in the behavioral manifestations of a neuroteratogen.

'Normal' non-treated animals during this time-span exhibit ontogenetic alterations in locomotor activity when tested in isolation. Campbell and associates have observed that the locomotor activity of isolated rat pups begins to increase around 12 days postnatally, peaks at 15 days of age, and returns to approximately the levels seen in 10 day old animals by 25 days of age (Campbell et al., 1969; Moorcroft et al., 1971; Campbell and Mabry, 1972). 6-OHDA-treated animals also exhibit an inverted U-shaped function of locomotor activity across this age span, although the amount of locomotor activity they exhibit during the transient ontogenetic period of increased activity is significantly greater than that of untreated control animals. Thus, it is approximately during this period of normal ontogenetic 'hyperactivity' that rat pups neonatally treated with 6-OHDA are significantly more active than control age-mates.

There have been several explanations of the ontogenetic increase and decrease in activity that has been observed in intact animals during this age period. Originally,

Table 14.1. Transient hyperactivity induced by neonatal treatment with 6-OHDA and DMI

Symbols: ↑, hyperactive when compared with controls; 0, no significant difference in activity when compared with controls; –, animals not tested at that postnatal age; P, postnatal day; ic, intracisternal.

Ref.	Treatment	Testing days						
		P8–10	P12	P15–16	P19–20	P22	P25–26	P29–30
Pappas et al. (1982)	P1–2; 6-OHDA (50 μg total) intrastriatum and DMI	0	–	↑	–	–	0	–
Concannan and Schechter (1982)	P5, 6-OHDA (100 μg) ic and DMI	–	–	0	↑	–	0	0
Pappas et al. (1980)	P1–2; 6-OHDA (50 μg total) lat. ventricles and DMI	0	–	↑	↑	–	0	0
Shaywitz et al. (1977)	P5; 6-OHDA (100 μg) ic and DMI	0	0	↑	↑	↑	0	0
Shaywitz et al. (1976a)	P5; 6-OHDA (100 μg) ic and DMI	0	↑	↑	↑	↑	0	0
Shaywitz et al. (1976b)	P5; 6-OHDA (100 μg) ic and DMI	0	0	↑	↑	↑	↑	–

Campbell and associates attributed the age-related increase in activity peaking at 15 days postnatally to the gradual maturation of excitatory catecholaminergic systems, and the decrease in activity observed after this peak to the maturation of inhibitory forebrain serotonergic and cholinergic systems (Campbell et al., 1969; Fibiger et al., 1970; Campbell and Mabry, 1973; Mabry and Campbell, 1974). Later, Campbell and associates suggested that this transient ontogenetic increase in activity was a function of testing animals in isolation away from siblings and the home nest; they observed that locomotor activity remained fairly constant over this age period if pups were tested in the presence of an anesthetized adult (Randall and Campbell, 1976) or odors from the home nest (Campbell and Raskin, 1978). From such data, they concluded that "these findings...raise serious questions about the ontogenetic sequence of excitation followed by inhibition postulated by Campbell and his associates" (Randall and Campbell, 1976, p. 458), yet they declined to replace this theoretical formulation with another directly addressing the issue of why isolation should produce differential effects on locomotor activity across age. Whatever the physiological mechanisms subserving the inverted U-shaped function of locomotor activity across age, one could postulate that such mechanisms are not disrupted in animals treated with 6-OHDA and DMI because a similar nonmonotonic function is seen in treated animals, although the levels of their locomotor activity are even greater than that of control animals during the 'hyperactive' phase.

Miller et al. (1981) have argued that the postweaning dissipation of hyperactivity seen in rats neonatally treated with 6-OHDA and DMI is related to the extent of DA depletion is not seen after administration of substantial doses of 6-OHDA into the forebrain ventricles. After injections of 6-OHDA into the lateral ventricles following DMI pretreatment on postnatal days 3 and 6, they observed that animals treated with a total of 50 or 70 μg tivity peaking at 16–20 days of age. The locomotor activity of the animals treated with these doses of 6-OHDA was significantly greater than that of control age-mates by 16–18 days of age and had largely returned to control levels by 24–30 days of age, thus presenting a similar profile of transient hyperactivity to that observed in the studies outlined in Table 14.1. At higher doses of 6-OHDA, a different ontogenetic profile of locomotor activity was observed. Rats treated with a total of 100 or 200 μg of 6-OHDA on postnatal days 3 and 6 showed an increase in locomotor activity at 16–18 days of age that was similar to that seen after the lower doses of 6-OHDA. However, the locomotor activity in these animals treated with the higher doses of 6-OHDA remained elevated and was not characterized by the post-weaning decline typical of both vehicle control animals and animals treated with lower doses of 6-OHDA. In these animals neonatally treated with 100–200 μg 6-OHDA, hyperactivity was first evident at 18 days of age, and they continued to be more active than control animals throughout the remaining test period (until 32 days of age). Other animals neonatally injected with these same doses of 6-OHDA were tested in adulthood (postnatal days 56–62). Only the animals given 200 μg 6-OHDA neonatally were still hyperactive in adulthood. From these results, Miller et al. (1981) concluded that the duration of hyperactivity was greatest in animals that experienced the largest depletion of DA.

Similar results were reported in another study by the same group (Erinoff et al., 1979). Animals pretreated with DMI and injected with a total of 200 μg 6-OHDA into the lateral ventricles on postnatal days 3 and 6 failed to show the ontogenetic decline in locomotor activity normally seen in control animals around the time of weaning, and were still hyperactive when compared with age-mate controls when tested between 46 and 62 days of age. In that study, the effects of age at the time of 6-OHDA treatment were also examined. Injection of a total of 200 μg 6-OHDA into the lateral ventricles over two injection days was reported to induce hyperactivity in adulthood if the injections were given at 3 and 6, 11 and 14, or 20 and 23 days postnatally, although no hyperactivity was seen if the injections were given at 46 and 48 days of age. From these results the investigators concluded that the decline in locomotor activity seen ontogenetically around the time of weaning may be dependent on dopaminergic functioning, and furthermore "that DA depletion per se does not lead to increased locomotor activity, but rather it is the removal of dopaminergic fibers before the normal period of locomotor suppression which results in elevated locomotor activity" (Erinoff et al., 1979, p. 204).

Weaning as being a critical age for catecholaminergic maturational processes is also seen in another quite different example concerning the ontogenetic manifestations of neonatal treatment with 6-OHDA. In adult animals, 6-OHDA injections have been reported to decrease post-decapitation convulsions in rats (e.g. Fukuda et al., 1975). Saari et al. (1978) examined the ontogeny of this response after subcutaneous administration of 6-OHDA on the first day of life. While 6-OHDA-treated subjects displayed an increased latency to convulse and a decreased number of convulsive kicks neonatally as well as in adulthood, there were no differences between 6-OHDA-treated subjects and vehicle controls in either measure at 20 days of age. Thus, with these post-decapitation convulsions as well as with locomotor activity, testing animals around the age of weaning may produce a different pattern of manifestations of the effects of 6-OHDA when compared with that seen earlier or later in life, perhaps in part due to maturational events occurring in the catecholaminergic systems during that period in ontogeny.

The influence of age at the time of assessing locomotor activity after neonatal 6-OHDA illustrates how ontogenetic patterns in the manifest behavioral effects of neuroteratogens can further understanding of the role of nascent brain systems in the mediation of ontogenetic behaviors. These data suggest that the typical ontogenetic increase in locomotor activity seen in pre-weanling animals is not dependent on normal dopaminergic levels, although the ontogenetic decline in locomotor activity seen in post-weanling animals may indeed be dependent upon adequate dopamine levels during that period of life. These suggestions derived from teratological investigations of 6-OHDA are markedly different from those originally hypothesized after work with intact animals. As discussed previously, Campbell and associates initially suggested, on the basis of studies examining the acute response of intact animals to psychoactive drugs during ontogeny, that the ontogenetic increase in locomotor activity seen at approximately 15 days postnatally was a result of catecholaminergic maturational processes, with the decline in activity seen in weanling animals being a function of maturation of serotonergic and cholinergic inhibitory systems (Campbell et al., 1969; Fibiger et al., 1970; Campbell and Mabry, 1973; Mabry and Campbell, 1974). Thus, teratological studies in which animals are tested across a wide age-span may provide information about nascent brain systems that are difficult to examine in the intact animal, and thus may valuably augment conceptualization of neuronal functioning and its ontogeny derived from other research approaches.

Testing age as a critical variable in assessing the effects of chronic haloperidol treatment during development

Several years ago, my laboratory became interested in assessing the effects of chronic pre- and postnatal administration of the dopaminergic antagonist, haloperidol, on behavioral and psychopharmacological sensitivity later in life. In our initial work in this area, female rats were given twice daily subcutaneous injections of 0.25 mg/kg per ml haloperidol from the first day of gestation until the weaning of their offspring on postnatal day 21 (Spear et al., 1980). Haloperidol is a lipophilic drug that crosses the placental barrier and is rapidly partitioned into milk (Lundborg and Ross, 1974; Ziv et al., 1974; Goldberg and DiMascio, 1978); thus, pups received the drug both prenatally and postnatally via the maternal female.

Although the pups were tested for catalepsy during the preweaning period, we were interested primarily in the behavior of the pups after termination of the drug treatment regime at weaning. To assess whether age at the time of testing was a critical variable in determining the effects of this chronic treatment, different groups of offspring were tested at various times after treatment termination: postnatal days (P) 23–30, P35–42 and P47–54. On the first two testing days, offspring were given a 10 min test in an open field-hole poke apparatus. On the third day during each testing interval, offspring were given drugs prior to open field testing (including doses of 2, 5 or 10 mg/kg *dl*-amphetamine or saline). On the last day of each testing interval (one week after the first day of open field testing), offspring were given a catalepsy test every 30 min for 4 h after the intraperitoneal administration of saline, 0.5, 1 or 2 mg/kg haloperidol.

We hypothesized that the offspring would be most profoundly influenced by the chronic treatment when tested shortly after treatment termination, and that they might exhibit progressively fewer behavioral symptoms with time after termination of the treatment. As an alternative but intuitively less appealing hypothesis, we postulated that the effects of the chronic developmental drug treatment would instead become more pronounced with time, the so-called 'growing into one's deficits' seen after some types of brain damage early in infancy (e.g. Isaacson, 1975).

Much to our surprise, the effects we observed were not consistent with either of these two initial hypotheses. Haloperidol-treated animals tested during the immediate post-weaning period (P23–30) or as young adults (P47–54) were hyperactive in the open field-hole poke apparatus, and exhibited an increase in hole poke behavior when compared with control age-mates. They were also less sensitive to amphetamine when measured in terms of increases in open field activity and were more sensitive to the cataleptic effects of a test dose of haloperidol when compared with age-mate control animals. In marked contrast, however, haloperidol-treated offspring tested during the periadolescent period (P35–42) did not vary significantly from control age-mates in amount of locomotor behavior, nor in responsivity to amphetamine or haloperidol. At this age, haloperidol-treated offspring differed significantly from control age-mates only in the hole poke response measure where they exhibited a decrease in hole poke behavior, a pattern of response opposite to that observed with this behavior in haloperidol-treated animals tested as weanlings or as young adults. As can be seen in the summary of this data presented in Table 14.2, the manifest behavioral effects of early chronic administration of haloperidol appeared to be largely ameliorated in a temporary fashion during the periadolescent period.

This age-specific attenuation seen during periadolescence of the behavioral alterations induced by ontogenetic administration of haloperidol is remarkably similar to the ontogenetic patterns reported by Nomura and Segawa (1978) following administration of the catecholaminergic neurotoxin 6-hydroxydopa at birth, and by Monder (1978) following chronic prenatal administration of amphetamine. In the Nomura and Segawa (1978) study, for example, 6-hydroxydopa-treated animals were more sensitive than control age-mates to the stimulant effects of apomorphine at 14, 20 and 50 days postnatally, but were less sensitive than controls when tested at 30 days of age

322

Table 14.2. Influence of age at the time of testing on the manifest behavioral effects of chronic
haloperidol treatment during development
Summary of data from Spear et al. (1980).

Behavior response measure	Age at testing		
	P23–30	P35–42	P47–54
Locomotor activity	hyperactive	no difference	hyperactive
Hole-poke behavior	increased	decreased	increased
Response to amphetamine	attenuated	no difference	possibly attenuated
Response to haloperidol	accentuated	no difference	accentuated

and were not different from control animals at 40 days postnatally. The results of these
studies suggest that some developmental phenomena occurring around adolescence
may temporarily mask, in animals tested at this age, the consequences of early chronic
treatment with drugs influencing the catecholaminergic systems.

There is also some suggestion that the effects of neonatal 6-OHDA on locomotor
activity may also be different during the periadolescent period than earlier or later
in life. As discussed previously, neonatal treatment with 6-OHDA has been shown to
produce transient hyperactivity that is evident between roughly 15 and 22 days postnatally after moderate depletions of DA (see Table 14.1 for references), and hyperactivity that is also evident in adulthood with more extensive DA depletions (Erinoff et
al., 1979; Miller et al., 1981). Yet, Smith et al. (1973) reported that intracisternal administration of 100 μg 6-OHDA in combination with DMI pretreatment on postnatal
day 7 produces *hypo*activity when animals are tested during the periadolescent period
(age at the time of testing for locomotor activity was not precisely detailed in the original article although in a subsequent article by the same group (Mueller et al., 1980)
they mentioned that the testing in this earlier study had occurred on postnatal day
42). Although these comparisons by necessity involve cross-laboratory comparisons
and thus are subject to numerous confounds, the markedly different profile of locomotor activity induced by neonatal 6-OHDA seen during the periadolescent period as
compared with testing earlier or later in life is reminiscent of other marked ontogenetic
discontinuities seen at that age in the manifestation of the effects of neuroteratogens
influencing the catecholaminergic systems.

We (Spear and Brake, 1983) have reviewed the behavior and psychopharmacological sensitivity of rats during the periadolescent period (from approximately 30 to 42
days postnatally). It appears that, when compared with other-aged rats, periadolescents are hyperactive and engage in more conspecific play behavior (Baenninger,
1967; Bronstein, 1972, 1973; Lanier and Isaacson, 1977; Spear et al., 1980; Meaney
and Stewart, 1981; Panksepp, 1981). Periadolescents also exhibit enhanced performance of simple active-avoidance learning tasks, but perform more poorly in more
complex appetitive and avoidance learning tasks when compared with other-aged rats
(e.g. Bronstein and Spear, 1972; Campbell et al., 1974; Amsel and Chen, 1976; Bur-

dette et al., 1976; Myslivecek and Hassamannova, 1979; Bauer, 1980; Brake et al., 1980; Niemi and Thompson, 1980), perhaps as a result of age-specific alterations in selective attention or stimulus processing. Periadolescence is also associated with an attenuated sensitivity to catecholaminergic agonists along with an accentuated sensitivity to the catecholaminergic antagonist haloperidol (e.g. Bauer and Duncan, 1975; Lanier and Isaacson, 1977; Infurna and Spear, 1979; Spear and Brick, 1979; Shalaby and Spear, 1980; Spear et al., 1980). Evidence is presented in this review to support the hypothesis that a negative feedback system in the form of dopamine autoreceptors may become functionally mature in mesolimbic brain regions during the periadolescent period (i.e. Shalaby and Spear, 1980; Shalaby et al., 1981; Scalzo and Spear, 1982), and that maturation of these self-inhibitory autoreceptors might result in a temporary decrease in the efficacy of mesolimbic dopamine projections, perhaps contributing to the psychopharmacological and behavioral characteristics of periadolescent animals.

Consequently, the periadolescent period appears to be characterized by both an age-specific alteration in catecholaminergic activity as well as a temporary amelioration of, or alteration in, the manifest effects of early chronic administration of drugs affecting the catecholaminergic systems. This suggests the tentative possibility that perhaps the temporary alterations seen during periadolescence in the manifest effects of early chronic treatment with neurobehavioral teratogens are a function of developmental events, such as autoreceptor development in dopaminergic mesolimbic terminal regions, occurring in the catecholaminergic systems during that period in ontogeny. Regardless of the ultimate veracity of this tentative hypothesis, it is clear from this example that the effects of neurobehavioral teratogens cannot be considered in isolation; the manifest effects of a neurobehavioral teratogen at any particular age must be embedded upon the functional constitution of the nervous system at that particular point in the life span.

Summary and Discussion

Two different types of examples of ontogenetic discontinuities in the appearance of behavioral effects after neuroteratological insults influencing the catecholaminergic systems have been presented to illustrate the importance of age at the time of testing as a variable in neurobehavioral teratological research. In the first case, an example was given of a transient appearance of behavioral alterations following developmental administration of a catecholaminergic neurotoxin. In the second case, a temporary amelioration of, or alteration in, the behavioral manifestations of neurobehavioral teratogens influencing the catecholaminergic systems was seen during the periadolescent period. As illustrated in these examples, the underlying maturational state of the nervous system presumably influence in a profound manner the manifest behavioral effects of a neuroteratogen when assessed at any particular point in ontogeny.

324

When examining a neurobehavioral teratogen with known or suspected effects upon a particular neurotransmitter system, it appears to be critical to assess its long-term effects not only in adulthood, but also during and surrounding ontogenetic periods when there may be important developmental events occurring in the potentially affected neurotransmitter system. For instance, in the examples presented in this chapter, it appears that normal developmental processes occurring within the catecholaminergic systems at certain ages may contribute to the ontogenetic discontinuities observed in the manifest behavioral effects of neuroteratogens. Consequently, it appears that systematic consideration of such age periods would be particularly important when working with neurobehavioral teratogens that influence catecholaminergic neuronal function or maturation.

In cases where it is unclear what effects a particular neurobehavioral teratogen has on a neurotransmitter system(s), the time course of behavioral alterations induced by the neuroteratogen may provide suggestive evidence as to which neurotransmitter systems are influenced by the teratogen. For example, there is some evidence that lead may alter dopaminergic functioning after chronic administration during development (e.g. Lucchi et al., 1981). Yet, there has been no systematic examination of lead-treated subjects during age periods when there appear to be developmental modifications in catecholaminergic neuronal functioning. However, Zenick et al. (1979) tested lead-treated and control animals in an open field longitudinally, beginning before the periadolescent period and extending into the first few days of periadolescence. Lead-treated animals were observed to be hyperactive only on the last few days of open field testing, i.e. during the periadolescent period. While other factors could of course contribute to the appearance of hyperactivity at this time (e.g. the longitudinal testing design), these results are intriguing in that they might possibly reflect that periadolescence is a 'sensitive' period for assessing the effects of early chronic lead treatment, perhaps as a function of alterations in dopaminergic activity occurring at that ontogenetic age. This suggestion needs to be more systematically examined by testing different groups of lead-treated and control animals before, during and after the periadolescent period.

While the examples used in this chapter to illustrate the importance of testing age in neurobehavioral teratological research have focused on chemical insults influencing the catecholaminergic systems, similar ontogenetic discontinuities in the manifest behavioral effects of neuroteratogens may also occur with drugs influencing other neurotransmitter systems. As only one illustrative example, neonatal administration of a serotonergic neurotoxin, 5,7-dihydroxytryptamine, has been reported to induce hyperactivity in 14 day old animals (Breese et al., 1978), while having no influence on locomotor activity at 19 days of age (Isaacson et al., 1977), and inducing hypoactivity when animals are tested at 28 (Breese et al., 1978) or 34 (Isaacson et al., 1977) days of age. Are there critical maturational events occurring during this ontogenetic time span in the serotonergic system that may provide an altering ontogenetic baseline of serotonergic activity upon which the long-term effects of this neurotoxin are embedded? Are similar profiles of behavioral discontinuities seen after administration of other drugs influencing the serotonergic systems early in development? Further research is needed to address these questions, the answers to which may provide important information regarding serotonergic maturation valuable to research in neurobehavioral teratology and developmental psychobiology in general.

A new approach being emphasized in the field of developmental psychobiology involves a consideration of age-specific behaviors, or what Oppenheim calls 'ontogenetic adaptations' (e.g. Henderson, 1981; Oppenheim, 1980, 1981). According to this approach, infant behaviors, rather than being viewed as inadequate, fractional antecedents of adult behaviors, are viewed as perfectly adequate behaviors specifically adapted evolutionarily to the animal's age-specific ethological niche. The behavior of the developing organism is unique, and the developing nervous system may play a significant role in these behaviors quite apart from its incidental maturational course en route to the control of adult behavior. Behavioral development according to this view is not always progressive and continuous, but rather is sometimes characterized by age-specific quantitative of qualitative alterations resulting from the moment-to-moment interplay between nascent and established neural systems during ontogeny. Consideration of this interplay occurring in the nervous system during development is important for research in neurobehavioral teratology in that this normal ontogenetic background provides a changing matrix upon which the long-term effects of teratogens are embedded. It is quite possible that the observed behavioral effects of teratogens may be either more pronounced or less evident at certain points in the lifespan than at other ages as a result of the functional constitution of the nervous system at that age. Research using a developmental approach to examine systematically the ontogenetic appearance of behavioral effects induced by neuroteratogens has the potential to reveal a great deal about the processes of normal neural maturation and how they are altered by chemical insults early in life.

Acknowledgments

This work was supported in part by grants 1R01MH33215 and 1R01MH35761 from the National Institute of Mental Health.

References

Adams, J. and Buelke-Sam, J. (1981) Behavioral assessment of the postnatal animal: testing and methods development. In: Developmental Toxicology (Kimmel, C.A. and Buelke-Sam, J., eds.) Raven Press, New York, pp. 233–258.

Amsel, A. and Chen, J.S. (1976) Ontogeny of persistence: immediate and long-term persistence in rats varying in training age between 17 and 65 days. J. Comp. Physiol. Psychol. 90, 808–820.

Baenninger, L.P. (1967) Comparison of behavioral development in socially isolated and grouped rats. Anim. Behav. 15, 312–323.

Bauer, R.H. (1980) Shuttlebox avoidance in Norway rats from infancy to maturity. Bull. Psychon. Soc. 15, 15–17.

Bauer, R.H. and Duncan, D.L. (1975) Differential effects of d-amphetamine in mature and immature rats. Physiol. Psychol. 3, 312–316.

Brake, S.C., Burdette, D.R., Chen, J.S. and Amsel, A. (1980) Retention of response persistence in weanling and adolescent rats. J. Comp. Physiol. Psychol. 94, 1060–1068.

Breese, G.R., Vogel, R.A. and Mueller, R.A. (1978) Biochemical and behavioral alterations in developing rats treated with 5,7-dihydroxytryptamine. J. Pharmacol. Exp. Ther. 205, 587–595.

Bronstein, P.M. (1972) Open field behavior of the rat as a function of age. J. Comp. Physiol. Psychol. 80, 335–341.

Bronstein, P.M. (1973) Replication report: age and open-field activity of rats. Psychol. Rep. 32, 403–406.

Bronstein, P.M. and Spear, N.E. (1972) Acquisition of a spatial discrimination by rats as a function of age. J. Comp. Physiol. Psychol. 78, 206–212.

Burdette, D.R., Brake, S.C., Chen, J.S. and Amsel, A. (1976) Ontogeny of persistence: immature extinction effects in preweanling and weanling rats. Anim. Learn. Behav. 4, 131–138.

Campbell, B.A. and Mabry, P.D. (1972) Ontogeny of behavioral arousal: a comparative study. J. Comp. Physiol. Psychol. 81, 371–379.

Campbell, B.A. and Mabry, P.D. (1973) The role of catecholamines in behavioral arousal during ontogenesis. Psychopharmacologia, 31, 253–264.

Campbell, B.A. and Raskin, L.A. (1978) Ontogeny of behavioral arousal: the role of environmental stimuli. J. Comp. Physiol. Psychol. 92, 176–184.

Campbell, B.A., Lytle, L.D. and Fibiger, H.C. (1969) Ontogeny of adrenergic arousal and cholinergic inhibitory mechanisms in the rat. Science 166, 635–637.

Campbell, B.A., Misanin, J.R., White, B.C. and Lytle, L.D. (1974) Species differences in the ontogeny of memory: indirect support for neutral mediation as a determinant of forgetting. J. Comp. Physiol. Psychol. 87, 193–202.

Concannon, J.T. and Schechter, M.D. (1982) Failure of amphetamine isomers to decrease hyperactivity in developing rats. Pharmacol. Biochem. Behav. 17, 5–9.

Erinoff, L., MacPhail, R.C., Heller, A. and Seiden, L.S. (1979) Age-dependent effects of 6-hydroxydopamine on locomotor activity in the rat. Brain Res. 164, 195–205.

Fibiger, H.C., Lytle, L.D. and Campbell, B.A. (1970) Cholinergic modulation of adrenergic arousal in the developing rat. J. Comp. Physiol. Psychol. 72, 384–389.

Fukuda, T., Araki, Y. and Suenaga, N. (1975) Inhibitory effects of 6-hydroxydopamine on the clonic convulsions induced by electroshock and decapitation. Neuropharmacology 14, 579–583.

Goldberg, H.L. and DiMascio, A. (1978) Psychotropic drugs in pregnancy. In: Psychopharmacology : A Generation of Progress (Lipton, M.A., DiMascio, A. and Killam, K.R., eds.) Raven Press, New York, pp. 1047–1055.

Henderson, N.D. (1981) Genetic influences on locomotor activity in 11-day-old house mice. Behav. Genet. 11, 209–225.

Infurna, R.N. and Spear, L.P. (1979) Developmental changes in amphetamine-induced taste aversions. Pharmac. Biochem. Behav. 11, 31–35.

Isaacson, R.L. (1975) The myth of recovery from early brain damage. In: Aberrant Development in Infancy: Human and Animal Studies (Ellis, N.R., ed.) Lawrence Erlbaum Associates, Potomac, MD, pp. 1–26.

Isaacson, R.L., Fish, B.F., Lanier, L.P. and Dunn, A. (1977) Serotonin reduction early in life and its effects on behavior. Life Sci. 21, 213–222.

Lanier, L.P. and Isaacson, R.L. (1977) Early development changes in the locomotor response to amphetamine and their relation to hippocampal function. Brain Res. 126, 567–575.

Lucchi, L., Memo, M, Airaghi, M.L., Spano, P.F. and Trabucchi, M. (1981) Chronic lead treatment induces in rat a specific and differential effect on dopamine receptors in different brain regions. Brain Res. 213, 397–404.

Lundborg, P. and Ross, B.E. (1974) Increased concentration of homovanillic acid in the brains of infant rabbits after administration of haloperidol to their nursing mothers. J. Pharm. Pharmacol. 26, 816–818.

Mabry, P.D. and Campbell, B.A. (1974) Ontogeny of serotonergic inhibition of behavioral arousal in the rat. J. Comp. Physiol. Psychol. 86, 193–201.

Meaney, M.J. and Stewart, J. (1981) A descriptive study of social development in rat (Rattus norvegicus). Anim. Behav. 29, 34–45.

Miller, F.E., Heffner, T.G., Kotake, C. and Seiden, L.S. (1981) Magnitude and duration of hyperactivity following neonatal 6-hydroxydopamine is related to the extent of brain dopamine depletion. Brain Res. 229, 123–132.

Monder, H. (1978) Effects of prenatal amphetamine on the development of behavior in rats. Doctoral dissertation, SUNY-Binghamton, New York.

Moorcroft, W.H., Lytle, L.D. and Campbell, B.A. (1971) Ontogeny of starvation-induced behavioral arousal in the rat. J. Comp. Physiol. Psychol. 75, 59–67.

Mueller, R.A., Mailman, R.B. and Breese, G.R. (1980) Behavioral and monoaminergic consequences of exposure to neurotoxins during development. In: Biogenic Amines in Development (Parvez, H. and Parvez, S., eds.) Elsevier/North-Holland Biomedical Press, Amsterdam, pp. 617–639.

Myslivecek, J. and Hassamannova, J. (1979) Ontogeny of active avoidance in the rat: learning and memory. Dev. Psychobiol. 12, 169–186.

Niemi, R.R. and Thompson, W.R. (1980) Pavlovian excitation, internal inhibition, and their interaction with free operant avoidance as a function of age in rats. Dev. Psychobiol. 79, 61–76.

Nomura, Y. and Segawa, T. (1978) Apomorphine-induced locomotor stimulation in developing rats treated with 6-hydroxydopamine. Eur. J. Pharmacol. 50, 153–156.

Oppenheim, R.W. (1980) Metamorphosis and adaptation in the behavior of developing organisms. Dev. Psychobiol. 13, 353–356.

Oppenheim, R.W. (1981) Ontogenetic adaptations and retrogressive processes in the development of the nervous system and behavior: A neuroembryological perspective. In: Maturation and Development: Biological and Psychological Perspectives (Connolly, K.J. and Prechtl, H.F.R., eds.) Lippincott, Philadelphia, PA, pp. 73–109.

Panksepp, J. (1981) The ontogeny of play in rats. Dev. Psychobiol. 14, 327–332.

Pappas, B.A., Gallivan, J.V., Dugas, T., Saari, M. and Ings, R. (1980) Intraventricular 6-hydroxydopamine in the newborn rat and locomotor responses to drugs in infancy: no support for the dopamine depletion model of minimal brain dysfunction. Psychopharmacology, 70, 41–46.

Pappas, B.A., Vickers, G., Buxton, M. and Pusztay, W. (1982) Infant rat hyperactivity elicited by home cage bedding is unaffected by neonatal telecephalic dopamine or norepinephrine depletion. Pharmacol. Biochem. Behav. 16, 151–154.

Randall, P.K. and Campbell, B.A. (1976) Ontogeny of behavioral arousal in rats: effect of maternal and sibling presence. J. Comp. Physiol. Psychol. 90, 453–459.

Saari, M., Ings, R. and Pappas, B.A. (1978) Ontogeny of the post-decapitation convulsion in the rat: effects of neonatal systemic 6-hydroxydopamine. Neuropharmacology 17, 873–877.

Scalzo, F. and Spear, L.P. (1982) The functional ontogeny of dopamine autoreceptors in the nucleus accumbens, olfactory tubercles and striatum in the rat. Paper presented at the Meeting of the Society for Neuroscience, Minneapolis, November, 1981.

Schmidt, R.H. and Bhatnagar, R.K. (1979) Assessment of the effects of neonatal subcutaneous 6-hydroxydopamine on noradrenergic and dopaminergic innervation of cerebral cortex. Brain Res. 166, 309–319.

Shalaby, I.A. and Spear, L.P. (1980) Psychopharmacological effects of low and high doses of apomorphine during ontogeny. Eur. J. Pharmacol. 76, 451–459.

Shalaby, I.A., Dendel, P.S. and Spear, L.P. (1981) Differential functional ontogeny of dopamine presynaptic receptor regulation. Devel. Brain Res. 1, 434–439.

Shaywitz, B.A., Yager, R.D. and Klopper, J.H. (1976a) Selective brain dopamine depletion in developing rats: an experimental model of minimal brain dysfunction. Science 191, 305–308.

Shaywitz, B.A., Klopper, J.H., Yager, R.D. and Gordon, J.W. (1976b) Paradoxical response to amphetamine in developing rats treated with 6-hydroxydopamine. Nature 261, 153–155.

Shaywitz, B.A., Gordon, J.W., Klopper, J.H. and Zelterman, D.A. (1977) The effect of 6-hydroxydopamine on habituation of activity in the developing rat pup. Pharmacol. Biochem. Behav. 6, 391–396.

Smith, R.D., Cooper, B.R. and Breese, G.R. (1973) Growth and behavioral changes in developing rats treated intracisternally with 6-hydroxydopamine: evidence for involvement of brain dopamine. J. Pharmacol. Exp. Ther. 185, 609–619.

Spear, L.P. and Brake, S.C. (1983) Periadolescence: age-dependent behavior and psychopharmacological responsivity in rats. Dev. Psychobiol. 16, 83–109.

Spear, L.P. and Brick, J. (1979) Cocaine-induced behavior in the developing rat. Behav. Neural. Biol. 26, 401–415.

Spear, L.P., Shalaby, I.A. and Brick, J. (1980) Chronic administration of haloperidol during development: behavioral and psychopharmacological effects. Psychopharmacology 70, 47–58.

Spyker, J.M. (1975) Assessing the impact of low level chemicals on development: behavioral and latent effects. Fed. Proc. 34, 1835–1844.

Zenick, H., Ward, J., Rodriquez, W., Aragon, P. and Scrivseth, R. (1979) Offspring open field performance following maternal lead exposure: a question of dosage and nutritional status. Pharmacol. Biochem. Behav. 11, Suppl., 35–38.

Ziv, G., Shani, J., Givant, Y., Buchman, O. and Sulman, F.G. (1974) Distribution of tritiated haloperidol in lactating and pregnant cows and ewes. Arch. Int. Pharmacodyn. Ther. 212, 154–163.

Section V

HORMONES AND VITAMINS

SEE also the discussion on neuropeptides by Swaab and Mirmiran, Chapter 2 in Section I.

Neurobehavioral Teratology
edited by Joseph Yanai
© Elsevier Science Publishers BV 1984

15

EFFECTS OF THYROID HORMONES ON CENTRAL NERVOUS SYSTEM DEVELOPMENT

Jacques Legrand

Laboratoire de Physiologie comparée I, Université des Sciences et Techniques du Languedoc, ERA 955 du CNRS, Neurobiologie du Développement et Endocrinologie, 34060 Montpellier Cédex, France

IN the infant suffering from congenital hypothyroidism ('sporadic cretinism' as occurs in cases of thyroid dysgenesis and inborn errors of thyroid hormone synthesis), neurological troubles and mental retardation progressively appear within the first six months of postnatal life. Both the severity and the timing of the onset of thyroid hormone deficiency seem to play an important role in the degree and reversibility of the disorders. Timing of the onset of adequate substitution therapy is also crucial for the prevention of mental retardation. From the information available, it appears that hypothyroidism starting after 2–3 years of age exerts only slight effects on mental development, in the sense that the level of mental performance achieved is relatively good. On the other hand, the sooner hypothyroidism is present during fetal development, the higher the probability that the subsequent neurological and mental disorders be severe and irreversible, even if treatment is started within 4–6 months of birth (Smith et al., 1957). Indeed, hormonal replacement before 3 months of age has long been considered essential for substantially increasing the probability of therapeutic success as regards intelligence (Klein et al., 1972). Today, babies with congenital hypothyroidism may be identified by neonatal screening programmes and immediately treated. It is presently considered that adequate thyroid hormone treatment must be started before the end of the first postnatal month to prevent irreversible brain damage (Wolter et al., 1980).

Adequate treatment of thyroid dysfunction acquired late in infancy, or after, is accompanied by a return to normal mental performance. Furthermore, the functional abnormalities of the nervous system observed in acquired hypothyroidism of the adult can easily be corrected by thyroid treatment at any time.

All these clinical observations indicate that congenital hypothyroidism leads to brain structure abnormalities at an early period of development. In other words, this indicates that thyroid hormones play an important role during development of the nervous system.

Information regarding the gross anatomy and histology of the brain of human cretins, from which one may try to extrapolate back to a possible cause of mental retardation in congenital hypothyroidism, is very poor (Brasel and Boyd, 1975). It is obvious that any attempt to advance our knowledge of the underlying mechanisms requires the use of experimental animals.

The general scheme of neurodevelopmental events is the same for man and all mammalian species studied up to now. The main difference resides in the growth-speed characteristic of the species and in the timing of neurodevelopmental events in relation to the moment of birth. In man, thyroid function starts at the end of the first trimester of gestation (10–12 gestational weeks). The brain growth spurt, i.e. the period during which there is a particularly rapid increase in brain weight, begins at about the 19th gestational week and continues long after birth (into the second and perhaps into the third year). In the rat, which is the most widely used species for studying the effects of altered thyroid state on the developing central nervous system, thyroid function starts on the 18th gestational day, i.e. 4–5 days before birth, and the growth spurt of the brain is almost entirely postnatal and ends about 4 weeks after birth. From the point of view of neurodevelopmental events, the newborn rat may be compared with a human fetus in the second trimester of pregnancy and the newborn human baby to a 6–10 day old rat. Thus, in man as in the rat (and in other species), the brain growth spurt begins well after the onset of thyroid function. Numerous studies have also shown that it coincides with a span of life when the brain is particularly vulnerable to various environmental modifications and specifically an altered thyroid state.

Of course, the preceding description of the brain growth spurt is oversimplified. In fact, the different parts of the brain do not develop simultaneously. For example, the period of active neurogenesis and the growth spurt start much later in the cerebellum than in the forebrain. In the forebrain itself, the hippocampus and the olfactory bulbs exhibit intense neurogenesis long after neuron formation has ceased in the somatosensory cerebral cortex. This must be borne in mind when considering the differential morphogenetic effects of altered thyroid state on the different parts of the brain (in terms of the sensitivity of the nervous structures to thyroid hormone, and in terms of the severity and nature of the disturbances observed in altered thyroid state).

Use of the rat as an animal model has provided considerable information concerning the influence of congenital thyroid deficiency and neonatal hyperthyroidism on the development of the central nervous system. The rat is very immature at birth, so the effects of thyroid hormone deprivation or excess can be studied with relative ease in this species. The main experimental studies which have been carried out in the rat to try to gain insight into the organizing action of thyroid hormones and to try to correlate thyroid hormone deprivation or excess with the behavioural deficits observed in adulthood will be described in a first step. In a second step, attention will mainly be focused on the relatively homogenous cerebellum, to find out at which of the stages of cell formation, migration, maturation, and death, thyroid hormones have their effect.

Structural, functional and behavioural consequences of altered thyroid state during infancy

Studies on the forebrain

Effects of thyroid deficiency   Eayrs and his colleagues have made the first detailed histological studies of the influence of neonatal thyroid deficiency on the somatosensory cerebral cortex of the developing rat. The cerebral cortex was first chosen for such studies, owing to mental and intellectual deficiencies characteristic of human congenital hypothyroidism and to the prevalent idea that higher brain functions are likely associated with the cerebral cortex.

In the cerebral cortex of 24 day old rats made hypothyroid from birth by radiothyroidectomy or daily administration of methylthiouracil, the density of nerve cell bodies is increased and their mean size is reduced (Eayrs and Taylor, 1951), the capillary blood vessels are less numerous and their mean diameter is increased (Eayrs, 1954). Probably more significant are the abnormalities in the development of cell processes. The density of axons is decreased, especially in layer IV which receives specific thalamic afferents. There is also a reduction in growth and abnormalities in branching of the dendrites of pyramidal neurons (Eayrs, 1955; Eayrs and Horn, 1955). From these histologic observations, Eayrs estimated that the dendritic and axonal deficiencies possibly lead to a greater than 50% decrease in the probability of dendritic and axonal interaction (review in Eayrs, 1971; see also Hamburgh, 1969). Actually, a reduction in the number of nerve terminals associated with each neuron of the visual cortex was later demonstrated by electron microscopy (Cragg, 1970). Inhibition of dendritic arborization, decreased numbers of dendritic spines, a reduced complexity of axonal plexuses and persistent disturbances in synaptogenesis have also been reported in the rat caudate nucleus (Lu and Brown, 1977a, b). Lastly, a decreased density and abnormal distribution of the dendritic spines on the apical shaft of pyramidal cells (which constitute sites of synaptic contacts) have been observed in Golgi preparations of the cerebral visual cortex (Sanchez-Toscano et al., 1977; Ruiz-Marcos et al., 1979) and the auditory cortex (Ruiz-Marcos et al, 1978) in rats rendered severely hypothyroid at 10 days of age.

Changes in the electroencephalogram are observed in hypothyroid children (Lenard and Bell, 1973) and in rats thyroidectomized at birth (Bradley et al., 1960) which are not found again in animals thyroidectomized when adult. In the rat, neonatal thyroid deficiency is also accompanied by changes in the evoked potential cortical response to stimulation of thalamic structures which can be related to disturbances in axon and dendritic development (Bradley et al., 1961, 1964).

The histological and electrophysiological disturbances which have just been briefly described are accompanied by a retardation of several innate behavioural responses (Eayrs and Lishman, 1955). The capacity for adaptive behaviour is also delayed and/or impaired in the rat made hypothyroid at birth and some behavioural changes seem to be persistent (Eayrs and Lishman, 1955; Eayrs, 1961; Eayrs and Levine, 1963; Davenport and Dorcey, 1972; Davenport and Hennies, 1976; Schalock et al., 1977; Johanson et al., 1980). In fact, the behavioural deficits observed by Eayrs and others in rats made hypothyroid at birth appear to be more or less severe depending on the difficulty of the problem submitted to the animals. Roughly, the severity of impairment of the capacity for adaptive behaviour is inversely proportional to the time interval between birth and onset of thyroid deficiency. Furthermore, replacement therapy in animals made hypothyroid at birth seems to be completely effective only when started before the end of the second postnatal week. These studies establish that in the rat, as in man, thyroid deficiency during the brain growth spurt results in severe and irreversible impairment of brain function, and that substitution therapy must be instituted well before the end of the growth spurt in order that the capacity for adaptive behaviour may return to near normal.

However, when rats made hypothyroid at birth are given thyroxine from the age of 24 days only, they recover an apparently normal cortical structure at 2 months (Horn, 1955) but still display behavioural abnormalities (Eayrs, 1971; see also Davenport and Hennies, 1976). It is possible either that more subtle structural changes than those already detected or that irreversible functional deficiencies due to some permanent biochemical disturbances, whose detection would need very specific methods of investigation, are also effective. Indeed, in rats thyroidectomized at 10 days, the effects of thyroxine treatment on the number and distribution of pyramidal cell spines depend on the age when the treatment is started. When started at 12 days of age, the number and distribution of spines are similar to that of age-paired intact rats, but the treatment is no longer completely effective when started at 30 days of age (Ruiz-Marcos et al., 1982).

On the other hand, disturbances in the development of dendritic spines of pyramidal neurones have been found in rats thyroidectomized as late as 40 days of age (Ruiz-Marcos et al., 1980). These observations show that for the normal development of the brain, thyroid hormones are not only particularly important during the first two postnatal weeks, but also conserve some morphogenetic action in later life. However, it is likely that this late action has relatively less functional significance with respect to the ultimate capacity for adaptive behaviour. In agreement with the latter view is the finding that when thyroxine treatment is delayed for 25 days in rats thyroidectomized at 40 days of age both the number and distribution of spines tend to revert to normal values, whereas this has no ameliorating effect in rats thyroidectomized at 10 days (Ruiz-Marcos et al., 1981).

The developmental pattern of DNA in the entire forebrain of the hypothyroid rat is not affected (Balázs et al., 1968; Patel et al., 1976). This lack of effect of thyroid deficiency on cell formation in the forebrain contrasts with its marked effect on multiplication of cerebellar cells (see section on cell formation). Since in the total forebrain there is no significant formation of neurons after birth, whereas in the cerebellum most of the interneurons are formed postnatally, this suggests that altered thyroid state especially interacts with neuron formation. Indeed, another factor which may contribute to the impaired capacity to adapt to changes in the environment is the action of thyroid deficiency in reducing cell formation in those regions of the forebrain such as the hippocampus and the olfactory bulbs which undergo significant postnatal acquisition of neurons (Patel et al., 1976; Rabié et al., 1979). The final cell number (DNA content) is permanently decreased in the hippocampus and olfactory bulbs of hypothyroid rats. In the olfactory bulbs, even if there is a final reduced cell number, the mitotic activity is not significantly affected, indicating that the deficit of cells results from disturbances in migration of the cells originating in the germinative periventricular layer (Patel et al., 1976). In the caudate nucleus, the neuron density is below normal during the first postnatal month. At 30 days of age, it attains a plateau in controls, whereas active neuron acquisition is still taking place in the hypothyroid rat. In the latter, the dissolution of the germinal subependymal layer is retarded and cell migration from this layer to the caudate nucleus is delayed (Lu and Brown, 1977b). Since the developmental pattern of the total DNA content of the forebrain is not changed in the thyroid-deficient rat, the lasting deficit in the final number of neurons in the olfactory bulbs and the hippocampus must be compensated in other parts of the brain by some hyperplasia (perhaps implying glia). Lastly, no significant effect of thyroid deficiency has been observed on the cell cycle parameters in the germinative zones of the brain (Lewis et al., 1976). Lack of thyroid hormone seems to affect the maturation and migration of cells rather than their replication.

The reduction in cell numbers in the hippocampus is accompanied by a decrease in the dimensions of this structure. Furthermore, the dimensions and morphology of the hippocampus are relatively more affected than those of the entire forebrain (Rabié et al., 1979). Thus, thyroid deficiency results not only in a reduction in the overall growth of the brain but also the dimensions of the brain are ultimately distorted.

Effects of thyroid hormone excess   Neonatal hyperthyroidism in the rat (induced by thyroxine treatment of the normal newborn) transiently accelerates the morphologic development of cortical pyramidal neurons and particularly the ontogenesis of their dendritic spines (Schapiro et al., 1973; see however Hodge et al., 1976). Thyroxine treatment of newborn rats has also been found to lead to an accelerated develop-

336

ment of the mossy fiber tract in the hippocampus and to produce an ectopic infrapyramidal bundle of mossy fibers in stratum oriens of field CA 3 a–b of Ammon's horn. This effect is more or less intense depending on the anatomical level studied in the hippocampus. The appearance of ectopic fibers is dose-dependent and long-lasting, indicating that the mossy fiber-pyramidal cell circuitry is permanently altered. Lastly, the critical period for the production of ectopic infrapyramidal mossy fibers in hyperthyroidism coincides with the first three postnatal weeks, i.e. with the main period of granule cell formation and mossy fiber development (Lauder and Mugnaini, 1980).

In rats given relatively high doses of triiodothyronine during infancy, active cell formation in the forebrain ceases earlier than in controls, causing a persistent reduction in total cell number (Balázs et al., 1971b). The degree of the final deficit of cells in the total brain seems to be related to the dose of thyroid hormone used (Grave et al., 1973). So far as we know, the effects of thyroid hormone excess on cell formation in the different parts of the forebrain (for example the hippocampus and the olfactory bulbs) have not yet been studied. In the cerebellum, neonatal hyperthyroidism leads to a marked reduction in the number of granule cells (see further on). It is likely that the same situation occurs in the hippocampus and the olfactory bulbs. Estimates of cell proliferation kinetics and cell death in the lateral ventricular subependymal layer show no apparent abnormality in the hyperthyroid brain (Patel et al., 1979). Like those of thyroid deficiency, the effects of thyroid hormone excess do not appear to concern cell replication.

Initially, thyroxine treatment accelerates the appearance of several automatic and innate responses (Eayrs, 1964 in the rat; Hamburgh and Vicari, 1957; Hamburgh, 1958 in the mouse) and improves locomotor coordination and learning abilities. Despite this initial precocity, adult rats made hyperthyroid at birth do not perform better and often perform less well than littermate controls (Eayrs, 1964, 1971; Davenport and Gonzales, 1973; Davenport et al., 1975; Stone and Greenough, 1975; Murphy and Nagy, 1976; Sjöden, 1976; Sjöden and Söderberg, 1976a, b).

It must be noted that early exposure to excess thyroid hormone induces many profound and permanent alterations of the neuroendocrine regulations, known as the 'neo-T4 syndrome', including a relative state of thyroid deficiency (Pascual-Leone et al., 1976; Phelps and Leathem, 1976; see however Sjöden and Södenberg, 1976a). Whether the behavioural troubles observed result from impaired brain organization or neuroendocrine functional disturbances is still unclear.

Studies on the cerebellum
Owing to the relative simplicity and homogeneity of its structure and to its relatively late development compared with those of the cerebral cortex, the cerebellar cortex is more convenient for studying the morphogenetic action of thyroid hormone on the central nervous system. In the rat, which is born in a very immature state, about 97% of the cerebellar cells are formed during postnatal life and most of them are interneu-

rons originating from the external granular layer (or germinative layer), from which they migrate down to the molecular or the internal granular layer. This provides a convenient opportunity for studying the effects of thyroid dysfunction on the formation, maturation and migration of neurons.

At present there is much documentation showing that alterations of the thyroid state lead to perturbations in these three developmental processes. The cerebellum is probably not the critical part of the central nervous system with respect to adaptive behaviour. Rather, its main role is the control of locomotor activity, which is permanently impaired in congenital hypothyroidism. However, changes occurring in the developing cerebellar cortex are also likely to take place in other parts of the brain.

Cell formation and final cellular composition

(i) Effects of thyroid deficiency   In the rat rendered hypothyroid from the end of gestation or from birth, the external granular layer persists beyond the normal age of 21 days (Legrand et al., 1961; Hamburgh et al., 1964; Legrand, 1967a). The rate of cell acquisition is decreased. However, as a result of the lengthening of the proliferative phase, the final number of cerebellar cells is normal (Balázs et al., 1968; Nicholson and Altman, 1972a; Patel et al., 1976; Legrand et al., 1976). More precisely, in the thyroid-deficient cerebellum, the rate of in vivo DNA synthesis is reduced during the second week only. Cell proliferation, in terms of DNA synthesis, is even greater at day 21 than at day 12, when in the cerebellum of controls, cell division reaches its maximum rate. Therefore, cell replication carries on for a relatively long time in the cerebellar external granular layer of hypothyroid rats, resulting in full restoration of a normal cell number (Patel et al., 1976). As mentioned above, these observations have subsequently focused attention on the regions of the forebrain such as the hippocampus and the olfactory bulbs, which, like the cerebellum, are characterized by an intense postnatal acquisition of neurons. In these forebrain regions, there are no powerful compensatory mechanisms able to restore a normal number of cells as in the cerebellum, probably because most of the cell deficit results from disturbances in the migration of the cells originating in the germinal periventricular layer, i.e. relatively far from their final localization.

As in the germinative sites of the forebrain, thyroid hormone deprivation has an influence on cell production in the cerebellar external granular layer by affecting the germinal pool size, probably through the retention of daughter cells in this layer, rather than by altering the replication rate of dividing cells (Lewis et al., 1976; see however Lauder, 1977). Another factor which can decrease the rate of cell acquisition in the hypothyroid cerebellum is the increased proportion of degenerating cells in the internal granular layer. A detailed analysis of this phenomenon will be given in a further section. Lastly, an increased density of pyknoses has been observed in the external granular layer itself, in 13 day old hypothyroid rats, and this can also contribute to the reduction of the germinal pool size (Clos, 1980).

Even if the total number of cells is finally normal in the hypothyroid cerebellum, the final cellular composition of the organ is modified (Nicholson and Altman, 1972a; Clos and Legrand, 1973). The number of Purkinje cells, which are formed relatively early during fetal life (before the onset of fetal thyroid function), is not changed. The number of internal granule cells, which originate from the external granular layer and whose formation extends over a long period (at least up to the 22nd postnatal day in controls and the 29th day in the hypothyroid animals), is normal or slightly elevated. The effect of thyroid deficiency on the number of inhibitory interneurons also originating from the external granular layer appears to be different depending on the date of birth and/or the duration of the period of formation of these neurons. The basket cells, which are formed during a relatively short period at the end of the first postnatal week (Altman, 1969), are less numerous, whereas the number of later-forming stellate cells is increased. There are also more astrocytes in both the ganglionic layer (Bergmann glia cells) and the internal granular layer (internal astrocytes). Bergmann glia cells are formed during the perinatal period but they remain able to divide, even when already well differentiated, for a long period, to give birth to internal astrocytes (Basco et al., 1977). Lastly, the number of oligodendrocytes in the white matter is normal (Vitiello et al., 1980; Clos et al., 1982b).

Less severe disturbances in the formation of cerebellar granule cells are still observable when hypothyroidism is induced during the second postnatal week, but changes are no longer observed when thyroid deficiency starts later (Legrand, 1963, 1967b).

(ii) Effects of thyroid hormone excess   Tusques (1956) was the first to report briefly the precocious disappearance of the external granular layer in the cerebellum of rats given thyroxine at birth. It was shown later that thyroxine treatment during the early postnatal period leads to a marked but transient increase in the rate of cell acquisition in the rat cerebellum during the first postnatal week (Gourdon et al., 1973; Weichsel Jr., 1974; Legrand et al., 1976). This effect is not observed in the forebrain. In the cerebellum, the build-up of cell numbers in the external granular layer seems to be due to a transient retardation in cell migration from this layer rather than to an acceleration of cell replication, since cell cycle parameters remain normal (Patel et al., 1979). Later in development, from day 12, active cell formation ceases earlier than in controls in the cerebellum of hyperthyroid rats, causing a persistent reduction in total cell number, as in the forebrain (Balázs et al., 1971b; Nicholson and Altman, 1972a; Gourdon et al., 1973; Legrand et al., 1976). Advancement of cellular maturation appears to be mainly involved in this phenomenon.

The final deficit of cells in the hyperthyroid cerebellum predominantly involves the granule cells (Nicholson and Altman, 1972a; Rabié et al., 1977). The numbers of basket cells, astrocytes and oligodendrocytes are also decreased (Nicholson and Altman, 1972a; Vitiello et al., 1980; Clos et al., 1982a and b). Contrary to what has been reported in the total brain (Grave et al., 1973), the final deficit of cells in the cerebellum does not appear to depend on the severity of neonatal hyperthyroidism (Legrand et al., 1976; Rabié et al., 1977).

Effects of thyroid deficiency on nerve cell maturation and death

(i) Nerve cell maturation The histological maturation of Purkinje cell bodies, particularly the organization of their endoplasmic reticulum and ribosomes into Nissl bodies, is delayed for several days in the rat made hypothyroid by propylthiouracil treatment or surgically thyroidectomized at birth (Legrand, 1967a). The transient perisomatic processes of Purkinje cells and their axosomatic synapses with the climbing fibres persist for a longer time (Hajós et al., 1973). In other words, the translocation of the synapses with the climbing fibres, from the perisomatic processes of Purkinje cells to their dendrites, is retarded. At the same time, additionally, the regression of the multiple innervation of Purkinje cells by climbing fibres and the establishment of the one-to-one relationship between them are delayed for several days (Crépel et al., 1981). Still more striking is the severe retardation in growth and branching of Purkinje cell dendritic arborizations (Legrand, 1967a). The ontogenesis of the dendritic spines of Purkinje cells is also delayed (Legrand and Bout, 1970) and their dendritic branchlets display regions where spines are absent (Brown et al., 1976). Although the dendritic tree of Purkinje cells continues to grow with age as in controls, it presents a permanent degree of hypoplasia. Moreover the base of the dendritic tree displays permanent morphological abnormalities. In particular, there is an abnormal lengthening of the primary dendrite(s) (Rebière and Legrand, 1972a; Brown et al., 1976). The length of parallel fibres (Crépel, 1975; Lauder, 1978) and the density of synapses between parallel fibres and Purkinje cell dendritic spines are also considerably and permanently reduced (Nicholson and Altman, 1972b; Rebière and Legrand, 1972b).

A very important feature of the hypothyroid cerebellum is that the dendritic tree of Purkinje cells remains very hypoplastic after the cessation of the formation and deposition of granule cells (Legrand, 1967a; Rebière and Legrand, 1972a). Finally, besides transient troubles such as the retarded laying down of granule cells and the delayed maturation of Purkinje cell bodies, more persistent abnormalities in growth and branching of neuronal processes are found, resulting in the disappearance of the normal synchrony between the main processes of cerebellar cortex histogenesis. In this way, thyroid hormone deprivation might result not only in reduced but also in ultimate abnormal connectivity.

A quantitative ultrastructural study of large areas of cerebellar molecular layer in 14 day old thyroid-deficient rats (Vincent et al., in press) has confirmed that the retardation in synaptogenesis between Purkinje cell dendritic spines and varicosities of parallel fibres is related to the marked hypoplasia of Purkinje cell dendritic arborizations and to the delayed development of parallel fibres, rather than to the delay in the deposition of granule cells and their axons. Furthermore, the decrease in the synaptic density is more marked in the inner than in the outer part of the molecular layer. The normal 'march' of synaptogenesis in the molecular layer, from the bottom of the layer outwards, is therefore distorted, and the synaptic organization (in terms of the distribution of synapses in space) is finally affected by thyroid hormone deprivation both quantitatively and qualitatively. Lastly, thyroid hormone deprivation seems to affect synaptogenesis by interacting with growth and branching of neuronal processes rather than with the differentiation of structural specializations forming the synapses (see also Hajós et al., 1973; Lauder, 1978).

The cerebellar glomeruli, which are complex synaptic structures in the internal granular layer between granule and Golgi cells and mossy fibre terminals, also differentiate several days later than in controls and their development is abnormal (Legrand, 1967a; Hajós et al., 1973). Thus, in the hypothyroid animal, the immature wiring pattern characterized by predominance of the climbing fibre-Purkinje cell circuit persists for a longer time and the inadequate establishment of the mossy fibre-Purkinje cell-granule cell circuit still favours the immature climbing fibre-Purkinje cell circuit.

These developmental abnormalities have functional correlates: the adult spontaneous activity of Purkinje cells is considerably delayed and their activation responses exhibit a deficit after stimulation of their afferents. Accentuated inhibition responses can be observed at the same time (Crépel, 1972, 1974; Crépel and Legrand, 1974). The electrophysiological studies of Crépel (1976) lead to the conclusion that in the cerebellum of adult rats made hypothyroid during the first five postnatal weeks, the bioelectric properties of neuronal membranes are normal, and that the only persistent functional deficits concern neuronal connectivity.

(ii) Nerve cell death   The pyknotic index in the internal granular layer, i.e. the ratio of dying granule cells to the total number of granule cells (Lewis, 1975), is dramatically increased in 12 day old hypothyroid rats (Lewis et al., 1976). The authors have proposed that as in the staggerer mutant mouse (Sotelo and Changeux, 1974b), the increase in histogenetic cell death results from a greater proportion of granule cells failing to make adequate connections with Purkinje cells. However, an increased death of granule cells could be due in part to a reduced rate of removal of chromatin debris and this may be more important in hypothyroid animals where the general metabolism in the brain is retarded. The increase of the pyknotic index is not in fact due to a decreased rate of removal of chromatin debris but rather to increased mortality of granule cells (Patel and Rabié, 1980). The maximal increase in the pyknotic index is observed during the second postnatal week, when the retardation in the morphologic maturation of Purkinje cells is most striking. At 21 days, when Purkinje cells display relatively more normal morphologic features, the number of dying granule cells is not increased to the same extent as seen during the second postnatal week (Rabié et al., 1977). The granule cells which die at 14 days are formed on day 9 (Rabié et al., 1980a) and are those which are actively engaged in the process of establishing synaptic connections with Purkinje cells. Their axons are localized in the inner parts of the molecular layer, just where the deficit of synapses between parallel fibres and Purkinje cell dendritic spines is greatest (Vincent et al., in press). The granule cells which are formed earlier (at 6 days) do not die (Lewis et al., 1976; Patel and Rabié, 1980).

Thus, at the end of the second postnatal week, the survival of the newly formed and differentiating cells is preferentially compromised in the thyroid-deficient cerebellum. Such a discrimination between cells which have already established, and cells which are in the process of establishing synaptic connections, is consistent with the hypothesis that increased death of granule cells is a consequence of the limited availability of synaptic contact sites, due to the hypoplasia of Purkinje cells.

However, although probably less important, other factors may be involved in increased granule cell death. As pointed out above, the length of parallel fibres is decreased and this results in a reduced number of Purkinje cells which one granule cell can contact. Death of granule cells may not only be due to their failure to make contact with Purkinje cells but also to their failure to contact a sufficient number of Purkinje cells. Another factor which may be involved in the increased granule cell death is the reduction in the number of basket cells. There are good reasons for suspecting that cell death occurs in those neurons which form connections with specific postsynaptic targets and are unable to make connections elsewhere if these targets are not present or are unavailable. This is the case for granule cells which contact both Purkinje cells and basket cells.

Corrective effects of thyroid hormone in the hypothyroid animal   In propylthiouracil-treated young rats, the disappearance of the external granular layer can be obtained in the normal delay and the morphologic abnormalities of Purkinje cells can be entirely corrected only if thyroxine is given before the end of the second postnatal week. However, when given later, the hormone can still promote some growth of Purkinje cell dendrites but in this case the anomalies of the base of Purkinje cell dendritic trees persist (Legrand, 1967b). The length of parallel fibres (Crépel, 1975; Lauder, 1978) and the density of synapses in the molecular layer (Rebière and Legrand, 1972b) remain permanently reduced in the rat treated with propylthiouracil during the first three to five postnatal weeks, though the thyroid gland again becomes functional in these animals.

In 14 day old propylthiouracil-treated rats given a small and constant daily dose of thyroxine from birth, the increase in granule cell death occurs only when the dose of hormone administered is too low and when the normal synchrony between the development of Purkinje cell dendritic arborizations and the laying down of granule cells remains disturbed (Rabié et al., 1977). This observation emphasizes the importance of maintaining this synchrony for subsequent normal development of the cerebellum.

The postnatal development of thyroid function in the rat is now relatively well known (Vigouroux, 1974; 1976; Fisher et al., 1977) and the doses of thyroxine which can be considered as physiologic depending on the age of the animals can be calculated. In animals treated with propylthiouracil, administration from birth of a progressively increasing daily dose of thyroxine nearly equal to half the amount of hormone excreted on the corresponding day by the thyroid of the normally developing rat corrects all the disturbances in the structural (in terms of cell formation, migration, maturation and death) and functional maturation of the cerebellum (Clos et al., 1974; Legrand et al., 1976; Vincent et al., 1979; Rabié et al., 1979). It is likely that the very low doses of thyroxine we consider as physiologic and which result in normal plasma concentration of hormone only within a short time after the injection cannot completely correct all the biochemical troubles due to continued propylthiouracil treatment. The action of the hormone on the structural and functional maturation of the cerebellum therefore appears to be permissive. In any case, physiologic levels of thyroxine, even only transiently attained once per day, are capable of reversing the maturational delays and abnormalities observed in the cerebellum of the hypothyroid rat if the hormone is administered at an early age.

Owing to the adverse effects of hyperthyroidism on the developing cerebellum (see p. 343), the demonstration of the physiologic nature of the doses of thyroxine used is an important condition for validating the experimental procedure employed to determine the latency and sequence of appearance of the corrective effects of the hormone on the main processes of cerebellar development. Young rats treated with propylthiouracil from the end of fetal life have daily received a progressively increasing physiologic dose of hormone from diverse stages of development and their cerebella have been studied on day 14 (Rabié et al., 1979). The effect of thyroxine on cell formation (estimated from the mitotic index in the external granular layer) appears after 2 days, in agreement with previous results showing that thyroxine excess accelerates the rate of cell acquisition. With the same latency, thyroxine induces migration of the newly formed granule cells. It is interesting to note that among the various parameters studied the most rapidly corrected is the number of dying granule cells in the internal granular layer. The pyknotic index in the layer is reduced by half after only one day and returns entirely to normal within four days. The corrective effects of thyroxine on granule cell death thus occur more rapidly than those on granule cell formation. Since granule cell survival depends on their degree of maturation and on that of Purkinje cells, more precisely on the possibility the two kinds of cells have of establishing synaptic contacts, these observations strongly suggest that the primary effect of thyroid hormone is on growth of neuronal processes and synaptogenesis rather than on cell formation. Indeed, the first detectable effect of a single physiologic dose of thyroxine injected into the propylthiouracil-treated rat 24 h before killing consists in the rapid maturation of parallel fibres and in the appearance of new parallel fibre varicosities accompanied by a slight increase in the density of synapses between parallel fibres and Purkinje cells. This results mainly from a rapid lengthening of the existing parallel fibres rather than from the appearance of new ones. The Purkinje cell dendritic spines respond to the hormone more slowly than the parallel fibres and their varicosities. Two days of hormonal treatment are necessary to allow the Purkinje cells to develop numerous spines on a dendritic tree which remains very hypoplastic. The same treatment markedly augments the density of synapses between Purkinje cells and parallel fibres. Lastly, four days of hormone treatment (from day 10 to day 13) entirely return to normal the development of Purkinje cell dendritic trees, as well as the density of synapses between Purkinje cells and parallel fibres and the number of degenerating granule cells in the internal granular layer (Vincent et al., in press).

Thus the granule cells which are formed in great number and are rapidly maturing during the second postnatal week are very sensitive to thyroid hormone level. Purkinje cells which are formed during fetal life and mature more slowly but over a longer period respond less rapidly to the hormone. However, only three very low doses of thyroxine administered on days 7, 8 and 9 to propylthiouracil-treated rats are sufficient to prevent the increase in granule cell death not only at 14 days but also up to 22 days, when the animals are once more severely hypothyroid and the granule cells respond again to thyroid hormone deprivation (as seen by the persistence of the external granular layer at 22 days) (Rabié et al., 1980b). Therefore, the hormone prevents the death of the granule cells which are not formed at the time of its administration and also of the granule cells which are formed late when thyroid deficiency has come back. These observations indicate that during the second postnatal week, thyroid hormone exerts an organizing action on Purkinje cells, rendering them definitively able to make a sufficient number of contacts with parallel fibres, and thus allowing the granule cells to survive. In other words, the fate of granule cells (in terms of survival) is not entirely dependent on direct action of the hormone. However, from the second postnatal week, Purkinje cells seem to play a special directing role. Most likely, this is one of the reasons why the second postnatal week is so important with regard to the requirement of thyroid hormone for subsequent normal development of the cerebellum.

Effects of thyroid hormone excess on nerve cell maturation   Neonatal thyroid hormone excess accelerates the disappearance of the cerebellar external granular layer (Tusques, 1956) and the morphogenesis of Purkinje cells including ontogenesis of their dendritic spines (Legrand, 1965, 1967b; Turques et al., 1967; Legrand and Bout, 1970), without leading to morphologic abnormalities of Purkinje cells (Rebière and Legrand, 1972a; see however Nicholson and Altman, 1972b). It stimulates transiently parallel fibre growth without changing the density of varicosities along the parallel fibres (Lauder, 1978). The transient increase in length of these axons produces a transient increase in the total number of synaptic sites per parallel fibre, reflected in the transient increase of the synaptic density in the inner molecular layer early in the postnatal period, followed by a transient early increase of the density of synapses in the outer molecular layer (Nicholson and Altman, 1972b). This pattern of synaptogenesis is commensurate with the accelerated development of parallel fibres, with the accelerated transition in parallel fibre length in the two halves of the molecular layer, combined with accelerated development of the Purkinje cell dendritic tree. These observations are consistent with the view that excess thyroid hormone does not cause the disappearance of the normal synchrony between the formation, deposition and maturation of granule cells, and the morphogenesis of Purkinje cells (Rebière and Legrand, 1972a). However, the effects of early thyroid hormone excess on the development of the cerebellar cortex seem to be different depending on the part of the cortex studied (Lauder, 1978). In this way neonatal hyperthyroidism, therefore, might lead to dysharmonies in the development of the whole cerebellum.

A normal synaptic density is achieved in the adult cerebellar molecular layer of the rat made hyperthyroid at birth. However, due to the early cessation of granule cell formation and to the final deficit of granule cells, early hyperthyroidism causes a terminal deficit of synapses in the cerebellar molecular layer (Nicholson and Altman, 1972b).

It is of particular interest to notice that daily administration to propylthiouracil-treated rats of a constant dose of thyroxine as low as 0.20 μg, i.e. a dose much lower than all those generally employed to create hyperthyroidism in the newborn rat, is sufficient to accelerate the structural maturation of the cerebellar cortex and moreover leads to a deficit in the final number of cerebellar cells (Rabié et al., 1977). Since neonatal hyperthyroidism leads to a reduced learning ability in adulthood, such observations must be taken into consideration for comprehending the consequences of perinatal hyperthyroidism and for the treatment of congenital thyroid deficiency.

An increased density of synapses has been reported at birth in the rat cerebellum after in utero administration of excess thyroxine to the foetus (Legrand et al., 1982). To our knowledge, except for the action of thyroid hormone on the histological structure of fetal bone (Legrand, 1969), this constitutes the most precocious morphogenetic effect of the hormone described up to the time of writing during development in the rat. It is of interest that this early stimulation of synaptogenesis is associated with an augmentation in the density of nerve terminals, again indicating that it is probably mediated through an acceleration of neurite outgrowth.

Thyroid hormones and biochemical maturation of the central nervous system

Nucleic acid and protein metabolism

The study of the developmental pattern of the DNA concentration and ratios of the wet weight, RNA and protein contents of the cerebrum and the cerebellum to DNA shows that cell maturation (in terms of mean cell wet weight, RNA and protein contents) is permanently affected by thyroid deficiency, and only transiently accelerated by hyperthyroidism. In the hypothyroid rats, the persistent lower weight of the organ is due to smaller mean cell size. In the hyperthyroid animals, on the other hand, the final mean cell size is normal and the final lower weight of the cerebrum and the cerebellum results from the deficit in the number of cells (Balázs et al., 1968, 1971a and b); Geel and Timiras, 1967a; Gourdon et al., 1973; Legrand et al., 1976; Pasquini et al., 1967).

Considerable evidence exists that thyroid hormones stimulate in vivo protein synthesis in the tissues whose metabolism is increased by these hormones (Michels et al., 1963; Tata and Widnell, 1966). This may be transiently the case for the nervous tissue (Fazekas et al., 1951; Reiss et al., 1956; Hamburgh et al., 1964; see however Schwartz and Oppenheimer, 1978). In vivo incorporation of leucine or phenylalanine into the cerebral or cerebellar proteins is transiently reduced in the hypothyroid young rat (Geel et al., 1967; Balázs et al., 1968; Dainat et al., 1970a, b; Szijan et al., 1971; Jarlsted and Norström, 1972) and transiently increased in the hyperthyroid animal (Dainat and Legrand, 1971; Macho et al., 1972). Neonatal thyroidectomy does not affect cerebral RNA synthesis in 25 to 35 day old rats (Balázs et al., 1968, 1971a; Geel, 1975; Geel and Gonzales, 1975; Geel and Timiras, 1970, 1971; Geel and Valcana, 1971; see however Kohl, 1972). However, it leads to a significant decrease in the synthesis of rapidly labelled cerebral RNA on day 10, accompanied by an altered transport of RNA out of the nucleus (Duvilanski et al., 1975; Gómez et al., 1971). As noticed by Hamburgh and Flexner (1957), the inhibition of the development of numerous enzyme activities sensitive to thyroid hormone deprivation (see further) coincides with the period of major increase in these enzyme activities and in total protein in the brain of controls. Undoubtedly, thyroid deficiency leads to reduced synthesis of specific proteins in the developing brain. However, the spectrum of proteins affected by thyroid state may be sufficiently broad to be detectable when total protein synthesis is measured.

Further evidence for a specific effect on growth of neuronal processes
The proteins which are specifically affected in altered thyroid state appear to be mainly localized in neuronal processes and nerve terminals, thus confirming the structural data reported above. For example, the increase in synaptosomal proteins is slowed or accelerated to a greater extent than that of total proteins in the cerebellum of hypothyroid or hyperthyroid young rats, and the synaptosomal proteins are especially sensitive to very low doses of thyroxine in the thyroid-deficient animals (Rabié and Legrand, 1973). In vitro analysis of certain metabolic aspects of synaptosomes isolated from both the cerebellum and the cerebrum has also provided indices of synaptic deficiency in hypothyroidism (Verity et al., 1976; Battie and Verity, 1982). In the same context, it is interesting to mention that the increased conversion of glucose into aminoacids during development, which reflects the increase in the metabolic compartments associated with neuronal processes during maturation (Balázs et al., 1973), is accelerated or retarded as a consequence of hyper- or hypothyroidism (Cocks et al., 1970; Gómez and Ramirez De Guglielmone, 1967).

As detailed in a subsequent section, the synthesis of tau-proteins, which act as assembly promoting factors of microtubules, is dependent on thyroid hormones (Francon et al., 1977; Fellous et al., 1979; Nunez et al., 1980). Since growth of neuronal processes necessitates the integrity of their microtubular apparatus, this finding constitutes a strong argument in favour of a specific effect of thyroid hormones not only on the synthesis of specific proteins, but also on neurite outgrowth.

The developmental patterns of several enzyme activities associated with nerve endings have been shown to be specifically altered by neonatal hypothyroidism in the rat. For example, in the hypothyroid rat cerebral cortex, the activity of succinate dehydrogenase, which is mainly associated with the mitochondria of synaptosomes, and that of glutamate decarboxylase (a constituent of nerve endings) are decreased (Garcia-Argiz et al., 1967; Hamburgh and Flexner, 1957), whereas the activities of lactate dehydrogenase, a cytoplasmic enzyme, and glutamate dehydrogenase, an enzyme located in mitochondria of neuronal bodies and glia, are less affected (Balázs et al., 1971a; Balázs et al., 1968). Cortical succinate dehydrogenase activity, which remains low in rats thyroidectomized at birth, can return to normal levels if thyroxine is given from the age of 10 days. But the hormone has no effect if given only after the age of 15 or 20 days (Hamburgh and Flexner, 1957). In the thyroid-deficient or hyperthyroid rat cerebellar cortex, the changes in distribution of succinate dehydrogenase activity in the molecular layer mainly reflect the delayed or accelerated appearance of synaptic contacts between varicosities of parallel fibres and dendritic spines of Purkinje cells; those in the internal granular layer mainly reflect the retardation or the advance in the development of cerebellar glomeruli (Legrand, 1965, 1967a, c). The finding of Hamburgh and Flexner (1957) probably has similar morphologic correlates in the cerebral cortex.

Transmitter systems

Cholinergic systems   In the cerebellum of hypothyroid rats, the developmental increase of total cholinesterase activity (expressed per mg protein) is retarded (Clos, 1972; Clos et al., 1974). That of specific acetylcholinesterase is not changed when expressed per organ but is higher than normal when expressed per mg protein (Clos, 1980). In the rat cerebral cortex and hypothalamus, the development of acetylcholinesterase activity (per g of tissue) is retarded by thyroid deficiency (Geel and Timiras, 1967b; Hamburgh and Flexner, 1957; Valcana, 1971) and accelerated by neonatal administration of thyroxine (Schapiro, 1968).

In the cerebellum of thyroxine-treated and thyroid-deficient rats, respectively, the advance and the delay in the acquisition of the adult normal distribution of acetylcholinesterase activity within the internal granular layer (Clos, 1972, 1980; Clos et al., 1974; Lefranc et al., 1968) mainly reflect the acceleration or the retardation in the growth of mossy fibers and in the development of cerebellar glomeruli.

The ontogenetic increase in choline acetyltransferase activity of the rat brain (expressed per g of tissue, Ladinsky et al., 1972; Valcana, 1971) and the cerebellum (expressed per organ, Clos, 1980) is retarded in thyroid deficiency. In the cerebellum, the final normal decrease in choline acetyltransferase activity (expressed per g of tissue, Valcana, 1971, or per mg protein, Clos, 1980) is also retarded. The activity expressed per mg protein, however, is finally depressed in the hypothyroid cerebellum (Clos, 1980).

In the forebrain, the normal increase in the density of muscarinic cholinergic receptors is slightly advanced in hyperthyroidism from day 12, while it is transiently delayed in hypothyroidism. In the cerebellum, the development of cholinergic receptors is more markedly influenced by thyroid disorders: the rate of decrease in receptor density is accelerated by hyperthyroidism and retarded in thyroid deficiency. In comparison with controls, the density of muscarinic receptors in the cerebellum is 30% lower in the hyperthyroid rat (at day 21) and 40% higher in the thyroid-deficient animal (at day 35) (Patel et al., 1980b). It is worth mentioning that in the thyroid-deficient cerebellum both the high density of cholinergic receptors and the cholinesterase activity of Purkinje cells (Clos, 1972) persist for a longer time. Similarly, the high initial choline acetyltransferase activity (per g of tissue or mg protein) persists longer in the cerebellum of hypothyroid rats (Valcana, 1971; Clos, 1980). Thus, the development of the cholinergic system in the brain is affected in altered thyroid state.

Monoaminergic systems   Changes in the sensitivity to catecholamines accompany abnormal thyroid states. Thyroid deficiency results in a retardation of the developmental increase of β-adrenergic receptors in the rat forebrain and cerebellum. Replacement therapy from birth restores nearly to normal the density of β-adrenergic receptors in the brain. However, treatment of normal rats with an excess of thyroid hormone has no significant effect upon the age course of the receptor concentration (Smith et al., 1980). It has been reported that in the brain of hypothyroid rats the developmental increase in the concentration of monoamines and the activities of tyrosine hydroxylase and tryptophan hydroxylase, the rate limiting enzymes of monoamine synthesis, are depressed, while these enzyme activities are increased in hyperthyroidism (Rastogi and Singhal, 1976; Rastogi et al., 1976). Reports of Schwark and Keesey (1975, 1976) concerning the effect of neonatal thyroid deficiency on the concentration of monoamines are at variance with these results. However, Schwark and Keesey (1975, 1976) have observed that the apparent turnover rates of serotonin in three brain regions, and of noradrenaline in the hypothalamus only, are reduced under this condition. More information is required to establish the influence of thyroid state on the development of monoaminergic systems in the CNS. It seems to depend on the brain region studied (Vaccari et al., 1977) and undoubtedly it is more complex than that on the noradrenergic system seen in the periphery, where it is clear that hyperthyroidism and hypothyroidism, respectively, accelerate and slow the time course of development of sympathetic nerves and sympathetic function (see for example Lau and Slotkin, 1982). Central aminergic systems develop earlier than cholinergic ones. Thus, they may partly escape the morphogenetic action of thyroid hormone. Nevertheless, morphological evidence from intraocular grafting experiments for thyroxine dependency of the developing noradrenergic neurons of the locus coeruleus (Seiger and Granholm, 1981; Granholm and Seiger, 1981a) and of dopamine-containing neurons of substantia nigra (Granholm and Seiger, 1981b) has been reported.

GABAergic systems   The increase in the density of GABA receptors with age is very small in the normal rat forebrain relative to the marked rise in the cerebellum. In the forebrain, thyroid state has no significant effect on this development. In contrast, the development of the GABAergic system in the cerebellum is a sensitive indicator of the action of thyroid hormone. The ontogenesis of cerebellar GABA receptors is advanced by thyroid hormone treatment and retarded in thyroid deficiency. However, by day 35, receptor density is normal in both conditions (Patel et al., 1980b).

The data available concerning the effects of altered thyroid state on the development of catecholaminergic, cholinergic and GABAergic systems including the transmitter receptors strongly suggest that distortions rather than synchronized shifts occur in the relative development of the central transmitter systems. Such an imbalance between the different interacting neuronal systems can more easily explain the lasting functional anomalies associated with thyroid disorders in early life than synchronized shifts in overall development (see Patel et al., 1980a).

Effects of thyroid hormones on the microtubule apparatus of neurons

From the structural and biochemical data available, it appears that thyroid hormones interact with cell maturation rather than with cell replication, and that their maturational effect on neurons mainly consists in a stimulating action on growth of neuronal processes, since the final configuration of synapses does not seem to be affected in the thyroid-deficient or the hyperthyroid animal. The hormone might modulate some molecular mechanism(s) responsible for control of nerve cell maturation including growth of neuronal processes. Neurite outgrowth and the formation of nerve connections depend on the integrity of the cell microtubular apparatus (Yamada et al., 1970; Spiegelman et al., 1979). Using in vitro experiments with crude supernatants of whole rat brain, it has been shown that during the critical period of development of the brain, thyroid hormones are absolutely necessary for the normal appearance and development of tau factors, i.e. of microtubule associated proteins which act as assembly promoting factors of microtubules (Francon et al., 1977; Fellous et al., 1979; Nunez et al., 1980). The microtubules isolated from the brain of young hypothyroid rats are much shorter and polydispersed when analyzed in sucrose gradient ultracentrifugation (Francon et al., 1982). In electron micrographs of the cerebellar cortex the microtubules of Purkinje cell dendrites are wavy and shorter than normal. They are also not so abundant and not so well axially oriented as in controls. On the other hand, the density of microtubules in the cross sections of granule cell axons is not changed. As a result of their persistent immaturity, the parallel fibres are larger and consequently contain a greater number of microtubules (Vincent et al., in press). In cross sections of the Purkinje cell dendritic tree, it has been found that the density of microtubules is reduced by half in the largest dendritic shafts, while it is not significantly changed in the small ramifications (Faivre et al., 1983). These observations indicate that the effects of thyroid hormone deprivation on the microtubular apparatus are different depending on the size of the cell processes involved. The smallest ones require a normal density of microtubules for their stabilization and elongation. On the other hand, the severe reduction in the number of microtubules in the largest dendritic shafts of Purkinje cells might decrease considerably their possibilities of branching, and might explain the striking hypoplasia of the Purkinje cell dendritic arborization, characteristic of thyroid deficiency.

As described above, the first detectable effect of a single physiological dose of thyroxine injected 24 h before sacrificing the hypothyroid animal at 14 days consists in the rapid elongation of parallel fibres, reflected in the reduction of their cross-sectional area. Concomitantly, the density of microtubules in parallel fibres transiently becomes lower than normal, indicating a very rapid remodelling of their microtubular apparatus under the influence of the hormone (Vincent et al., in press).

In Purkinje cell dendrites, the corrective effects of thyroxine on the development of the microtubular apparatus are also obvious after only one day and complete after four days. The morphological effects of hypothyroidism on mitochondria are relatively weak when compared to those on microtubules. However, mitochondria respond more rapidly than microtubules to thyroxine treatment (Faivre et al., 1983). These observations suggest that beside more general effects on the maturation of neurons, thyroid hormone may control growth and branching of dendrites by an action on microtubules mediated through local stimulation of mitochondria. Microtubule heterogeneity is now well documented. Several reports in the literature show that several categories of microtubules coexist in the central nervous system, differing through their composition and their biochemical properties in vitro (Connolly and Kalnins, 1980a, b; Sandoval and Vandekerkhove, 1981; Job et al., 1981, 1982) or their distribution in axons and dendrites (Matus et al., 1981; Vallee, 1982). Beside their stimulating action on the synthesis of tau factors during brain development, thyroid hormones might lead to subtle changes in the composition and properties of microtubules, including their sensitivity to temperature and Ca^{2+}. The activity of tubulin-tyrosine ligase is also decreased in neonatally hypothyroid mice (Lakshmanan et al., 1981), indicating a biochemical disorder of a-tubulin metabolism. Thus, microtubules are probably the target of multiple molecular changes in altered thyroid state.

Effects of thyroid hormones on glia development and myelination

It is recognized that the development of glia occurs earlier than was generally stated and to a large extent concomitantly with neuron formation and maturation. The morphologic and biochemical data reported above may suggest that in the central nervous system, lack or excess of thyroid hormone affects the formation and maturation of neurons only. Indeed, neurons are not the only cells affected in thyroid dysfunction. Increasing evidence indicates that the development of glia is also altered.

Astroglia

Effects of thyroid deficiency   As mentioned above, thyroid deficiency leads to changes in the final cellular composition of the cerebellum. The astrocytes in the ganglionic layer (Bergmann glial cells) and in the internal granular layer (internal astrocytes) are more numerous (Clos and Legrand, 1973; Nicholson and Altman, 1972a). Astroglial hyperplasia is accompanied by a glial hypertrophy in the molecular layer (Clos et al., 1973) which is more marked in the inner parts of the layer (Vincent et al., in press). A glial hypertrophy is also observed in the internal granular layer around the cerebellar glomeruli (Hajós et al., 1973).

The Bergmann astrocytes are formed relatively early during the late gestational and neonatal period (Clos et al., 1980; Basco et al., 1977; Ghandour et al., 1981). Their cell bodies are located in the vicinity of Purkinje cells and their processes (Bergmann fibres) closely surround the Purkinje cell dendrites in the molecular layer. Their morphologic (as seen in Golgi preparations and electron micrographs) and biochemical maturation (estimated from the dosage of S100 protein, a specific astroglial marker in the cerebellum (Legrand et al., 1981)) are retarded in the hypothyroid rat (Clos et al., 1980, 1982). This causes a prolongation of the period of astroblast multiplication and results in an increased final number of astrocytes.

To what extent these astroglial hyperplasia and hypertrophy constitute a simple reactive response to the important reduction of the neuronal compartment is unknown. Changes in the development of Bergmann fibres may influence the formation, survival, migration and deposition of interneurons (Rákic, 1971a, b; Rákic and Sidman, 1973; Sotelo and Changeux, 1974a). Glial hypertrophy may also influence the establishment of synapses by decreasing the neuronal surface available. For example, the synaptic density is most decreased in the innermost part of the molecular layer. The dendritic tree of Purkinje cells is the most abnormal and the hypertrophy of glial processes the most marked in the same region (Vincent et al., 1983). These facts are undoubtedly correlated.

Effects of thyroid hormone excess   In thyroxine-treated rats the whole maturation process of Bergmann glial cells is accelerated until each cell attains the most mature form (Clos et al., 1980). Acceleration of maturation after thyroxine treatment causes a reduction in the duration of the period during which astrocytes multiply and, because of this, the final number of astrocytes in the cerebellum is reduced (Nicholson and Altman, 1972a). The accelerated maturation of astroglia in the thyroxine-treated animals is reflected in the amount and concentration of S100 protein which are higher than in normal animals during the first three postnatal weeks. The final smaller number of astrocytes is shown by the lower content of S100 protein per cerebellum at 40 days. The S100 protein concentration at 40 days is similar to that in controls. This suggests that the decreased amount of S100 protein, hence the decrease in astrocyte population, is proportional to the reduction in cerebellum size in the thyroxine-treated animals (Clos et al., 1982).

Again, it is not known to what extent these disturbances in Bergmann glia development may influence the maturation of neurons in the hyperthyroid animal.

Oligodendroglia and myelination

Myelination   The formation of a myelin sheath around the axon is one of the most obvious features of the morphological maturation of the neuron. The critical period of the development of the central nervous system coincides with the start of active myelination. Myelinogenesis is retarded and the amount of myelin deposited in the nervous system of rats made thyroid deficient at birth is decreased. However, the final quality of the myelin deposited does not appear to be markedly impaired, indicating that the metabolism of oligodendroglial cells is not greatly abnormal. Conversely a transient and slight advance in myelination can be observed in rats given excess thyroid hormone neonatally. However, in vivo the final myelin content of the brain is reduced in these animals (for a review, see Legrand, 1980). In cultures of rat cerebellum, the most consistent effect of thyroxine is the accelerated appearance of myelin (Hamburgh, 1966). Dissociated brain cells from embryonic mice grown in the presence of hypothyroid calf serum show a diminished synthesis of myelin-associated glycolipids; adding triiodothyronine at physiological concentration in the medium restores to normal the synthesis of cerebrosides and sulfatides (Bhat et al., 1979). It appears that the hormone has differential effects on the development of enzyme activities and exerts a specific inductive effect on certain enzymes directly involved in the process of myelinogenesis (review in Legrand, 1980; see also Clos, 1980; Bhat et al., 1981).

Oligodendroglia   It is generally admitted that oligodendrocytes in the central nervous system are responsible for myelination. Disturbances in this process may therefore result from perturbations in the formation and/or maturation of the former. Disturbances in the migration of glial cells from the subependymal germinative layer up to the cerebral cortex, smaller numbers of well-differentiated oligodendrocytes and hypomyelination in the subcortical white matter have been reported in rats radiothyroidectomized at birth and sacrificed at 50 days of age (Bass and Young, 1973). In the white matter of the hypothyroid rat cerebellum, the number of oligodendrocytes is normal at 35 and 160 days of age, and it is in animals rendered hyperthyroid neonatally that the number of oligodendrocytes is reduced at 35 days (Vitiello et al., 1980; Clos et al., 1982b).

2',3'-Cyclic nucleotide 3'-phosphohydrolase (CNP) is believed to be present in oligodendroglia membranes and is generally considered as a myelin-associated enzyme. The development of the enzyme (in terms of specific activity) is significantly enhanced in the spinal cord of 5 day old rats receiving triiodothyronine injections soon after birth; conversely, in the propylthiouracil-treated rat, the spinal cord has a diminished enzyme activity, which however gradually approaches that of controls by day 23 (Wysocki and Segal, 1972). In cultures of cells dissociated from brains of embryonic mice, CNP activity has been found to be triiodothyronine dependent (Bhat et al., 1981). Carbonic anhydrase (CA form II) is now considered to be another good marker of oligodendrocytes and myelin in the developing cerebellum. In the hypothyroid cerebellum, in comparison with control, the total and specific activities of CAII and CNP are markedly and permanently reduced (Vitiello et al., 1978, 1980; Clos, 1980; Clos et al., 1982b). Since there is no final deficit of oligodendrocytes, it appears that there is a lasting retardation in the maturation of oligodendroglia. In the hyperthyroid cerebellum, the total and specific CAII activities are transiently higher but finally below normal. As for the deficit of myelin, this may be related to the reduction in the final number of oligodendrocytes (Vitiello et al., 1980; Clos, 1980; Clos et al., 1982b).

To summarize, in neonatal hyperthyroidism, myelin and oligodendrocyte markers accumulate at an earlier age than in controls in the cerebellum. The fact that the final number of oligodendrocytes in adulthood is below normal argues in favour of the idea that the hormone acts by switching the glial precursor cells from a proliferating into a differentiating state (as occurs for granule cells). On the other hand, thyroid deficiency retards both the formation and maturation of oligodendrocytes in the cerebellum, without causing a reduction in their final number (as again occurs for granule cells). In the central nervous system, the effect of hypothyroidism on myelin appears to be greater than its effects on the structural and metabolic maturation of oligodendrocytes. This apparent discrepancy may perhaps be explained by the control that the axon exerts on the process of myelination. Lastly, it is not yet known to what extent the effects of altered thyroid state on glia development are direct or mediated through its marked and precocious effects on neurons.

Concluding remarks

From the findings reported above, mainly acquired in vivo, the following conclusions can be drawn for actions within the CNS.

The regions which mature late are the most severely affected in altered thyroid state and are also those which acquire a significant number of late-forming interneurons.

Thyroid hormones affect cell maturation (including cell migration) rather than cell replication in the germinative zones.

The maturational effect of thyroid hormones on neurons mainly consists in a stimulation of the growth and branching of their axon and dendrites. This, in turn, involves an effect on the edification of their microtubular apparatus.

The disturbances in growth of neuronal processes observed in various parts of the hypothyroid or hyperthyroid brain not only lead to final deficits of synapses but can also result in alterations of the synaptic organization (in terms of the distribution of synapses in space).

Owing to its differential effects on the different parts of the brain on the one hand, and to the qualitative and quantitative alterations of neuronal circuitry in various brain regions on the other hand, altered thyroid state may lead to abnormal connectivity.

Physiologic levels of thyroid hormones during an early period of development which covers the main part of the brain growth spurt and may be considered as a critical period, are necessary to allow normal maturation of neurons (and secondarily their normal formation and the establishment of normal interactions between them).

Even when adequate thyroid hormone therapy starts late during development of thyroid-deficient animals, it can still promote some growth of neuronal processes. The number of synapses remains permanently below normal and the synaptic organization (in terms of neuronal circuitry) is irreversibly affected in this condition.

The formation and maturation of glial cells, both astrocytes and oligodendrocytes, are also altered in thyroid dysfunction, as is myelination.

Finally, thyroid hormones appear to be potent factors of nerve and glial cell maturation and of synchronization of the different processes of histogenesis leading to a normal and complex synaptic organization. Even though they may conserve some morphogenetic action after the end of the critical period of development of the central nervous system, their organizing role is particularly obvious during this period. Precise correlations between these findings and the persistent and often irreversible behavioural abnormalities observed in subjects suffering from early acquired hypo- or hyperthyroidism are not yet established.

Several in vitro systems (tissue culture, cultures of dissociated cells, aggregating cell cultures in serum free, chemically defined media) are available for studying the effects of hormones on the development of neurons. As reported above, they have already led to significant results with regard to the action of thyroid hormone on myelination. They may also be useful for identifying specific hormonal effects on individual neurotransmitter systems and for approaching the mechanism of hormone action. The main findings of in vitro studies presently available, mostly on postmitotic neurons from various regions of the central nervous system, seem to show that thyroid hormones at physiologic concentration mostly act on neurite elongation. In addition, they appear to inhibit the development of astrocytes and modulate certain neuron specific enzymes such as choline acetyltransferase (see for example, Puymirat et al., 1982; Tixier-Vidal et al., 1982). On the whole, the findings are consistent with the in vivo observations described above.

Postnatal growth and development of the rat brain are accompanied at the cellular level by changes in the binding properties of the specific nuclear and cytosolic receptors to triiodothyronine. The affinity of the receptors during the period of brain maturation and the number of binding sites in the nuclei tend to diminish with age (Geel, 1977; Valcana and Timiras, 1978; Schwartz and Oppenheimer, 1978; Dozin, 1982). In the rat, plasma thyroxine and triiodothyronine concentrations progressively increase from birth to the third postnatal week and then decrease to attain the value characteristic of the adult (Vigouroux, 1974, 1976; Fisher et al., 1977). Free thyroid hormone concentrations in the plasma show the same developmental pattern as the total hormonal pool of the plasma (Walker et al., 1980). Concomitantly with this stimulation of thyroid function, the captation and utilization (deiodination) of exogenous thyroxine by the brain are greater at 10 than at 30 days (Eberhardt et al., 1976; Vigouroux et al., 1979; Valcana, 1981). Furthermore, in rats maintained in isotopic equilibrium with ^{125}I, the amount of endogenous hormonal iodine is 4 to 6 times higher in the immature neurons isolated in bulk from the brain of 10 day old rats than in the neurons isolated from 30 day old animals. At 10 days, thyroxine and triiodothyronine represent respectively 30 and 60% of the total iodine in the neuronal fraction, suggesting that the metabolism of thyroid hormone is particularly intense in immature neurons (Vigouroux et al., 1979). All these observations may explain the particular sensitivity of the developing brain to thyroid hormones. They are consistent with the generally accepted idea that thyroid hormones, beside other effects, can initiate their maturational effects by augmenting the transcription of genetic information.

Acknowledgements

The main part of the work performed in our group (Drs. J. Clos, C. Faivre, Ch. Legrand, A. Rabié, J. Vincent, Pr.E. Vigouroux and myself) and described in this chapter was supported by grants from DGRST and INSERM. I wish to thank Mrs. C. Aimar for her assistance in preparing this article and for secretarial help.

References

Altman, J. (1969) Autoradiographic and histological studies of postnatal neurogenesis. III. Dating he time of production and onset of differentiation of cerebellar microneurons in rats. J. Comp. Neurol. 136, 269–294.

Balázs, R., Cocks, W.A., Eayrs, J.T. and Kovács, S. (1971a) Biochemical effects of thyroid hormones on the developing brain. In: Hormones in Development (Hamburgh, M. and Barrington, E.J.W., eds.) Appleton Century Crofts, New York, pp. 357–379.

Balázs, R., Kovács, S., Cocks, W.A., Johnson, A.L. and Eayrs, J.T. (1971b) Effect of thyroid hormone on the biochemical maturation of rat brain. Postnatal cell formation. Brain Res. 25, 555–570.

Balázs, R., Kovács, S., Teichgräber, P., Cocks, W.A. and Eayrs, J.T. (1968) Biochemical effects of thyroid deficiency on the developing brain. J. Neurochem. 15, 1335–1349.

Balázs, R., Patel, A.J. and Richter, D. (1973) Metabolic compartments in the brain: their properties and relation to morphological structures. In: Metabolic Compartmentation in the Brain (Balázs, R. and Cremer, J.E., eds.) Macmillan, London, pp. 167–184.

Basco, E., Hajós, F. and Fülöp, Z. (1977) Proliferation of Bergmann glia in the developing rat cerebellum. Anat. Embryol. 151, 219–222.

Bass, N.H. and Young, E. (1973) Effects of hypothyroidism on the differentiation of neurons and glia in developing rat cerebrum. J. Neurol. Sci. 18, 155–173.

Battie, C.A. and Verity, M.A. (1982) Morphology of developing cerebral cortical synaptosomal fractions isolated from eu- and hypothyroid rats. Dev. Brain Res. 3, 219–228.

Bhat, N.R., Sarliève, L.L., Subba Rao, G. and Pieringer, R. (1979) Investigations on myelination in vitro. Regulation by thyroid hormone in cultures of dissociated brain cells from embryonic mice. J. Biol. Chem. 254, 9342–9344.

Bhat, N.R., Subba Rao, G. and Pieringer, R.A. (1981) Investigations on myelination in vitro. Regulation of sulfolipid synthesis by thyroid hormone in cultures of dissociated brain cells from embryonic mice. J. Biol. Chem. 256, 1167–1171.

Bradley, P.B., Eayrs, J.T., Glass, A. and Heath, R.W. (1961) The maturational and metabolic consequences of neonatal thyroidectomy upon the recruiting response in the rat. Electroenceph. Clin. Neurophysiol. 13, 577–586.

Bradley, P.B., Eayrs, J.T. and Richards, N.M. (1964) Factors influencing potentials in normal and cretinous rats. Electroenceph. Clin. Neurophysiol. 17, 308–313.

Bradley, P.B., Eayrs, J.T. and Schmalback, K. (1960) The EEG of normal and hypothyroid rats. Electroenceph. Clin. Neurophysiol. 12, 467–477.

Brasel, J.A. and Boyd, B. (1975) Influence of thyroid hormone on fetal brain growth and development. In: Perinatal Thyroid Physiology and Disease (Fisher, D.A. and Burrow, G.N., eds.) Raven Press, New York, pp. 59–71.

Brown, W.J., Verity, M.A. and Smith, R.L. (1976) Inhibition of cerebellar dendrite development in neonatal thyroid deficiency. Neuropathol. Appl. Neurobiol. 2, 191–207.

Clos, J. (1972) Etude histochimique et biochimique des effets de la déficience thyroïdienne et de la thyroxine sur le développement de l'activité cholinestérasique dans le cervelet du jeune rat. C.R. Acad. Sci. (Paris) 275, 2917–2920.

Clos, J. (1980) Influence de l'état thyroïdien et de la sous-alimentation sur les interactions cellulaires au cours du développement du cervelet du rat. Analyse morphologique, histochimique et biochimique. Thèse de Doctorat-ès-Sciences, Université Montpellier II.

Clos, J., Crépel, F., Legrand, C., Legrand, J., Rabié, A. and Vigouroux, E. (1974) Thyroid physiology during the postnatal period in the rat: a study of the development of thyroid function and of the morphogenetic effects of thyroxine with special reference to cerebellar maturation. Gen. Comp. Endocrinol. 23, 178–192.

Clos, J. and Legrand, J. (1973) Effects of thyroid deficiency on the different cell populations of the cerebellum in the young rat. Brain Res. 63, 450–455.

Clos, J., Legrand, C. and Legrand, J. (1980) Effects of hypothyroidism and hyperthyroidism on the development of cerebellar Bergmann glia. Dev. Neurosci. 3, 199–208.

Clos, J., Legrand, C., Legrand, J., Ghandour, M.S., Labourdette, G., Vincendon, G. and Gombos, G. (1982a) Effects of thyroid state and undernutrition on S100 protein and astroglia development in rat cerebellum. Dev. Neurosci. 5, 285–292.

Clos, J., Legrand, J., Limozin, N., Dalmasso, C. and Laurent, G. (1982b) Effects of abnormal thyroid state and undernutrition on carbonic anhydrase and oligodendroglia development in the rat cerebellum. Dev. Neurosci. 5, 243–251.

Clos, J., Rebière, A. and Legrand, J. (1973) Differential effects of hypothyroidism and undernutrition on the development of glia in the rat cerebellum. Brain Res. 63, 445–449.

Cocks, J.A., Balázs, R., Johnson, A.L. and Eayrs, J.T. (1970) Effect of thyroid hormone on the biochemical maturation of rat brain: conversion of glucose carbon into aminoacids. J. Neurochem. 17, 1275–1285.

Connolly, J.A. and Kalnins, V.I. (1980a) The distribution of tau and HMW associated proteins in different cell types. Exp. Cell Res. 127, 341–350.

Connolly, J.A. and Kalnins, V.I. (1980b) Tau and HMW microtubule associated proteins have different microtubule binding sites in vivo. Eur. J. Cell Biol. 21, 296–300.

Cragg, B.G. (1970) Synapses and membranous bodies in experimental hypothyroidism. Brain Res. 18, 297–307.

Crépel, F. (1972) Maturation of the cerebellar Purkinje cells. II. Hypothyroidism and ontogenesis of cerebellar Purkinje cell spontaneous firing. Exp. Brain Res. 14, 472–479.

Crépel, F. (1974) Excitatory and inhibitory processes acting upon cerebellar Purkinje cells during maturation in the rat; influence of hypothyroidism. Exp. Brain Res. 20, 403–420.

Crépel, F. (1975) Consequences of hypothyroidism during infancy on the function of cerebellar neurons in the adult rat. Brain Res. 85, 157–160.

Crépel, F. (1976) Développement du cervelet chez le Rat; influence des hormones thyroïdiennes et rôle des interactions cellulaires. Thèse de Doctorat-es-Sciences, Université Paris VI. No. CNRS: AO 12327.

Crépel, F., Delhaye-Bouchaud, N. and Dupont, J.L. (1981) Fate of the multiple innervation of cerebellar Purkinje cells by climbing fibers in immature control, X-irradiated and hypothyroid rats. Dev. Brain Res. 1, 59–71.

Crépel, F. and Legrand, J. (1974) Electrophysiological and structural correlates of the effects of thyroid deficiency on the cerebellum of the young rat. In: Ontogenesis of the Brain, Vol. 2 (Jilek, L. and Trojan, S., eds.) Charles University, Prague, pp. 259–270.

Dainat, J., Gourdon, J. and Legrand, J. (1970a) Variations avec l'âge de l'incorporation de la leucine dans les protéines du cervelet après traitement par le propylthiouracile chez le rat. C.R. Soc. Biol. 164, 1550–1554.

Dainat, J. and Legrand, J. (1971) Influence de l'hyperthyroïdisme néonatal sur l'incorporation in vivo de la L-^{3}H-leucine dans les protéines du cervelet chez je jeune rat. C.R. Soc. Biol. 169, 1377–1381.

Dainat, J., Rebière, A. and Legrand, J. (1970b) Influence de la déficience thyroïdienne sur l'incorporation in vivo de la L-^{3}H-leucine dans les protéines du cervelet chez le jeune rat. J. Neurochem. 17, 581–586.

Davenport, J.W. and Dorcey, T.P. (1972) Hypothyroidism: learning deficit induced in rats by early exposure to thiouracil. Hormones Behav. 3, 97–112.

Davenport, J.W. and Gonzales, L.M. (1973) Neonatal thyroxine stmulation in rats: accelerated behavioral maturation and subsequent learning deficit. J. Comp. Physiol. Psychol. 85, 397–408.

Davenport, J.W., Hagquist, W.W. and Hennies, R.S. (1975) Neonatal hyperthyroidism: maturational acceleration and learning deficit in triiodothyronine-stimulated rats. Physiol. Psychol. 3, 231–236.

Davenport, J.W. and Hennies, R.S. (1976) Perinatal hypothyroidism in rats. Persistent motivational and metabolic effects. Dev. Psychobiol. 9, 67–82.

Dozin, B. (1982) Les récepteurs des hormones thyroïdiennes dans le cerveau. Etude chez le rat au cours du développement et à l'âge adulte. Thèse de Doctorat-ès-Sciences, Université catholique de Louvain.

Duvilanski, B.H., Soto, A.M., Ramirez De Guglielmone, A.E. and Gomez, C.J. (1975) Age dependent changes of uridine nucleotide and RNA metabolism in the brain of normal and hypothyroid rats. Acta Physiol. Lat. Am. 25, 165–171.

Eayrs, J.T. (1954) The vascularity of the cerebral cortex in normal and cretinous rats. J. Anat. 88, 164–173.

Eayrs, J.T. (1955) The cerebral cortex of normal and hypothyroid rats. Acta Anat. 25, 160–183.

Eayrs, J.T. (1961) Age as a factor determining the severity and reversibility of the effect of thyroid deprivation in the rat. J. Endocrinol. 22, 409–419.

Eayrs, J.T. (1964) Effect of neonatal hyperthyroidism on maturation and learning in the rat. Anim. Behav. 12, 195–199.

Eayrs, J.T. (1971) Thyroid and developing brain: anatomical and behavioural effects. In: Hormones in Development (Hamburgh, M. and Barrington, E.J.W., eds.) Appleton Century Crofts, New York, pp. 345–355.

Eayrs, J.T. and Horn, G. (1955) The development of cerebral cortex in hypothyroid and starved rats. Anat. Rec. 121, 53–61.

Eayrs, J.T. and Levine, S. (1963) Influence of thyroidectomy and subsequent replacement therapy upon conditioned avoidance in the rat. J. Endocrinol. 25, 503–513.

Eayrs, J.T. and Lishman, W.A. (1955) The maturation of behaviour in hypothyroidism and starvation. Brit. J. Anim. Behav. 3, 17–24.

Eayrs, J.T. and Taylor, S.H. (1951) The effect of thyroid deficiency induced by methylthiouracil on the maturation of the central nervous system. J. Anat. 85, 350–358.

Eberhardt, N.L., Valcana, T. and Timiras, P.S. (1976) Hormone-receptor interactions in brain: uptake and binding of thyroid hormone. Psychoneuroendocrinology 1, 399–409.

Faivre, C., Legrand, C. and Rabié, A. (1983) Effects of thyroid deficiency and corrective effects of thyroxine on microtubules and mitochondria in cerebellar Purkinje cell dendrites of developing rats. Dev. Brain Res. 8, 21–30.

Fazekas, J.F., Graves, F.B. and Alman, R.W. (1951) The influence of the thyroid on cerebral metabolism. Endocrinology 48, 169–174.

Fellous, A., Lennon, A.M., Francon, J. and Nunez, J. (1979) Thyroid hormones and neurotubule assembly in vitro during brain development. Eur. J. Biochem. 101, 365–376.

Fisher, D.A., Dussault, J.H., Sack, J. and Chopra, I.J. (1977) Ontogenesis of hypothalamic-pituitary-thyroid function and metabolism in man, sheep and rat. Rec. Prog. Horm. Res. 33, 59–107.

Francon, J., Fellous, A., Lennon, A.M. and Nunez, J. (1977) Is thyroxine a regulatory signal for neurotubule assembly during brain development. Nature 266, 188–190.

Francon, J., Lennon, A.M., Fellous, A., Marek, A., Pierre, M. and Nunez, J. (1982) Developmental changes in MAPs heterogeneity and the effects of thyroid hormones on microtubule assembly. Third International Meeting of the International Society for Developmental Neurosciences, Patras. Abstr.

Garcia-Argiz, C.A., Pasquini, J.M., Kaplún, B. and Gómez, C.J. (1967) Hormonal regulation of brain development. II. Effect of neonatal thyroidectomy on succinate dehydrogenase and other enzymes in developing cerebral cortex and cerebellum of the rat. Brain Res. 6, 635–646.

Geel, S.E. (1975) Neonatal hypothyroidism: enhanced incorporation of precursors into cerebral RNA in vivo and normalizing effect of a semi-acute injection of thyroxine. Life Sc. 17, 539–544.

Geel, S.E. (1977) Development-related changes of triiodothyronine binding to brain cytosol receptors. Nature 269, 428–430.

Geel, S.E. and Gonzales, L.K. (1975) In vitro studies of cerebral cortical RNA and nucleotide metabolism in hypothyroidism. J. Neurochem. 25, 377–385.

Geel, S.E. and Timiras, P.S. (1967a) The influence of neonatal hypothyroidism and of thyroxine on the ribonucleic acid and deoxyribonucleic acid concentrations of rat cerebral cortex. Brain Res. 4, 135–142.

Geel, S.E. and Timiras, P. S. (1967b) Influence of neonatal hypothyroidism and of thyroxine on the acetylcholinesterase and cholinesterase activities in the developing central nervous system of the rat. Endocrinology 80, 1069–1074.

Geel, S.E. and Timiras, P.S. (1970) Influence of growth hormone on cerebral cortical RNA metabolism in immature hypothyroid rats. Brain Res. 22, 63–72.

Geel, S.E. and Timiras, P.S. (1971) The role of thyroid and growth hormones on RNA metabolism in the immature brain. In: Hormones in Development (Hamburgh, M. and Barrington, E.J.W., eds.) Appleton Century Crofts, New York, pp. 391–401.

Geel, S.E. and Valcana, T. (1971) Cerebral RNA metabolism and thyroid function in early life. In: Influence of Hormones on the Nervous System (Ford, D.H., ed.) Karger, Basel, pp. 165–173.

Geel, S.E., Valcana, T. and Timiras, P.S. (1967) Effect of neonatal hypothyroidism and of thyroxine on (^{14}C)leucine incorporation in protein in vivo and the relationship to ionic levels in the developing brain of the rat. Brain Res. 4, 143–150.

Ghandour, M.S., Labourdette, G., Vincendon, G. and Gombos, G. (1981) A biochemical and immunohistological study of S100 protein in developing rat cerebellum. Dev. Neurosci. 4, 98–109.

Gómez, C.J. and Ramirez De Guglielmone, A.E. (1967) Influence of neonatal thyroidectomy on glucoseaminoacids interrelations in developing rat cerebral cortex. J. Neurochem. 14, 1119–1128.

Gómez, C.J., Ramirez De Guglielmone, A.E. and Duvilanski, B. (1971) Effect of neonatal thyroidectomy on ribonuecleic acid synthesis in developing rat brain. Acta Physiol. Lat. Am. 21, 152–155.

Gourdon, J., Clos, J., Coste, C., Dainat, J. and Legrand, J. (1973) Comparative effects of hypothyroidism, hyperthyroidism and undernutrition on the protein and nucleic acid contents of the cerebellum in the young rat. J. Neurochem. 21, 861–871.

Granholm, A.C. and Seiger, Å (1981a) Thyroid hormone dependency in immature but not mature grafted locus coeruleus neurons. Evidence from intraocular innervation of iris transplants. Med. Biol. 59, 51–57.

Granholm, A.C. and Seiger, Ä (1981b) Thyroxine dependency of the developing substantia nigra. Evidence from intraocular grafting experiments in rats. Neurosci. Lett. 22, 279–284.

Grave, G.D., Satterthwaite, S., Kennedy, C. and Sokoloff, L. (1973) Accelerated postnatal development of D(−) β-hydroxybutyrate deshydrogenase (EC 1.1.1.30) activity in the brain in hyperthyroidism. J. Neurochem. 20, 495–501.

Hajós, F., Patel, A.J. and Balázs, R. (1973) Effects of thyroid deficiency on the synaptic organization of the rat cerebellar cortex. Brain Res. 50, 387–401.

Hamburgh, M. (1958) Effects of thyroid hormone on the maturation of the central nervous system. Am. J. Dis. Child. 96, 521–522.

Hamburgh, M. (1966) Evidence for a direct effect of temperature and thyroid hormone on myelinogenesis in vitro. Dev. Biol. 13, 15–30.

Hamburgh, M. and Flexner, L.B. (1957) Biochemical and physiological differentiation during morphogenesis. XXI. Effect of hypothyroidism and hormone therapy on enzyme activities of the developing cerebral cortex of the rat. J. Neurochem. 1, 279–288.

Hamburgh, M., Lynn, E. and Weiss, E.P. (1964) Analysis of the influence of thyroid hormone on prenatal and postnatal maturation of the rat. Anat. Rec. 150, 147–162.

Hamburgh, M. and Vicari, E. (1957) Effect of thyroid hormone on nervous system maturation. Anat. Rec. 127, 302 (Abstr.).

Hodge, G.K., Butcher, L.L. and Geller, E. (1976) Hormonal effects on the morphologic differentiation of layer VI cortical cells in the rat. Brain Res. 104, 137–141.

Horn, G. (1955) Thyroid deficiency and inanition: the effects of replacement therapy on the development of the cerebral cortex of young albino rats. Anat. Rec. 121, 63–79.

Jarlstedt, J. and Norström, A. (1972) Effect of neonatal hypothyroidism and hyperthyroidism on aminoacid incorporation into proteins of subcellular fractions from developing brain tissue. Exp. Neurol. 34, 51–63.

Job, D., Fischer, E.H. and Margolis, R.L. (1981) Rapid disassembly of cold-stable microtubules by calmodulin. Proc. Natl. Acad. Sci. USA 78, 4679–4682.

Job, D., Rauch, C.T., Fischer, E.H. and Margolis, R.L. (1982) Recycling of cold-stable microtubules: evidence that cold stability is due to substoichiometric polymer blocks. Biochemistry 21, 509–515.

Johanson, I.B., Turkewitz, G. and Hamburgh, M. (1980) Development of home orientation in hypothyroid and hyperthyroid rat pups. Dev. Psychobiol. 13, 331–342.

Klein, A.H., Meltzer, S. and Kenny, F.M. (1972) Improved prognosis in congenital hypothyroidism treated before age three months. J. Pediatr. 81, 912–915.

Kohl, H.H. (1972) Depressed RNA synthesis in the brains and livers of thyroidectomized, normal and hormone injected rats. Brain Res. 40, 445–458.

Ladinsky, H., Consolo, S., Peri, G. and Garattini, S. (1972) Acetylcholine, choline and choline acetyltransferase activity in the developing brain of normal and hypothyroid rats. J. Neurochem. 19, 1947–1952.

Lakshmanan, J., Mansfield, H., Weichsel, M.E., Hoath, S., Scott, S., Shapsak, P. and Fisher, D.A. (1981) Neonatal hypothyroidism. A biochemical disorder of α-tubulin metabolism. Bioch. Biophys. Res. Comm. 100, 1587–1596.

Lau, C. and Slotkin, T.A. (1982) Maturation of sympathetic neurotransmission in the rat heart. VIII. Slowed development of noradrenergic synapses resulting from hypothyroidism. J. Pharmacol. Exp. Ther. 220, 629–636.

Lauder, J.M. (1977) The effects of early hypo- and hyperthyroidism on the development of rat cerebellar cortex. III. Kinetics of cell proliferation in the external granular layer. Brain Res. 126, 31–51.

Lauder, J.M. (1978) Effects of early hypo- and hyperthyroidism on development of rat cerebellar cortex. IV. The parallel fibers. Brain Res. 142, 25–39.

Lauder, J.M. and Mugnaini, E. (1980) Infrapyramidal mossy fibers in the hippocampus of the hyperthyroid rat. A light and electron microscopic study. Dev. Neurosci. 3, 248–265.

Lefranc, G., George, Y. and Tusques, J. (1968) Etude de l'activité acétylcholinestérasique du cortex cérébelleux du rat nouveau-né au cours de sa maturation sous l'action de la thyroxine. C.R. Soc. Biol. 162, 219–221.

Legrand, C. (1969) Influence de l'hypothyroïdisme sur la croissance en longueur et la différenciation histologique du fémur chez le foetus de rat en fin de gestation. Arch. Anat. Microsc. Morphol. Exp. 58, 291–310.

Legrand, C., Clos, J. and Legrand, J. (1982) Influence of altered thyroid and nutritional states on early histogenesis of the rat cerebellar cortex with special reference to synaptogenesis. Reprod. Nutr. Dev. 22, 201–208.

Legrand, C., Clos, J., Legrand, J., Langley, O.K., Ghandour, M.S., Labourdette, G., Gombos, G. and Vincendon, G. (1981) Localization of S100 protein in the rat cerebellum: an electron microscope study coupled to immunoperoxidase technique. Neuropathol. Appl. Neurobiol. 7, 299–306.

Legrand, J. (1963) Maturation du cervelet et déficience thyroïdienne: données chronologiques. Arch. Anat. Microsc. Morphol. Exp. 52, 205–214.

Legrand, J. (1965) Influence de l'hypothyroïdisme sur la maturation du cortex cérébelleux. C.R. Acad. Sci. (Paris) 261, 544–547.

Legrand, J. (1967a) Analyse de l'action morphogénétique des hormones thyroïdiennes sur le cervelet du jeune rat. Arch. Anat. Microsc. Morphol. Exp. 56, 205–244.

Legrand, J. (1967b) Variations, en fonction de l'âge, de la réponse du cervelet à l'action morphogénétique de la thyroïde chez le Rat. Arch. Anat. Microsc. Morphol. Exp. 56, 291–307.

Legrand, J. (1967c) La maturation du cervelet chez le rat blanc hypothyroïdien. In: Regional Development of the Brain in Early Life (Minkowski, A., ed.) Blackwell Scientific Publications, Oxford, pp. 485–493.

Legrand, J. (1980) Effects of thyroid hormone on brain development, with particular emphasis on glial cells and myelination. In: Multidisciplinary Approach to Brain Development (di Benedetta, C., Balázs, R., Gombos, G. and Porcellati, G., eds.) Elsevier/North-Holland Biomedical Press, Amsterdam, pp. 279–292.

Legrand, J. and Bout, M.C. (1970) Influence de l'hypothyroïdisme et de la thyroxine sur le développement des épines dendritiques des cellules de Purkinje dans le cervelet du jeune Rat. C.R. Acad. Sci. (Paris) 271, 1199–1202.

Legrand, J., Kriegel, A. and Jost, A. (1961) Déficience thyroïdienne et maturation du cervelet chez le Rat blanc. Arch. Anat. Microsc. Morphol. Exp. 50, 507–519.

Legrand, J., Selme-Matrat, M., Rabié, A., Clos, J. and Legrand, C. (1976) Thyroid hormone and cell formation in the developing rat cerebellum. Biol. Neonate 29, 368–380.

Lenard, H.G. and Bell, E.F. (1973) Bioelectric brain development in hypothyroidism. A quantitative analysis with EEG power spectra. Electroenceph. Clin. Neurophysiol. 35, 545–549.

Lewis, P.D. (1975) Cell death in the germinal layers of the postnatal rat brain. Neuropathol. Appl. Neurobiol. 1, 21–29.

Lewis, P.D., Patel, A.J., Johnson, A.L. and Balázs, R. (1976) Effect of thyroid deficiency on cell acquisition in the postnatal rat brain. A quantitative histological study. Brain Res. 104, 49–62.

Lu, E.J. and Brown, W.J. (1977a) An electron microscopic study of the developing caudate nucleus in euthyroid and hypothyroid states. Anat. Embryol. 150, 335–364.

Lu, E.J. and Brown, W.J. (1977b) The developing caudate nucleus in the euthyroid and hypothyroid rat. J. Comp. Neurol. 171, 261–284.

Macho, L., Štrbák, V. and Hromadová, M. (1972) The effect of thyroxine on aminoacid incorporation into protein during ontogenesis in rat. Hormones 3, 354–360.

Matus, A., Bernhardt, R. and Hugh-Jones, T. (1981) High molecular weight microtubule-associated proteins are preferentially associated with dendritic microtubules in brain. Proc. Natl. Acad. Sci. USA 78, 3010–1014.

Michels, R., Cason, J. and Sokoloff, L. (1963) Thyroxine: effects on amino acid incorporation into protein in vivo. Science 140, 1417–1418.

Murphy, J.M. and Nagy, Z.M. (1976) Neonatal thyroxine stimulation accelerates the maturation of both locomotor and memory processes in mice. J. Comp. Physiol. Psychol. 90, 1082–1091.

Nicholson, J.L. and Altman, J. (1972a) The effects of early hypo- and hyperthyroidism on the development of rat cerebellar cortex. I. Cell proliferation and differentiation. Brain Res. 44, 13–23.

Nicholson, J.L. and Altman, J. (1972b) The effects of early hypo- and hyperthyroidism on the development of the rat cerebellar cortex. II. Synaptogenesis in the molecular layer. Brain Res. 44, 25–36.

Nunez, J., Francon, J., Lennon, A.M., Fellous, A. and Marek, A. (1980) The role of MAPs in microtubule assembly. In: Microtubules and Microtubule Inhibitors (de Brabander, M. and de Meys, J., eds.) Elsevier/North-Holland, Amsterdam, pp. 213–225.

Pascual-Leone, A.M., Garcia, M.D., Hervas, F. and Morreale de Escobar, G. (1976) Decreased pituitary growth hormone content in rats treated neonatally with high doses of L-thyroxine. Horm. Metabol. Res. 8, 215–217.

Pasquini, J.M., Kaplún, B., Garcia-Argiz, C.A. and Gómez, C.J. (1967) Hormonal regulation of brain development. I. The effect of neonatal thyroidectomy upon nucleic acids, protein and two enzymes in developing cerebral cortex and cerebellum of the rat. Brain Res. 6, 621–634.

Patel, A.J., Balázs, R., Smith, R.M., Kingsbury, A.E. and Hunt, A. (1980a) Thyroid hormone and brain development. In: Multidisciplinary Approach to Brain Development (di Benedetta, C., Balázs, R., Gombos, G. and Porcellati, G., eds.) Elsevier/North-Holland Biomedical Press, Amsterdam, pp. 261–277.

Patel, A.J., Lewis, P.D., Balázs, R., Bailey, P. and Lai, M. (1979) Effects of thyroxine on postnatal cell acquisition in the rat brain. Brain Res. 172, 57–72.

Patel, A.J. and Rabié, A. (1980) Thyroid deficiency and cell death in the rat cerebellum during development. Neuropathol. Appl. Neurobiol. 6, 45–49.

Patel, A.J., Rabié, A., Lewis, P.D. and Balázs, R. (1976) Effects of thyroid deficiency on postnatal cell formation in the rat brain. A biochemical investigation. Brain Res. 104, 33–48.

Patel, A.J., Smith, R.M., Kingsbury, A.E., Hunt, A. and Balázs, R. (1980b) Effects of thyroid state on brain development: muscarinic acetylcholine and gaba receptors. Brain Res. 198, 389–409.

Phelps, C.P. and Leathem, J.H. (1976) Effects of postnatal thyroxine administration on brain development, response to postnatal androgen and thyroid regulation in female rats. J. Endocrinol. 69, 175–182.

Puymirat, J., Barret, A., Faivre-Bauman, A., Loudes, C. and Tixier-Vidal, A. (1982) Effect of triiodothyronine (T3) on the development of mouse fetal hypothalamic cells in vitro. EMBO Workshop, the Molecular Mechanisms of Nervous System Development, Strasbourg (Abstr.).

Rabié, A., Clavel, M.C. and Legrand, J. (1980a) Analysis of the mechanisms underlying increased histogenetic cell death in the developing cerebellum of the hypothyroid rat: determination of the time required for granule cell death. Brain Res. 190, 409–414.

Rabié, A., Favre, C., Clavel, M.C. and Legrand, J. (1977) Effects of thyroid dysfunction on the development of the rat cerebellum, with special reference to cell death within the internal granular layer. Brain Res. 120, 521–531.

Rabié, A., Favre, C., Clavel, M.C. and Legrand, J. (1979a) Sequential effects of thyroxine on the developing cerebellum of rats made hypothyroid by propylthiouracil. Brain Res. 161, 469–479.

Rabié, A., Favre, C., Clavel, M.C. and Legrand, J. (1980b) Thyroid hormone and cell death in the developing rat cerebellum. In: Multidisciplinary Approach to Brain Development (di Benedetta, C., Balázs, R., Gombos, G. and Porcelatti, G., eds.) Elsevier/North-Holland Biomedical Press, Amsterdam, pp. 317–318.

Rabié, A. and Legrand, J. (1973) Effects of thyroid hormone and undernourishment on the amount of synaptosomal fraction in the cerebellum of the young rat. Brain Res. 61, 267–278.

Rabié, A., Patel, A.J., Clavel, M.C. and Legrand, J. (1979b) Effect of thyroid deficiency on the growth of the hippocampus in the rat. A combined biochemical and morphological study. Dev. Neurosci. 2, 183–194.

Rakic, P. (1971a) Guidance of neurons migrating to the fetal monkey neocortex. Brain Res. 33, 471–476.

Rakic, P. (1971b) Neuron-glia relationship during granule cell migration in developing cerebellar cortex. A Golgi and electron microscopic study in Macacus rhesus. J. Comp. Neurol. 141, 283–312.

Rakic, P. and Sidman, R.L. (1973) Sequence of developmental abnormalities leading to granule cell deficit in cerebellar cortex of Weaver mutant mice. J. Comp. Neurol. 182, 103–132.

Rastogi, R.B., Lapierre, Y. and Singhal, R.L. (1976) Evidence for the role of brain biogenic amines in depressed motor activity seen in chemically thyroidectomized rats. J. Neurochem. 26, 443–449.

Rastogi, R.B. and Singhal, R.L. (1976) Influence of neonatal and adult hyperthyroidism on behavior and biosynthetic capacity for norepinephrine, dopamine and 5-hydroxytryptamine in rat brain. J. Pharmacol. Exp. Ther. 198, 609–618.

Rebière, A. and Legrand, J. (1972a) Effets comparés de la sous-alimentation, de l'hypothyroïdisme et de l'hyperthyroïdisme sur la maturation histologique de la zone moléculaire du cortex cérébelleux chez le jeune Rat. Arch. Anat. Microsc. Morphol. Exp. 61, 105–126.

Rebière, A. and Legrand, J. (1972b) Données quantitatives sur la synaptogenèse dans le cervelet du rat normal et rendu hypothyroïdien par le propylthiouracile. C.R. Acad. Sci. (Paris) 274, 3581–3584.

Reiss, J.M., Reiss, M. and Wyatt, A. (1956) Action of thyroid hormones on brain metabolism of newborn rats. Proc. Soc. Exp. Biol. Med. 93, 19–22.

Ruiz-Marcos, A., Sala, J., Sanchez-Toscano, F. and Morreale de Escobar, G. (1978) Influence of neonatal hypothyroidism on the pyramidal cells of the rat auditory cortex. Ann. Endocrinol. (Paris) 39, 15A (Abstr.).

Ruiz-Marcos, A., Sanchez-Toscano, F., Escobar Del Rey, F. and Morreale de Escobar, G. (1979) Severe hypothyroidism and the maturation of the rat cerebral cortex. Brain Res. 162, 315–329.

Ruiz-Marcos, A., Sanchez-Toscano, F., Escobar Del Rey, F. and Morreale de Escobar, G. (1980) Reversible morphological alterations of cortical neurons in juvenile and adult hypothyroidism in the rat. Brain Res. 185, 91–102.

Ruiz-Marcos, A., Sanchez-Toscano, F., Escobar Del Rey, F. and Morreale de Escobar, G. (1981) Maturation of pyramidal cells of the cerebral cortex in hypothyroidism. In: Fetal Brain Disorders-Recent Approaches to the Problem of Mental Deficiency (Hetzel, B.S. and Smith, R.M., eds.) Elsevier/North-Holland Biomedical Press, Amsterdam, pp. 205–226.

Ruiz-Marcos, A., Sanchez-Toscano, F., Obregon, M.J., Escobar Del Rey, F. and Morreale de Escobar, G. (1982) Thyroxine treatment and recovery of hypothyroidism-induced pyramidal cell damage. Brain Res. 239, 559–574.

Sanchez-Toscano, F., Escobar Del Rey, F., Morreale de Escobar, G. and Ruiz-Marcos, A. (1977) Measurement of the effects of hypothyroidism on the number and distribution of spines along the apical shaft of pyramidal neurons of the rat cerebral cortex. Brain Res. 126, 547–550.

Sandoval, I.V. and Vandekerckhove, J.S. (1981) A comparative study of the in vitro polymerization of tubulin in the presence of the microtubule associated proteins MAP2 and tau. J. Biol. Chem. 256, 8795–8800.

Schalock, R.L., Brown, W.J. and Smith, R.L. (1977) Neonatal hypothyroidism: behavioral, thyroid hormonal and neuroanatomical effects. Physiol. Behav. 19, 489–491.

Schapiro, S. (1968) Some physiological, biochemical and behavioural consequences of neonatal hormone administration: cortisol and thyroxine. Gen. Comp. Endocrinol. 10, 214–228.

Schapiro, S., Vukovich, K. and Globus, A. (1973) Effects of neonatal thyroxine and hydrocortisone administration on the development of dendritic spines in visual cortex of rats. Exp. Neurol. 40, 286–296.

Schwark, W.S. and Keesey, R.R. (1975) Thyroid hormone control of serotonin in developing rat brain. Res. Comm. Chem. Pathol. Pharmacol. 10, 37–50.

Schwark, W.S. and Keesey, R.R. (1976) Influence of thyroid hormone on norepinephrine metabolism in rat brain during maturation. Res. Comm. Chem. Pathol. Pharmacol. 13, 673–683.

Schwartz, H.L. and Oppenheimer, J.H. (1978) Ontogenesis of 3,5,3′-triiodothyronine receptors in neonatal rat brain: dissociation between receptor concentration and stimulation of oxygen consumption by 3,5,3′-triiodothyronine. Endocrinology 103, 943–948.

362

Seiger, Å and Granholm, A.C. (1981) Thyroxin dependency of the developing locus coeruleus. Evidence from intraocular grafting experiments. Cell Tissue Res. 220, 1–15.

Sjöden, P.O. (1976) Effects of neonatal thyroid hormone stimulation and differential preweaning rearing on spatial discrimination learning in rats. Physiol. Psychol. 4, 515–520.

Sjöden, P.O. and Söderberg, U. (1976a) Effects of neonatal thyroxine stimulation on adult open-field behaviour and thyroid activity in rats. Physiol. Psychol. 4, 50–56.

Sjöden, P.O. and Söderberg, U. (1976b) Effects of neonatal thyroid hormone stimulation and differential preweaning rearing on open-field behavior in rats. Dev. Psychobiol. 9, 413–424.

Smith, D.W., Blizzard, R.M. and Wilkins, L. (1957) The mental prognosis in hypothyroidism of infancy and childhood. A review of 128 cases. Pediatrics 19, 1011–1022.

Smith, R.M., Patel, A.J., Kingsbury, A.E., Hunt, A. and Balázs, R. (1980) Effects of thyroid state on brain development: β-adrenergic receptors and 5'-nucleotidase activity. Brain Res. 198, 375–387.

Sotelo, C. and Changeux, J.P. (1974a) Bergmann fibers and granular cell migration in the cerebellum of homozygous Weaver mutant mouse. Brain Res. 77, 484–491.

Sotelo, C. and Changeux, J.P. (1974b) Transynaptic degeneration 'en cascade' in the cerebellar cortex of staggerer mutant mice. Brain Res. 77, 519–526.

Spiegelman, B.N., Lopata, M.A. and Kirschner, M.W. (1979) Aggregation of microtubule initiation sites preceding neurite outgrowth in mouse neuroblastoma cells. Cell 16, 253–263.

Stone, J.M. and Greenough, W.T. (1975) Excess neonatal thyroxine: effects on learning in infant and adolescent rats. Dev. Psychobiol. 8, 479–488.

Szijan, I., Kalbermann, L.E. and Gómez, C.J. (1971) Hormonal regulation of brain development. IV. Effect of neonatal thyroidectomy upon incorporation in vivo of L^{3}H phenylalanine into proteins of developing rat cerebral tissues and pituitary gland. Brain Res. 27, 309–318.

Tata, J.R. and Widnell, C.C. (1966) Ribonucleic acid synthesis during the early action of thyroid hormones. Biochem. J. 98, 604–619.

Tixier-Vidal, A., Faivre-Bauman, A., Loudes, C. and Puymirat, J. (1982) Effect of hormones on neuron survival and development in culture. Third International Meeting of the International Society for Developmental Neurosciences, Patras, Abstr.

Tusques, J. (1956) Recherches expérimentales sur le rôle de la thyroïde dans le développement du système nerveux. Biol. Méd. 45, 395–413.

Tusques, J., Lefranc, G. and George, Y. (1967) Analyse par la technique de Golgi-Cox de la maturation du cortex cérébelleux sous l'influence de la thyroxine chez le rat nouveau-né. C.R. Soc. Biol. 161, 2256–2260.

Vaccari, A., Valcana, T. and Timiras, P.S. (1977) Effects of hypothyroidism on the enzymes for biogenic amines in the developing rat brain. Pharmacol. Res. Comm. 9, 763–780.

Valcana, T. (1971) Effect of neonatal hypothyroidism on the development of acetylcholinesterase and choline acetyltransferase activities in the rat brain. In: Influence of Hormones on the Nervous System (Ford, D.H., ed.) Karger, Basel, pp. 174–184.

Valcana, T. (1981) Conversion and binding of tetraiodothyronine in developing rat brain. Neurochem. Res. 6, 743–753.

Valcana, T. and Timiras, P.S. (1978) Nuclear triiodothyronine receptors in the developing rat brain. Mol. Cell. Endocrinol. 11, 31–41.

Vallee, R.B. (1982) A taxol-dependent procedure for the isolation of microtubules and microtubule associated proteins (MAPs). J. Cell. Biol. 92, 435–442.

Verity, M.A., Brown, W.J., Cheung, M., Huntsman, H. and Smith, R. (1976) Effects of neonatal hypothyroidism on cerebral and cerebellar synaptosome development. J. Neurosci. Res. 2, 323–335.

Vigouroux, E. (1974) Développement de la fonction thyroïdienne chez le jeune Rat. Thèse de Doctorat-ès-Sciences, Université Paris VI, No. CNRS: AO 10057.

Vigouroux, E. (1976) Dynamic study of postnatal thyroid function in the rat. Acta Endocrinol. 83, 752–762.

Vigouroux, E., Clos, J. and Legrand, J. (1979) Uptake and metabolism of exogenous and endogenous thyroxine in the brain of young rats. Horm. Metabol. Res. 11, 228–232.

Vincent, J., Legrand, C., Rabié, A. and Legrand, J. (1983) Effects of thyroid hormone on synaptogenesis in the molecular layer of the developing rat cerebellum. J. Physiol. (Paris), in press.

Vincent, J., Rabié, A. and Legrand, C. (1979) Thyroxine et synaptogenèse dans le cervelet du Rat. J. Physiol. (Paris) 75, 25A (Abstr.).

Vitiello, F., Clos, J., Legrand, J., Ghandour, M.S., Filippi, D., Limozin, N., Laurent, G. and Vincendon, G. (1980) Myelination and oligodendroglia development in the rat cerebellum: effects of undernutrition and thyroid state. In: Multidisciplinary Approach to Brain Development (di Benedetta, C., Balázs, R., Gombos, G. and Porcellati, G., eds.) Elsevier/North-Holland Biomedical Press, Amsterdam, pp. 329–330.

Vitiello, F., Ghandour, M.S., Clos, J., Legrand, J., Vincendon, G. and Gombos, G. (1978) Effects of neonatal hypothyroidism on rat cerebellum ontogenesis. Second Meeting of the European Society for Neurochemistry, Gottingen (Abstr.).

Walker, P., Dubois, J.D. and Dussault, J.H. (1980) Free thyroid hormone concentrations during postnatal development in the rat. Pediatr. Res. 14, 247–249.

Weichsel Jr., M.E. (1974) Effect of thyroxine on DNA synthesis and thymidine kinase activity during cerebellar development. Brain Res. 78, 455–465.

Wolter, R., Noël, P., De Cock, P., Craen, M., Ernould, C.H., Malvaux, P., Verstraeten, F., Simons, J., Mertens, S., Van Broek, N. and Vanderschueren-Lodewyckx, M. (1980) Neuropsychological study in treated thyroid dysgenesis. Acta Pediatr. Scand. 277, 41–46.

Wysocki, S.J. and Segal, W. (1972) Influence of thyroid hormones on enzyme activities of myelinating rat central nervous tissues. Eur. J. Biochem. 28, 183–189.

Yamada, K.M., Spooner, B.S. and Wessels, N.K. (1979) Axon growth: roles of microfilaments and microtubules. Proc. Natl. Acad. Sci. USA 66, 1206–1212.

Neurobehavioral Teratology
edited by Joseph Yanai
© Elsevier Science Publishers BV 1984

16

GLUCOCORTICOID INDUCED TERATOLOGIES
OF THE NERVOUS SYSTEM

Martha C. Bohn

Department of Neurobiology and Behavior, State University of New York at Stony Brook,
Stony Brook, NY 11794, USA

ALTHOUGH steroid hormones influence the differentiation of many tissues, their influence on the developing nervous system is particularly interesting since alterations in steroid levels during development may permanently affect behavior, homeostatic control mechanisms and brain morphology. In the case of steroids produced by the gonads, these effects are well known and it is evident that the maintenance of physiological levels of gonadal steroids is important for the normal development of sex-related behavior and the control of gonadotrophic hormone secretion (for reviews see McEwen, 1982; McEwen et al., 1982). In contrast, the physiological role(s) of glucocorticoids in brain development is less clear, although numerous studies have demonstrated behavioral abnormalities in rodents following neonatal glucocorticoid treatment (Table 16.1)

Glucocorticoids have specific effects on various stages of cell differentiation in both neurons and glial cells. Our studies and those of others have demonstrated that glucocorticoids affect (1) the rate of cell proliferation in various germinal zones in the brain, (2) the kinetics of cell generation and the number of cells generated, (3) phenotypic expression and development of neuronal and glial antigens, (4) myelination, and (5) dendritic and axonal growth. Studies demonstrating these effects will be reviewed here with the perspective that the pharmacological treatment of developing rodents with glucocorticoids may elucidate conditions which could lead to behavioral, biochemical or morphological teratologies of the nervous system in humans, and suggest mechanisms which, in the future, may lead to an understanding of the physiological role played by glucocorticoids in the development of the nervous system.

Table 16.1. Effects of neonatal glucocorticoid treatment on the development of behavior
[a]Rat; [b]mouse; [c]ducklings; F, cortisol; B, corticosterone; DEX, dexamethasone.

Effect	Steroid and dose	Age at treatment	Reference
Decreased activity in openfield test in adults[a,b]	F[a], 1 mg; B[b], pellet	day 1	Schapiro, 1968; Howard and Granoff, 1968
High activity in openfield test[a]	B, 250 mg/kg	day 6	Turner and Taylor, 1975
Delayed development of startle response[a]	F, 1 mg	day 1	Schapiro, 1971a
Delayed development of swimming response	F, 0.5–1 mg	day 1	Schapiro, 1971b; Anderson and Schanberg, 1975
Delayed ontogeny of cortical evoked potential response to light, sound and sciatic nerve stimulation[a]	F, 1 mg	day 1	Salas and Schapiro, 1970
Decreased voluntary running in activity wheels and fine motor coordination[b]	B, pellet	day 1	Howard and Granoff, 1968
Increased rearing activity[b]	B, 500 μg	days 3–5	Nyakas, 1977
Impaired acquisition of 2-way, but not 1-way, active avoidance[a]	B, pellet	day 2	Olton et al., 1974
Delayed development of tonic-clonic seizure response[a]	F, 10 mg/kg	days 4–7	Vernadakis and Woodbury, 1963
Accelerated development of tonic-clonic seizure response[a]	F, 10 mg/kg	days 8–12 or 13–16	Vernadakis and Woodbury, 1963
Lengthened estrous cycle[a]	F, 0.5 mg; DEX, 1 μg	day 3	Cost and Mann, 1976
Low lordosis quotients and altered estrous cycles	B, 250 mg/kg	day 3, 6, 12 or 18	Turner and Taylor, 1977
Suppression of circadian rhythm of plasma B at 30 days[a]	F, 0.5 mg; DEX, 1 μg	days 2 or 4	Krieger, 1972
Delayed development of plasma B rhythm at 30 days with establishment at 70 days[a]	F, 0.5 mg; DEX, 1 μg	day 3	Cost and Mann, 1976
Altered pituitary adrenal function[a]	B, 250 mg/kg	days 3, 6, 12 or 18	Turner and Taylor, 1976
Decreased stress response at 20–25 days due to increased feedback sensitivity to circulating corticosteroids[a]	F, 0.1–1 mg	day 1	Erskine et al., 1979, 1981
Delayed onset of corticosterone rhythm[a]	DEX, 100 μg	day 1	Poland et al., 1981a
Altered circadian rhythm of plasma TSH[a]	DEX, 100 μg	day 1	Poland et al., 1981b
Inhibited approach and following response[c]	B, 500 ng	day 1	Martin, 1978
Facilitation of following response[c]	antiserum to B	day 1	Martin, 1978

Effects on cell proliferation in brain

High levels of glucocorticoids inhibit the rate of cell proliferation in most developing tissues and cells in cultures (Chen et al., 1977; Fodge and Rubin, 1975; Frankfurt, 1968; Grasso and Johnson, 1977; Henderson and Loeb, 1974; Wright et al., 1974). Similarly, treatment of newborn rodents with cortisol or corticosterone inhibits body and brain growth producing permanent decreases in brain weight and DNA content in adult animals (Table 16.2). These deficits are particularly marked in the cerebellum where most neurogenesis takes place during the postnatal period. The incorporation of tritiated thymidine ([³H]T) into DNA is inhibited in cerebellum, whole cerebrum, hippocampus and olfactory bulb during the period of glucocorticoid treatment (Coterrell et al., 1972; Szijan and Burdman, 1973; Bohn, 1980) suggesting that this growth retardation results from an interference with the rate of cell formation rather than cell destruction. To investigate the neuromorphological consequences of glucocorticoids, we undertook a series of autoradiographic studies of cell proliferation and genesis in three germinal zones in the brain of the postnatal rat treated with cortisol: (1) the external granular layer (EGL) of the cerebellum, (2) the hilus of the dentate gyrus in the hippocampal formation, and (3) the subventricular zone of the lateral ventricle.

Table 16.2. Glucocorticoid effects on cell proliferation and DNA synthesis in brain
[a]Rat; [b]mouse; EGL, cerebellar external granular layer; [³H]T, tritiated thymidine; ODC, ornithine decarboxylase; SVZ, subventricular zone; TK, thymidine kinase

Effect	Treatment	Reference
Decreased cerebral and cerebellar DNA content[a,b]	B pellet, day 2	Howard, 1968; Howard, 1973
Inhibited incorporation of [³H]T into DNA during treatment and decreased DNA in cerebellum, cerebrum and olfactory bulb at 35 days[a]	F, 200 µg/day days 1–4	Cotterell et al., 1972
Decreased incorporation of [³H]T into DNA in hippocampus[a]	F, 200 µg/day days 1–4	Bohn, 1980
Decreased DNA content in cerebellum and cerebrum and increased mean cell territory[a]	F, various treatments	Clos et al., 1975
Inhibited incorporation of [³H]T into DNA and decreased leucine incorporation into chromatin proteins[a]	F, 60 µg/g, day 6 or 20	Szijan and Burdman, 1973; Burdman, 1975
Decreased labeling index in EGL, dentate gyrus and SVZ; Decreased mitotic index in EGL[a]	F, 200 µg/day days 1–4	Bohn and Lauder, 1978; Bohn, 1979, 1980
Altered genesis of different types of neurons[a]	F, 200 µg/day days 1–4 or 10 µg/g, days 7–18	Bohn and Lauder, 1978, 1980; Bohn, 1980
Prolonged genesis of oligodendrocytes in optic nerve[a]	F, 10 µg/g, days 7–18	Bohn and Friedrich, 1982
Decreased TK activity at 3 and 6 days and increased activity at 12 and 15 days[a]	F, 0.6 mg at birth	Weichsel, 1974
Altered ontogeny of ODC activity	F, 0.5 mg at birth or DEX, 1 mg/kg days 1–4	Anderson and Schanberg, 1975; Slotkin et al., 1982

Cell proliferation in the cerebellum

The rodent cerebellar cortex is an elegant structure for developmental studies since it consists of a few, easily identified cell types (Paley and Chan-Palay, 1974) whose genesis and differentiation have been described in detail in normal animals (Altman, 1969, 1972a,b,c). Most of the neurons comprising the cerebellar cortex are formed from a secondary germinal zone, the EGL which arises prenatally from the rhombic lip at the junction of the alar and basal plates of the neural epithelium and forms a sheet of cells covering the surface of the cerebellum (Harkmark, 1954; Altman, 1972a). In the newborn rat, the EGL is only one to two cells thick, but it increases in thickness during the first ten postnatal days due to a rapid rate of cell division. As the EGL grows, waves of cells become postmitotic, migrate out of the EGL and differentiate into cerebellar microneurons of the molecular layer (the basket and stellate cells) and the internal granular layer (granule cells). The EGL then gradually dissipates and disappears around postnatal day 24.

We compared the effects of glucocorticoids on cerebellar development at two different stages by treating with cortisol immediately after birth (days 1–4) or from days 7 to 18. These two paradigms were chosen since previous studies had suggested that 'early' and 'late' postnatal cortisol treatments have opposite effects on neural development (Vernadakis and Woodbury, 1963). When cortisol treated rats reach adulthood the size of the cerebellum and the number of microneurons are reduced with the deficits greater in rats receiving the late treatment (Fig. 16.1; Bohn and Lauder, 1978, 1980). The number of granule and stellate cells in the late treated rats is reduced by 40% and 30%, respectively (Bohn and Lauder, 1980). While the early treatment results in cerebellar weight and neuronal deficits in the range of only 20%, this treatment has a more dramatic effect than the late treatment on the shape of the cerebellum since it markedly changes the development of foliation producing malformed lobules in the adult (Figs. 16.1 and 2).

A number of observations suggest that treatment during either stage inhibits cell proliferation in the EGL. As mentioned before, the incorporation of [³H]T into DNA is inhibited by the early treatment (Cotterell et al, 1972). We have observed that the mitotic index, the labeling index, the number of EGL cells and EGL size are all

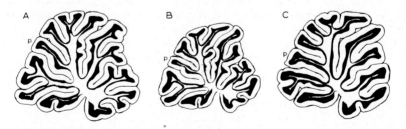

Fig. 16.1. Midsagittal sections of the cerebellar vermis (72 days of age). A. control. B. Hydrocortisone acetate (HCA) on days 7–18. C. Hydrocortisone (HCA) on days 1–4. p = pyramis (lobule VIII). By permission of S. Karger, Basel.

369

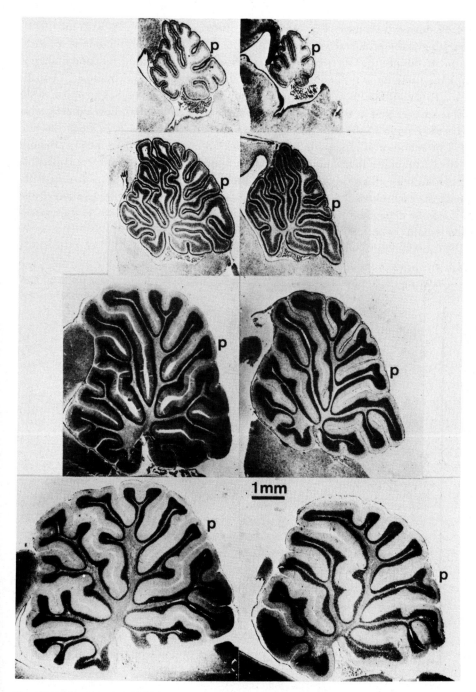

Fig. 16.2. Effect of cortisol (HCA) treatment on days 1–4 on cerebellar folication. A. 5-day control. B. 5-day HCA. C. 10-day control. D. 10-day HCA. E. 21-day control. F. 21-day HCA. G. 72-day control. H. 72-day HCA. p = pyramis (lobule VIII). By permission of S. Karger, Basel.

reduced during treatment (Figs. 16.3 and 4; Bohn and Lauder, 1978; Bohn, 1979). Interestingly, cell proliferation in the EGL rebounds following termination of the early treatment, but not the late treatment. This rebound is similar to the rebound in thymidine kinase activity in the cerebellum observed after glucocorticoid treatment (Weichsel Jr., 1974). Although this rebound is insufficient to produce a full complement of cells, it appears that at early stages, but not at late stages, of EGL development most EGL cells remain in the cell cycle or can re-enter the cell cycle even when the rate of cell proliferation is inhibited. Since both the mitotic and labeling indices rebound above control levels following termination of glucocorticoid treatment, it is possible that the decrease in glucocorticoid levels following termination of treatment actually stimulates cell proliferation. Consequently, a normal rate of cell proliferation in the EGL may be dependent on physiological levels of these steroids. However, this speculation remains to be proven.

Cell proliferation in the hippocampus
In considering the action of glucocorticoids on brain development, their effects on hip-

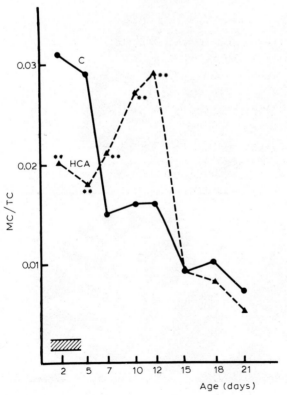

Fig. 16.3. Mitotic index in the external granular layer (EGL) of cerebellar lobule VIII (number of mitotic cells divided by the total number of cells; MC/TC); C = control; HCA = cortisol; Hatched inset indicates treatment period; **$p \leqslant 0.01$; by permission of S. Karger, Basel.

pocampal development is particularly interesting for two reasons. First, the hippocampus is another brain region in which most of the microneurons, the granule cells in
the dentate gyrus, are formed after birth (Bayer and Altman, 1974; Schlessinger et al.,
1975). Secondly, glucocorticoid receptors are more highly concentrated in the hippocampus than any other brain region (Stumpf, 1971; McEwen et al., 1975). As anticipated, cortisol treatment on days 1–4 was observed to inhibit cell proliferation in the
hippocampus as revealed by the decreased incorporation of [³H]T into DNA (Fig.
16.5; Bohn, 1980). This inhibition was particularly evident in the ventral hippocampus
where the number of [³H]T labeled cells was severely reduced in the hilus of the dentate gyrus, a secondary germinal zone giving rise to granule cells (Fig. 16.6; Bohn,
1980; Bayer and Altman, 1974; Schlessinger et al., 1975). Similar to observations made
in the cerebellum, cell proliferation in the dentate gyrus of rats receiving cortisol on
days 1–4 rebounds during the second postnatal week (Fig. 16.5). However, in contrast
to the cerebellum, the size of the granular layer in the hippocampus is not significantly
decreased in adult rats treated with cortisol at birth in spite of the severe inhibition
of cell proliferation during treatment (Bohn, 1980).

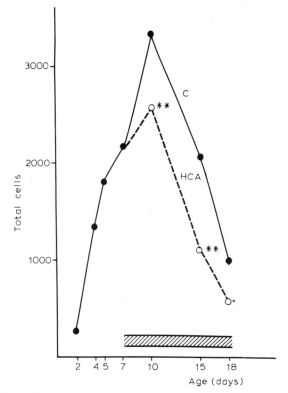

Fig. 16.4. Total number of cells in the external granular layer (EGL) at various ages in sagittal sections
of lobule VIII in C, control and HCA, cortisol treated; hatched insert indicates treatment period; *$p \leqslant 0.05$;
**$p \leqslant 0.01$; by permission of S. Karger, Basel.

Cell proliferation in the subventricular zone

Postnatal neurogenesis in the cerebrum is minimal except in the dentate gyrus, whereas most cerebral gliogenesis occurs postnatally. Since glucocorticoid treatment at birth reduces cerebral weight and DNA content, it has been suggested that glucocorticoids may inhibit gliogenesis thus reducing glial cell number in the adult cerebrum (Howard and Benjamins, 1975). This suggestion is also supported by observations that the division of glial cells in culture is inhibited by glucocorticoids (Grasso and Johnson, 1977). To investigate the effects of cortisol on cell proliferation of glial cells in vivo, I determined the labeling index in the subventricular zone of the lateral ventricle, a germinal zone producing glial cells (Privat and Leblond, 1972). As observed in the cerebellar EGL and hippocampal dentate gyrus, cortisol treatment on days 1–4 transiently inhibits cell proliferation in the subventricular zone (Fig. 16.7). Consequently, it appears that both neurogenesis and gliogenesis are vulnerable to increased glucocorticoid levels during the early postnatal period.

Effects on neurogenesis

In addition to reducing the number of cells generated, neonatal glucocorticoid treatment has other consequences on neurogenesis. The time courses over which various types of microneurons are generated ('neuronal birthdays') are also altered. Glucocorticoid treatment on postnatal days 1–4 delays the peak of granule cell production in both the cerebellum and hippocampus (Bohn and Lauder, 1978; Bohn, 1980). This is probably a consequence of the rebound in cell proliferation following the inhibition

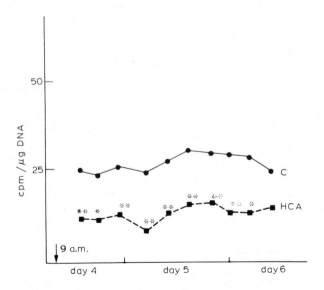

Fig. 16.5. Incorporation of [³H]thymidine into DNA in the hippocampus in cpm/μg DNA in C, control and HCA, cortisol treated; arrow indicates last cortisol injection; *$p \leqslant 0.05$; **$p \leqslant 0.01$; by permission of Pergamon Press, New York.

produced during glucocorticoid treatment. In addition, a larger proportion of basket and granule cells are generated during the period of glucocorticoid treatment than in normal animals, suggesting that high levels of glucocorticoids can permanently turn off cell division in some cells. This effect is more obvious in rats treated with glucocorticoids on days 7–18 where the peak birthdays of cerebellar stellate and granule cells and hippocampal granule cells occur earlier than in controls (Fig. 16.8; Bohn and Lauder, 1980; Bohn, 1979). Consequently, the altered patterns of neuronal birthdays resulting from glucocorticoid treatment arise from three effects: (1) a precocious cessation of cell division in some stem cells, probably those near their last cell division at the time of treatment, (2) an inhibition of cell proliferation leading to a decreased production of cells during treatment, and (3) a rebound in cell proliferation above control levels following cessation of treatment, resulting in delayed genesis of some cells.

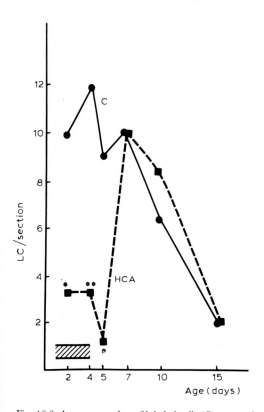

Fig. 16.6. Average number of labeled cells (C) per section in the dentate gyrus of the ventral hippocampus one hour after [³H]thymidine injection plotted as a function of age in C, control and HCA, cortisol treated; hatched insert indicates treatment period; *$p \leqslant 0.05$; **$p \leqslant 0.01$; by permission of Pergamon Press, New York.

Effects of glucocorticoids on neurotransmitter phenotypic expression and development

There are a number of discrete stages during the differentiation of neurons which lend themselves to study of factors involved in normal and/or aberrant development. Above, I discussed the effects of glucocorticoids on the event of cessation of division in neurons. Another important event in the lifetime of neurons is the expression and development of neurotransmitter systems. Alterations in glucocorticoid levels have also been observed to affect this stage of neuronal differentiation and in particular, to affect the development of the monoamine systems. In general, glucocorticoid treatment during specific limited periods in development causes precocious increases in the activity of a number of enzymes involved in monoamine synthesis (Table 16.3). However, in only two instances has it been demonstrated that normal development of neurotransmitter related enzymes requires physiological levels of glucocorticoids. The development of tryptophan hydroxylase (TPH) in postnatal rat midbrain and the prenatal development of phenylethanolamine N-methyltransferase (PNMT) in the embryonic

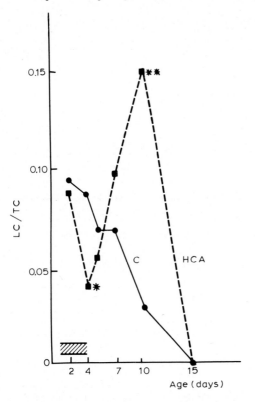

Fig. 16.7. Number of labeled cells/total cells (LC/TC) 1 h after [³H]thymidine injection in the subventricular zone of the ventral horn of the lateral ventricle plotted as a function of age in C, control and HCA, cortisol treated; $*p \leqslant 0.05$; $**p \leqslant 0.01$; hatched area indicates treatment period.

Table 16.3. Developmental effects of glucocorticoids on monoamine systems

[a]Rat; [b]mouse; [c]chick; ADX, adrenalectomy; B, corticosterone; CA, catecholamines; CAT, choline acetyltransferase; DEX, dexamethasone; E, epinephrine; F, cortisol; 5 HT, serotonin; NE, norepinephrine; PC12, pheochromocytoma; PNMT, phenylethanolamine N-methyltransferase; SCG, superior cervical ganglion; TAC, triamcinolone; TH, tyrosine hydroxylase; TPH, tryptophan hydroxylase

Effect	Steroid dose	Treatment	Reference
Precocious rise in TPH activity in midbrain[a]	B, 5 mg/kg	days 6–12 only	Sze, 1980
Rise in TPH abolished[a]		ADX (reversed by B replacement)	Sze, 1980
Increased TPH in whole brain during second week[a]	F, 1 mg	day 1	Yuwiler et al., 1978
Delayed maturation of blood-brain barrier to tryptophan[a]	F, 1 mg	day 1	Yuwiler et al., 1978
Precocious rise in TH activity in pons[b]	B, 20 mg/kg twice daily	days 7–12	Markey et al., 1980
Increased NE and 5 HT in hindbrain at 4 months[a]	B, 500 μg	days 3–5	Nyakas, 1977
Increased NE and 5 HT levels in hypothalmus at 30 days[a]	F, 1 mg	day 1	Ulrich et al., 1975
Increased TH activity in whole brain[b]	F, 20 mg/kg	days 7–10	Diez et al., 1982
Increased TH in pons-medulla at 8 and 14 days in adrenal at 8 days and in striatum of adults[a]	B, 3 μmoles	days 3–5 (ADX had no effect)	Nyakas et al., 1980
Prolonged expression of TH and CA in embryonic gut cells[a]	F, pellet	Maternal treatment E11.5–14.5	Jonakait et al., 1981
Increased number of CA containing cells[a,c]	F, 100 mg/l[c] F, 20 mg/kg[a]	in vitro[c] days 1–5[a]	Hervonen and Enranko, 1975; Costa et al., 1974
Decreased ratio of CAT to TH in neonatal SCG in vitro[a]	DEX (10^{-7} M) B (10^{-6} M)	14 days in vitro	McLennan et al., 1980
Decreased ability of heart conditioned medium to cause adrenergic to cholinergic switch in sympathetic neurons in vitro[a]	F, 10^{-5}–10^{-7} M	24 h	Fukada, 1980
Increased TH activity in neuroblastoma[b]	DEX, F, TAC	3–9 days in vitro	Williams et al., 1981
Increased TH activity in PC12 cells	B, 5×10^{-6} M DEX, 10^{-6} M	72 hours in vitro	Lucas and Thoenen, 1977
mRNA for TH increased in PC12	DEX, 10 μM	3 days in vitro	Baetge et al., 1981
Increased PNMT activity and E content in postnatal adrenal[a]	DEX, 10–100 μg	maternal treatment E12–21	Parker and Noble, 1967
Decreased PNMT activity and immunofluoresc. in fetal adrenal[a]		Fetal decapitation (reversed by F)	Margolis et al., 1966; Bohn et al., 1981
Increased PNMT immunofluorescence in fetal adrenal[a]	F, pellet	maternal treatment E14.5–18.5	Bohn et al., 1981
Increased PNMT activity and protein in fetal adrenal in vitro[a]	DEX, 10^{-5} M	2–9 days in vitro	Teitelman et al., 1980
Increased PNMT activity and immunofluorescence and E content in SCG[a]	DEX, 0.1–0.5 μg/g B, pellet	days 2–3	Gianutsos and Moore, 1977; Bohn et al., 1982; Phillipson and Moore, 1975; Luizzi et al., 1977; Koslow et al., 1975
Increased PNMT activity and immunofluorescence in extra-adrenal chromaffin tissue and SCG[a]	DEX, 1 mg/kg	days 1–6	Moore and Phillipson, 1975

376

rat adrenal are abolished by lowering glucocorticoid levels either by adrenalectomy in the case of TPH or by fetal decapitation in the case of PNMT (Sze, 1980; Margolis et al., 1966; Bohn et al., 1981). The effects on both enzymes are reversed by glucocorticoid replacement.

Teratologies at the level of neurotransmitter expression have also been observed following glucocorticoid treatment. During the fetal period, glucocorticoids have transplacental effects on phenotypic expression in the fetus. For example, in the embryonic gut, tyrosine hydroxylase (TH) is normally expressed during a brief period from gestation day 11.5 to 13.5 and then disappears (Cochard et al., 1978; Jonakait et al., 1979). Treatment of pregnant rats with cortisol during this period prolongs TH expression in these embryonic gut cells (Jonakait et al., 1980, 1981). This effect may be related to two interesting observations made in vitro on the effects of glucocorticoids on TH activity: (1) that the proportion of messenger RNA specifically coding for TH in pheochromocytoma is increased by glucocorticoids (Baetge et al., 1981) and (2) that

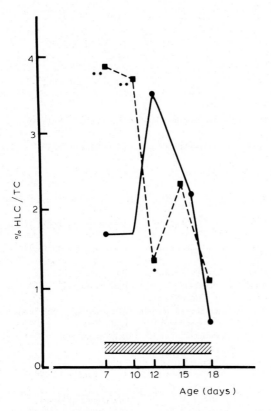

Fig. 16.8. Granule cell birthdays in lobule VIII of the cerebellum. Control (C) or cortisol treated (HCA) rats were injected with [³H]thymidine at ages indicated on x-axis and killed at 72 days of age. The number of heavily labeled granule cells (HLC) is plotted as percent of total granule cells (TC) versus age at time of [³H]thymidine injection; hatched area indicates treatment period; *$p \leqslant 0.05$; **$p \leqslant 0.01$; by permission of S. Karger, Basel.

glucocorticoids appear to affect TH activity in dissociated sympathetic neurons by acting indirectly through non-neuronal cells (Fukada, 1980). Whether these mechanisms also apply in vivo is an intriguing area for future investigation.

Glucocorticoid effects on PNMT development are not limited to the adrenal, but have also been observed in other cells derived from the neural crest (for a review, see Bohn, 1982). We have observed that glucocorticoid treatment of pregnant rats late in gestation increases PNMT immunofluorescence in the fetal adrenal and causes the appearance of PNMT immunofluorescent cells in fetal sympathetic ganglia (Fig. 16.9; Bohn et al., 1981, 1982). Treatment of newborn rats with dexamathasone or corticosterone also causes the appearance of PNMT immunofluorescent cells in sympathetic

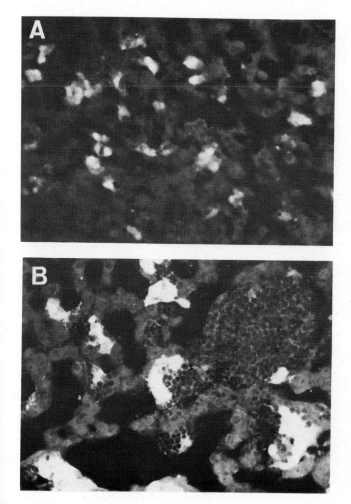

Fig. 16.9. Transverse sections of E18.5 adrenals demonstrating PNMT immunofluorescence in (A) control fetus and (B) fetus from mother treated with cortisol from E14.5. Note that the number of cells staining for PNMT and the intensity of staining is increased by cortisol treatment. (× 80).

ganglia and extra-adrenal chromaffin tissue (Fig. 16.10). These morphological observations are supported by biochemical studies showing that PNMT activity and epinephrine levels are increased in various areas of the peripheral nervous system following neonatal glucocorticoid treatment (Koslow et al., 1975; Liuzzi et al., 1977; Moore
and Phillipson, 1975; Gianutsos and Moore, 1977; Phillipson and Moore, 1975). In
contrast to these effects which are short-lived and apparent only in the late gestation
fetus or neonatal rat, we have observed one long term effect of glucocorticoids on
PNMT. When newborn rats are treated transiently (days 1–6) with dexamethasone
and then allowed to mature, PNMT immunofluorescence appears in a few cells in the
superior cervical ganglion (SCG) following a second dexamethasone treatment at 30

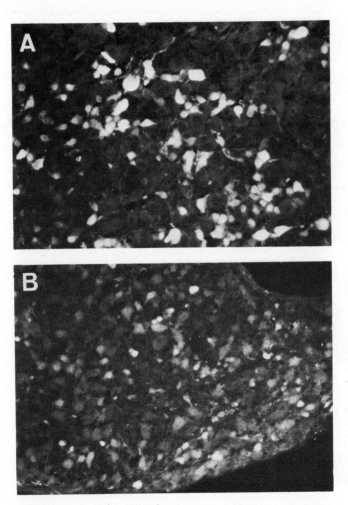

Fig. 16.10. PNMT immunofluorescence in 7 day old rat treated with dexamethasone (0.5 μg/g) from birth
in (A) superior cervical ganglion and (B) the organ of Zuckerkandl; by permission of Academic Press, New
York (A, × 390; B, × 150).

days (Fig. 16.11; Bohn et al., 1982). PNMT containing cells are never observed in normal adult rats or adult rats treated with dexamethasone. Although the mechanisms involved in this aberrant development remain unexplained, it appears that glucocorticoid treatment during the neonatal period alters the normal developmental fate of these cells.

Effects of glucocorticoids on later aspects of neuronal and glial differentiation

A change in hormonal levels has the potential of affecting different cells at different times in development depending on which vulnerable processes are ongoing during the insult. Above, I discussed the effects of glucocorticoids on some early aspects of cell differentiation. Although at any one moment during the development of the nervous system, there is a complex arrangement of cells in various stages of differentiation, certain aspects of differentiation are known to occur generally later than those already considered. For example, axonal and dendritic growth, synaptogenesis and myelination occur after the cells involved have ceased division. Unfortunately, studies of the effects of glucocorticoids on such processes are few in number. However, increased levels of glucocorticoids have been reported to inhibit the growth of processes and the formation of dendritic spines (Table 16.4).

Myelination of central tracts is vulnerable to glucocorticoid treatment (Table 16.4). We have observed that when rats are treated during the period when most oligodendrocytes are formed in the optic nerve (days 7–18; Skoff et al., 1976a,b) there is a significant reduction of myelin in the optic nerve (Fig. 16.12; Bohn and Friedrich, 1982). Interestingly, myelin formation recovers following termination of the cortisol treat-

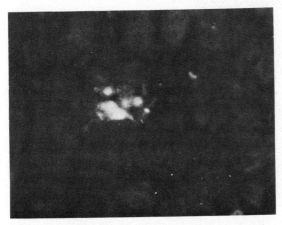

Fig. 16.11. Cluster of small cells containing immunofluorescence to PNMT in the superior cervical ganglion at 30 days in rat treated with dexamethasone on days 0–6 and 24–30; by permission of Academic Press, New York (× 570).

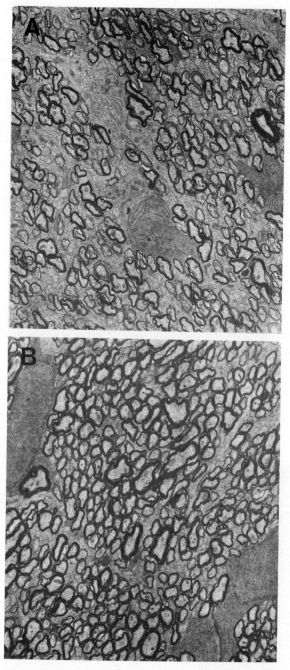

Fig. 16.12. Cross-section of the optic nerve at 21 days of age from (A) a rat treated with cortisol on postnatal days 7 to 18 and (B) a normal rat. Whereas most axons in the normal nerve are surrounded by compact myelin, many groups of axons remain unmyelinated in the treated rat; by permission of Williams and Wilkins Co., Baltimore. (× 4800).

Table 16.4. Morphological effects of glucocorticoids on 'Late' aspects of differentiation
Abbreviations as in Table 16.3.; NGF, nerve growth factor.

Effect	Treatment	Reference
Delayed development of dendritic spines on pyramidal cells in visual cortex	1 mg F on day 1	Schapiro et al., 1973
Altered dendritic development in parietal cortex	800 μg prednisone on day 6, 9 or 12	Oda and Huttenlocher, 1974
Inhibited NGF induced neurite outgrowth in dissociated adrenal cells	10^{-5}–10^{-7} M DEX	Unsicker et al., 1978
Decreased reactive sprouting in dentate gyrus after entorhinal lesions	0.2 mg/day	Scheff et al., 1980
Delayed lining up of Purkinje cells and altered growth of the Purkinje dendritic tree	F, 200 μg/day days 1–4	Bohn, 1979
Permanent myelin decrease in the pryramidal tracts	800 μg prednisone on day 6	Gumbinas et al., 1973
Transient deficit in myelin in the optic nerve	F, 10 μg/g, days 7–18	Bohn and Friedrich, 1982
Decreased sprouting of lesioned serotonin fibers in adult rat brain	adrenalectomy	Zhou and Azmitia, 1982

ment, and the optic nerve of adult treated rats is normal in the amount of myelin and the number of glial cells. One possibility accounting for the initial myelin deficit may be that fewer oligodendrocytes are formed during cortisol treatment (Bohn and Friedrich). This possibility would be in agreement with the effects of glucocorticoids on cell division in the subventricular zone, as discussed above, and in glioma cell cultures (Grasso and Johnson, 1975). Oligodendrocytes in the optic nerve and Schwann cells in sympathetic ganglia and sciatic nerve contain glucocorticoid receptors (Meyer et al., 1982; Warembourg et al., 1981) and glucocorticoids affect the activity of a number of glial specific enzymes (DeVellis and Inglish, 1973; Dawson and Kernes, 1979; Juurlink et al., 1981; Waziri and Saku, 1980; Mandel et al., 1976; Pishak and Phillips, 1980; Volpe and Marsala, 1976). Therefore, it is possible that glucocorticoids may also affect myelin synthesis. Although the mechanisms underlying the glucocorticoid inhibition of myelination have not yet been defined, this effect has obvious relevance to some of the behavioral modifications outlined in Table 16.1 in which the maturation of various sensory and seizure parameters are delayed by glucocorticoid treatment.

Future research directions

The literature reviewed here demonstrates that, in rodents, increased levels of glucocorticoids act on diverse processes to alter the differentiation of both neurons and glial cells. Furthermore, transient glucocorticoid treatment of rats at birth produces behavorial consequences in adult animals. In a few studies, the requirement for physiological levels of glucocorticoids in normal development has been elucidated. Future research in this area should focus on the effects of decreased levels and dose-dependent effects of glucocorticoids in order to gain a better understanding of the physiological role of these steroids in the development of the nervous system. Such knowledge would be helpful in elucidating the possible side effects of steroid treatment during the prenatal period and in pediatrics (see Bacon and Spencer, 1975). In addition, some of the well-known effects of these steroids, such as the regulation of adrenal PNMT, should be investigated at the molecular level to determine whether these steroids directly regulate messenger RNA coding for PNMT and at the cellular level to determine whether such effects are indirectly mediated by action on other cell types, as has been observed for TH activity in dissociated sympathetic neurons (Fukada, 1980). In conjunction with this, the development of specific high-affinity glucocorticoid receptors in different cell types in the nervous system should be followed.

The transplacental effects on fetal neural development following steroid treatment of pregnant rats are probably the most interesting effects reviewed here. Although these observations have possible significance in human prenatal care, little is known about placental transfer of steroids in humans, or even rodents for that matter. Knowledge concerning the efficacy of transfer of various synthetic glucocorticoids and endogenous steroids, especially following stress-induced increases, at various times in gestation would, therefore, be valuable.

Glucocorticoid action on glial cells and myelination certainly deserve further attention. Glucocorticoids are routinely used clinically as anti-inflammatory agents and to prevent brain edema in cases of malignancies or trauma. They are often prescribed for multiple sclerosis even though positive effects on this disease have not been demonstrated. On the contrary, glucocorticoids may actually inhibit glial cell division and remyelination if their action in humans resembles that in rodents.

Finally, the importance of proper hormonal milieu in development of the nervous system must be stressed. The effects of altered levels of glucocorticoids in vivo cannot be dissociated from their effects on the development of other hormonal systems. For example, glucocorticoid treatment alters circulating levels of adrenocorticotrophic hormone, growth hormone, growth hormone-releasing factor and thyroid stimulating hormone (Sawano et al., 1969). Any one developmental process, such as the rate of cell proliferation in neural germinal zones or the rate of neuronal process elongation, may be vulnerable to multiple hormonal action (see Lauder and Bohn, 1980).

Acknowledgements

This chapter was written while the author was supported by NIH grants NS 18420 and a Research Career Development Award NS 00713. The author thanks Mrs. Bettye Mayer and Ms. Elise Grossman for typing the manuscript.

References

Altman, J. (1969) Autoradiographic and histological studies of postnatal neurogenesis.III. Dating the time of production and onset of differentiation of cerebellar microneurons in rats. J. Comp. Neurol. 136, 269–294.

Altman, J. (1972a) Postnatal development of the cerebellar cortex in the rat. I. The external germinal layer and the transitional molecular layer. J. Comp. Neurol. 145, 353–398.

Altman, J. (1972b) Postnatal development of the cerebellar cortex in the rat. II. Phases in the maturation of Purkinje cells and of the molecular layer. J. Comp. Neurol. 145, 399–464.

Altman, J. (1972c) Postnatal development of the cerebellar cortex in the rat. III. Maturation of the components of the granular layer. J. Comp. Neurol. 145, 465–514.

Anderson, T.R. and Schanberg, S.M. (1975) Effect of thyroxine and cortisol on brain ornithine decarboxylase activity and swimming behavior in development. Biochem. Pharmacol. 24, 495–501.

Bacon, G.E. and Spencer, M.L. (1975) Pediatric uses of steroids. In: Steroid Therapy (Azarnoff, D.L., ed.) Saunders Philadephia, PA.

Baetge, E.E., Kaplan, B.B., Reis, D.J. and Joh, T.H. (1981) Translation of tyrosine hydroxylase from poly(A)-mRNA in pheochromocytoma cells is enhanced by dexamethasone. Proc. Natl. Acad. Sci. USA 78, 1269–1273.

Bayer, S.A. and Altman, J. (1974) Hippocampal development in the rat. Cytogenesis and morphogenesis examined with autoradiography and low-level X-irradiation. J. Comp. Neurol. 158, 55–80.

Bohn, M.C. (1979) Effects of hydrocortisone on neurogenesis in the neonatal rat brain: a morphological and autoradiographic study. Ph.D. Dissertation, University of Connecticut, Storrs.

Bohn, M.C. (1980) Granule cell genesis in the hippocampus of rats treated neonatally with hydrocortisone. Neuroscience 5, 2003–2012.

Bohn, M.C. (1982) Role of glucocorticoids in expression and development of phenylethanolamine N-methyltransferase (PNMT) in cells derived from the neural crest. Psychoneuroendocrinology (in press).

Bohn, M.C. and Lauder, J.M. (1978) The effects of neonatal hydrocortisone on rat cerebellar development. Dev. Neurosci. 1, 250–266.

Bohn, M.C. and Lauder, J.M. (1980) Cerebellar granule cell genesis in the hydrocortisone-treated rat. Dev. Neurosci. 3, 81–89.

Bohn, M.C., Goldstein, M. and Black I.B. (1981) Role of glucocorticoids in expression of the adrenergic phenotype in rat embryonic adrenal gland. Develop. Biol. 82, 1–10.

Bohn, M.C., Goldstein, M. and Black, I.B. (1982) Expression of phenylethanolamine N-methyltransferase in rat sympathetic ganglia and extra-adrenal chromaffin tissue. Develop. Biol. 89, 299–308.

Bohn, M.C. and Friedrich Jr., V.L. (1982) Recovery of myelination in rat optic nerve after development retardation by cortisol. J. Neurosci. 2, 1292–1298.

Burdman, J.A., Jahn, G.A. and Szijan, I. (1975) Early events in the effect of hydrocortisone acetate on DNA replication in the rat brain. J. Neurochem. 24, 663–666.

Ciaranello, R.D. and Axelrod, J. (1975) Effect of dexamethasone on neurotransmitter enzyme in chromaffin tissue of the newborn rat. J. Neurochem. 24, 775–778.

Ciaranello, R.D., Jacobowitz, D. and Axelrod, J. (1973) Effect of dexamethasone on phenylethanolamine N-methyltransferase in chromaffin tissue of the neonatal rat. J. Neurochem. 20, 799–805.

Chen, T.L., Aronow, L. and Feldman, D. (1977) Glucocorticoid receptors and inhibition of bone cell growth in primary culture. Endocrinology 100, 619–628.

Clos, J., Selme-Matrat, M., Rabie, A. and Legrand, J. (1975) Effets du cortisol sur la proliferation et la maturation cellulaires dans le cerveau et le cervelet du rat J. Physiol. 70, 207–218.

Cochard, P., Goldstein, M. and Black, I.B. (1978) Ontogenetic appearance and disappearance of tyrosine hydroxylase and catecholamines in the rat embryo. Proc. Natl. Acad. Sci. USA 75, 2986–2990.

Cost, M.G. and Mann, D.R. (1976) Neonatal corticoid administration: retardation of adrenal rhythmicity and desynchronization of puberty. Life Sci. 19, 1929–1936.

Costa, M., Eranko, O. and Eranko, L. (1974) Hydrocortisone-induced increase in the histochemically demonstrable catecholamine content of sympathetic neurons of the newborn rat. Brain Res. 67, 457–466.

Cotterrell, M., Balazs, R. and Johnson, A.L. (1972) Effects of corticosteroids on the biochemical maturation of rat brain: postnatal cell formation. J. Neurochem. 19, 2151–2167.

Dawson, G. and Kernes, S.M. (1979) Mechanism of action of hydrocortisone potentiation of sulfogalactosylaramide synthesis in mouse oligodendroglioma clonal cell lines. J. Biol. Chem. 254, 163–167.

DeVellis, J. and Inglish, D. (1973) Age-dependent changes in the regulation of glycerolphosphate dehydrogenase in the rat brain and in a glial cell line. Prog. Brain Res. 40, 321–330.

Diez, J.A., Sze, P.Y. and Ginsburg, B.E. (1977) Effect of hydrocortisone and electric foot shock on mouse brain tyrosine hydroxylase activity and tyrosine levels. Neurochem. Res. 2, 161–170.

Erskine, M.S., Geller, E. and Yuwiler, A. (1979) Effects of neonatal hydrocortisone treatment on pituitary and adrenocortical response to stress in young rats. Neuroendocrinology 29, 191–199.

Erskine, M.S., Geller, E. and Yuwiler, A. (1981) Modification of pituitary-adrenal feedback sensitivity in young rats by neonatal treatment. Acta Endocrinol. 96, 252–257.

Fodge, D.W. and Rubin, H. (1975) Differential effects of glucocorticoids on DNA synthesis in normal and virus-transformed chick embryo cells. Nature 257, 804–806.

Frankfurt, O.S. (1968) Effect of hydrocortisone, adrenalin and actinomycin D on transition of cells to the DNA synthesis phase. Exp. Cell Res. 52, 220–232.

Fukada, K. (1980) Hormonal control of neurotransmitter choice in sympathetic neurone cultures. Nature 287, 553–555.

Gianutsos, G. and Moore, K.E. (1977) Effects of pre- or post-natal dexamethasone, adrenocorticotrophic hormone and environmental stress on phenylethanolamine N-methyltransferase activity and catecholamines in sympathetic ganglia of neonatal rats. J. Neurochem. 28, 935–940.

Grasso, R.J. and Johnson, C.E. (1977) Dose-response relationships between glucocorticoids and growth inhibition in rat glioma monolayer cultures. Proc. Soc. Exp. Biol. Med. 154, 238–241.

Gumbinas, M., Oda, M. and Huttenlocker, P. (1973) The effects of corticosteroids on myelination of the developing rat brain. Biol. Neonate 22, 355–366.

Harkmark, W. (1954) The rhombic lip and its derivatives in relation to the theory of neurobiotaxis. In: Aspects of Cerebellar Anatomy, (Jensen, J. and Brodal, A., eds.) Johan Grundt and Tanum Forlag, Oslo.

Henderson, I.C. and Loeb, J.N. (1974) Hormone-induced changes in liver DNA synthesis: effects of glucocorticoids and growth hormone on liver growth and DNA polymerase. Endocrinology 94, 1637–1643.

Hervonen, H. and Eranko, O. (1975) Fluorescence histochemical and electron microscopic observations on sympathetic ganglia of the chick embryo cultures with and without hydrocortisone. Cell Tissue Res. 156, 145–166.

Howard, E. (1968) Reduction in size and total DNA of cerebrum and cerebellum in adult mice after corticosterone treatment for infancy. Exp. Neurol. 22, 191–208.

Howard, E. (1973) Hormonal effects on the growth and DNA content of the developing brain. In: Biochemistry of the Developing Brain (Himwich, W., ed.), Marcel Dekker, New York, pp. 1–68.

Howard, E. and Benjamins, J.A. (1975) DNA, ganglioside and sulfatide in brain of rats given corticosterone in infancy, with an estimate of cell loss during development. Brain Res. 92, 73–87.

Howard, E. and Granoff, D.M. (1968) Increased voluntary running and decreased motor coordination in mice after neonatal corticosterone implantation. Exp. Neurol. 22, 661–673.

Jonakait, G.M., Wolf, J., Cochard, P., Goldstein, M. and Black, I.B. (1979) Selective loss of noradrenergic phenotypic characters in neuroblasts of the rat embryo. Proc. Natl. Acad. Sci. USA 76, 4683–4686.

Jonakait, G.M., Bohn, M.C. and Black, I.B. (1980) Maternal glucocorticoid hormones influence neurotransmitter phenotypic expression in embryos. Science 210, 551–553.

385

Jonakait, G.M., Bohn, M.C., Markey, K., Goldstein, M. and Black, I.B. (1981) Elevation of maternal glucocorticoid hormone alters neurotransmitter phenotypic expression in embryos. Dev. Biol. 88, 288–296.

Juurlink, B.H., Schousboe, A., Jorgensen, O.S. and Hertz, L. (1981) Induction by hydrocortisone of glutamine synthetase in mouse primary astrocyte cultures. J. Neurochem. 36, 136–142.

Koslow, S.H., Bjegovic, M. and Costa, E. (1975) Catecholamines in sympathetic ganglia of rat: effects of dexamethasone and reserpine. J. Neurochem. 24, 277–283.

Krieger, D.T. (1972) Corticosteroid periodicity: critical period for abolition by neonatal injection of corticosteroid. Science 178, 1205–1207.

Lauder, J.M. and Bohn, M.C. (1980) Thyroid hormones and corticosteroids as temporal regulators of postnatal neurogenesis in the cerebellum and hippocampus. In: Progress in Psychoneuroendocrinology (Brambilla, F., Racagni, G. and De Wied, D., eds.), Elsevier/North-Holland Biomedical Press, Amsterdam, pp. 603–620.

Liuzzi, A., Foppen, F.H., Saavedra, J.M., Jacobowitz, D. and Kopin, I.J. (1977) Effect of NGF and dexamethasone on phenylethanolamine N-methyltransferase (PNMT) activity in neonatal rat superior cervical ganglia. J. Neurochem. 28, 1215–1220.

Lucas, C.A. and Thoenen, H. (1977) Selective induction by glucocorticoids of tyrosine hydroxylase in organ cultures of rat pheochromocytoma. Neuroscience 2, 1095–1101.

Mandel, P., Farooqui, A.A. and Elkowy, A. (1978) Effects of hydrocortisone and thyroxine on arylsulphatase and β-galactosidase of primary cell cultures of neural and glial types. J. Neurochem. 30, 1613–1615.

Margolis, F.L., Raffi, J. and Jost, A. (1966) Norepinephrine methylation in fetal rat adrenals. Science 154, 275–276.

Markey, K.A., Towle, A.C. and Sze, P.Y. (1980) Glucocorticoid effects on brain tyrosine hydroxylase. Soc. Neurosci. 6, 144.

Martin, J.T. (1978) Imprinting behavior, pituitary-adrenocortical modulation of the approach response. Science 200, 563–567.

McEwen, B.S. (1982) Sexual differentiation of the brain: gonadal hormone action and current concepts of neuronal differentiation. In: Molecular Approaches to Neurobiology (Brown, I., ed.), Academic Press, New York.

McEwen, B.S., Gerlach, J.L. and Micco, D.J. (1975) Putative glucocorticoid receptors in hippocampus and other regions of the rat brain. In: The Hippocampus, Vol. I, (Isaacson, R.L. and Pribram, K.L., eds.) Plenum Press, New York, pp. 375–391.

McEwen, B.S., Biegon, A., Davis, P.G., Krey, L.C., Luine, V.N., McGinnis, M.Y., Paden, C.M., Parsons, B. and Rainbow, T.C. (1982) Steroid hormones: humoral signals which alter brain cell properties and functions. Rec. Prog. Hormone Res. 38, 41–92.

McLennan, I.S., Hill, C.E. and Hendry, I.A. (1980) Glucocorticosteroids modulate transmitter choice in developing superior cervical ganglion. Nature 283, 206–207.

Meyer, J.S., Leville, P.J., DeVellis, J., Gerlach, J.L. and McEwen, B.S. (1982) Evidence for glucocorticoid target cells in the rat optic nerve. Hormone binding and glycerol phosphate dehydrogenase induction. J. Neurochem. 39, 423–433.

Moore, K.E. and Phillipson, O.T. (1975) Effects of dexamethasone on phenylethanolamine N-methyltransferase and adrenaline in the brains and superior cervical ganglia of adult and neonatal rats. J. Neurochem. 25, 289–294.

Nyakas, C. (1977) Effect of neonatal corticosterone treatment on brain monoamines and rearing activity in rats. Acta Physiol. Acad. Sci. Hung. 50, 127–130.

Nyakas, C., Viltsek, J. and Endroczi, E. (1980) Sensitivity of catecholamine neuron systems to corticosterone and ACTH 4–10 in newborn rats. Studies on brain and adrenal tyrosine hydroxylase. In: Catecholamines and Stress: Recent Advances, (Udsin, E., Kvetnansky, I. and Kopin, I., eds). Elsevier/North Holland, Amsterdam, p.p. 375–380.

Oda, M.A.S. and Huttenlocher, P.R. (1974) The effect of corticosteroids on dendritic development in the rat brain. Yale J. Biol. Med. 3, 155–165.

Olton, D.S., Johnson, C.T. and Howard, E. (1974) Impairment of conditioned active avoidance in adult rats given corticosterone in infancy. Dev. Psychobiol. 8, 55–61.

Palay, S.L. and Chan-Palay, V. (1974) Cerebellar Cortex, Springer-Verlag, New York.

Parker, L.N. and Noble, E.P. (1967) Prenatal glucocorticoid administration and the development of the epinephrine-forming enzyme. Soc. Exp. Biol. Med. 126, 734–737.

Pishak, M.P. and Phillips, A.T. (1980) Glucocorticoid stimulation of glutamine synthetase production in cultured rat glioma cells. J. Neurochem. 34, 866–872.

Phillipson, O.T. and Moore, K.E. (1975) Effects of dexamethasone and nerve growth factor on phenyletha-nolamine N-methyltransferase and adrenaline in organ cultures of newborn rat superior cervical ganglion. J. Neurochem. 25, 295–298.

Poland, R.E., Weichsel Jr., M.E. and Rubin, R.T. (1981a) Neonatal dexamethasone administration. I. Temporary delay of development of the circadian serum corticosterone rhythm in rats. Endocrinology 108, 1049–1054.

Poland, R.E., Rubin, R.T. and Weichsel Jr., M.E. (1981b) Neonatal dexamethasone administration. II. Persistent alteration of circadian serum anterior pituitary hormone rhythms in rats. Endocrinology 108, 1055–1059.

Privat, A. and Leblond. C.P. (1972) The subependymal layer and neighboring region in the brain of the young rat. J. Comp. Neurol. 146, 277–302.

Rotundo, R. (1976) The effects of handling on the development of the adrenal medulla in the rat. Ph.D. Dissertation, University of Connecticut, Storrs.

Salas, M. and Schapiro, S. (1970) Hormonal influences upon the maturation of the rat brain's responsiveness to sensory stimuli. Physiol. Behav. 5, 7–11.

Sawano, S., Arimura, A., Schally, A.V., Redding, T.W. and Schapiro, S. (1969) Neonatal corticoid administration: effect upon adult pituitary growth hormone and hypothalamic growth hormone-releasing hormone activity. Acta Endocrinology 61, 57–67.

Schapiro, S. (1968) Some physiological, biochemical and behavioral consequences of neonatal hormone administration of cortisol and thyroxine. Gen. Comp. Endocrinol. 10, 214–228.

Schapiro, S. (1971a) Hormonal and environmental influences on rat brain development and behavior. In: Brain Development and Behavior, (Sherman, M.B.S., McGinty, D.J. and Adinolfi, A.M., eds.) Academic Press, New York, pp. 307–339.

Schapiro, S. (1971b) Influence of hormones and environmental stimulation on brain development. In: Influence of Hormones on the Nervous System, Proc. Int. Soc. Psychoneurochem., Karger, Basel, pp. 63–73.

Schapiro, S., Vakovich, K. and Globus, A. (1973) Effects of neonatal thyroxine and hydrocortisone administration on the development of dendritic spines in the visual cortex of rats. Exp. Neurol. 40, 286–296.

Scheff, S.W., Benardo, L.S. and Cotman, C.W. (1980) Hydrocortisone administration retards axon sprouting in the rat dentate gyrus. Exp. Neurol. 68, 195–201.

Schlessinger, A.R., Cowan, W.M. and Gottlieb, D.I. (1975) An autoradiographic study of the time of origin and the pattern of granule cell migration in the dentate gyrus of the rat. J. Comp. Neurol. 159, 149–176.

Skoff, R.P., Price, D.L. and Stocks, A. (1976a) Electron microscopic autoradiographic studies of gliogenesis in rat optic nerve. J. Comp. Neurol. 169, 313–333.

Skoff, R.P., Price, D.L. and Stocks, A. (1976b) Electron microscopic autoradiographic studies of gliogenesis in rat optic nerve. J. Comp. Neurol. 169, 291–312.

Slotkin, T.A., Barnes, G., Lau, E., Seidler, F.J., Trepanier, P., Weigel, S.J. and Whitmore, W.L. (1982) Development of polyamine and biogenic amine systems in brain and hearts of neonatal rats given dexamethasone: role of biochemical alterations in cellular maturation for production of deficits in ontogeny of neurotransmitter levels, uptake, storage and turnover. J. Pharmacol. Exp. Ther. 221, 686–692.

Stumpf, W.E. (1971) Autoradiographic techniques and the localization of estrogen, androgen and glucocorticoid receptors in the pituitary and brain. Am. Zool. 11, 725–739.

Sze, P.Y. (1980) Glucocorticoids as a regulatory factor for brain tryptophan hydroxylase during development. Dev. Neurosci. 3, 217–223.

Szijan, I. and Burdman, J.A. (1973) The relationship between DNA synthesis and the synthesis of nuclear protein in rat brain. Effect of hydrocortisone acetate. Biochim. Biophys. Acta 299, 344–353.

Teitelman, G., Joh. T.H., Park, D., Brodsky, M., New, M. and Reis, D.J. (1982) Expression of the adrenergic phenotype in cultured fetal adrenal medullary cells: role of intrinsic and extrinsic factors. Dev. Biol. 89, 450–459.

Turner, B.B. and Taylor, A.N. (1975) Postnatal corticosterone treatment: effects on reproductive development and open-field behavior. Fed. Proc. 34, 302.

Turner, B.B. and Taylor, A.N. (1976) Persistent alteration of pituitary-adrenal function in the rat by prepuberal corticosterone treatment. Endocrinology 98, 1–9.

Turner, B.B. and Taylor, A.N. (1977) Effects of postnatal corticosterone treatment on reproductive development in the rat. J. Reprod. Fertil. 51, 309–314.

Turner, B.B., Katz, R.J. and Carroll, B.J. (1979) Neonatal corticosteroid permanently alters brain activity of epinephrine-synthesizing enzyme in stressed rats. Brain Res. 166, 426–430.

Ulrich, R., Yuwiler, A. and Geller, E. (1975) Effects of hydrocortisone on biogenic amine levels in the hypothalamus. Neuroendocrinology 19, 259–268.

Unsicker, K.B., Krisch, U., Otten, U. and Thoenen, H. (1978) Nerve growth factor-induced fiber outgrowth from isolated rat adrenal chromaffin cells: impairment by glucocorticoids. Proc. Natl. Acad. Sci. USA 75, 3498–3502.

Vernadakis, A. and Woodbury, D.M. (1963) Effect of cortisol on the electroshock seizure thresholds in developing rats. J. Pharmacol. Exp. Ther. 139, 110–113.

Volpe, J.J. and Marasa, J.C. (1976) Regulation of palmitic acid synthesis in cultured glial cells: effects of glucocorticoids on fatty acid synthetase, acetyl-CoA carboxylase, fatty acid and sterol synthesis. J. Neurochem. 27, 841–845.

Warembourg, M., Otten, U. and Schwab, M.E. (1981) Labelling of Schwann and satellite cells by ^{3}H-dexamethasone in a rat sympathetic ganglion and sciatic nerve. Neuroscience 6, 1139–1143.

Waziri, R. and Saku, S.K. (1980) Induction of 2',3'-cyclic nucleotide 3'-phosphohydroxylase and morphological alterations in C_6 glioma cells by dexamethasone,(3-butoxy-4-methoxybenzyl)-2-imidazocinone and prostaglandin E_1. In Vitro 16, 97–102.

Weichsel Jr., M.E. (1974) Glucocorticoid effect upon thymidine kinase in the developing cerebellum. Pediatr. Res. 8, 843–847.

Williams, L.R., Sandquist, D., Black, A.C. and Williams, T.H. (1981) Glucocorticoids increase tyrosine hydroxylase activity in cultured marine neuroblastoma. J. Neurochem. 36, 2057–2062.

Wright, N.A., Appleton, D.R. and Morley, A.R. (1974) Effect of dexamethasone on cell population kinetics in the adrenal cortex of the prepubertal male rat. J. Endocrinol. 62, 527–536.

Yuwiler, A., Simon, M., Bennett, B., Plotkin, S., Wallace, R., Brammer, G. and Ulrich, R. (1978) Effect of neonatal corticoid treatment on tryptophan and serotonin metabolism. Endrocinol. Exp. 12, 21–32.

Zhou, F.C. and Azmitia, E.C. (1982) Effects of adrenalectomy on axonal sprouting of hippocampal 5-HT fibers. Soc. Neurosci. Abstr. 8, 749.

Neurobehavioral Teratology
edited by Joseph Yanai
© Elsevier Science Publishers BV 1984

17

THE POSSIBLE AETIOLOGICAL EFFECTS OF VITAMIN SUPPRESSING DRUGS

Howard S. Cuckle

ICRF Cancer Studies Unit, Nuffield Department of Clinical Medicine, University of Oxford, Radcliffe Infirmary, Oxford OX2 6HE, UK

THE suggestion that vitamin (in particular, folic acid) supplementation during the peri-conceptual period (say, plus or minus 2 months of conception) may prevent neural tube defects (NTDs) has wide-ranging implications (Smithells, 1981a,b.) Not the least of these is the possibility that drugs which suppress the activity of vitamins may cause some cases of NTD if taken during this period. Furthermore, using the argument of Klingberg and his colleagues (see Chapter 3), these drugs should be considered when studying the aetiology of the less obvious neurobehavioural defects which are present at birth.

The purpose of this chapter is to review critically the evidence for the aetiological effect of vitamins, to suggest further studies and to draw general conclusions regarding the procedures necessary for answering such questions in the future. Before proceeding with this, some background information is required on the sort of drugs which are vitamin suppressive on the one hand and the general epidemiology of NTDs on the other.

Drugs which suppress vitamin capacity

The list of drugs which have some effect on vitamin nutrition is growing, so that a comprehensive review is not possible here. However, it may be enlightening to consider

the range of relatively common drugs that have been classically associated with vitamin deficiency.

The use of oral contraceptives has been shown to reduce the plasma, erythrocyte
and urinary levels of most soluble vitamins. Notable is pyridoxine which has come
under close scrutiny because of the complex mechanism by which this may come
about. Deficiencies of folate, riboflavin and ascorbic acid have also been established.
Fat soluble vitamins have also been shown to be affected by oral contraceptive use
but in the case of vitamin A this results in an actual increase in plasma levels. From
the point of view of teratology it is of interest that oral contraceptives have been associated with some birth defects, not only in women continuing to take the pill after
becoming pregnant but also some months after stopping. Whilst a carry over effect
of vitamin deficiency may be involved in such cases this is unlikely. With regard to
NTDs, the balance of evidence is against any causal connection in non-breakthrough
pregnancies (Cuckle and Wald, 1982).

Alcohol has been known for its effect on vitamin status by accelerating the use of
vitamins such as riboflavin and ascorbic acid which are involved in its metabolism.
Further effects are brought about by damping appetite, through the provision of calories without vitamins, minerals or proteins, and by impairing the efficiency of digestion
or by reducing absorption through its doing damage to intestinal linings.

Turning to medications that might be used in early pregnancy, many common ones
have side effects relating to vitamin depression. Various mechanisms are involved.
Amphetamines bring about these effects simply by depressing appetite, whereas meth-
otrexate and pyrmethamine specifically block the activation of folic acid. Another
group of drugs which is particularly relevant to the present discussion is comprised of
certain anti-convulsants, namely phenytoin, primidone, phenobarbitone and,
recently, valproic acid (Bjerkedal et al., 1982). Maternal epilepsy is associated with
the risk of central nervous system defects and it is not clear whether the disease itself
or the use of the drugs is responsible. It is difficult in such cases to distinguish the two.
For example, the observation that the risk in epileptics who take anticonvulsants is
greater than in those who do not need drug control is of little help since the former
tend to have a more severe form of epilepsy which may of itself be related to a greater
risk than that found among epileptics in general.

Other drugs reduce the absorption of all vitamins (e.g. phenolphthalein) or specific
ones (e.g. paraaminosolicyclic acid for cobalamin), others increase excretion (e.g. hyd-
ralazine for vitamin pyridoxine).

The need for folate

The folates are necessary for many metabolic processes and especially in the production of new cells. Therefore it is reasonable to assume that the requirement may be
increased during pregnancy at time of rapid tissue growth. Animal experiments have

shown that the folate antagonist aminopterin is capable of producing abortions as well as a range of malformations including NTDs. However, this work was done against a background of folate deficiency in the test animals and it remains essentially unknown whether the available folate in pregnant women with even the lowest blood levels should be regarded as a deficiency.

Neural tube defects

Defects of the neural tube are one of the largest single groups of congenital malformations in most countries. Their cause is not known and the only proven method of preventing the birth of affected infants is antenatal detection and subsequent abortion. Three main types of neural tube defect can be identified, namely: anencephaly, spina bifida and encephalocele. Antenatal diagnosis is possible by amniocentesis for 100%, 80% and 10% of these cases, respectively (Collaborative AChE Study, 1982).

The stimulus behind much of the research into the methods for antenatal detection has been the great distress associated with the delivery of an anencephalic child or, worse, the delivery of one with spina bifida or encephalocele who is likely to be severely handicapped and subject to frequent medical procedures. The extent of this burden of handicap depends partly on the medical tretment given to affected children; active intervention increases the survival rate but also raises the proportion of survivors who are severely handicapped. In the absence of any medical treatment the proportion that survive beyond a few months of life is small.

Opinion on how much medical treatment should be given to affected infants differs, and hence so does opinion on the value of antenatal detection. In general most people would probably regard the termination of a foetus thought to have an NTD less distressing than withholding treatment from a live-born affected child, provided of course that the probability of the foetus being normal (or having only a minor defect) was small. It is on this premise that antenatal detection has been developed and is now offered as a service in many countries.

The prevalence of NTDs in the UK is about 4 per thousand births and is approximately equal for anencephaly and spina bifida. Encephalocele is rare, accounting for only about 5% of all NTDs. The frequency of NTDs in the rest of the world tends generally to be lower; in the USA it is 1 to 2 per thousand births. Studies on immigrants show that the prevalence of the condition can change within the first and second generation after migration, suggesting that environmental factors are important in its aetiology.

Incidence of foetal NTDs is increased about 10-fold (about 40 per thousand births in the UK) among women who have previously had one affected child, 20-fold among those who have had two affected children, and 40-fold among those who have had three affected children However, in spite of these high risks of recurrence about 95% of the infants with NTDs are born to women who have not previously had affected children.

In Oxford, immediately prior to the introduction of antenatal screening when a policy of selective treatment for infants with spina bifida was generally adopted, just over one third of infants with detectable (open) lesions survived for 5 years (Althouse and Wald, 1980). Using a standard set of criteria to classify the extent of handicap, about 85% of those who survived for at least 5 years were severely handicapped, 10% were moderately handicapped, and only 5% had no handicap. On average they spent over half the year in hospital during the first 5 years of their life and had 6 surgical operations.

Vitamins and NTDs

A link between vitamins and NTDs in humans was found in a study which showed that among 35 women whose pregnancies were affected by defects of the central nervous system (including NTDs) 24 women (79%) had a positive forminoglutamic acid excretion test, indicating impaired folate absorption or metabolism, compared with 6 out of 35 matched controls (17%) (Hibbard and Smithells, 1965). In addition, the study of first trimester blood samples from 6 women who subsequently delivered NTDs showed lower than average levels in their blood of folate, ascorbic acid, cobalamin and riboflavin (Smithells et al., 1976). This result could have arisen if women who deliver NTD infants have diets that are generally deficient (not just in vitamins) and one study suggests that this is so. Prospective dietary assessments were performed on 186 pregnant women who had previously delivered an NTD infant (Laurence et al., 1980). The quality of the mother's diet was considered to be poor in all 8 cases subsequently found to be affected by NTD, compared with 37 out of the 178 (20%) who delivered or miscarried unaffected infants.

Experiments on animals have shown non-specific teratogenic effects of several vitamins when a deficient state has been brought about. These include retinol, calciferol, riboflavin, niacin, thiamine, folic acid and pentothenic acid. Other experiments using whole embryo cultures have shown little effect of vitamins. The only significant finding is that inocitol, a substance similar to a vitamin, has been associated with NTD malformation.

Direct human evidence
In the main study Smithells and his colleagues (1981a,b) invited women who had previously given birth to infants with neural tube defects to take multivitamin and mineral supplementation immediately before and until shortly after conception. Women who agreed to take the treatment and who complied with it are the cases of this study and they number 348. Only three (0.7%) subsequently delivered or had terminated a foetus with a neural tube defect. The control group comprised women invited to take the treatment but who refused or who were already pregnant at the time of invitation. In all 493 such women formed the control group and 23 of them

(4.7%) subsequently delivered an NTD infant. This difference is statistically significant and has been subject to several types of statistical analysis. The conclusion is that on the face of it there is a difference between outcome in the two groups caused by the vitamin supplementation, but there is reason to believe that this difference has been brought about by the selective nature in which cases were recruited to the study. The extent to which such self selection may have affected the results is difficult to quantify. However, it is worth considering the way in which self selection has affected other studies.

The effect of self selection

A classic example (cited by Wald (1983)) is in the use of clofibrate among patients with coronary heart disease. In one of the trials of this drug (the Coronary Drug Project Research Group, 1980) the patients who took the drug regularly, taken to be 80% or more prescribed over a particular period, are considered separately from those who took the drug less often. The former had a statistically significant lower short-term mortality (only 15% and almost 25% for the latter). This is particularly interesting since the same finding is found amongst the controls who were taking placebo and not active drugs at all (15% for those not complying with the placebo compared with 28% for those compliant persons.) The conclusion that must be drawn is that some strong selective influence is involved both in the taking of the drugs and in survival. It is not too difficult to hypothesise factors which may be related to this. In fact the Coronary Drug Project have collected enough information to be able to allow for some of these factors in the analysis. They in fact allowed for 40 different factors and nonetheless the compounding factors were not identified since the statistically significant differences persisted even after adjustment.

Non-randomised controls

Quite apart from self-selection, other factors arising from the use of non-randomised controls were probably involved in the Smithells study. The extent to which other factors can play a part is no less than self-selection and no easier to detect.

The effect of using non-randomised controls can be simply seen by comparing the magnitude of differences that can arise between the results of nominally similar treatment protocols when they are given in successive trials. The explanation may involve unnoticed changes in patient selection criteria, in supportive care, or in either the vigour or caution with which treatment is given. However, whatever the explanation, the phenomenon has important implications for the methodology that is appropriate for the evaluation of new treatments. Such treatments are sometimes 'evaluated' not by randomisation but by switching over at a particular time from routine use of some standard protocol to routine use of that same protocol plus the new factors. The idea is that the new factor can be assessed by comparing the prognosis of the more recent patients with that of the earlier patients. An interesting example arises in the Medical Research Council's Acute Myelocytic Leukaemia Trials (MCR, 1983). In these trials one of the protocols (Barts 3) has been used with slight modifications in four different trials. The differences in survival in patients who took Barts 3 in each of these four trials is statistically significant, that is, there is a strong tendency for later trials with Barts 3 to show better prognosis than in early trials. The magnitude of this difference, this improvement in survival, is greater than that found between the different treatments being compared in the individual trials. Thus some selective effects whatever they are have been greater than the actual effects from active treatments. Given this background improvement in treatment any historically controlled comparison would have been unreliable in these centres over this period. New treatments introduced in this period and compared historically would have produced significant positive effects which were in fact spurious. Likewise the evaluation of new factors by comparing the patient outcome at centres that have been elected to use it routinely with that at other centres is presumably also potentially misleading if the chief cause of the trend seen in the AML trials is indeed some change in the style of patient management. In comparing centres that do elect routinely to include some particular factor in their protocols with centres that do not, the difference in other respects of their styles of management may differ by at least as much as did the styles which similar centres administered Barts 3 in the four AML trials reviewed.

Where there is doubt as to whether or not some particular component of a treatment confers any material benefit on patients, and that component is one with respect to which it is practical to randomise large numbers of patients, it would therefore seem advisable to do so, for both historical controls and most other forms of non-randomised evaluation appear to contain potential biases which may have been of the same order of magnitude as the effect one might reasonably hope to discover.

Evidence for bias due to self-selection in the Smithells study
There are two selective factors which may have led to the controls having a higher recurrence risk of neural tube defects than the cases. These are social class and previous history of miscarriages. Controls in the Smithells study were of lower social class and for more of them the immediately preceding pregnancy was a miscarriage compared with the cases. The lower social class in the controls is presumably due to the pattern of availability of medical services and the extent to which drug compliance was maintained. More controls than cases had previous miscarriages for the simple reason that miscarriages are generally followed more quickly by a pregnancy than are births. Thus those eligible to be cases by virtue of the fact that they were planning to become pregnant were less likely to include women who had just had a miscarriage than those who where ineligible because they were already pregnant. It has long been observed that low social class is associated with an increased risk of neural tube defect and in the last ten years it has also been observed that a miscarriage in an immediately preceding pregnancy is a risk factor for neural tube defects (Clarke et al., 1975). More recently, data have been presented to show that these associations are also present in women who have previously had one or more NTDs (Nevin, 1980; Cuckle, 1983). Inter-

estingly enough, the relative risk of neural tube defect given these risk factors is the same in women who have previously had a neural tube defect as for pregnant women in general. Since the social class of all the women in Smithell's study and the number of previous miscarriages is documented, it is possible to allow for these factors in the analysis. An allowance for social class has already been made in one of the papers of the study, and an allowance for miscarriage can be simply performed: both of these adjustments, however, do not radically alter the results of Smithell's study.

Social class is a rather crude statistical variable. It has been derived in these studies by asking the women for the occupation of their husband. Presumably the underlying factor which is related to social class and to the degree of compliance to be expected from a patient will be measured very poorly by the occupation of the husband. To an even greather extent the underlying association which relates social class to neural tube defect incidence will be even more poorly related to occupation. Clearly any re-analysis of the data, however sophisticated, will not overcome this problem nor will the collection of an even larger series of data. The only purpose of repeating this study with the same study design would be to take account of random variability. With the data already collected we can see that the observed effect is very unlikely to be due to chance and must be due either to a real benefit of multivitamins or to the self-selection which we have described.

To conclude, therefore, the study of Smithells and his colleagues is suggestive and requires confirmation by using a large randomised clinical trial (RCT) design.

Possible randomised study

The randomisded study would be a trial of prevention versus intervention, that is, a regime aimed at reducing the frequency of NTD conceptions would be offered to one group of women as a primary measure, whereas the controls would be offered antenatal diagnosis and selective abortion as the primary approach. Obviously the treatment group would be offered antenatal diagnosis as a back-up, but if their regime was effective they would have a reduced chance of needing a therapeutic abortion on account of the diagnosis of an affected foetus.

Such a trial is only practical (and ethical, see below) among women who have had one or more affected infants, and a number of study designs are possible. The first would be to interview all women who had a previous NTD pregnancy to see if they intend to have a further pregnancy and if so if they are willing to enter a randomised study. Another design would be to identify the same group of women, randomise them before approaching them individually, and contact personally only those randomised to the treatment group. The controls could be simply informed about possible antenatal diagnosis. In the first type of design compliance would be expected to be high because potential non-compliers will have been selected out before the time of randomisation. The second approach, though simple and avoiding a painfully difficult inter-

396

view, is likely to lead to a large degree of non-compliance. Because of the design it is necessary to analyse the results of the trial according to the intention to take the drug rather than compliance with taking the drug. This will lead to a low power for the study, that is, the ability of the study to identify an effect, if one existed, would be relatively small.

An optimal design might be to combine the two approaches so that once having identified the women at high risk they would be sent a letter asking them if they were interested in services available for antenatal diagnosis of foetal neural tube defects. Those that respond to this query would be then eligible for the trial and would be randomised.

A simple calculation would provide some indication of the numbers that might be needed for such a trial. In the UK we can assume a response rate of 20% to the initial enquiry (i.e. they would like to comply and are not now in fact pregnant and are planning a future pregnancy) and the recurrence risk is 4%. For every 1000 women who are approached, the 200 who respond would be randomised, 100 into a supplemented group and 100 not supplemented. The former would deliver two NTDs and the latter four if the effect of multivitamins was to halve the NTD recurrence rates. In order to have a good chance of detecting a significant difference at the 5% level, if there is a difference, at least 5000 women would need to be studied. Since only 2500 women deliver children with NTDs each year in a country the size of the UK, a large multi-centre international study would be required to answer this question.

A randomised trial of folic acid has already been performed. This was done by Professor Laurence and his colleagues (1981) and was double blind. 60 women were randomised to receive folic acid and 51 into the group who were to take a placebo. Two of the former and four of the latter pregnancies ended in a neural tube defect birth. Thus there has already been a small randomised trial which yielded an apparently 50% reduction in the risk of neural tube defects following folic acid supplementation. However, the difference is not statistically significant and is in itself of little value.

It is interesting that in the original analysis of the study an attempt was made separately to analyse women according to whether they had in fact taken the tablets. This was done by both asking the women and by chemical analysis, namely, serum folic acid levels. Of the 44 women believed to have taken the tablets regularly, none of them produced infants with neural tube defects, whereas in the remaining women 6 (9%) did have affected infants. Thus the recurrence rate in women who, though allocated to take the treatment, did not comply is 2/16 (12%), that is higher than women in the placebo group.

The MRC trial

A large multicentre international trial on these lines has now been started by the MRC in the U.K. An interesting aspect of the MRC trial is the way in which it is attempting to evaluate the effect of both folic acid and the multivitamin preparation used by Smithells in the same study, that is, doing two studies in one. This design, the so-called 2 by 2 design, is to randomise all women into four groups, one to take the multivitamin preparation without folic acid, another the multivitamin preparation with folic acid, another folic acid alone, and another placebo group (all receive mineral dose). This means that half the women randomised will be taking folic acid and half not, or looking at it another way half the women will be taking the multivitamin preparation and half not, though these will be different groups of women. This trial design is optimal provided that folic acid and multivitamins do not both work or rather that if they do then the effect of taking multivitamins alone or folic acid alone will be less than taking both together.

Other approaches

If a randomised trial were unacceptable in this area then another approach would have to be taken. It is probably better to carry out some investigations rather than none at all and provided these are not biased then they will contribute some information. The first suggested approach would be to offer multivitamin preparations to all women who had a previous infant with a neural tube defect who want genetic counselling. If this were done over a specified period of time and the outcomes of pregnancy compared with the recurrence risk in the period immediately preceding the period of study then this historical comparison might be expected to show an effect. However, the publicity generated by the results of Smithells' study probably means that the type of women who now present for genetic counselling (and multivitamin supplementation) will be in some way different from those who did so in a previous historical period. Moreover, there is some evidence to believe that the incidence of neural tube defects is declining in Western countries, so that a historical comparison would be subject to this trend. The recurrence risk of neural tube defects is related in all studies so far analysed to the background incidence of the disease. Therefore, one might expect that with a background of a reducing incidence in the general population the recurrence risk would be reduced also. Thus the results of the proposed trial would be subject to this downward trend and women recruited in the trial period would have a lower recurrence risk than those in the preceding period. The former objection to this trial design could be overcome by having a very active publicity campaign in an attempt to get all eligible women into the trial and thus make some impact on the overall incidence of neural tube defects. Even so, only a small proportion of infants with neural tube defects are born to women with previous NTDs and even a 100% reduction in the risk among these women would have only a relatively small effect on total incidence especially against a background of declining general population incidence. However, the second objection is paramount. Even any attempt to estimate the rate of decline of the incidence of the disease is made difficult by the unknown impact of antenatal diagnosis. Furthermore, it is quite possible that the incidence patterns of neural tube defects are cyclical rather than declining at this moment, as they have been throughout the century in the UK for example, and that the incidence might in the trial period actually increase, so that even if the vitamins were effective this might still be obscured by the cyclical increase.

Ethical questions

The randomised clinical trial has been used in cancer research for some years and is now becoming more popular in other areas, particularly in the treatment of coronary heart disease. The randomised trial has not been used to any great extent in obstetrics. There is therefore some resistance to its use in the particular case cited above. The ethical basis of the randomised clinical trial is that a priori the potential benefits of one regime are equal to those of another. In practice this usually means that if a clinician is presented with a particular disease, it is only a matter of chance rather than clinical judgement which leads him to use one of the two treatments concerned in the trial. Whilst no individual clinician may divide a case between one type of treatment or another, two hypothetically identical colleagues may be such that one preferred one treatment and the other preferred the other treatment. The purpose of the trial in this case is to come to an unbiased conclusion as to the efficacy of one treatment over the other, by formalising the doubt which exists in the world over whether there is any real difference between the two. The situation which we are considering here is slightly different insofar as an existing treatment is available, that is, doing nothing, and the new treatment giving multivitamins is to be introduced. Since vitamins are on the face of it normal dietary consistuents there appears to be no reason why there should be any doubt, since the vitamins can be assumed to be potentially harmless and at best of some great benefit. That is to say that there is no good reason not to intervene with the vitamin treatment. This is unfortunately a spurious argument since only a small harmful effect of vitamins could eliminate any benefit that may be derived from them. Since the MRC design envisages prenatal diagnosis for all those receiving a placebo treatment as well as those receiving the active drugs, the net benefit on NTD births would be (even if the drugs were 100% effective) the prevention of the 10% of neural tube defects which cannot be detected by prenatal diagnosis because they are closed defects. Therefore the actual benefit for 1000 women treated would be 2 closed NTDs prevented in those who took the drug ($10\% \times 4\% \times 500$). Should the use of multivitamins cause only two infants to have defects not subject to antenatal diagnosis, then the benefit will be equal to the extra risk imposed. Such adverse outcomes of the use of multivitamin preparations are not far fetched since some of the components of the preparations are known to be teratogenic. High doses of retinol and calciferol have been shown to be teratogenic in animals.

Implications of the MRC trial

If the MRC trial demonstrates a role for vitamin supplementation it cannot be concluded that all women should take multivitamins in the periconceptual period, and that vitamin suppressing drugs should be avoided at that time. There are two reasons for this. Firstly, women with more than one affected pregnancy may be a group particularly susceptible to the teratogenic effects of vitamin depletion. Whilst that is possible, it is not likely and given that vitamin supplements are relatively cheap it would be prudent to assume that this were not so. The second reason relates to the fact that the risk of NTD among women with a previous affected pregnancy is about ten times greater than that in the general population. Thus a small harmful effect of vitamins may not have been important in the MRC trial but would be if the general population was exposed. Moreover, the trial would be too small to discover such an effect unless it was great. Thus once again a randomised clinical trial would be required to decide the issue, this time in the general population and in which many tens of thousands of women would need to be tested because of the low background risks.

Conclusions regarding the use of RCTs

The case we have been considering is exemplary of how not to proceed with research. All would agree that the question considered by Smithells et al. was an important one but the method used to answer it was designed neither to optimise the chance of discovering the correct answer nor to convince other workers, clinicians and general population of the veracity of the answer once found. In fact the opposite has occurred. The results have led to an uncertainty which will take many years to settle. Further research has been limited and large numbers are perhaps being exposed to dangers. Only a large randomised control trial, analysed and interpreted with caution, could have avoided this.

The kind of question involved here is not atypical, and is particularly apposite to neurobehavioural teratology, where we are trying to discover small effects. The order of magnitude for a trial in these circumstances is greater than might be anticipated using common sense. For example, ten thousand subjects might be required in order to have an 80% chance of discovering the effect if one exists when commonsense might have suggested less than a thousand. Not only is a small trial unlikely to discover the effect if there is one, it is likely to appear to show an effect even when there is not one. The former fault constitutes a waste of time and resources for the investigators whilst the latter is likely to stimulate waste, anxiety and danger in the work of others.

The need for very large numbers often leads to collaborative studies being considered between different centres and in different countries. There are no doubt practical difficulties with multi-centre collaboration but they need not be formidable. One apparent problem is that medical or diagnostic facilities may differ from centre to

400

centre. If this is so then it is a reason for collaboration rather than against it because the trial will then reflect the true state of affairs in general practice rather than what would happen in a large specialist academic centre. That is, the conclusions will be more generally applicable and acceptable. All this assumes, of course, that there is a reasonable balance and the results are analysed having stratified the data by centre. A more serious problem is that compromise on design reached between the different parties will lead to a lowest common denominator being adopted. This can only be avoided by being aware of the problem but nevertheless there is likely to be some such effect. The incentive to collaborate can be enhanced in several practical ways, by reducing complexity. Simple, minimal form filling, relaxation of exclusion criteria, unstratified allocation of treatment, and allowing extra complexity as an option are possible ways.

Conclusion

There are insufficient grounds for believing that vitamin deficiency is a major cause of neural tube defects whether brought about by poor diet or vitamin suppressive drugs. Moreover, if there is an effect it will take some years to establish, by the use of a randomised controlled trial. Such trial designs should be the first choice when intervention is being considered with a new drug or diet which may have teratological implications.

References

Althouse, R. and Wald, N.J. (1980) Survival and handicap of infants with spina bifida. Arch. Dis. Child. 55, 845–850.
Bjerkedal, T., Czeizel, A., Goujard, J., Kallen, B., Mastroiacova, P., Nevin, N., Oakley, G. and Robert, E. (1982) Valproic acid and spina bifida. Lancet ii, 1096.
Cuckle, H. (1983) Recurrence risk of neural tube defect following a miscarriage. Prenatal Diagnosis (in press).
Clarke, C., Hobson, D., McKendrick, O.M., Rogers, S.C. and Sheppard, P.M. (1975) Spina bifida and anencephaly: miscarriage a possible cause. Brit. Med. J. 4, 743–746.
Cuckle, H. and Wald, N.J. (1982) Evidence against oral contraceptives as a cause of neural tube defects. Brit. J. Obstet. Gynaecol. 89, 547–549.
Collaborative AChE Study (1981) Amniotic fluid acetylcholinesterase electrophoresis as a secondary test in the diagnosis of anencephaly and open spina bifida in early pregnancy. Lancet ii, 321–324.
Coronary Drug Project Research Group (1980) Influence of adherence to treatment and response of cholesterol on mortality in the Coronary Drug Project. New Engl. J. Med. 303, 1038–1041.
Hibbard, E.D. and Smithells, R.W. (1965) Folic acid metabolism and human embryopathy. Lancet i, 1254.
Laurence, K.M., James N., Miller, M. and Campbell, H. (1980) Increased risk of recurrence of pregnancies complicated by fetal neural tube defects in mothers receiving poor diets, and possible benefit of dietary counselling. Brit. Med. J. 281, 1592–1594.
Laurence, K.M., James, N., Miller, M.H., Tennant, G.B. and Campbell, H. (1981) Double blind ran-

domised controlled trial of folate treatment before conception to prevent recurrence of neural tube defects. Brit. Med. J. 282, 1509–1511.

Medical Research Council (1983) Treatment of acute myeloid leukaemia in 1970 s. (in press)

Nevin, N.C. (1980) Recurrence risk of neural tube defects. Lancet i, 1302–1303.

Smithells, R.W., Sheppard, S. and Schorah C.J. (1976) Vitamin deficiencies and neural tube defects. Arch. Dis. Child. 51, 944–950.

Smithells, R.W., Sheppard, S., Schorah, C.J., Seller, M.J., Nevin, N.C., Harris, R., Read, A.P. and Fielding, D.W. (1981a) Apparent prevention of neural tube defects by periconceptual vitamin supplementation. Arch. Dis. Child. 56, 911–918.

Smithells, R.W., Sheppard, S., Schorah, C.J., Seller, M.J., Nevin, N.C., Harris, R., Read, A.P., Fielding, D.W. and Walker, S. (1981b) Vitamin supplementation and neural tube defects. Lancet ii, 1424–1425.

Wald, N. (1983) Possible prevention of neural tube defects by vitamin supplementation. In: Prevention of Spina Bifida and Other Neural Tube Defects (Dobbing, J., ed.), Academic Press, New York.

Section VI
HEAVY METALS

Neurobehavioral Teratology
edited by Joseph Yanai
© Elsevier Science Publishers BV 1984

18

Developmental Neuropathology and Behavioral Teratology of Methylmercury

Louis W. Chang[1] and Zoltan Annau[2]

[1]Department of Pathology, University of Arkansas for Medical Sciences, Little Rock,
AR 72205 and [2]Department of Environmental Health, Johns Hopkins University,
Baltimore, MD 21205, USA

SINCE the outbreak of Minamata disease in Japan during the early 1950s, methylmercury has been well recognized as a hazardous enviromental pollutant and a potent neurotoxicant (Kurland et al., 1960; Takeuchi, 1968). Outbreaks of methylmercury poisoning in Iraq (Amin-Zaki et al., 1974; Bakir et al., 1973) and the alarmingly high mercury levels in the waters of Canada (Takeuchi et al., 1977) clearly indicate that this compound still remains a serious and realistic threat to human health.

The toxic effects of methylmercury on adult organisms (humans as well as animals) have been extensively investigated and presented in several excellent reviews (Takeuchi, 1968; Chang, 1977, 1979, 1980, 1982; Chang and Reuhl, 1982) demonstrating toxic changes in the nervous systems, livers, kidneys and fetuses of the exposed animals. Several studies have indicated that the fetus accumulates more mercury than the maternal tissues, suggesting a 'trapping' phenomenon of mercury by the fetus and so presenting a much higher toxic risk to the fetus than the mother (Suzuki et al., 1967; Yang et al., 1972; Null et al., 1973; Garcia et al., 1974; Reynolds and Pitkin, 1975; King et al., 1976; Fujita and Takabatake, 1977). Indeed, it was reported in Japan that there were 19 cases of 'fetal Minamata disease' in the first 111 cases of confirmed methylmercury poisoning (Irukayama, 1969). Since an average population is unlikely to contain 17.3% of pregnant women, these figures strongly suggest that the unborn infant is at

406

much greater risk from methylmercury poisoning than the adult. By 1976, a total of 40 cases of fetal Minamata disease had been reported (Harada, 1976).

Despite the extensive investigations and conceptual development on the pathogenetic mechanisms of methylmercury poisoning in adult systems, attempts to understand the fetal toxicity of methylmercury are still relatively few and no comprehensive theory on the pathological events or mechanisms for such toxic effects have been proposed (Chang et al., 1980). It is our hope to summarize the major findings related to the developmental neuropathology and behavioral teratology of methylmercury in this chapter and to postulate a basic pathogenetic mechanism or pathway by which this toxicant affects fetal development.

Human studies of fetal Minamata disease

Clinical findings
The available clinical data concerning fetal methylmercury intoxication (fetal Minamata disease) are derived mainly from two major outbreaks of methylmercury poisoning: one in Japan in the 1950s and 1960s, the Minamata Bay and Niigata episodes, and one in Iraq during the early 1970s (Takeuchi, 1968; Harada, 1967, 1976, 1978; Tsubaki and Irukayama, 1977; Bakir et al., 1973; Al-Tikriti and Al-Mufti, 1976; Amin-Zaki et al., 1976; WHO Bulletin, 1976).

In both cases, gross malformation was rare. In Japanese cases, the major neurological signs consisted of mental disturbance, mental retardation, impairment of gait, speech and visual ability. Both spastic and flaccid paralysis, and delayed developmental mileposts such as grasping, crawling, and standing were frequently observed. The major symptomology of these patients is summarized in Table 18.1.

Similar observations were made in the Iraqi cases. Although total blindness was never reported in the Japanese cases, blindness was present in 5 of 15 cases in the Iraqi

Table 18.1. Prevalence of symptoms in 22 cases of prenatal methylmercury intoxication in Minamata
Visual fields and hearing not examined. (From Harada, 1968.)

Symptoms	Prevalance (%)
Mental disturbance	100
Ataxia	100
Impairment of gait	100
Disturbance in speech	100
Disturbance in chewing and swallowing	100
Brisk and increased tendon reflex	82
Salivation	77
Involuntary movement	73
Pathological reflexes	54
Forced laughing	27

episode. This discrepancy may be the result of much more acute exposure to methyl-mercury in the Iraqi incident than in the Japanese tragedy. Although motor uncoordination predominated in the early phase of infant development, mental disturbance and retardation became more severe as the victims matured. It was reported that 100% of these infants eventually developed mental or neurological disturbances in later life (Harada, 1976).

Neuropathology of human fetal Minamata disease

Again, the main literature of neuropathology of patients suffering from fetal Minamata disease stems from either the Japanese or the Iraqi episodes of methylmercury poisoning. Due to the different situations and conditions under which these patients were exposed to methylmercury, the Japanese cases may be considered as chronic toxic situations (lower dose of exposure and longer survival periods) and the Iraqi cases may be considered as acute toxic conditions (higher toxic exposure and shorter survival time).

Japanese cases   Although stillbirths were unusual, gross deformities such as microcephalia, asymmetric skull, enlarged fontanelle, atresia of auditory canal, strabismus, nystagmus, defective chorioretinal membrane and umbilical hernia were observed (Murakami, 1972). Cerebral palsy was a common occurrence. Generally the brains were atrophic with a markedly reduced brain weight as compared to age-matched specimens. Coronal sections of the brains revealed generalized thinning of the cortex, and reduced development of the basal ganglia, corpus callosum and white matter.

Microscopic examination demonstrated widespread neuronal damage throughout the cerebrum and cerebellum. This pattern of neural damage is markedly different from those observed in either adult or infantile cases of methylmercury poisoning, which showed considerably more anatomic or regional selectivity of damage (Fig. 18.1).

Many of the patients in Minamata episodes survived until 5–18 years of age. Autopsy materials demonstrated definitive and permanent damage to the nervous system. One of the most striking and prominent pathological findings was disruption of the

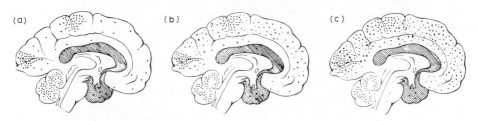

Fig. 18.1. Diagrammatic representation of the different neuropathological lesion distributions in (a) adult, (b) infantile and (c) fetal Minamata diseased brains. It is apparent that the younger the age of involvement, the more widespread the lesions. (After Takeuchi, 1968).

408

cytoarchitecture of both the cerebral and cerebellar cortices. Resting matrix cells still lining the periventricular region were observed. Extensive neuronal loss was evident throughout the cerebral cortex. Proliferation of microglial cells in the gray matter and thinning of myelination in the white matter were also observed.

The cerebellum, as a rule, was severely affected. The cerebellar hemispheres and vermis were grossly atrophic with thinning of both the granular and molecular layers. Extensive loss of granule cells, not only limited to the depth of the sulci, was observed (Fig. 18.2). However, areas of the cerebellum showing only minimal damage also existed. Degenerative changes of the Purkinje cells were also regional; while some folia showed extensive loss or derangement of Purkinje neurons, other folia showed only minor neuronal loss. Atopic and disorientation of Purkinje neurons (Fig. 18.3,4) were also found indicating severe migratory disturbance of these nerve cells during development. Disrupted development of the Punkinje dendritic processes (Fig. 18.5,6) and occasional swelling of these dendrites (Fig. 18.4,7) were also found. Although demyelination may not have occurred, poor myelination of areas of the cerebellar white matter, especially those near the apical folia, could be demonstrated. Damage to the parallel fibers and basket cells was also evident.

A recent study by Takeuchi et al. (1978) also revealed changes in the peripheral nerve fibers. Extensive loss of myelinated fibers, incomplete myelination and abnormal myelination were described.

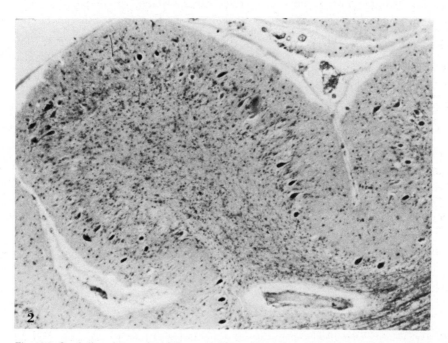

Fig. 18.2. Cerebellum, human fetal Minamata disease. Extensive loss of granule cells in a cerebellar folium. Patching loss and derangement of Purkinje neurons were also evident. × 250.

Iraqi cases   Only infant brains were examined. The brains were smaller than normal. Upon cutting heterotopic gray (patches of gray matter existed among the white matter) was found. Although there was an apparent reduction in the overall size of the white matter, the corpus callosum and basal ganglia were grossly normal.

Microscopically, disruption of the cytoarchitecture was also noted. Many nests of heterotopic or atopic neurons were seen in both the cerebrum and cerebellum. Areas of the cerebral cortex were described as having an 'undulating' pattern, and in these areas the overlying gyri were not developed. Despite the presence of large numbers of gemistocytic astrocytes in both gray and white matter, proliferation of reactive microglia was not observed. Despite the marked disruption of cellular organization in the cerebellum, necrotic changes of either the granule cells or Purkinje neurons were not remarkable.

Although there were some differences in the Japanese and Iraqi cases, patients from both episodes showed reduction in brain size and disturbances in cellular cytoarchitectures. It is reasonable to assume that such migratory, positional and orientational changes in the neurons will result in a disruption in synaptic formations and general neural circuitry of the brain which would precipitate some of the neurological problems and behavioral changes of these patients.

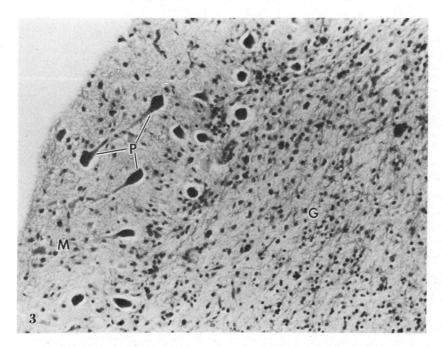

Fig. 18.3. Cerebellum, human fetal Minamata desease. Besides a massive reduction of granule cells in the granule layer (G), atopic and disoriented Purkinje neurons (P) were also found in the molecular layer (M). × 450.

Experimental fetal methylmercury poisoning

Placental transfer and fetal uptake of mercury

Although the placenta tends to 'filter' inorganic mercuric ions (Radaody-Ralarosy, 1938; Suzuki et al., 1967; Takahashi et al., 1971), methylmercury crosses readily the placental barrier (Suzuki et al., 1967; Mansour et al., 1973; Kelman, 1977; Kelman and Sasser, 1977). It was also demonstrated that brain mercury concentrations in the fetus were 2–4 fold higher than those in the mother (Null et al., 1973; King et al., 1976). However, the neonates were capable of clearing the mercury much faster than the adults, resulting in a brain concentration of about one-third that of the maternal level by day 21 of postnatal age (Casterline and Williams, 1972).

Teratogenic effects of methylmercury

The effects of mercury on fetal development have been studied in a variety of animal species, including mice (Spyker et al., 1972; Khera and Tabacova, 1973; Koller, 1975; Inouye and Murakami, 1975; Su and Okita, 1976b; Spyker and Spyker, 1977; Burton et al., 1977; Chang et al., 1977b; Olson and Massaro, 1977; Matsumoto and Spindle, 1982), rat (Nonaka, 1969; Newberne et al., 1972; Nolen et al., 1972; Casterline and Williams, 1972; Khera and Tabacova, 1973; Sobotka et al., 1974; Zenick, 1974; Ware et al., 1974; Olson and Boush, 1975; Inouye and Murakami, 1975; Chang and

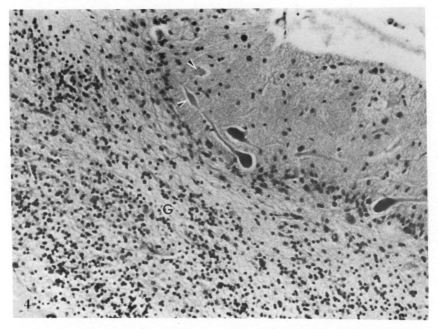

Fig. 18.4. Cerebellum, human fetal Minamata disease. Many Purkinje neurons show disorientation (oriented parallel to the granule layer (G) rather than perpendicular to it) and swelling of the dendrite (arrow heads). × 450.

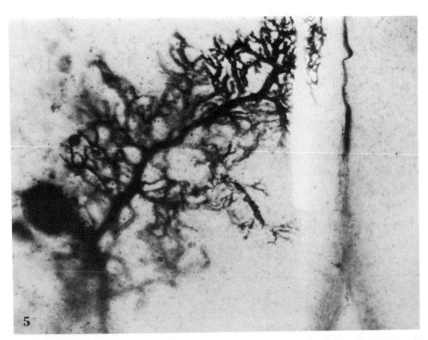

Fig. 18.5. Human cerebellum, normal. A Purkinje neuron showing normal dendritic spread and aberration. Golgi stain. × 1000.

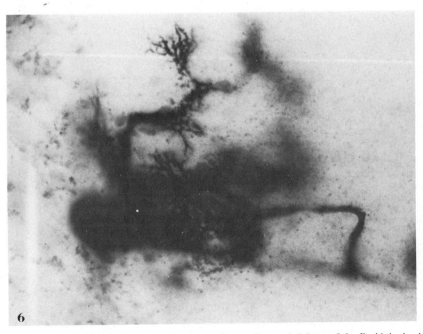

Fig. 18.6. Cerebellum, human fetal Minamata disease. Severe shrinkage of the Purkinje dendritic tree is noted. Golgi stain. × 1000.

Sprecher, 1976; Chang et al., 1977a), hamster (Gale and Ferm, 1971; Harris et al., 1972; Gale, 1974; Lamperti and Printz, 1973; Gale and Hanlow, 1976; Reuhl et al., 1981a,b), dog (Earl et al., 1973), pig (Earl et al., 1973), cat (Morikawa, 1961; Khera, 1973b; Khera et al., 1974), and monkey (Nordberg et al., 1970; Dougherty et al., 1974; Reynolds and Pitkin, 1975; Evans et al., 1977). Defects in limb development, cleft palate, hydrocephalus, and other anomalies have been reported (Harris et al., 1972; Spyker and Smithberg, 1972; Gilani, 1975; Su and Okita, 1976b; Olson and Massaro, 1977).

Since the toxic effects are greatly influenced by the species/strain of animals studied, the compounds of mercury tested, the dose and duration of intoxication, and the routes and gestational time of exposure, direct comparison should be made with care. The teratogenic effects of mercury have recently been reviewed (Khera, 1979) and will not be further emphasized here.

Biochemical and metabolic changes

By means of enzyme histochemistry, Khera and Nera (1971) demonstrated a suppression of DPN diaphorase, succinic dehydrogenase, cytochrome oxidase and ATPase activities in the cerebellum of mouse neonates treated with methylmercury. However, such enzymatic suppression was only transient and the levels eventually returned to

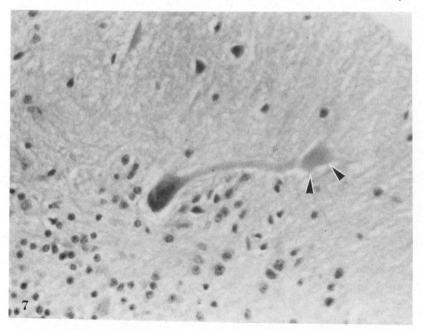

Fig 18.7. Cerebellum, human fetal Minamata disease. Swelling of a Purkinje dendrite (arrow heads) is demonstrated. × 650.

normal. Exposure to methylmercury of pregnant mice or hamsters failed to induce any significant changes in choline acetyltransferase, acetylcholinesterase, and cholinesterase activities in the brains of offspring (Spyker et al., 1972). Inhibition of lipid synthesis and metabolism in offspring, however, has been demonstrated following prenatal administration of methylmercury (Menon et al., 1978).

Biochemical studies by Taylor and DiStefano (1976) revealed an early postnatal effect on biogenic amines in rat pups. An early suppression and later elevation of serotonin levels, monoamine oxidase, tryptophan hydroxylase and animo acid tryptophan were found to be significantly reduced. These biochemical alterations may precipitate both behavioral and morphological consequences.

Utilizing whole fetuses, Olson and Massaro (1977) demonstrated a significant reduction of DNA and protein synthesis levels following methylmercury administration. Such biochemical deficits may contribute to the retarded growth and some of the developmental malformations that have been described.

Disturbance in carbohydrate metabolism in neonatal pups by methylmercury has also been reported (Snell et al., 1977). Biochemical analysis revealed decreased plasma glucose, liver glycogen, and hepatic glucose-6-phosphatase (G6Pase) activities. Impaired glycogen mobilization as well as severe protracted hypoglycemia were also observed in the neonates. Since the CNS is extremely sensitive to blood glucose levels and heavily dependent on carbohydrate metabolism, it is conceivable that severe hypoglycemia at critical developmental periods of the brain would precipitate changes in the nervous system.

Neuropathology of experimental fetal methylmercury poisoning
The neuropathology of experimental animals resulting from fetal methylmercury intoxication was initially studied by Japanese investigators (Moriyama, 1967; Tatetsu and Harada, 1968) and comprehensively reviewed by Murakami (1972). Loss of nerve cells and disruption of cytoarchitecture were noted in the cerebrum and cerebellum of rat pups prenatally exposed to methylmercury. Lesions in the internal capsule and caudate nucleus, small hemorrhage and cystic changes in both the gray and white matter were also found (Tatetsu and Harada, 1968; Fuyuta et al.,1978). Migratory disruption of the cerebellar granule cells with hypoplastic and atopic neurons have been reported in mice and cats (Khera and Tabacova, 1973; Khera, 1973a; Harada, 1967). Studies by Reuhl and co-workers (1981a,b) further documented delayed migration of the cerebellar granule neurons in hamsters prenatally treated with methylmercury (Fig. 13.8). Pyknotic changes were also prominent in the external granule layer. Astrogliosis, particularly in the molecular layer, could be observed in the cerebellum of these animals when they were allowed to survive to adulthood (Fig. 18.9.)

By means of electron microscopy, Chang and co-workers demonstrated both early and long-term effects on brains of mice, rats and hamsters prenatally exposed to methylmercury (Chang et al., 1977a,b; Reuhl et al., 1981a,b). Accumulations of lysosomes and shortening of the rough endoplasmic reticulum were observed in the cerebellar granule cells and Purkinje neurons. Large areas of focal cytoplasmic degradation (Fig. 18.10,11) and endothelial damages (Fig. 18.12) were some of the more prominent findings. Many dendrites also appeared to be swollen or degenerated (Fig. 18.13,14,15). Necrotic neurons were also observed (Fig. 18.16). Long-term studies (animals allowed to survive to adulthood) revealed abundance of lysosomal residual bodies (lipofuscin) in the neuronal processes (Fig. 18.17) and in the Purkinje cells. Degenerative changes in some myelinated axons (Fig. 18.18) were still evident. Accumulation of abnormal tubular structures in the neurons and their processes (Fig. 18.19,20), incomplete myelination (Fig. 18.21) and abnormal synaptic formations (Fig. 18.22,23) were also found. These findings clearly indicate that the prenatal toxic effects of methylmercury persist well into, and probably throughout, adult life. This finding is in good correlation with observations made in adult patients suffering from fetal Minamata disease. Such early trauma and long-term effects of methylmercury are responsible for the neurological problems and behavioral changes observed in both human patients and experimental animals.

Behavioral teratology of methylmercury

The first animal model of the congenital Minamata syndrome was initiated by Spyker et al. (1972). Using primiparous 129/SvSl mice, these authors administered 8.0 mg/kg methylmercury dicyandiamide on day 7 or 9 of pregnancy. The dose of mercury was

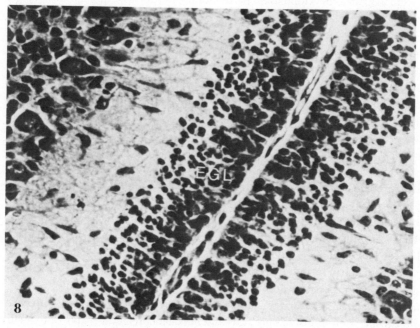

Fig. 18.8. Cerebellum, neonatal hamster, prenatally exposed to methylmercury (MeHg). Thickening of the external granule layer (EGL) as compared to age-control animals suggesting a delay in neuronal migration. × 650. (Reuhl et al., Environ. Res. 26, 1981a).

not toxic to the mothers or offspring as far as could be determined by litter size and weight. Behavioral testing was started on the offspring at 30 days of age. The tests consisted of two sessions in the open field for two minutes on each day and a swimming test in a tank for an undetermined period of time. The behavior of the mercury-exposed animals in the open field test revealed a series of differences between treated and control animals. Offspring of treated mothers had a longer latency in initiation of movement than controls, took more steps backward, and defecated and urinated significantly less than controls. The evaluation of the swimming task consisted of observing postural adjustments in the water as well as motor coordination. The mercury-exposed mice exhibited a significant increase in abnormal swimming movements and postures when compared to controls, although all animals could swim. An attempt by the authors to correlate neurochemical alterations with the behavioral data proved negative since no changes in choline acetyltransferase or cholinesterase were found in the brains of the mercury-treated animals.

Sobotka et al. (1974) exposed pregnant Charles River rats to 0, 0.1, 0.5 and 2.5 mg/kg methylmercury chloride orally from day 6 through 15 of gestation. None of the doses had an effect on number of offspring. Measures of toxicity were: neonatal weight; eye opening; righting reflex; clinging ability, as well as several neurochemical measures. At the 2.5 mg/kg dose, there was a significant reduction in the body weights of the pups by day 10 after birth that was maintained through day 28. Eye opening

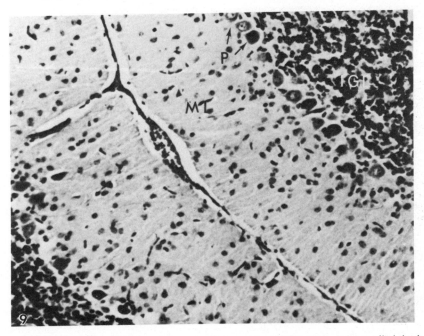

Fig. 18.9. Cerebellum, adult hamster, prenatally exposed to MeHg. Increased astrogliosis in the molecular layer (ML) was observed. Purkinje neurons (P), internal granular layer (IGL). × 650. (Reuhl et al., Environ. Res. 26, 1981b).

416

occurred significantly earlier in the 2.5 mg/kg group than in controls or other mercury groups. The righting reflexes were not altered by treatment. Clinging alibity was significantly enhanced at the 2.5 mg/kg dose on days 6 and 7. There were some alterations in brain neurochemistry, but these did not seem to be dose related.

The results of this experiment are interesting because they suggest that the mercury exposure may enhance neural development; i.e. earlier opening etc., although no alterations in thyroid weight were found. Since the experiments were terminated at 28 days postpartum, no long-term effects were observed.

In a more complex study, Zenick (1974) administered methylmercury chloride via the drinking water at the unusually high dose of 2.5 mg/kg per day to six treatment groups. Group G received mercury during gestation, group N during nursing, group PW at weaning from days 21 to 30, group CFN were untreated controls cross-fostered to group G mothers, group CFG were pups derived from group G mothers and cross-fostered to control mothers (group C). The behavioral task was a water escape T maze and the animals were first tested at 30 days of age for 4 days, and then retested for retention 21 days after completion of training. The results divided the animals into two distinct groups. Groups PW, CFG and G performed with significantly more errors both in the orginal testing and the retesting than groups CFN, N and C. There were no differences within these subgroups. Groups G and CFG had 7.07 and 6.36 μg/g brain weight of mercury at birth and these amounts were diminished to 0.4939 and

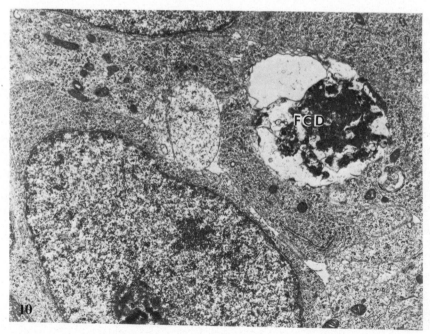

Fig. 18.10. Cerebellum, neonatal rat, prenatally exposed to MeHg. Large areas of focal cytoplasmic degradation (FCD) in a nerve cell, consisting of degenerated cytoplasmic and organelle debris were observed. × 20 000. (Chang et al., Environ. Res. 14, 1977a).

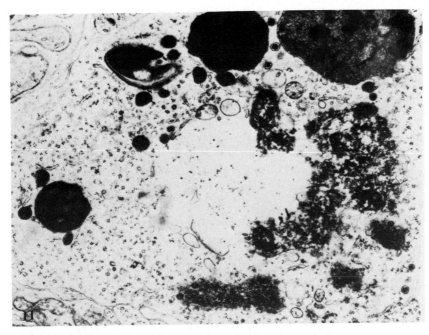

FIg. 18.11. Cerebellum, neonatal hamster, prenatally exposed to MeHg. Lysosomal accumulation and cytoplasmic degradation in a neuron. × 32 000.

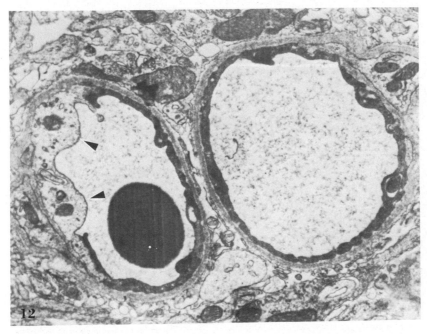

Fig. 18.12. Cerebellum, adult mouse, prenatally exposed to MeHg. Endothelial swelling (arrow heads) was observed in some cerebral capillaries. × 21 000. (Chang et al., Environ. Res. 13, 1977b).

0.352 μg/g respectively during nursing (exact day unspecified). While the high daily dosage of mercury is troublesome in this experiment, it shows the importance of the gestational exposure, and the fact that the behavorial deficits cannot be overcome by cross-fostering (results of group CFG). These results also suggest for the first time that the prenatal exposure has long-term consequences even when mercury is no longer detectable in the brain.

Olson and Boush (1975) fed one group of pregnant rats 'lyophilized and powdered Pacific Blue Marlin' containing 2 ppm methylmercury, a second group were fed 2 ppm methylmercury added to their laboratory chow as well as tuna, and the third group were fed control laboratory chow. The rats were maintained on these diets throughout pregnancy and the offspring continued on the diets after weaning. Early postnatal tests showed an effect of mercury on the righting reflex, and swimming ability by the marlin-fed rats. The marlin group also made significantly more errors on a maze-learning task than the other two groups. Data from these experiments are difficult to interpret sice the two mercury groups received the same dosage of mercury and yet only one of these groups showed behavioral effects. Since the animals were kept on the mercury diets after weaning, this study is a lifetime exposure rather than being, strictly speaking, a prenatal exposure study.

Using a greater number of mercury doses, Su and Okita (1976a,b) exposed 129/SvSl pregnant mice to 0, 6, 8 or 12 mg/kg methylmercury hydroxide on day 10

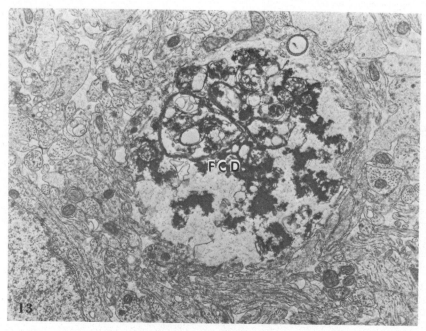

Fig. 18.13. Cerebral cortex, neonatal rat, prenatally exposed to MeHg. A large area of focal cytoplasmic degradation (FCD), presumably confined to a neuronal process, was observed. × 18 000. (Chang et al., Environ. Res. 14, 1977a).

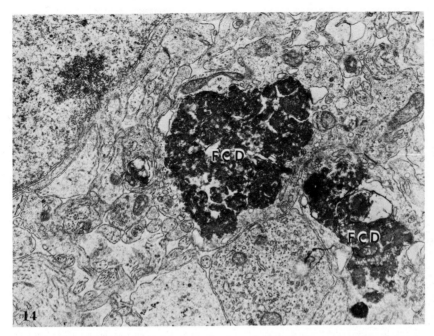

Fig. 18.14. Cerebellum, neonatal rat, prenatally exposed to MeHg. Large areas of focal cytoplasmic degradation (FCD) containing degenerated organelles were observed in neuronal processes, presumably dendrites. × 25 000. (Chang et al., Environ. Res. 14, 1977a).

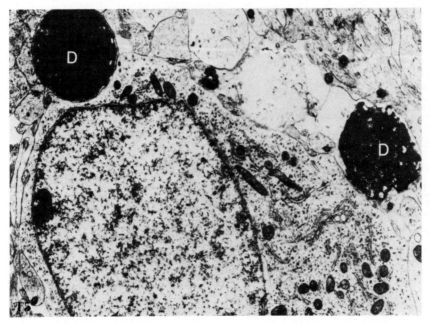

Fig. 18.15. Cerebellum, neonatal hamster, prenatally exposed to MeHg. Degenerated dendrites (D) filled with degradated debris were observed. × 25 000. (Reuhl et al., Environ. Res. 26, 1981a).

420

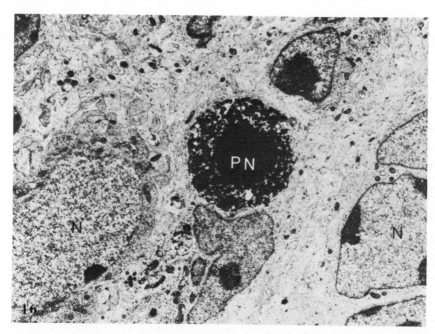

Fig. 18.16. Cerebellum, neonatal hamster, prenatally exposed to MeHg. A necrotic neuron (PN) with densely pyknotic nucleus and degenerated cytoplasm was observed among other granule neurons (N). × 15 000. (Reuhl et al., Environ. Res. 26, 1981a).

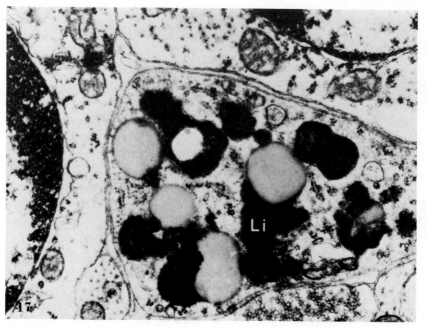

Fig. 18.17. Cerebellum, adult hamster, prenatally exposed to MeHg. Accumulation of lipofuscin (Li) in a dendritic process. × 50 000. (Reuhl et al., Environ. Res. 26, 1981b).

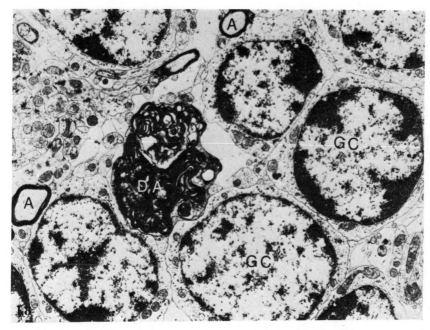

Fig. 18.18. Cerebellum, adult hamster, prenatally exposed to MeHg. A degenerated axon (DA) was observed among normally appearing axons (A) and granule cells (GC). × 15 000. (Reuhl et al., Environ. Res. 26, 1981b).

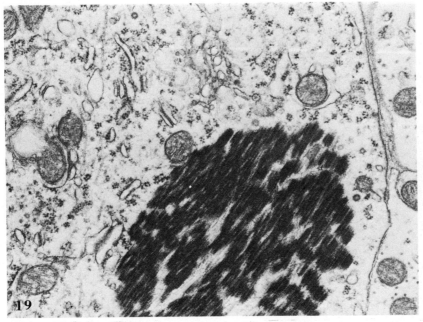

Fig. 18.19. Cerebellum, adult hamster, prenatally exposed to MeHg. Accumulation of abnormal tubular structures in a Purkinje neuron. × 50 000.

422

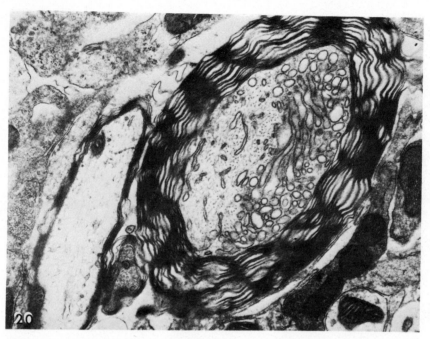

Fig. 18.20. Cerebellum, adult mouse, prenatally exposed to MeHg. Accumulation of smooth endoplasmic reticulum (SER)-like tubular structures was found in a myelinated axon. × 31 000. (Chang et al., Environ. Res. 13, 1977b).

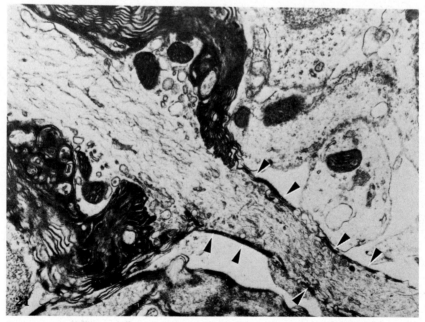

Fig. 18.21. Cerebellum, adult mouse, prenatally exposed to MeHg. Segmental thinning of myelination (arrow heads) was evident in a large myelinated axon. × 25 000. (Chang et al., Environ. Res. 13, 1977b).

of gestation and in a second experiment they administered 4 mg/kg on days 10, 11 and 12 of gestation. Both the 8 and the 12 mg/kg doses reduced the body weight of the offspring significantly up to postnatal day 33, with the repeated exposure group showing the greatest reduction. The highest dose also induced teratogenic effects in 15–20% of the offspring. Behavioral measures were carried out on the offspring and consisted of open field activity at 33 days of age and spontaneous locomotor activity by an automated device measuring the activity of two groups of two mice simultaneously for 30 min at 24, 44, and 64 days of age. Postnatal convulsive behavior induced by flurothyl was also evaluted.

In the open field test, the animals were placed in the center of the field and observed for two minutes. An analysis of variance revealed a significant treatment effect in the single dose experiments. This was due mainly to the significantly prolonged center field latency of the 12 mg/kg treatment group, an effect also seen with the repeated dose group. Subsequent *t*-tests revealed that several other behavioral measures also showed a significant difference between the 12 mg/kg groups and the controls. Locomotor activity was significantly decreased by both 8 and 12 mg/kg at 24 days of age, but this effect was only seen by the 12 mg/kg group at subsequent days of testing. Mercury treatment reduced the number of animals showing convulsive behavior as well as increasing the latency of the convulsive response.

The authors concluded that mercury causes subtle behavioral and biological abnor-

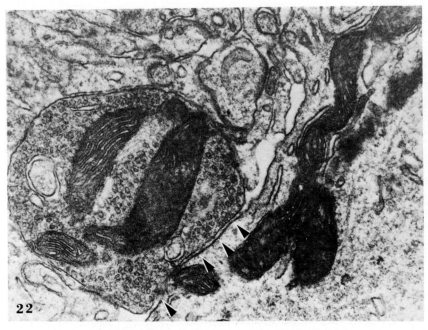

Fig. 18.22. Cerebellum, adult mouse, prenatally exposed to MeHg. A total lack of post-synaptic density formation (arrow heads) in a large synaptic junctional complex. × 55 000. (Chang et al., Environ. Res. 13, 1977b).

424

malities at doses that do not cause gross teratogenic malformations. It must be noted, however, that at the highest dose used in these studies (12 mg/kg), they were close to the range of maternal toxicity and mortality.

An experiment that indicated major differences in strain sensitivity to mercury was carried out by Hughes and Annau (1976). Using CFW mice, these authors administered 0, 1, 2, 3, 5 and 10 mg/kg methylmercury hydroxide perorally on day 8 of gestation. Starting at 3 mg/kg there was a dose dependent reduction in number of surviving pups at 24 hours after birth. Doses higher than 2 mg/kg also reduced the growth of the animals significantly although by the fourth week postpartum these weight differences disappeared. Analysis of variance indicated that this reduction in weight persisted even in cross-fostered groups of animals. Behavioral testing consisted of two way avoidance, passive avoidance, open field activity, conditioned suppression and a water escape test. Since the 10 mg/kg dose proved highly toxic, only the lower dose animals were used in the behavioral measures.

Avoidance conditioning was significantly retarded in animals exposed to 3 and 5 mg/kg on a measure of the number of avoidances in the first training session. Using number of trials to criterion (eleven consecutive avoidance responses), the 3 and 5 mg/kg groups took significantly longer to learn than controls, an effect also seen with the 5 mg/kg cross-fostered group (mercury-exposed animals reared by control females). The mothers exposed to 5 mg/kg showed no learning deficits and the progeny of the

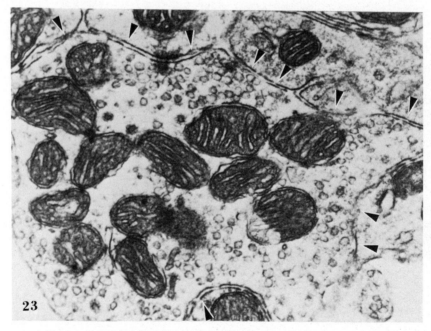

Fig. 18.23. Cerebellum, adult mouse, prenatally exposed to MeHg. A large mossy fiber terminal complex showing either a total lack of or reduced postsynaptic densities at all points of synaptic contact (arrow heads). × 55 000. (Chang et al., Environ. Res. 13, 1977b).

5 mg/kg males also showed no learning deficit. The cross-fostering experiment again indicated that exposure to mercury had to occur prenatally to affect behavior. Of the other measures used in this series of experiments, only the passive avoidance task showed a significant difference between animals exposed to 5 mg/kg and controls. Mercury exposure accelerated the extinction process in this task.

These experiments demonstrated that mercury doses that are clearly not toxic to the mother can cause significant learning deficits in the offspring and that the deficit arises from exposure to this agent during gestation and not during lactation as a result of mercury ingested through the mother's milk. Hughes and Annau (1976) used CFW mice instead of 129/SvSl and found significant effects at 2 mg/kg, indicating this strain to be far more sensitive to mercury toxicity. An intriguing hypothesis was proposed by Hughes and Sparber (1977) suggesting that the teratogenic effects of prenatal methylmercury intoxication may be revealed only under special circumstances. Pregnant rats were exposed to methylmercury on days 0, 7 or 14 of gestation. Their offspring were trained on a discrete trail autoshape task at six months of age and when performing at asymptote challenged with d-amphetamine. There was no difference in the performance of the groups before drug challenge. The amphetamine differentiated the groups, however, in that animals that had been exposed to mercury prenatally on day 0 or 7 were significantly less sensitive to amphetamine than nonexposed controls. Animals exposed to mercury on day 14 of gestation were not different from controls in their response to amphetamine. Thus, a 'normal' animal when challenged with a drug can reveal abnormal behavioral responses as a result of prenatal influences provided those prenatal influences occur during critical periods of development.

Two studies originating in Germany explored the effects of prenatal methylmercury exposure on operant behavior (Musch et al., 1978; Borshausen et al., 1980). The procedure in both studies was similar in that pregnant rats were intubated daily with 0.005, 0.01, 0.05 and 2.0 mg/kg per day on days 6,7, 8 and 9 of gestation. When 4 months old, the offspring were trained on a differential reinforcement of high rates schedule for food reinforcement. The results of these studies indicate that even at 0.01 mg/kg there are residual effects of the prenatal mercury exposure that can be measured with behavioral techniques. Unfortunately, since the authors did not indicate the original weights of the pregnant rats, it is impossible to determine the total dose of mercury administered, although assuming the female rat to be about 200 g, the total dose would be somewhere between 0.004 and 0.16 mg.

Eccles and Annau (1982a,b) examined the effect of two doses of methylmercury chloride administered at two different stages of gestation, days 8 and 15 in rats. Neonatal activity was determined at days 4, 7, 14 and 21 as well as two-way avoidance conditioning in the adult offspring and performance on a water reinforced differential reinforcement of low rates schedule (DRL). The mercury exposure altered the neonatal development of locomotor activity in the rats both as a function of dose and time of administration. Five mg/kg administered on day 8 of gestation significantly elevated activity on day 4, whereas 8 mg/kg administered on day 8 elevated activity on postnatal days 8 and 15. Mercury administered on day 15 of gestation at both doses resulted in enhanced activity on postnatal days 8 and 15. These behavioral alterations occurred without any signs of maternal or neonatal toxicity as evaluated by number of live births and growth curves. The mercury content of the brain of one day old pups as measured by ^{14}C-labeled methylmercury was 3.5 and 5.8 μg/g at 5 mg/kg administered on gestational day 8 and 6.5 and 9.2 μg/g at 8 mg/kg administered on day 15.

In the two-way avoidance task, the animals were trained to a criterion of 10 consecutive avoidances, extinguished and retrained to the original criterion. Methylmercury administered on day 8 of gestation did not alter significantly the avoidance training. During retraining, however, the animal exposed to 8 mg/kg required significantly more trials to criterion than controls. When given on day 15 of gestation, both doses of mercury prolonged training and retraining severely. A group of animals exposed to 8 mg/kg of mercury on day 8 of gestation and trained on a DRL-10 s task showed no consequences of mercury exposure. When challenged with two doses of d-amphetamine (0.5 and 1.0 mg/kg), the mercury animals showed a shift in the dose response curve in that they responded to the lower dose of amphetamine by increasing response rates and decreasing interresponse intervals just like the control animals, but at the higher dose of amphetamine the mercury-treated animals returned to the control, i.e. non-amphetamine performance. This biphasic response to amphetamine was also seen in activity measures taken during the DRL session. In the mercury-treated animals, activity first increased in response to 0.05 mg/kg of amphetamine and then returned to normal at 1.0 mg/kg.

These studies again point to the importance of developmental stage in the study of the prenatal administration of neurotoxic agents. The variability in the results obtained by different laboratories may be at least in part due to mercury affecting different developing cell populations, and thereby altering behavior differentially. The studies reviewed above illustrate the difficulties inherent in the field of neurotoxicity. While it is clear that prenatal exposure to methylmercury has deleterious effects on the subsequent behavior of the offspring, the threshold dose for this exposure has yet to be determined with certainty. Most investigators in this area have not tried to corroborate behavioral measures with mercury brain level determinations and the morphological analyses; when attempted, the results have been rudimentary. Thus there remains a suggestion that behavioral abnormalities can be seen following mercury ingestion without concomitant morphological or other neurobiological alterations. This type of reasoning, based largely on lack of evidence, leads researchers in the field to heated arguments as to whose methods are more sensitive in detecting neurotoxicity. As methodologies in neurotoxicology develop, it becomes increasingly clear that this is a futile argument. Behavior is the output of the nervous system and changes in the output are always associated with changes in the central processor, i.e. the brain, and if we look long enough we shall discover these changes.

427

Table 18.2. Schematic postulation of effects of methylmercury on the developing nervous system

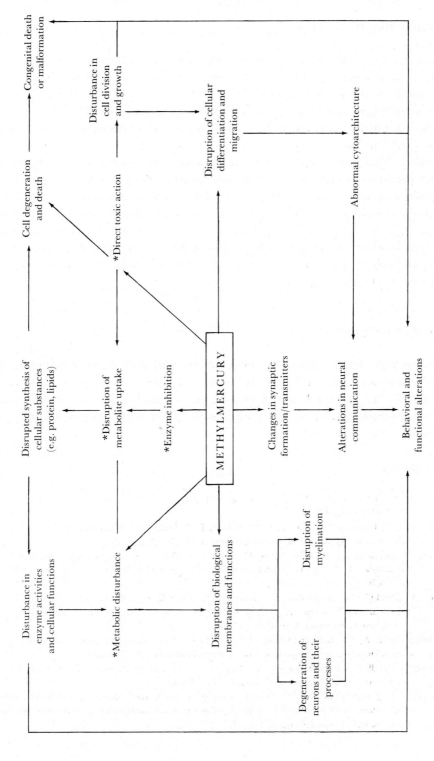

*Both placental and fetal.

Concluding remarks

Methylmercury, besides being a neurotoxicant to the adult animal, is also a potent fetotoxicant inducing toxic trauma, pathological lesions, and functional changes in the developing nervous system and animal. Since the fetal tissues, especially the brain, are known to behave as 'mercury traps' concentrating more mercury than the mother, the fetus is at much greater risk than the mother even when the mother is exposed to a low level of mercury.

Methylmercury is known to cross the placenta very readily, exerting both direct toxic insults and metabolic disturbances to the fetus. These actions subsequently precipitate a cascade of pathological events leading to both morphological and behavioral changes in the tissues and animals. The cascades of pathological consequences are constructed and presented in Table 18.2. It is our hope that we are successful in helping to elucidate the pathological events of fetal methylmercury poisoning and to put the various findings by different approaches (biochemical, morphological, behavioral) to date in their proper perspectives.

Acknowledgments

The authors wish to acknowlegde gratefully the pathology material on human fetal Minamata cases provided by Dr. T. Takeuchi of Kumamoto University, Japan. We would also like to thank Academic Press for their courtesy in allowing us to reuse some of the illustrations which we have previously published in *Environmental Research*.

References

Al-Tikriti, K. and Al-Mufti, A.W. (1976) An outbreak of organomercury poisoning among Iraqi farmers. Bull. WHO Suppl. 53, 15–21.

Amin-Zaki, L., Elhassani, S., Majeed, M.A., Clarkson, T.W., Doherty, R.A. and Greenwood, M.R. (1974) Intra-uterine methylmercury poisoning in Iraq. Pediatrics 54, 587–595.

Amin-Zaki, L., Elhassani, S., Majeed, M.A., Clarkson, T.W., Doherty, R.A., Greenwood, M.R. and Giovanoli-Jakubczak, T. (1976) Perinatal methylmercury poisoning in Iraq. Am. J. Dis. Child. 130, 1070–1076.

Bakir, F., Damluji, S.F., Aman-Zaki, L., Murtadha, M., Khalidi, A., Al-Rawi, N.Y., Tikriti, S., Dhahir, H.I., Clarkson, T.W., Smith, J.C. and Doherty, R.A. (1973) Methylmercury poisoning in Iraq – An interuniversity report. Science 181, 230–241.

Bornhausen, M., Musch, H.R. and Greim, H. (1980). Operant behavior performance changes in rats after prenatal methylmercury exposure. Toxicol. Appl. Pharmacol. 56, 305–310.

Burton, G.V., Alley, R.J., Rasmussen, G.L., Orton, P., Cox, V., Jones, P. and Graff, D. (1977) Mercury and behavior in wild mouse populations. Environ. Res. 14, 30–34.

Casterline Jr., J. and Williams, C.H. (1972) Elimination pattern of methylmercury from blood and brain of rats (dams and offspring) after delivery, following oval administration of its chloride salt during gestation. Bull. Environ. Contam. Toxicol. 7, 292–315.

Chang, L.W. (1977) Neurotoxic effects of mercury intoxication – A review. Environ. Res. 14, 329–373.

Chang, L.W. (1979) Pathological effects of mercury poisoning. In: Biogeochemistry of Mercury (Nriagu, J.O., ed.) Elsevier, New York, pp. 518–580.

Chang, L.W. (1980) Neurotoxic effects of mercury. In: Experimental and Clinical Neurotoxicology (Spencer, P.S. and Schaumberg, H.H., eds.) Williams and Wilkins, Baltimore, MD, pp. 508–526.

Chang, L.W. (1982) Pathogenetic mechanisms of the neurotoxicity of methylmercury. In: Mechanisms of Neurotoxic Substances (Prasad, K.N. and Vernadakis, A., eds.) Raven Press, New York, pp. 51–66.

Chang, L.W., Pounds, J.G., Reuhl, K.R. and Wade, P.R. (1980) Toxicity and pathology of heavy metals. In: Advances in Pharmacology and Chemotherapy, Vol. 17 (Farattini, S., Goldin, A., Hawking, F., Kopin, I.J. and Schnitzer, R.J., eds.) Academic Press, New York, pp. 195–231.

Chang, L.W. and Reuhl, K.R. (1982) Mercury effects on human and animal health. In: Trace Elements and Health (Rose, J., ed.). IPC Sci. Technol. Press, Ltd. (in press).

Chang, L.W., Reuhl, K.R. and Lee, G.W. (1977a) Electron microscopic evidence of degenerative changes in the developing nervous system as a result of in utero exposure to methylmercury. Environ. Res. 14, 414–423.

Chang, L.W., Reuhl, K.R. and Spyker, J.M. (1977b) Ultrastructural study of the long-term effects of methylmercury on the nervous system after prenatal exposure. Environ. Res. 13, 171–185.

Chang, L.W. and Sprecher, J.A. (1976) Degenerative changes in the neonatal kidney following in utero exposure to methylmercury. Environ. Res. 11, 392–406.

Dougherty, W.J., Coulston, F. and Goldberg, L. (1974) Toxicity of methylmercury in pregnant rhesus monkeys. Toxicol. Appl. Pharmacol. 29, 138.

Earl, F.L., Miller, E. and Van Loon, E.J. (1973) Teratogenic research in beagle dogs and miniature swine. In: The Laboratory Animal in Drug Testing (Spiegel, A., ed.) Gustav Fischer Verlag, Stuttgart, pp. 233–247.

Eccles, C.U. and Annau, Z. (1982a) Prenatal methylmercury exposure. I. Alterations in neonatal activity. Neurobehav. Toxicol. Teratol. 4, 317–376.

Eccles, C.U. and Annau, Z. (1982b) Prenatal methylmercury exposure. II. Alterations in learning and psychotropic drug sensitivity in adult offspring. Neurobehav. Toxicol. Teratol. 4, 377–382.

Evans, H.L., Garman, R.H. and Weiss, B. (1977) Methylmercury: Exposure duration and regional distribution as determinants of neurotoxicity in nonhuman primates. Toxicol. Appl. Pharmacol. 41, 15–33.

Fujita, M. and Takabatake, E. (1977) Mercury levels in human maternal and neonatal blood, hair and milk. Bull. Environ. Contam. Toxicol. 18, 205–209.

Fuyuta, M., Fujimoto, T. and Hirada, S. (1978) Embryotoxic effects of methylmercury chloride administered to mice and rats during organogenesis. Teratology 18, 362–366.

Gale, T. (1974) Embryopathic effects of different routes of mercuric acetate in the hamster. Environ. Res. 8, 207–213.

Gale, T.F. and Ferm, V.H. (1971) Embryopathic effects of mercuric salts. Life Sci. 10, 1341–1348.

Gale, T.F. and Hanlow, D.P. (1976) The permeability of the Syrian hamster placenta to mercury. Environ. Res. 12, 26–31.

Garcia, J.D., Yang, M.G., Wang, H.C. and Belo, P.S. (1974) Translocation and fluxes of mercury in neonatal and maternal rats treated with methyl mercuric chloride during gestation. Proc. Soc. Exp. Biol. Med. 174, 224–231.

Gilani, S.H. (1975) Congenital abnormalities in methylmercury poisoning. Environ. Res. 9, 128–134.

Harada, M. (1976) Intrauterine poisoning. Clinical and epidemiological studies and significance of the problem. Bull. Inst. Constit. Med. Kumamoto Univ. Suppl. 25, 1–60.

Harada, Y. (1967) Congenital Minamata Disease. In: Minamata Disease – Methylmercury poisoning in Minamata and Niigata, Japan (Tsubaki, T. and Irukayama, K., eds.) Elsevier, New York.

Harada, Y. (1978) Clinical investigations of Minamata disease. C. Congenital (or fetal) Minamata disease. In: Minamata Disease (Kutsuna, M., ed.) Kumamoto University, Japan, pp. 93–117.

Harris, S.B., Wilson, J.G. and Printz, R.H. (1972) Embryotoxicity of methylmercuric chloride in golden hamster. Teratology 6, 139–142.

430

Hughes, J.A. and Annau, Z. (1976) Postnatal behavioral effects in mice after prenatal exposure to methyl-mercury. Pharmacol. Biochem. Behav. 4, 385–391.

Hughes, J.A. and Sparber, S. (1977) d-Amphetamine unmasks postnatal consequences of exposure to meth-ylmercury in utero: Methods for studying behavioral teratogenesis. Pharmacol. Biochem. Behavior 8, 365–375.

Inouye, M. and Murakami, U. (1975) Teratogenic effect of orally administered methylmercuric chloride in rats and mice. Congen. Anom. Senten Ijo 15, 1–9.

Irukayama, K. (1969) The pollution of Minamata Bay and Minamata disease. Adv. Pollut. Res. 3, 153–159.

Kelman, B.J. (1977) Inorganic mercury movements across the perfused guinea pig placenta in late ges-tation. Toxicol. Appl. Pharmacol. 41, 659–665.

Kelman, B.J. and Sasser, L.B. (1977) Methylmercury movements across the perfused guinea pig placenta in late gestation. Toxicol. Appl. Pharmacol. 39, 119–127.

Khera, K.S. (1973a) Reproductive capability of male rats and mice treated with methylmercury. Toxicol. Appl. Pharmacol. 24, 167–177.

Khera, K.S. (1973b) Teratogenic effects of methylmercury in the cat: Note on the use of this species as a model for teratogenicity studies. Teratology 8, 293–304.

Khera, K.S. (1979) Teratogenic and genetic effects of mercury toxicity. In: Biogeochemistry of Mercury in the Environment (Nriagu, J.O., ed.) Elsevier/North-Holland, Amsterdam, pp. 503–518.

Khera, K.S., Iverson, F., Hierlihy, L., Tanner, R. and Trivett, G. (1974) Toxicity of methylmercury in neonatal cats. Teratology 10, 69–76.

Khera, K.S. and Nera, E.A. (1971) Maternal exposure to methylmercury and postnatal cerebellar develop-ment in mice. Teratology 4, 233.

Khera, K.S. and Tabacova, S.A. (1973) Effects of methylmercuric chloride on the progency of mice and rats treated before or during gestation. Food Cosmet. Toxicol. 11, 245–254.

King, R.B., Robkin, M.A. and Shepard, T.H. (1976) Distribution of ^{203}Hg in pregnant and fetal rats. Tera-tology 13, 275–280.

Koller, L.D. (1975) Methylmercury: Effect on oncogenic and nononcogenic viruses in mice. Am. J. Vet. Res. 36, 1501–1504.

Kurland, L.T., Faro, S.N. and Siedler, H. (1960) Minamata disease. The outbreak of a neurologic disorder in Minamata, Japan, and its relationship to the ingestion of seafood contaminated by mercuric com-pounds. World Neurol. 1, 370–395.

Lamperti, A.A. and Printz, R.H. (1973) Effects of mercuric chloride on the reproductive cycle of the female hamster. Biol. Reprod. 8, 378–387.

Mansour, M.M., Dyer, N.C., Hoffman, L.H., Schulert, A.R. and Brill, A.B. (1973) Maternal-fetal transfer of organic and inorganic mercury via placenta and milk. Environ. Res. 6, 479–484.

Matsumoto, N. and Spindle, A. (1982) Sensitivity of early mouse embryos to methylmercury toxicity. Toxi-col. Appl. Pharmacol. 64, 108–117.

Menon, N., Lopez, R.R. and Kark, R.A.P. (1978) Effects of mild methylmercury poisoning on the lipid metabolism of the developing rat brain. Society for Neuroscience. Abstracts of 8th Annual Meetings. A. 1020, November.

Morikawa, N. (1961) Pathological studies of organic mercury poisoning. II. Experimental production of congenital cerebellar atrophy by bis-ethyl-mercuric sulfide in cats. Kumamoto Med. J. 14, 87.

Moriyama, H. (1967) A study on the congenital Minamata disease. J. Kumamoto Med. Soc. 41, 506.

Murakami, U. (1972) The effect of organic mercury on intrauterine life. Adv. Exp. Med. Biol. 27, 301–336.

Musch, H.R., Bornhausen, M., Kriegel, H. and Greim, H. (1978) Methylmercury chloride induces learning deficits in prenatally treated rats. Arch. Toxicol. 40, 103–108.

Newberne, P.M., Glaser, O., Friedman, L. and Stillings, B.R. (1972) Chronic exposure of rats to methyl-mercury in fish protein. Nature 237, 40–41.

Nolen, G.A., Bohne, R.L. and Buehler, E.V. (1972) Effects of trisodium nitrilotriacetate, trisodium citrate and a trisodium nitrilotriacetate-ferric chloride mixture on cadmium and methylmercury toxicity and teratogenesis in rats. Toxicol. Appl. Pharmacol. 23, 238–250.

Nonaka, I. (1969) An electron microscopical study on the experimental congenital Minamata disease in rat. Kumamoto Med. J. 22, 27–40.

Nordberg, G.F., Berlin, M.H. and Grant, C.A. (1970) Methylmercury in the monkey – autoradiographical distribution and neurotoxicity. In: Proc. 16th Int. Congr. Occup. Health, Tokyo.

Null, D.H., Gartside, P.S. and Wei, E. (1973) Methylmercury accumulation in brains of pregnant, non-pregnant and fetal rats. Life Sci. 12, 65–72.

Olson, K. and Boush, C.M. (1975) Decreased learning capacity in rats exposed prenatally and postnatally to low doses of mercury. Bull. Environ. Contam. Toxicol. 13, 73–79.

Olson, F.C. and Massaro, E.J. (1977) Pharmacodynamics of methylmercury in the murine maternal/embryo: fetal unit. Toxicol. Appl. Pharmacol. 39, 263–273.

Radaody-Ralarosy, M.P. (1938) Recherches histochimiques sur le passage de l'arsenic et du mercure dans le placenta. Arch. Soc. Sci. Med. Biol. 19, 22–26.

Reuhl, K.R., Chang, L.W. and Townsend, J.W. (1981a) Pathological effects of in utero methylmercury exposure on the cerebellum of the golden hamster. I. Early effects upon the neonatal cerebellar cortex. Environ, Res. 26, 281–306.

Reuhl, K.R., Chang, L.W. and Townsend, J.W. (1981b) Pathological effects of in utero methylmercury exposure on the cerebellum of the golden hamster. II. Residual effects on the adult cerebellum. Environ. Res. 26, 307–327.

Reynolds, W.A. and Pitkin, R.M. (1975) Transplacental passage of methylmercury and its uptake by primate fetal tissues. Proc. Soc. Exp. Biol. Med. 184, 523–526.

Snell, K., Ashby, S.L. and Barton, S.J. (1977) Disturbances of perinatal carbohydrate metabolism in rats exposed to methylmercury in utero. Toxicology 8, 277–283.

Sobotka, T.J., Cook, M.P. and Brodie, R.E. (1974) Effects of perinatal exposure to methylmercury on functional development neurochemistry. Biol. Pshychiat. 8, 307–320.

Spyker, D.A. and Spyker, J.M. (1977) Response model analysis for cross-fostering studies: prenatal versus postnatal effects on offspring exposed to methylmercury dicyandiamide. Toxicol. Appl. Pharmacol. 40, 511–527.

Spyker J.M. and Smithberg, M. (1972) Effects of methylmercury on prenatal development in mice. Teratology 5, 181–190.

Spyker, J.M., Sparber, S.B. and Goldberg, A.M. (1972) Subtle consequences of methylmercury exposure: behavioral deviations in offspring of treated mothers. Sci. Abstr. 177, 621–623.

Su, M.Q. and Okita, G.T. (1976a) Behavioral effects on the progeny of mice treated with methylmercury. Toxicol. Appl. Pharmacol. 38, 195–205.

Su, M.Q. and Okita, G.T. (1976b) Embryocidal and teratogenic effects of methylmercury in mice. Toxicol. Appl. Pharmacol. 38, 207–216.

Suzuki, T., Matsumoto, N., Miyama, T. and Katsunuma, H. (1967) Placental transfer of mercuric chloride, phenyl mercury acetate and methylmercury acetate in mice. Indust. Health 5, 149–155.

Takahashi, T., Kimura, T., Jato, Y., Shiraki, H. and Ukita, T. (1971) Time dependent distribution of 203 Hg-Mercury compound in cat and monkeys as studied by whole body autoradiography. J. Hyg. Chem. 17, 93–107.

Takeuchi, T. (1968) Pathology of Minamata disease. From Minamata Disease (Organic Mercury Poisoning) Study group of Minamata disease. Kumamoto Univ., Japan.

Takeuchi, T. (1977) Pathology of fetal Minamata disease. Pediatrician 6, 69–87.

Takeuchi, T., Eto, K., Oyanag, S. and Miyajima, H. (1978) Ultrastructural changes of human sural nerves in the neuropathy induced by intrauterine methylmercury poisoning (so-called fetal Minamata disease) Virchows Arch. B. Cell. Pathol. 27, 137–154.

Tatetsu, S. and Harada, M. (1968) Mental deficiency resulting from intoxication in the prenatal period. Adv. Neurol. Sci. 12, 181–190.

Taylor, L.L. and DiStefano, V. (1976) Effects of methylmercury on brain biogenic amines in the developing rat pup. Toxicol. Appl. Pharmacol. 38, 489–497.

432

Tsubaki, T. and Irukayama, T. (1977) Minamata Disease – Methylmercury Poisoning in Minamata and Niigata, Japan. Elsevier, New York.

Ware, R.A., Chang, L.W. and Burkholder, P.M. (1974) Ultrastructural evidence for fetal liver injury induced by in utero exposure to small doses of methylmercury. Nature 251, 236–237.

World Health Organization (1976) Conference on intoxication due to alkylmercury-treated seed. Supplement to Vol. 53, WHO. Geneva, Switzerland.

Yang, M.G., Krawford, K.S., Garcia, J.D., Wang, J.H. and Lei, K.Y. (1972) Deposition of mercury in fetal and maternal brain. Proc. Soc. Exp. Biol. Med. 141, 1004–1007.

Zenick, H. (1974) Behavioral and biochemical consequences in methylmercury chloride toxicity. Pharmacol. Biochem. Behav. 2, 709–713.

Neurobehavioral Teratology
edited by Joseph Yanai
© Elsevier Science Publishers BV 1984

19

BEHAVIORAL TERATOLOGY OF LEAD

Ellen K. Silbergeld

Environmental Defense Fund, 1525 18th St., NW, Washington DC 20036, USA

LEAD is an element still in widespread economic use throughout the world. As a consequence, much of the world's population in industrialized countries and elsewhere is continuously exposed to lead, usually as an inorganic salt (NAS, 1980). Lead is now generally recognized as a neurotoxin with effects, dependent upon dose and chronicity of exposure, which range from specific dysfunctions in learning and fine motor function to central and peripheral neuropathy, seizures and death. Several reviews have discussed the clinical and experimental neurotoxicity of lead (Bornschein et al., 1980; Silbergeld and Hruska, 1980; Silbergeld, 1981; Needleman and Landrigan, 1981). This topic will not be reviewed here. The purpose of this chapter is to discuss the evidence concerning actions of lead as a neurobehavioral teratogen. In support of this hypothesis, it is known that lead is a neurotoxin whose adverse effects are greater in the young; that lead can gain access to the developing fetus in utero; and that lead can exert toxic effects on several functional aspects of reproduction.

It has been recognized for a long time that the young organism, including the human child, is more susceptible than the adult to lead toxicity, particularly with respect to the central nervous system (Lin-fu, 1973). This differential response involves increased absorption and retention, decreased renal excretion, and a relatively greater concentration of lead in brain in the young as compared to the mature organism. In addition, the immature nervous system is generally more sensitive to many types of xenobiotics during the perinatal period of rapid brain growth, synaptogenesis, and arborization (Dobbing, 1968).

Humans may be exposed to lead through all the prenatal stages of early development, including preconceptional exposure of gonads and germ cells of the parents. Lead appears to accumulate specifically in testis and seminal fluid (Gunn and Gould, 1970; Plechaty, et al., 1977). After embryonic growth begins, lead can gain access through the placenta. Measurements of fetal : maternal blood lead levels appear to be relevant indicators of ambient lead levels encountered by the mother during pregnancy (Needleman et al., 1982).

The reproductive toxicity of lead has been recently reviewed (Rom, 1976; Thomas and Brogan, 1982; Silbergeld, 1982). As will be discussed below, prenatal exposure to lead can be lethal to the fetus and newborn. Nevertheless, it is not presently clear that lead is a teratogenic neurotoxin, exerting effects on the CNS during the period of organogenesis. In part, this may be because of the difficulty in clearly distinguishing prenatal exposure. Even after exposure of the mother is ended, offspring will continue to be exposed through the mothers' milk, since nursing mothers will deliver lead, mobilized from bone, via their milk, at potentially higher concentrations than maternal blood (Lorenzo et al., 1977). Many infants may grow up in leaded environments, breathing contaminated air and mouthing objects coated with leaded dust so that their exposure continues through the perinatal period. Furthermore, although neurotoxic consequences have been reported in animals and some human cases following in utero exposure, the mechanisms of actions of lead in these cases are not clear. Behavioral teratology must be defined as distinct from either mutagenicity or toxicity resulting from continuing internal exposure to lead remaining in the developing brain after cessation of external exposure.

This chapter will review evidence for neurotoxic sequelae associated with prenatal exposure to lead, and attempt to distinguish teratologic, mutagenic, and toxic bases for the types of neurotoxicity observed. It should be noted that, notwithstanding the mechanisms involved, identification of a significant neurotoxic effect of low-level lead exposure of the fetus has important implications for public health. Several large-scale surveys indicate the prevalence of elevated blood lead concentrations in pregnant women: in the US, a population of urban women was found in 1971 to have a mean blood lead concentration of 22 μg/100 ml (Scanlon, 1972), while a decade later mean umbilical concentrations were reported to 7μg/100 ml (Rabinowitz and Needleman, 1982); in Belgium, a group of 474 women was reported to have a mean blood lead concentration of 13 μg/100 ml (Lauwerys et al., 1978); in Zambia, mothers living near an active lead mine were found to have mean blood leads of 41 μg/100 ml (Clark, 1977); in England, urban women were found to have blood levels of 16 μg/100 ml, 4 μg/100 ml higher than similar subjects living in rural areas (Alexander and Delves, 1981). Thus, establishment of adverse effects of lead at these levels of internal dose on the fetus would indicate that potentially large numbers of unborn children may be at risk.

General effects of prenatal lead exposure

Lead is a reproductive toxin, in that high levels of parental exposure can be shown to be associated with infertility, fetal death, spontaneous abortion, stillbirth and early childhood death (Rom, 1976). Since these effects have been observed after either parent was occupationally exposed to lead, it may be more accurate to consider lead a gametotoxin.

There are reports that lead levels are elevated in placental tissue obtained from stillbirths (Wibberley et al., 1977) but this is not resolved, since site of sampling and storage appear to influence analytical results (Khera et al., 1980).

Experimentally, lead has measurable teratogenic effects in chicks and rodents. In chicks, lead administered once on the fourth day after fertilization at doses as low as 5 μg/embryo produced congenital malformations including localized teratogenic damage to brain (DeGennaro, 1978; Gilani, 1973). In rodents, exposure to lead during the first half of pregnancy also produced malformations of the spinal cord (Carpenter and Ferm, 1977; Jacquet and Gerber, 1979). These are consequent to relatively high discrete doses, after which internal exposure undoubtedly continues throughout pregnancy. Somewhat lower doses produce reductions in litter size and birthweight, and reduced rate of survival to weaning (Stowe and Goyer, 1971). Results of such studies are summarized in Table 19.1. In rodents, lead exposures initiated around day 8 of gestation appear most frequently associated with malformations. In human pregnancy this would correspond to exposure during the second trimester.

Exposure later in gestation (day 15 and after) is associated with brain hemorrhage and hydrocephaly (Hackett et al., 1978; Minsker et al., 1982). However, it should be noted that these effects also occur postnatally in neonatal rats given relatively high doses of lead (Pentschew and Garro, 1966; Goldstein et al., 1974). Thus, these effects may not result from specifically teratogenic effects of lead, but rather from toxic effects, in that patterns of development are not disrupted although sensitivity of the same targets for dysoria is greater.

Prenatal lead exposure can inhibit fetal heme synthesis, expressed biochemically as reduced activity of the enzyme δ-aminolevulinic dehydrase and elevations in tissue levels of porphyrin precursors (Hubermont et al., 1976; Jacquet et al., 1977). This is also an aspect of lead toxicity not unique to the fetus, although there is evidence to suggest that fetal hematopoietic systems respond more sensitively to circulating levels of lead, as compared to maternal systems (Roels et al., 1976).

Neurotoxicity of sublethal prenatal lead exposure

Clinical evidence suggests that low levels of exposure to lead in utero may affect the mental development of the child. In those children from homes served with water containing relatively high lead levels, a higher rate of mental retardation was found com-

Table 19.1. Effects of prenatal exposure to lead on the offspring of rodents

Species	Test agent	Dose[b] and mode	Timing[c]	Effect of the offspring[a]			Reference
				D	F	M	
Rat	Lead acetate	10000 ppm in diet	all	−	−	?	Stowe and Goyer, 1971
	Lead acetate	15.9 mg/kg, ip	9	+	+	+	Zegarska et al., 1974
	Lead acetate	45.5 mg/kg per day, po	6–8	+	+	−	Kennedy et al., 1975
	Lead nitrate	31.3 mg/kg, iv	8	−	+	+	McClain and Becker, 1975
		31.3 mg/kg, iv	9 or 16	+	+	+	
		31.3 mg/kg, iv	10, 11, 12, 13, 14, 15	+	+	−	
	Lead nitrate	0.63 ppm in water	all	−	−	?	Hubermont et al., 1976
		6.26 ppm in water	all	−	+	?	
	Lead (aerosol)	10 mg/m^3, inhaled	1–21	?	+	?	Prigge and Greve, 1977
	Lead nitrate	3.13 mg/kg, iv	9 or 15	−	−	?	Hackett et al., 1978
		15.6 mg/kg, iv	9	+	+	+	
	Lead acetate	0.32–159 ppm in water	all	−	+	−	Kimmel et al., 1980
	Lead acetate	31.9–47.8 mg/kg per day, po	all	?	+	?	Miller et al., 1982
	Lead acetate	255–478 mg/kg per day, water	all	?	+	?	Murray et al., 1978
	Lead nitrate	3.13 mg/kg, iv	17	−	+	−	Minsker et al., 1982
		15.6 mg/kg, iv	17	+	+	?	
Mouse	Lead acetate	637–3185 ppm in diet	1–18	+	+	?	Maisin et al., 1978
	Lead acetate	1593 ppm in diet	1–16, 17, or 18	+	+	−	Jacquet and Gerber, 1979
		3185 ppm in diet	1–16, 17, or 18	+	+	−	—
	Lead acetate	45.3 mg/kg per day, po	6–16	+	+	−	Kennedy et al., 1975
		455 mg/kg per day, po	6–8	+	+	−	
	Lead acetate	3185 ppm in diet	1–7	+	±	?	Jacquet, 1977
	Lead acetate	1593–6370 ppm in diet	7–16, 17, or 18	?	+	?	Gerber and Maes, 1978
	Lead acetate	1595–3185 ppm in diet	7–16, 17, or 18	?	+	?	Gerber et al., 1978
	Lead acetate	9.56–22.3 mg/kg, ip	8	−	+	+	Jacquet and Gerber, 1979
		9.56 mg/kg, ip	9	+	+	+	
		22.3 mg/kg, ip	9	+	+	+	
		22.3 mg/kg, ip	10 or 12	+	−	+	
Hamster	Lead nitrate	31.3 mg/kg, iv	7, 8, or 9	?	?	+	Ferm and Carpenter, 1967
	Lead acetate or chloride	31.9 or 37.3 mg/kg, iv	8	?	?	+	
	Lead nitrate	31.3 mg/kg, iv	8	+	+	+	Carpenter and Ferm, 1977
	Lead nitrate	31.3 mg/kg, iv	8	+	+	+	Gale, 1978

D = mortality, F = fetotoxicity, M = malformations.

[a] + = effect present, − = effect not seen, ± = effect ambiguous, ? = effect not examined or insufficient data.

[b] As elemental lead.

pared to a matched control group. Analyses of blood taken from these children soon after birth also showed a higher lead concentration in the retarded children (Moore et al., 1977).

Few experimental studies have been designed to expose the fetus to lead specifically during gestation in order to examine neurological endpoints. It is clear that lead exposure, initiated during gestation and *continued* during the early postnatal period (in most studies until weaning, at approximately day 20 or 30, respectively, in mice and rats) can produce neurotoxicity, that is, morphological and behavioral alterations in offspring.

As shown in Table 19.2, most studies have continued exposure over the perinatal period, encompassing pre- and postnatal exposure. Under such conditions, both ethological, that is spontaneously expressed, and learned behaviors show deficits related to lead exposure. These effects are associated with relatively low blood lead concentrations in the offspring, at the time at which behavioral toxicity was observed. For example, in a study in which rats were exposed only in utero, the mean blood lead concentration of the exposed pups at day 21 was 15 μg/100 ml, as compared to 5 μg/100 ml in control pups (Crofton et al., 1980). One of the most sensitive aspects of behavior appears to be the appearance of the maturational pattern of locomotion in pups, that is, the normal rise and fall in daytime activity which occurs over the first 20 days of life. This pattern is usually delayed by lead exposure, so that pups express increased motor activity as compared to age-matched controls (Reiter et al., 1975). Acquisition and extinction of operant tasks are also sensitive to perinatal and prenatal exposure (Carson et al., 1974; Brady et al., 1976; Zenick et al., 1978, 1978b).

Perinatal exposure to lead also affects the CNS morphologically and biochemically. Reduced number of dendritic spines, alterations in spine shape, decreased synapse formation, and changes in energy metabolism have been reported after relatively low-level lead exposure during gestation and suckling (Murray et al., 1978; McCauley et al., 1979). Two important factors make it difficult to define these studies as indicative of prenatal lead toxicity, however mediated. First, as mentioned in the introduction, lead exposure initiated during gestation will produce elevated lead concentrations in brain which persist after cessation of exposure. This point is important since most of the neurobehavioral and neurochemical studies are conducted well after brain organogenesis, so it is difficult to rule out postnatally mediated effects of lead absorbed by the brain prenatally. Second, the effects which have been described consequent to prenatal exposure are not unique to that time period. Decreases in synaptogenesis, energy metabolism and myelin synthesis have all been described in rodents exposed only *after* parturition (Silbergeld and Hruska, 1981), as well as the range of behavioral effects shown in Table 18.2. It is difficult to assume that there is a particular prenatal neurotoxicity of lead, especially since the first days after parturition are a critical period for the neurotoxic effects of lead (Brown, 1974). There is at present insufficient evidence to determine if prenatal exposure to lead, even if similar in consequence to postnatal exposure, produces effects at significantly lower doses.

Table 19.2. Effects of perinatal lead exposure on animal learning

Reference	Lead exposure			Blood lead (pg/dl)		Learning performance
	Species	Period[a]	Level[c]	Peak	At test	
Brady, et al. (1975)	Rat	PG, G, L	500[c] GAV	?	?	Impaired
Driscoll and Stegner (1976)	Rat	PG, G, L	2070[d] DT	?	?	Impaired
Winneke, et al. (1977)	Rat	PG, G, L	745[d] DT	29, 42	5, 9	Impaired
Carson et al. (1974)	Sheep	G	2.3, 4.5[c], DT	17–25	9–14	No effect
Gross-Selbeck (1979)	Rat	G&L	1 g/kg Pb(Ac)$_2$- DT (dam PbB: 20 µg/dl)	?	'normal'	Pre- and neonatally Pb-exposed Ss showed significantly higher respiration rates than controls on DRH schedule; Ss exposed postnatally did not differ from controls
				?	'normal'	
Gross-Selbeck (1979)	Rat	G&L	Dam's PbB: 20 pg/dl or 60 µg/dl	?	'normal'	Pre- and neonatally low-exposure Ss significantly increased resp. rate; high exposure Ss significantly decreased resp. rate
Zenick et al. (1979)	Rat	G-L, G-PW	750 pg/kg Pb(AC)$_2$	–		Impaired
Flynn et al. (1979)	Rat	G-L	0.5% Pb(AC)$_2$	Brain Pb at 3 days: Pb: 0.174 pg/g C: 0	–	No significant difference between Pb Ss and controls
		G	–W			
			0.2%			
			–W			
		L	225 mg/kg	Brain Pb at 75–76 Pb: 1.85 pg/g C: 0.13		No significant differences in trials to criterion; significantly fewer tentative approaches in Pb Ss suggesting tendency to avoid or ignore shock area
			–GAV			
		PW	0.25%			
			–W			
		G	0.2%			
		W	–W			
		L	90 mg/kg			No significant differences
		PW	–GAV			
		(21–33)	–W			

[a] PG = equals pregestation period, external exposure to dam. G = Gestation period, external to dam.
L = lactation period, external exposure to dam. PW = Post weaning period, external exposure to pup.
[b] DT = Diet. GAV = Gavage. IP = Intraperitoneal. W = Drinking water.
[c] mg/kg per day.
[d] ppm.

Mechanisms of action

Lead affects the developing fetus by several mechanisms; pregestational effects on the parents, including gonadotoxicity; gametotoxicity and mutagenic effects; hormonal effects (parental and fetal); teratogenic and fetotoxic effects; and maternal toxicity.

Pregestationally, lead reduces sperm count and alters sperm morphology in humans and rats (Lancranjan et al., 1978). Experimentally, morphological alterations in corpora lutea have also been described in females exposed during development (Stowe and Goyer, 1971). While these effects are usually cited with reference to endpoints of fertility, they may also have implications for the quality of reproductive outcomes, occurring under conditions of reduced but not completely suppressed fertility.

Lead is a positive mutagen in several in vitro assays for mutagenic activity (see review by Silbergeld, 1982). Clinically, mutagenic effects of lead have been reported in both males and females, primarily in association with occupational exposure, in cases with blood lead levels below 40 μg/100 ml (Thomas and Brogan, 1982). Several experimental studies, using seminal cytology as an assay for genetic mutations, have found increased numbers of abnormal appearing sperm in rodents exposed semichronically (Varma, 1975; Eyden et al., 1978) or even acutely (Bruce and Heddle, 1979). Even more potent mutagenic activity has been reported for the organometal compounds trimethyllead and tetraethyllead (Grandjean et al., 1982). However, there is no evidence to indicate that mutagenic activity of lead is directly related to any deformities or abnormalities in offspring.

After gestation begins, its progress is very sensitive to lead through hormonal mechanisms. The ability of lead to interfere with implantation of the fertilized blastocyst involves an alteration of the maternal progesterone/estrogen interactions critical for this process to occur (Wide, 1980; Jacquet, 1978). Although serum levels of maternal estradiol were normal on day 5 after fertilization, exposure to lead blocked the subsequent rise in progesterone. In addition, receptor response to hormones may be altered by lead, as suggested by a study of androgen receptors in mouse prostate (Thomas and Brogan, 1982). Hormonal effects in the mother may also have important implications for fetal neurological development. Maternal-fetal hormonal patterns are critical for supporting appropriate prenatal brain development, particularly of the hypothalamus and those areas which contain cytosolic hormone receptors and appear to respond to presence or lack of hormonal stimulation (Gorski, 1971). No studies have been done to investigate whether early lead exposure affects hormone-regulated brain development and behavior, which are responsive to levels of sex hormones (such as estrogen-induced changes in open field behavior) (Stewart and Cygan, 1980).

Fetal hormone metabolism may also be affected by fetotoxic effects of lead, specifically the effects of lead on hepatic heme-dependent drug metabolism. Young children have been shown to be sensitive to this effect of lead (Alvarez et al., 1975), and, while there is no direct evidence of such effects in infants exposed prenatally, the studies on hematopoietic toxicity of lead in mother-infant pairs, cited above, should indicate a probability that such effects occur. Interference with hepatic drug metabolism would reduce the enzymatic catabolism of estrogen and progesterone, which might lead to higher circulating levels in the fetus, with possible neurotoxic consequences.

Fetotoxic effects may be difficult to distinguish from maternal toxicity, since similar systems are affeted. The effects of lead on heme metabolism, as discussed above, may compromise metabolism of endogenous substances, with toxic consequences. In addition, this inhibition produces increases in potentially toxic intermediates in both maternal and fetal tissue. Some evidence now exists to suggest that the increased levels of the heme precursor δ-aminolevulinic acid (ALA) may be involved in the neurotoxicity of lead observed in the neonate and adult (Silbergeld et al., 1982). ALA produced by maternal tissues may cross the placental barrier; this has not been specifically investigated, but the ability of ALA to cross the blood-brain barrier suggests that it probably has no impediment to equilibration (Silbergeld and Lamon, 1980). ALA is able to displace weakly the neurotransmitter γ-aminobutyric acid (GABA) from its synaptic receptors in rat brain tissue (see Fig. 19.1) (Silbergeld and Lamon, 1980). It is also a potent inhibitor of GABA release in vitro (Brennan and Cantrill, 1979). These actions may be not only neurotoxic, resulting in disruptions of GABAergically mediated neurotransmission, in the postnatally exposed organisms, but also in the developing organism they may be of increased significance. GABA, like other transmitters, per-

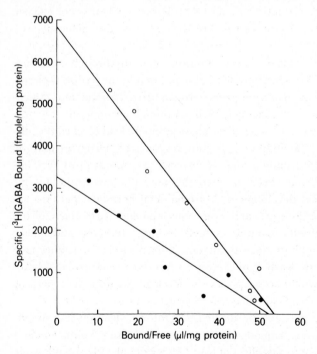

Fig. 19.1. Effects of chronic exposure to lead acetate on [³H]GABA binding in rat cerebellar tissue. Exposure was initiated after parturition; animals were studied 40–50 days later. Details from Silbergeld et al. (1980).

forms a neurotrophic role prior to the establishment of a network in which neurotransmitters mediate cell-cell information transfer. Disruptions in neurochemistry during the period of neural pathway formation can produce long-lasting alterations in brain structure. The ability of lead exposure to increase the number of GABAergic receptors (Silbergeld et al., 1982) suggests that neurotrophic actions of this animo acid may be sensitive to lead.

Other toxic actions of lead which may impact upon the developing fetus relate exclusively to maternal toxicity. These may include alterations in nutrient supply via the placenta; lead has been shown to reduce the transport of aminoisobutyrate, a tracer amino acid, across the placenta in lead-exposed pregnant rats (Gerber et al., 1978). The complications of undernutrition in the experimental study of lead toxicity are well known (Mahaffey and Michaelson, 1980); however, if these nutritional effects are highly specific to lead, then they should be considered part of lead toxicity and not as a complicating factor.

Summary

Neurotoxic effects of lead are known to be qualitatively more severe, and occur at lower doses, in the young as compared to the mature organism. Behavioral effects of lead appear to precede overt morphological damage of the CNS or its capillary endothelial cell barrier, and are probably correlated with significant neurochemical changes. The sensitivity of the young brain to lead strongly suggests that lead may be a neurobehavorial teratogen. Certainly neurotoxic sequelae can be discerned after prenatal exposure in animals and in some clinical case studies.

The persistence after birth of lead in the brain of prenatally exposed offspring makes precise differentiation difficult, even in cross-fostering experiments. Moreover, the mechanisms of these effects may not be teratogenic or unique to the prenatal period. Mutagenesis can result from lead exposure, in vivo and in vitro, and appears to include effects on male germ cells; however, there is no demonstration that these mutational and chromosomal events are related to neurotoxicity. Experimental teratogenesis can occur after high-dose lead exposure, and there is evidence in humans for an increased incidence of minor malformations (Needleman, personal communication). Retarda-

Table 19.3. The effect of lead on pregnancy (Oliver, 1911)

	No. of abortions and stillbirths per 1000 females	No. of neonatal deaths (first year) per 1000 females
Housewives	43.2	150
Female workers (mill work)	47.6	214
Females exposed to lead premaritally	86.0	157
Females exposed to lead after marriage	133.5	271

tion has been reported in children from homes with heavily leaded water. In some instances the foci of teratogenic events suggests sensitivity of neuronal cells or spinal cord or cerebral vasculature. In most cases the types of neurological terata observed are not distinct from the types of neurotoxicity produced by early postnatal exposure. However, the perinatal effects of lead may be defined as teratogenic, since the nervous system continues to develop during the period of maximal lead effects on neurophysiology, chemistry or behavior.

The most interesting studies on the prenatal toxicity of lead suggest that *pregestational* exposure may be toxic and perhaps specifically neurotoxic. If this is the case, then lead may be a neurobehavioral gametotoxin or possibly mutagen, rather than a teratogen, whose effects by definition are confined to those aspects of reproduction consequent to implantation of the fertilized zygote. This was suggested long ago, as shown in Table 19.3 (Oliver, 1911). In terms of clinical medicine, it is clear that exposure of the fetus to lead carries at least the same risk of toxic consequences as does exposure of the young child. In addition, potentially large numbers of children remain at risk from such lead exposure, which may have to include those conceived by parents exposed before reproduction.

References

Alexander, F.W. and Delves, H.T. (1981) Blood lead levels during pregnancy. Int. Arch. Occup. Environ. Health 48, 35–39.

Alvarez, A.P., Kapelner, S., Sassa, S. and Kappas, A. (1975) Drug metabolism in normal, lead poisoned children, and normal adults. Clin. Pharmacol. Ther. 17, 179–183.

Bornschein, R., Pearson, D. and Reiter, L. (1980) Behavioral effects of moderate lead exposure in children and animal models. CRC Crit. Rev. Toxicol. 8, 43–152.

Brady, K., Herrera, Y. and Zenick, H. (1975) Influence of parental lead exposure on subsequent learning ability of offspring. Pharmacol. Biochem. Behav. 3, 561–566.

Brennan, M.J.W. and Cantrill, R.C. (1979) d-Aminolevulinic acid is a potent agonist of GABA autoreceptors. Nature 280, 514–515.

Brown, D.R. (1975) Neonatal lead exposure in the rat: decreased learning as a function of age and blood lead concentrations. Toxicol. Appl. Pharmacol. 32, 628–637.

Bruce, W.R. and Heddle, J.A. (1979) The mutagenic activity of 61 agents as determined by the micronucleus, salmonella, and sperm abnormality assays. Can. J. Genet. Cytol. 21, 319–334.

Carpenter, S.J. and Ferm, V.H. (1977) Embryopathic effects of lead in the hamster a morphologic analysis. Lab. Invest. 37, 369–385.

Carson, T.L., Van Gelder, G.A., Karas, G.S. and Buck, W.B. (1974) Slowed learning in lambs prenatally exposed to lead. Environ. Health Persp. 7, 17–25.

Clark, A.R.L. (1977) Placental transfer of lead and its effects on the newborn. Postgrad. Med. J. 53, 67–678.

Crofton, K.M., Taylor, D.H., Bull, R.J., Sivulka, D.J. and Lutkenhoff, S.D. (1980) Developmental delays in exploration and locomotor activity in male rats exposed to low level lead. Life Sci. 26, 823–831.

De Gennaro, L.D. (1978) The effects of lead nitrate on the central nervous system of the chick embryo. I. Observations of light and electron microscopy. Growth 42, 141–155.

Dobbing, J. (1968) Development of the brain. In: Applied Neurochemistry (Davison, A.N. and Dobbing, J., eds.) Davis Publishing, Philadelphia, PA, 287–316.

Driscoll, J.W. and Stegner, S.E. (1976) Behavioral effects of chronic lead ingestion of laboratory rats. Pharmacol. Biochem. Behav. 4, 411–417.

Eyden, B.P., Maisin, J.R. and Mattelin, G. (1978) Long-term effects of dietary lead acetate on survival, body weight and seminal cytology in mice. Bull. Environ. Contam. Toxicol. 19, 266–272.

Ferm, V.H. and Carpenter, S.J. (1967) Developmental malformations resulting from the administration of lead salts. Exp. Mol. Pathol. 7, 208–213.

Flynn, J.C., Flynn, E.R. and Patton, J.H. (1979) Effects of pre-and postnatal lead on affective behavior and learning in the rat. Neurbehav. Toxicol. 1, 93–103.

Gale, T.F. (1978) A variable embryotoxic response to lead in different strains of hamsters. Environ. Res. 17, 325–333.

Gerber, G.B. and Maes, J. (1978) Heme synthesis in the lead-intoxicated mouse embryo. Toxicol. 9, 173–179.

Gerber, G., Maes, J. and Deroo, J. (1978) Effect of dietary lead on placental blood flow and on fetal uptake of a-amino isobutyrate. Arch. Toxicol. 41, 125–131.

Gilani, S.H. (1973) Congenital anomalies in lead poisoning. Am. J. Obstet. Gynecol. 41, 265–269.

Goldstein, G.W., Asbury, A.K. and Diamond I. (1974) Pathogenesis of lead encephalopathy. Arch. Neurol. 31, 382–389.

Gorski, R.A. (1971) Gonadal hormones and the perinatal development of neuroendocrine function. In: Frontiers in Neuroendocrinology (Martini, C. and Ganong, W.F., eds.) New York, Oxford, pp. 237–290.

Grandjean, P., Wulf, H.C. and Niebuhr, E. (1982) Sister chromatid exchange in response to variations in occupational lead exposure. Environ. Res., in press.

Gross-Selbeck, E. (1979) Effects of prenatal and neonatal lead exposure at the accepted no-effect level on operant behavior in rats. Naunyn-Schmied. Arch. Pharmacol. 308, R46.

Gunn, S.A. and Gould, T.C. (1970) Cadmium and other mineral elements. In: The Testis, Vol. III, (Johnson, A.D., Gomes, W.R. and Vandemark N.L. eds.) Academic Press, New York, p. 411.

Hackett, P.L., Hess, J.O. and Sikov, M.R. (1978) Lead distribution and effects during development in the rat. In: Developmental Toxicology of Energy-Related Pollutants (Mahlum, D.D., Sikov, M.R., Hackett, P.L. and Andrew, F.D., eds.) NTIS, Springfield, VA.

Hubermont, G., Buchet, J.P., Roels, H. and Lauwerys, R. (1976) Effect of short-term administration of lead to pregnant rats. Toxicology 5, 379–384.

Jacquet, P. (1977) Early embryonic development in lead-intoxicated mice. Arch. Pathol. Lab. Med. 101, 641–643.

Jacquet, P. (1978) Influence de la progesterone et de l'estradiol exogenes sur le processus de l'implantation embryonnaire, chez la souris femelle intoxiquee par le plomb. C.R. Soc. Biol. 172, 1037–1040.

Jacquet, P. and Gerber, G.B. (1979) Teratogenic effects of lead in the mouse. Biomed. 30, 223–229.

Kennedy, G.L., Arnold, D.W. and Calandra, J.C. (1975) Teratogenic evaluation of lead compounds in mice and rats. Fd. Cosmet. Toxicol. 13, 629–632.

Kennedy, G.L., Arnold, D.W. and Calandra, J.C. (1979) Teratogenic evaluation of lead compounds in mice and rats. Fd. Cosmet. Toxicol. 31, 629–632.

Khera, A.K., Wibberley, D.G. and Dathan, J.G. (1980) Placental and still birth tissue lead concentrations in occupationally exposed women. Brit. J. Indust. Med. 37, 394–396.

Kimmel, C.A., Grant, L.D., Sloan, C.S. and Gladen, B.C. (1980) Chronic low-level lead toxicity in the rat. Toxicol. Appl. Pharmacol. 56, 28–41.

Lancranjan, I., Popescu, H.I., Gavanescu, O., Kelkepsch, I. and Servanescu, M. (1975) Reproductive ability of workmen occupationally exposed to lead. Arch Environ. Health 30, 396–401.

Lauwerys, R., Buchet, J.P., Roels, H. and Hubermont, G. (1978) Placental transfer of lead, mercury, cadmium and carbon monoxide in women. Environ. Res. 15, 278–289.

Lin-Fu, J.S. (1973) Vulnerability of children to lead exposure and toxicity. N. Engl. J. Med. 289, 1229–1233.

Lorenzo, A.V., Gewirts, M., Maher, C. and Davidowski, L.I. (1977) The equilibration of lead between blood and milk lactating rabbits. Life Sci. 21, 1679–1984.

Mahaffey, K. and Michaelson, I.A. (1980) Interaction between lead and nutrition. In: Low Level Lead Exposure, (Needleman, H.L., ed.) Raven Press, New York, pp. 159–200.

Maisin, J.R., Lambiet-Collier, M. and De Saint-Georges, L. (1978) Toxicite du plomb pour les embryons de la Souris. C.R. Soc. Biol. 172, 1041–1043.

McCauley, P.T., Bull, R.J. and Lutkenhoff, S.D. (1979) Association of alterations in energy metabolism with lead-induced delays in rat cerebral cortical development. Neuropharmacology 18, 93–101.

McClain, R.M. and Becker, B.A. (1975) Teratogenicity, fetal toxicity and placental transfer of lead nitrate in rats. Toxicol. Appl. Pharmacol. 31, 72–82.

Miller, C.D., Buck, W.B., Hembrough, F.B. and Cunningham, W.L. (1982) Fetal rat development as influenced by maternal lead exposure. Vet. Hum. Toxicol. 24, 163–166.

Minsker, D.H., Moskalski, N., Peter, C.P., Robertson, R.T. and Bokelman, D.L. (1982) Exposure of rats to lead nitrate in utero or postpartum: effects of morphology and behavior. Biol. Neonate 41, 193–203.

Moore, M., Meredith, P.A. and Goldberg, A. (1977) A retrospective analysis of blood lead in mentally retarded children. Lancet i, 717–719.

Murray, H.M., Guruk, M. and Zenick, H. (1978) Effects of lead exposure on the developing rat parietal cortex. In: Proceedings of the 17th Annual Hanford Biology Symposium. NTIS, Springfield, VA. pp. 520–535.

National Academy of Sciences. Lead in the Human Environment. NAS, Washington.

Needleman, H.L. and Landrigan, P.L. (1981) The health effects of low level exposure to lead. Annu. Rev. Public. Health 2, 277–298.

Oliver, T. (1911) Lead poisoning and the race. Brit. Med. J. I, 1096–1098.

Pentschew, A. and Garro, F. (1966) Lead encephalo-myelopathy of the suckling rat and its implications for the porthyrinopathic nervous diseases. Acta Neuropathol. 6, 266–278.

Plechaty, M.M., Noll, B. and Sunderman, W.F. (1977) Lead concentrations in semen of healthy men without occupational exposure to lead. Ann. Clin. Lab. Sci. 7, 515–518.

Prigge, E. and Greve, J. (1977) Effects of lead inhalation exposures alone and in combination with CO in nonpregnant and pregnant rats and fetuses. Bakt. Hyg. Orig. B165, 294–304.

Rabinowitz, M.B. and Needleman, H.L. (1982) Temporal trends in the lead concentrations of umbilical cord blood. Science 216, 1429–1431.

Reiter, L.W., Anderson, G.E., Laskey, J.W. and Cahill, D.F. (1975) Developmental and behavioral changes in the rat during chronic exposure to lead. Environ. Health Persp. 12, 199–124.

Roels, H., Buchet, J.P., Lauwerys, R., Hubermont, G., Bruax, P., Claeys-Thoreau, F., LaFontaine, A. and van Overshlede, J. (1976) Impact of air pollution by lead on the heme biosynthetic pathway in school-age children. Arch. Environ. Health. 31, 310–316.

Rom, W.M. (1976) Effects of lead on the female and reproduction: a review. Mt. Sinai J. Med. 43, 542–552.

Scanlon, J. (1972) Human fetal hazards from environmental pollution with certain non-essential trace elements. Clin. Pediatr. II, 135–141.

Silbergeld, E.K. (1982) Neurochemical and ionic mechanisms of lead neurotoxicity. In: Mechanisms of Actions of Neurotoxic Substances (Prasad, K.N. and Vernadakis, A., eds.) Raven Press, New York, pp. 1–25.

Silbergeld, E.K. (1983) Effects of lead on reproduction: review of experimental studies. In: Effects of Low Level Lead Exposure, (Rutter, M. and Russell-Jones, R., eds.) John Wiley, London, pp. 217–227.

Silbergeld, E.K. and Hruska, R.E. (1982) Neurochemical investigations of low level lead exposure. In: Low Level Lead Exposure. (Needleman, H.L., ed.) Raven Press, New York, pp. 135–157.

Silbergeld, E.K., Hruska, R.E., Bradley, D., Lamon, J.M. and Frykholm, B.C. (1983) Neurotoxic aspect of porphyrinopathies: lead and succinylacetone. Environ. Res. 29, 459–471.

Silbergeld, E.K., Hruska, R.E., Miller, L.P. and Eng, N. (1980) Effects of lead in vivo and in vitro on GABAergic neurochemistry. J. Neurochem. 34, 1712–1718.

Silbergeld, E.K. and Lamon, J.R. (1980) The role of altered heme synthesis in the neurotoxicity of lead. J. Occup. Med. 680–684.

Stewart, J. and Cygan, D. (1980) Ovarian hormones act early in development to feminize adult open-field behavior in the rat. Hormones Behav. 14, 20–32.

Stowe, H.D. and Goyer, R.A. (1971) The reproductive ability and progeny of F_1 lead toxic rats. Fert. Steril. 22, 755–760.

Thomas, J.A. and Brogan, W.C. (1982) Some actions of lead on the sperm and upon the male reproductive system. Am. J. Indust. Med. in press.

Varma, B. (1975) Embryonic death in mouse due to lead exposure. Experientia 31, 1312–1313.

Wibberley, D.G., Khera, A.K., Edwards, J.H. and Rushton, D.I. (1977) Lead levels in human placentae from normal and malformed births. J. Med. Gen. 14, 339–345.

Wide, M. (1980) Interference of lead with implantation in the mouse: effect of exogenous oestradiol and progesterone. Teratology 21, 187–191.

Winneke, G., Brockhaus, A. and Baltissen, R. (1977) Neurobehavioral and systemic effects of longterm blood lead elevation in rats. Arch. Toxicol. 37, 247–263.

Zegarska, Z., Kilkowska, K. and Romankiewics-Wozniczko, G. (1974) Developmental defects in white rats caused by acute lead poisoning. Folia Morphol. (Warsaw) 33, 23–28.

Zenick, H., Padlich, R., Tokarek, R. and Aragon, P. (1978) Influence of prenatal and postnatal lead exposure on discrimination learning in rats. Pharmacol. Biochem. Behav. 8, 347–350.

Zenick, H., Rodriguez, W., Ward, J. and Elkington, B. (1978) Deficits in fixed interval performance following prenatal and postnatal lead exposure. Dev. Psychobiol. 12, 509–514.

Subject Index

448

452